Neurology and Neurobiology

THE HIPPOCAMPUS
New Vistas

THE HIPPOCAMPUS
New Vistas

Editors

Victoria Chan-Palay

Department of Neurology
University Hospital
Zürich, Switzerland

Christer Köhler

Astra Research Center
Södertälje, Sweden

ALAN R. LISS, INC., NEW YORK

Library of Congress Cataloging-in-Publication Data

The Hippocampus : new vistas / editors, Victoria Chan-Palay, Christer Köhler.
 p. cm. — (Neurology and neurobiology ; v. 52)
 Includes bibliographies and index.
 ISBN 0-8451-2756-X
 1. Hippocampus (Brain)—Physiology. 2. Hippocampus (Brain)–
–Diseases. I. Chan-Palay, Victoria. II. Köhler, Christer.
III. Series.
 [DNLM: 1. Hippocampus. W1 NE337B v. 52 / WL 314 H667]
QP383.25.H56 1989
599'.01'88—dc19
DNLM/DLC
for Library of Congress   89-2517
             CIP

This book is dedicated to **Sanford Louis Palay,**
Bullard Professor of Neuroanatomy, Harvard Medical School,
mentor and friend, on the occasion of his retirement.

Contents

Contributors

Paola Bagnoli, Dipartimento di Fisiologia e Biochimica, Università di Pisa, 56100 Pisa, Italy **[379]**

Verner P. Bingman, Department of Psychology, University of Maryland, College Park, MD 20742 **[379]**

Eberhard H. Buhl, Max-Planck-Institut für Hirnforschung, D-6000 Frankfurt am Main 71, Federal Republic of Germany; present address: Vision, Touch and Hearing Research Centre, Department of Physiology and Pharmacology, University of Queensland, St. Lucia, Queensland 4067, Australia **[71]**

György Buzsáki, Department of Neurosciences, University of California at San Diego, La Jolla, CA 92093 **[237]**

Giovanni Casini, Dipartimento di Scienze del Comportamento Animale, Università di Pisa, Pisa, Italy **[379]**

Victoria Chan-Palay, Department of Neurology, University Hospital, CH-8091 Zürich, Switzerland **[xvii, 145, 171, 513]**

Graham L. Collingridge, Department of Pharmacology, The School of Medical Sciences, The University of Bristol, Bristol BS8 1TD, England **[329]**

Marina Del Fiacco, Dipartimento di Citomorfologia, University of Cagliari, 09124 Cagliari, Italy **[131]**

Michael Frotscher, Institute of Anatomy, Johann Wolfgang Goethe University, D-6000 Frankfurt am Main 70, Federal Republic of Germany **[85]**

Fred H. Gage, Department of Neurosciences, University of California at San Diego, La Jolla, CA 92093 **[237]**

Christine Gall, Department of Anatomy and Neurobiology, University of California at Irvine, Irvine, CA 92717 **[153]**

Peter Germroth, Max-Planck-Institut für Hirnforschung, D-6000 Frankfurt am Main 71, Federal Republic of Germany **[71]**

R.W. Greene, Harvard Medical School and Veterans Administration Medical Center, Brockton, MA 02401 **[347]**

The numbers in brackets are the opening page numbers of the contributors' articles.

H.L. Haas, II. Physiologisches Institut, Johannes Gutenberg-Universität, D-6500 Mainz, Federal Republic of Germany [347]

Kristen M. Harris, Neuroscience Department, Children's Hospital, Boston, MA 02115 [33]

Mathias Höchli, Neurology Clinic, University Hospital, CH-8091 Zürich, Switzerland [513]

Bradley T. Hyman, Departments of Neurology and Anatomy, University of Iowa College of Medicine, Iowa City, IA 52242 [499]

Paolo Ioalè, Dipartimento di Scienze del Comportamento Animale, Università di Pisa, Pisa, Italy and Centro di Studio per la Faunistica ed Ecologia Tropicali del C.N.R., Firenze, Italy [379]

Frances E. Jensen, Neuroscience Department, Children's Hospital, Boston, MA 02115 [33]

Christer Köhler, Astra Research Center, Södertälje S-15185, Sweden [xvii, 171, 513]

Peter Kugler, Department of Anatomy, University of Würzburg, D-8700 Würzburg, Federal Republic of Germany [119]

Dennis D. Kunkel, Department of Neurological Surgery, University of Washington, Seattle, WA 98195 [287]

Jean-Claude Lacaille, Centre de Recherche en Sciences Neurologiques, Département de Physiologie, Université de Montréal, Montréal, Québec H3C 3J7, Canada [287]

Csaba Leránth, Section of Neuroanatomy, Yale University School of Medicine, New Haven, CT 06510 [85]

H.-P. Lipp, Institute of Anatomy, University of Zürich, CH-8057 Zürich, Switzerland [395]

M.A. Lynch, National Institute for Medical Research, London NW7 1AA, England [363]

H. McLennan, Department of Physiology, University of British Columbia, Vancouver, British Columbia V6T 1W5, Canada [317]

G. Mengod, Preclinical Research, Sandoz Ltd., CH-4002 Basel, Switzerland [207]

Lynn Nadel, Department of Psychology, University of Arizona, Tucson, AZ 85721 [17]

J. Victor Nadler, Department of Pharmacology, Duke University Medical Center, Durham, NC 27710 [463]

Robert Nitsch, Institute of Anatomy, Johann Wolfgang Goethe University, D-6000 Frankfurt am Main 70, Federal Republic of Germany [85]

J. O'Keefe, MRC Cerebral Functions Group, Department of Anatomy and Developmental Biology, University College, London WC1E 6BT, England [425]

David S. Olton, Department of Psychology, Johns Hopkins University, Baltimore, MD 21218 [411]

O.P. Ottersen, Anatomical Institute, University of Oslo, N-0162 Oslo 1, Norway [97]

J.M. Palacios, Preclinical Research, Sandoz Ltd., CH-4002 Basel, Switzerland [207]

Gary M. Peterson, Department of Anatomy and Cell Biology, East Carolina University, Greenville, NC 27858 [483]

Marina Quartu, Dipartimento di Citomorfologia, University of Cagliari, 09124 Cagliari, Italy [131]

Charles E. Ribak, Department of Anatomy and Neurobiology, University of California, Irvine, California College of Medicine, Irvine, CA 92717 [483]

Philip A. Schwartzkroin, Departments of Neurological Surgery and of Physiology and Biophysics, University of Washington, Seattle, WA 98195 [287]

H. Schwegler, Zentrum für Morphologie, J.-W.-Goethe-Universität, Frankfurt, Federal Republic of Germany [395]

Walter K. Schwerdtfeger, Max-Planck-Institut für Hirnforschung, D-6000 Frankfurt am Main 71, Federal Republic of Germany [71]

Menahem Segal, The Center for Neuroscience, The Weizmann Institute of Science, 76100 Rehovot, Israel [307]

Robert S. Sloviter, Neurology Research Center, Helen Hayes Hospital, New York State Department of Health, West Haverstraw, NY 10993 and Departments of Pharmacology and Neurology, College of Physicians and Surgeons, Columbia University, New York, NY 10032 [443]

Torben Sørensen, Institute of Neurobiology, University of Aarhus, DK-8000 Aarhus C, Denmark [257]

A. Speakman, MRC Cerebral Functions Group, Department of Anatomy and Developmental Biology, University College, London WC1E 6BT, England [425]

J. Storm-Mathisen, Anatomical Institute, University of Oslo, N-0162 Oslo 1, Norway [97]

Scott M. Thompson, Brain Research Institute, University of Zürich, CH-8029 Zürich, Switzerland; present address: Department of Neurology, College of Physicians and Surgeons, Columbia University, New York, NY 10032 [225]

Niels Tønder, Institute of Neurobiology, University of Aarhus, DK-8000 Aarhus C, Denmark [257]

Beatrice H. Tsao, Neuroscience Department, Children's Hospital, Boston, MA 02115 [33]

Thomas van Groen, Department of Cell Biology and Anatomy, University of Alabama at Birmingham, Birmingham, AL 35294; present address: Department of Pharmacology, University of Edinburgh, Edinburgh EH8 9JZ, Scotland [1]

Gary W. Van Hoesen, Departments of Neurology and Anatomy, University of Iowa College of Medicine, Iowa City, IA 52242 [499]

Jeffrey White, Division of Endocrinology, Department of Medicine, State University of New York, Stony Brook, NY [153]

Jeffrey Willner, Department of Psychology, University of Arizona, Tucson, AZ 85721 [17]

Menno P. Witter, Department of Anatomy, Vrije Universiteit, 1081 BT Amsterdam, The Netherlands [53]

J. Michael Wyss, Department of Cell Biology and Anatomy, University of Alabama at Birmingham, Birmingham, AL 35294 [1]

Karl Zilles, Anatomical Institute, University of Cologne, D-5000 Cologne 41, Federal Republic of Germany [189]

Jens Zimmer, Institute of Neurobiology, University of Aarhus, DK-8000 Aarhus C, Denmark [257]

Introduction

A book on the hippocampus is always a timely event. During the last decade this "simple" cortical region has invited an increasing number of scientists to explore its structure and function. The major achievements have also been documented in several volumes devoted to different aspects of hippocampal anatomy, physiology, and function.

Two factors have come to play pivotal roles in promoting the rapid progress that has been witnessed with regard to our understanding of hippocampal function in health and disease: First, the apparent simplicity of the hippocampal neuronal circuitry has attracted scientists from different disciplines of neurobiology, including anatomy, physiology, pharmacology, and molecular biology. Since in many instances the hippocampal formation has been used merely as a model system from which to answer more general questions, this has generated a multidisciplinary approach to hippocampal studies.

Second, investigations in recent years have suggested that the human hippocampus may affect mnemonic processes, as well as some neurodegenerative diseases (e.g., Alzheimer's disease) and certain pathological conditions (e.g., epilepsy, ischemia). This realization of the possible roles of the hippocampus has encouraged deepening analyses of neurotransmitters, receptors, and peptide and protein mRNAs in hippocampal tissues obtained from the postmortem human brain.

The purpose of this book is to highlight areas of hippocampal research where advances are particularly rapid, where state-of-the-art techniques are being used, and where experimental findings are most intriguing. At the same time we hope that the book reflects truly multidisciplinary approaches characteristic of hippocampal research today.

To reach this goal we have depended on the contribution of chapters from a large number of the leading neuroscientists exploring hippocampal biology. In general terms the chapters of this book can be grouped into eight major areas: *anatomy*, including developmental biology (Wyss and van Groen; Nadel and Willner; Harris et al.; Witter; Buhl et al.); *chemical iden-*

tity of pathways (Frotscher et al.; Ottersen and Storm-Mathisen; Kugler; Del Fiacco and Quartu); *expression of transmitter mRNAs* and other gene products (Chan-Palay; Gall and White); *receptor localization* (Köhler and Chan-Palay; Zilles; Palacios and Mengod); *plasticity* (Thompson; Gage and Buzsáki; Zimmer et al.); *physiology* (Lacaille et al.; Segal; McLennan; Collingridge; Greene and Haas; Lynch); *function* (Bingman et al.; Lipp and Schwegler; Olton; Speakman and O'Keefe); and *disease* (Sloviter; Nadler; Peterson and Ribak; Hyman and Van Hoesen; Chan-Palay et al.).

Victoria Chan-Palay
Switzerland

Christer Köhler
Sweden

The Hippocampus—New Vistas, pages 1–16
© 1989 Alan R. Liss, Inc.

1
Development of the Hippocampal Formation

J. MICHAEL WYSS AND THOMAS VAN GROEN
Department of Cell Biology and Anatomy, University of Alabama at Birmingham, Birmingham, Alabama

INTRODUCTION

The hippocampus and fascia dentata have been employed frequently as a model system for the study of neurobiological questions, including basic developmental ones, because of their simple and regular structure. Studies have revealed that in the rodent (Angevine, 1965; Bayer, 1980a,b; Caviness, 1973; Hine and Das, 1974; Schlessinger et al., 1978), guinea pig (Altman and Das, 1967), rabbit (Fernandez and Bravo, 1974), and monkey (Nowakowski and Rakic, 1981; Rakic and Nowakowski, 1981) the neurons of the hippocampal region are generated in an orderly manner and according to several spatiotemporal gradients. Pyramidal neurons tend to be born earlier than granule neurons, and within the dentate gyrus neurons in the hidden (suprapyramidal) blade undergo neurogenesis prior to those in the exposed (infrapyramidal) blade. Two radial gradients of production exist. The neurons in Ammon's horn and the parahippocampal cortex are positioned according to the inside-out gradient that typifies production in other regions of the cortex (Angevine, 1965). In contrast, the granule cells of the dentate gyrus are generated according to an outside-in gradient. Other gradients are present in some animals. Schlessinger et al. (1975, 1978) and Bayer (1980a,b) both report gradients along the temporoseptal axis, and Bayer also reports what she terms "sandwich gradients." While the findings of the previous studies are complementary, some differences are present, and these most often are attributed to either species or methodological differences.

In the first part of this review we summarize our studies on the development of cat hippocampal formation (Wyss et al., 1983; Wyss and Sripanidkulchai, 1985). Since gestation in the cat (62 ± 3 days in our study) is three times longer than that in the rat, these studies facilitate a higher resolution investigation of the spatiotemporal gradients that have been reported to be present in the development of the rodent hippocampal formation (Schlessinger et al., 1978; Bayer, 1980a). The primate has an even longer gestation period than the cat, but studies of hippocampal development in the primate focus on a limited septotemporal segment. Conversely, our study examines the entire rostrocaudal extent of the hippocampal formation, thus making it possible to characterize a temporoseptal gradient in the production of neurons. Second, we compare and contrast the development of the hippocampal formation in various species. Third, we consider the production gradients that define the development of the hippocampal formation and the hypotheses that attempt to explain the importance of these production gradients. Finally, the role of early generated neurons is considered in relation to hippocampal formation development.

STUDIES OF THE DEVELOPMENT OF THE HIPPOCAMPAL FORMATION IN THE CAT

Prior to 1965 there existed a voluminous literature describing the anatomy, connections (see e.g. Hines, 1922; Ramón y Cajal, 1972), and physiology of the hippocampal formation (e.g. Kandel and Spenser, 1961), but an accurate description of the development of this region awaited the development of the autoradiographic method (Angevine, 1965). Since that time several laboratories have characterized the generation of neurons within the hippocampal formation by injecting [³H]thymidine into embryos, pups, or mothers at various gestational or postnatal ages. Mitotic cells actively incorporated the [³H]thymidine into newly synthesized DNA, thus permanently labeling the neurons and glia that were undergoing final division following an injection. In the cat, [³H]thymidine did not effectively cross the placental membrane, and thus, in our study, individual concepti were injected with the tracer and the mothers subsequently delivered the kittens naturally. For the following discussion of the cat, the time of coitus was defined as embryonic day 1 (E01).

The cytoarchitectural studies of Ramón y Cajal (1972) in the rat and rabbit and of Lorente de Nó (1934) in mouse and monkey defined the divisions of the hippocampus. Although these studies did not examine the structure of Ammon's horn in the cat, the structure and connections (Habets, 1980; Habets et al., 1980) in the cat were quite similar to those reported for the other mammalian species. Because the terminology of Lorente de Nó (1934) was the most widely used, it was employed in the following review, except for the term CA4 (i.e. cornu Ammonis area 4; Fig. 1).

In the rat, the region underlying the granule cell layer consisted of scattered neurons of differing morphology, which project to the inner one-third of the molecular layer of the dentate gyrus (e.g. Hjörth-Simonsen and Laurberg, 1977; Swamson et al., 1978; Zimmer, 1971). Lorente de Nó (1934) referred to this area as CA4; however, Ramón y Cajal (1972) viewed this region in the rodent as a polymorphic zone of the fascia dentata. The recent work of Amaral (1978) and the connectional studies of West et al. (1979) supported the latter view. Therefore, we referred to this area as the "polymorphic layer of the fascia dentata" (Fig. 1).

The divisions of the subicular cortex used in this study were essentially those described by Lorente de Nó (1934) (Fig. 1). The parasubiculum was medial and dorsal to the medial entorhinal cortex (MEA). It consisted of two layers of cells (lamina principalis interna and externa). The adjacent presubiculum consisted of the same two neuronal cell layers; however, the external lamina of the presubiculum was populated by smaller, more darkly stained, and more densely packed neurons than the same layer of the parasubiculum. The subiculum proper had only a single neuronal cell layer.

The cat entorhinal cortex appeared to be essentially the same as that of the rat (Blackstad, 1956; Steward, 1976; Wyss, 1981). The cat entorhinal cortex stretches from the hippocampal–amygdaloid junction (Krettek and Price, 1978) to the occipital pole of the cortex.

Analysis of Ammon's Horn and Fascia Dentata

Injections of [^{3}H]thymidine into animals from age E21 to postnatal day (P)14 heavily labeled some neurons and/or glial cells within the hippocampus and facia dentata. Whereas all subfields contained some heavily labeled neurons following E22 injections, most labeled cells resided within the granule cell layer and the polymorphic layer of the fascia dentata and in area CA3. Within the granule cell layer, the vast majority of neurons was located in the hidden blade, and only a few were in the exposed blade or in the crest region. Labeling in the polymorphic zone followed a similar pattern. The highest density of labeled neurons was below the hidden blade, and relatively few labeled neurons were adjacent to the exposed blade. Labeled CA3 neurons tended to be near the polymorphic zone, and few CA2 or CA1 neurons were labeled (Fig. 2).

Neurons generated on E28 tended to occupy a slightly different region than those generated earlier. In the fascia dentata granule cell layer, neurons produced on E28 were located primarily in the hidden blade and near the crest, and those in the hidden blade tended to be scattered much more deeply into the granule cell layer than on previous days. Conversely, the E28 neurons in the exposed blade were very close to the superficial border of the granule cell layer. Within the polymorphic layer, neurons born on E28 were located below both the hidden and exposed blade, and each segment displayed an approximately equal density of labeled cells. The E28 neurons that populated CA3 were on the average more superficially located than those generated previously, and labeled CA1 and CA2 neurons were located deeper than the labeled CA3 cells.

By E37, there was a sharp drop-off in the generation of neurons destined for CA3 and the polymorphic layer of the dentate gyrus. The few labeled neurons in the polymorphic zone were scattered below both blades of the granule cell layer. Within CA3 most labeled neurons were close to the superficial border of the pyramidal layer, with a slightly greater scatter of neurons near CA2. Within CA2 and CA1 labeled neurons were positioned somewhat more deeply; however, no labeled cells were found deep to the pyramidal layer in the stratum oriens, and few were observed within the deep half of the pyramidal cell layer. Within the granule cell layer many labeled neurons were present in both blades, and those in the hidden blade were positioned more deeply than those in the exposed blade.

E42 injections resulted in few labeled cells in the CA fields. Generally, the labeled cells were immediately deep to the superficial border of the pyramidal layer, and a slightly greater number was observed in CA1 than in CA3. Within

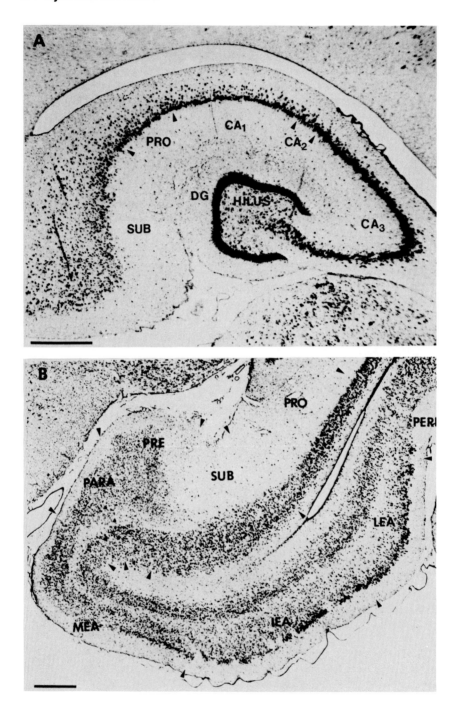

the fascia dentata only an occasional labeled neuron was observed in the polymorphic layer; however, the number of labeled granule cell neurons was similar to that observed on day E37. The two blades contained relatively equal numbers of labeled neurons, but the E42 neurons in the hidden blade were in a deeper radial position than those in the exposed blade.

Injections of [³H]thymidine made following E42 did not result in the labeling of any neurons in the hippocampus proper or in the polymorphic layer of the fascia dentata. Conversely, production of neurons destined for the granule cell layer of the fascia dentata continued for over 1 month. The neurons born on E55 were scattered in both blades of the granule cell layer rather equally. Many of cells born on E55 were at the deep border of the granule cell layer, and this became most prominent in the temporal portions of the hidden blade. By P7, production of neurons dramatically decreased at all levels of the granule cell layer. Relatively fewer neurons were labeled in the hidden than in the exposed blade at this stage, and the cells in the former tended to be more widely scattered (in the radial dimension). Injections of [³H]thymidine at later stages resulted in few labeled neurons in the fascia dentata.

Analysis of the Parahippocampal Gyrus

The first heavily labeled neurons in the parahippocampal cortex resulted from injections on E21 that labeled very few neurons in the deep part of layer VI and the subjacent white matter of the lateral and intermediate entorhinal areas (LEA and IEA, respectively; Fig. 2).

Injections on E22 resulted in the first heavy labeling of neurons within all parahippocampal regions (Fig. 2). The labeled neurons were primarily restricted to the deepest portion of each division. Within the LEA, a few labeled neurons were at the layer IV–V border; however, the median superficial to deep position of the labeled neurons was in the deepest portion of layer VI. A few labeled neurons were present in the molecular layer of the entorhinal cortex. The

---

Abbreviations for Figs. 1 and 2.

CA1,2,3	areas of Ammon's horn (cornu Ammonis)
DG	dentate gyrus
HILUS	polymorphic zone of the dentate gyrus
IEA	intermediate entorhinal area
LEA	lateral entorhinal area
MEA	medial entorhinal area
NEO	neocortex lateral to rhinal fissure
PARA	parasubiculum
PERI	perirhinal
PRE	presubiculum
PRO	prosubiculum
SUB	subiculum

Fig. 1. Bright-field photomicrographs of Nissl-stained coronal sections through the dorsal hippocampus (A) and ventral parahippocampal gyrus (B) of the cat to demonstrate the cytoarchitectonic divisions of this cortex. Bars = 500 μm and 1,000 μm in B.

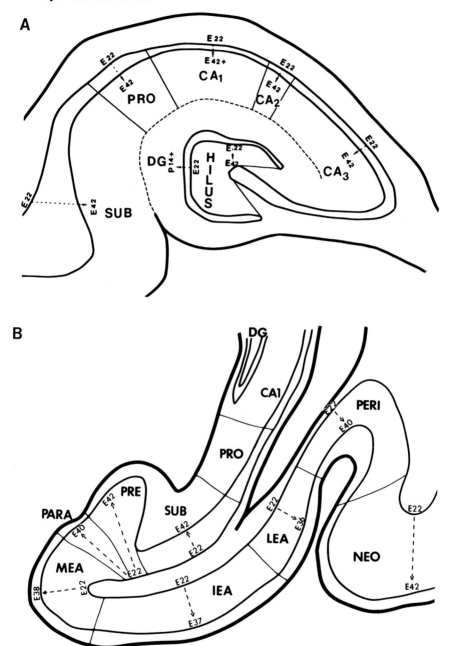

Fig. 2. Two line drawings to demonstrate the radial gradients of neuronal cell production in each region of the hippocampus (**A**) and parahippocampal gyrus (**B**) of the cat.

subicular fields contained relatively few labeled neurons, and these were in both the deep part of the deep neuronal layer and the underlying white matter.

Neurons that underwent their final mitosis on E32 had a more widespread superficial to deep distribution than those generated prior to this time. Within the entorhinal cortex, the LEA contained the most superficial, labeled neurons. The median labeled neuron in the IEA was somewhat more deeply situated than that in the LEA, while the median labeled neuron in the MEA was even more deeply situated. While the labeled neurons in the pre- and parasubiculum tended to be positioned more deeply than those in MEA, the labeled neurons in the subiculum were scattered throughout the full width of the pyramidal cell layer, with a few neurons located within the white matter. The subiculum proper contained a relatively high number of E32-generated neurons. An inspection of E30 and E31 animals led to the conclusion that the increase in the rate of neuron generation that began on E28 in the entorhinal cortex began in the subiculum around E32. This same increase began around E30 in the pre- and parasubiculum.

The distribution of neurons generated on E42 suggested that, by this date, nearly all neurons of the medial entorhinal area (MEA) and IEA (LEA proliferation ceased by day 38) had undergone their final mitosis. The rapid phase of neurogenesis of entorhinal neurons, which was initiated near E28, ceased by E36 in the LEA and by E38 in the MEA, and the remaining neuronal generation was at a much slower rate (i.e. fewer cells per day). The situation in the adjacent temporal neocortex was somewhat different. E42 injections label a rather large number of the layer III neurons, especially in the posterior half of this neocortical region. In this area of the neocortex neuronal production tapered off sharply by E50, and E55 injections resulted in no labeled neurons in this area. Production of subicular neurons still occurred at E42. In both subiculum and prosubiculum, the fast phase of cell production ceased around E38, and all neuronal production ceased shortly after E42. Despite the similarity in the ceasation of neuronal production in these regions, a entorhinosubiculum (i.e. rhinodentate) gradient of production was obvious.

RELATION OF HIPPOCAMPAL DEVELOPMENT IN CAT TO THAT IN OTHER SPECIES

The pattern of generation of neurons in the cat parahippocampal gyrus is quite similar to that described previously for the mouse (Angevine, 1965; Caviness, 1973), rat (Hine and Das, 1974; Bayer and Altman, 1974; Schlessinger et al., 1975, 1978; Bayer, 1980a,b), rabbit (Fernandez and Bravo, 1974), and monkey (Rakic and Nowakowski, 1981), but superimposed on this general pattern are alternations in the timing of neuron production within each of the previously reported gradients.

The production of parahippocampal neurons in the cat begins between E21 and E22 in all sectors of this cortex. Very few neurons are labeled in the LEA and IEA by E21 injections. On E22 more neurons are labeled in the LEA and IEA, and a significant number are labeled in all other regions of the parahippocampal gyrus. Thus, the initial slow phase of production begins nearly simultaneously in all regions (within 24 h). A fast phase of production begins slightly later, around E28. This fast phase begins first in the LEA, but within 24 h it has also begun in all other regions. Whereas both of these phases begin at nearly the same time, the end of production varies. By E36, the production of LEA neurons is nearly complete, with only a few caudal neurons produced on E37. IEA neuron production terminates approximately 24 h later. Production of MEA neurons continues up to E42. Subicular cortex neuron production also ends around E42.

The nearly simultaneous initiation of production in all parahippocampal sectors of the cat is similar to that seen in the monkey by Rakic and Nowa-kowski (1981). Further, the present observation that the initial tempo of pro-duction is markedly increased during a "fast phase" of production also agrees with these investigators; however, their finding that the date of initiation of the fast phase is significantly different in different areas with areas near the rhinal fissure entering this phase prior to those further removed was not ob-served in the cat parahippocampal cortex. The more limited time of neuronal production in these areas of the cat may preclude the detection of this gradient. In the cat, the slight gradient observed (LEA prior to MEA) in the onset of the fast phase is not significantly greater than that seen in the initiation of the slow phase.

One difference between the present timing analysis and that of Rakic and Nowakowski (1981) involves the subiculum and prosubiculum. In the latter study and in an independent study of the rat (Schlessinger et al., 1978), but apparently not in a study of the rabbit (Fernandez and Bravo, 1974), the sub-iculum is reported to be generated over a slightly shorter time period than other regions of the hippocampal cortex. This finding seems appropriate, since it is assumed that the subiculum (including the prosubiculum of the present analysis) is a phylogenetically older portion of the cortex than the more highly differential parts of the parahippocampal cortex (Swanson and Cowan, 1975; Meibach and Siegel, 1975; Rosene and van Hoesen, 1977; van Groen and Wyss, 1988). Further, since this region contains only a single neuronal cell layer that is continuous with the internal lamina of the presubiculum, it is logical to assume that subiculum neurons are born at a time similar to that of neurons in the internal lamina (and prior to that of the external lamina) of the pre-subiculum, thus resulting in a relatively short period of cell production. In the cat such a foreshortened period of neuronal production is not observed. In contrast, production is somewhat extended. Whether this reflects a species or a methodological difference cannot be concluded at this time; however, other aspects of subicular neuron generation are similar between the cat and the primate. For instance, as noted below, there is a lack of a clear inside-out gradient in the generation of primate subicular and prosubicular neurons in both species.

It is of interest to compare the relative embryonic period during which the parahippocampal gyrus is produced in different species (Table I). In the rodent (Angevine, 1965; Hine and Das, 1974) the period of parahippocampal neuron production is confined to the final one-third of gestation. Rakic and Nowa-kowski (1981) reported that in the monkey the production of parahippocampal

**TABLE I. Summary of Days on Which Neurons of a Given Region Are
Produced in Different Species**

Animal	Normal gestation	Granule cell layer fascia dentata	CA3	CA1	Subicular cortext	Entorhinal cortex
Mouse[1]	19	E10–P25+	E10–17	E10–17	E10–15	E10–16
Rat[2]	21	E14–P20+	E14–19	E14–19	E14–19	E13–18
Rat[3]	21	E16–P25+	E16–20	E16–20	E16–17	E15–17
Cat[4]	63	E22–P14+	E22–42	E22–42+	E22–42	E21–40
Monkey[5]	140	E38–P43+	E38–62	E38–70	E38–75	E36–70

The above data are from the following sources: 1, Angevine (1965); 2, Schlessinger et al. (1975, 1978); 3, Bayer (1980a,b); 4, Wyss et al. (1983) and Wyss and Sripanidkulchai (1985); 5, Rakic and Nowakowski (1981).

neurons is limited primarily to the second quarter of gestation, thus closely approximating the generation of the parahippocampal formation in humans (Humphrey, 1966). The cat appears intermediate in this respect, with production of parahippocampal neurons confined to the second one-third of gestation.

The production of neurons in the hippocampus proper and fascia dentata displays species differences similar to those noted above (Table I). Production of these neurons takes place close to the time of birth in the rodent, but in the monkey the CA neurons are generated near the middle of gestation. The cat is again intermediate. In the cat, neuronal production in all areas takes place over a period approximately two to four times longer than in the rat and 1.5 to 2.5 times shorter than in the monkey. Despite the timing differences, the relative production times between areas remains constant across species. As in the monkey, the period of production of hippocampal neurons in the cat is divided into slow and fast phases (Rakic and Nowakowski, 1981). Around E25 in CA3 and E32 in CA1 and CA2, production begins to accelerate dramatically. By day E42 production decreases significantly in all areas except the granule cell layer of the fascia dentata.

GRADIENTS OF CELL PRODUCTION

Four gradients of neurogenesis have commonly been observed within the hippocampal formation: 1) radial, 2) rhinodentate, 3) temporoseptal, and 4) sandwich. The most obvious gradient present is the radial (inside-out) gradient. This gradient, which is present in almost all areas of the cortex thus far studied, has been observed in the parahippocampal areas of the mouse (Angevine, 1965), rat (Hine and Das, 1974; Schlessinger et al., 1975; Bayer, 1980a), rabbit (Fernandez and Bravo, 1974), and monkey (Rakic and Nowakowski, 1981). In the cat, the subiculum and prosubiculum, which have a single neuronal layer, display less of an inside-out gradient than any of the other parahippocampal sectors. This lack of a sharp inside-out gradient has been previously noted in the monkey (Rakic and Nowakowski, 1981); however, that material indicated that the greatest lack of a gradient was present at the presubiculum–subiculum border, whereas in the cat the greatest lack of a gradient is in the region adjacent to the CA1 border.

An inside-out gradient also characterizes the production of neurons in the hippocampus proper; however, the gradient is less obvious than that present in the developing parahippocampal gyrus. This partial obscuring of the gradient likely results from the fact that Ammon's horn contains only a single, neuronal cell layer, and few neurons are present in the strata above and below that layer. The pyramidal layer is rather thin, and in some areas of CA1, the pyramidal layer is only two to three cells wide. The generation of neurons in the polymorphic layer of the facia dentata does not appear to be associated with any radial gradient. Neurons at all distances from the deep border of the granule cell layer are produced simultaneously throughout development.

In contrast to the inside-out gradient observed in most cortical regions, an outside-in gradient is present in granule cell layers of the fascia dentata of the rodent (Angevine, 1965; Bayer and Altman, 1974; Schlessinger et al., 1975), monkey (Rakic and Nowakowski, 1981), and cat (Wyss and Sripanidkulchai, 1985) in which, from E22 to P3, each successive wave of granule neurons generated assumes an increasingly deeper position in the layer. Neurons produced on P7 reside at the deepest portion of the layer; however, some of the granule neurons born on this and later days also take up positions in the center of the granule layer, thus diverging from the strict outside-in gradient. The fact that postnatal mitotic activity of granule neurons continues in the adult animal was first recognized by Altman (1963), and this finding has been confirmed repeatedly (Altman and Das, 1965, 1966; Bayer et al., 1982; Kaplan and Hinds, 1977). It seems likely that such late generated neurons either 1) increase the total population of granule neurons in the brain or 2) replace aberrant or dying granule neurons. Evidence for the first possibility is presented by Bayer et al. (1982), whose granule cell counts of the postnatally developing rat indicated a 35–43% accretion in number of neurons between postnatal days 30 and 365. If all of the late born neurons act to increase the total granule cell population, then one might expect that late born neurons would tend to lie close to the deep border of the granule layer and that a primitive stem cell population would also reside in this location. In the cat many late born neurons are located toward the center of the granule layer, suggesting that these cells may undergo mitosis within the layer but, more importantly, that these additional neurons may replace neurons in this location. Both propositions (i.e. increase and replacement) likely occur.

Studies in all species demonstrate that a production gradient proceeds away from the rhinal fissure and through the subiculum. Additionally, all studies report that the neurons in the hidden blade of the granule cell layer develop earlier than those in the exposed blade. Two exceptions exist. Our study in cat and the studies of Bayer (1980a) and Schlessinger et al. (1978) indicate that within Ammon's horn the neurons of the polymorphic area and CA3 tend to be born earlier than those of CA1. This finding is consistent with the general pattern of neurogenesis by which large cell production leads small cell production. Another exception to the rhinodentate production gradient is the development of the cat perirhinal cortex, which lags significantly behind that of the LEA, despite its position deep in the rhinal sulcus. This finding seems to differ from that reported for the rat (Schlessinger et al., 1978), in which the perirhinal cortex is considered to precede the LEA in development; however, a close inspection of the data of Schlessinger et al. (1978) shows that the MEA and perirhinal cortex are generated at nearly the same time, thus agreeing with the data from the cat.

A third production gradient (i.e. temporoseptal) is observed clearly in the entorhinal cortex of the cat and to a lesser extent in other regions of the hippocampal formation of the cat. A similar temporoseptal gradient is present in the rat dentate gyrus (Schlessinger et al., 1978), and Bayer (1980a) has reported a temporal to occipital pattern in the production of the rat dentate gyrus and parasubiculum. Previous studies did not find a temporoseptal neuronal production gradient in the other regions of the hippocampal/parahippocampal formation. Rakic and Nowakowski (1981) did not observe any temporal to septal gradients in the monkey. Several factors could account for these differences. Our analyses in the cat are based on the position of labeled cells within the inside-out gradient in each area at each level. The other studies are based on total number of cells produced on each day in each area at each level. Second, the longer production time of neurons in the cat (compared with that in the rat) entorhinal cortex may facilitate the observation of the temporoseptal gradients. Third, most of the previous reports deal mainly with the posterior half of the entorhinal cortex, and, even in the cat, the gradient is not as clear when only this portion is inspected.

Bayer (1980a; see also Bayer and Altman, 1987) indicates that in the rat the vast majority of neurons in the stratum radiatum and lacunosum-moleculare of Ammon's horn undergo final mitosis at a significantly earlier date than the neurons in most of the pyramidal layer, thus creating what she termed a "sandwich gradient," with deep and superficial neurons produced first and intermediate neurons (which account for over 80% of the neurons [our counts]) produced later. This pattern is present in other areas of the rat hippocampal formation, and, in general, this pattern is present in the monkey hippocampal formation (Rakic and Nowakowski, 1981) and in the cat parahippocampal gyrus (Wyss et al., 1983). In contrast, all of the superficial neurons of the CA fields in the cat are not produced at early stages; many of the most superficial continue to undergo mitosis rather late in gestation.

ROLE OF EARLY GENERATED NEURONS

Two types of neurons are born earlier than the appropriate gradients would suggest. The first of these are the molecular layer neurons, which are born between E22 and E27 in the cat and take up permanent residence in all parts of the parahippocampal cortex. Such early generated, molecular layer neurons have previously been reported in the mouse (Angevine, 1965), rat (Schlessinger et al., 1978; Bayer, 1980a), and monkey (Rakic and Nowakowski, 1981) parahippocampal cortex. These early born layer I neurons may be the remnant of the Cajal-Retzius neurons (Ramón y Cajal, 1891; Retzius, 1893). Although several authors have reported that Cajal-Retzius neurons do not survive into adult life (Noback and Purpura, 1961; Duckett and Pearse, 1968; Molliver and van der Loos, '70), others have suggested that they may be more permanent, either in their original form or in an altered morphology (Fox and Inman, 1966; Marin-Padilla, 1972). The present data demonstrate that some early generated neurons in the molecular layer of the parahippocampal cortex survive into young adulthood in the cat.

The second class of early generated neurons are those appearing in the transition zones. The data from the E22–E32 experiments in the cat indicate that neurons near the medial and lateral borders of all areas are situated somewhat more superficially than are neurons that were born on the same day but are situated nearer to the center of the specific area. Such a phenomenon is perhaps a varient of the "sandwich gradient" reported by Bayer (1980a) and may be similar to the observations of Rakic and Nowakowski (1981) concerning production of neurons at the subicular–presubicular border; however, neither of the later studies demonstrate this phenomenon at all transition zones.

Marin-Padilla (1970, 1972, 1978) suggested that early generated molecular layer neurons (Cajal-Retzius cells) are one of three classes (the other two are the Martinotti and pyramidal neurons of layer VI) of neurons that create the primordial cortical organization via their interrelationships with one another and by the receipt and holding of the first afferent connections to reach each area (see Konig et al., 1975; Raedler and Raedler, 1978; Rickmann et al., 1977). These neurons also may affect development by an ability to stop neuronal migration through a cell to cell interaction with the migrating neuron itself or with the radial glia directing the neuron's migration (Levitt et al., 1983; Sidman and Rakic, 1973). Whether these early generated neurons of the cat hippocampal formation are a remnant of such a functional class remains to be elucidated.

The relationship between the time of neuronal birthdate and the eventual afferent and efferent connections of hippocampal formation neurons remains unclear. Bayer and Altman (1987) reviewed the literature in this regard and suggested a strong correlation between birthdate and connections. For instance, the earliest born neurons in the entorhinal cortex (LEA) innervate the outer molecular layer of the dentate gyrus, whereas later born neurons innervate more proximal areas of the dentate granule cells. Despite this strong correlation, it seems unlikely that these factors alone could account for the very precise lamination of the entorhinal projections to the dentate gyrus (Hjörth-Simonsen and Zimmer, 1975; Steward, 1976; Wyss, 1981). The time of origin of the neuron or the time of axon arrival is more likely to play a role in the relative distribution of afferents within a restricted zone. For instance, the ipsilateral projection from cells of the dentate hilus to the dentate molecular layer is heaviest in the hidden (early generated) blade, but the commissural projection (later arriving) is densest in the outer (later generated) blade.

One further consideration relates to the recent finding of Stanfield et al. (1987) that demonstrates that the hippocampal formation sends out projections (i.e. a postmamillary projection) that are later retracted in favor of a more proximal collateral terminal field (i.e. the mamillary complex). The evidence for the temporal hypothesis must be considered in relation to these transient connections.

Although further studies in whole animal may elucidate the role of early generated neurons and neuronal production gradients in the development of connectivity in the hippocampal formation, it is likely that many of the answers will require the use of in vitro techniques to uncover the molecular signals that interact with mechanical and timing events to produce the exquisitely precise connections and physiology of the hippocampal formation (see e.g. Banker, 1980; Seifert et al., 1983).

ACKNOWLEDGMENTS

We thank Mrs. Maxine Rudolph for her secretarial assistance in the preparation of this manuscript. This study was supported by NIH grants NS 16592 and HL 34315.

REFERENCES

Altman, J. (1963) Autoradiographic investigation of cell proliferation in the brains of rats and cats. Anat. Rec. *145*:573–577.

Altman, J., and G. Das (1965) Autoradiographic and histological evidence of postnatal neurogenesis in rat. J. Comp. Neurol. *124*:319–336.

Altman, J., and G. Das (1966) Autoradiographic and histological studies of postnatal neurogenesis. I. A longitudinal investigation of the kinetics, migration and transformation of cells incorporating tritiated thymidine. J. Comp. Neurol. *126*: 337–390.

Altman, J., and G. Das (1967) Postnatal neurogenesis in the guinea pig. Nature (Lond.) *214*:1098–1101.

Amaral, D.G. (1978) A Golgi study of cell types in the hilar region of the hippocampus in the rat. J. Comp. Neurol. *182*:851–914.

Angevine, J.B. (1965) Time of neuron origin in the hippocampal region: An autoradiographic study in the mouse. Exp. Neurol. [Suppl.] *13(2)*:1–70.

Banker, G.A. (1980) Trophic interactions between astroglial cells and hippocampal neurons in culture. Science *209*:809–810.

Bayer, S.A. (1980a) Development of the hippocampal region in the rat. I. Neurogenesis examined with ^{3}H-thymidine autoradiography. J. Comp. Neurol. *190*:87–114.

Bayer, S.A. (1980b) Development of the hippocampal region in the rat. II. Morphogenesis during embryonic and early postnatal life. J. Comp. Neurol. *190*:115–134.

Bayer, S.A., and J. Altman (1974) Hippocampal development in the rat: Cytogenesis and morphogenesis examined with autoradiography and low-level X-irradiation. J. Comp. Neurol. *158*:55–80.

Bayer, S.A., and J. Altman (1987) Directions in neurogenic gradients and patterns of anatomical connections in the telencephalon. Prog. Neurobiol. *29*:57–106.

Bayer, S.A., J.W. Yackel, and P.S. Puri, (1982) Neurons in the rat dentate gyrus granular layer substantially increase during juvenile and adult life. Science *216*: 890–892.

Blackstad, T.W. (1956) Commissural connections of the hippocampal region in the rat, with special reference to their mode of termination. J. Comp. Neurol. *105:*417–537.

Caviness, V.S. Jr. (1973) Time of neuron origin in the hippocampus and dentate gyrus of normal and reeler mutant mice: An autoradiographic analysis. J. Comp. Neurol. *151:*113–120.

Duckett, S., and A.G.E. Pearse (1968) The cells of Cajal-Retzius in the developing human brain. J. Anat. *102:*183–187.

Fernandez, V., and H. Bravo (1974) Autoradiographic study of development of the cerebral cortex in the rabbit. Brain Behav. Evol. *9:*317–332.

Fox, M.W., and O. Inman (1966) Persistence of Cajal-Retzius cells in developing dog brain. Brain Res. *3:*192–194.

Habets, A.M.M.C. (1980) Projection of the Prepyriform Cortex to the Hippocampus in the Cat: A Multidisciplinary Study. Utrecht, The Netherlands: Institute of Medical Physics.

Habets, A.M.M.C., F.H. Lopes da Silva, and F.W. deQuartel (1980) Autoradiography of the olfactory-hippocampal pathway in the cat with special reference to the perforant path. Exp. Brain Res. *38:*257–265.

Hine, R.J., and G.D. Das (1974) Neuroembryogenesis in the hippocampal formation of the rat. An autoradiographic study. Z. Anat. Entwickl. Gesch. *144:*173–186.

Hines, M. (1922) Studies in the growth and differentiation of the telencephalon in man. The fissura hippocampal. J. Comp. Neurol. *34:*73–171.

Hjörth-Simonsen, A., and S. Laurberg (1977) Commissural connections of the dentate area in the rat. J. Comp. Neurol. *174:*591–605.

Hjörth-Simonsen, A., and J. Zimmer (1975) Crossed pathways from the entorhinal area to the fascia dentata. 1. Normal in rabbits. J. Comp. Neurol. *161:*57–70.

Humphrey, T. (1966) The development of the human hippocampal formation correlated with some aspects of its phylogenetic history. In R. Hassler and H. Stephan (eds): Evolution of the Forebrain. Stuttgart: Georg Thieme Verlag, pp. 104–116.

Kandel, E.R., and W.A. Spencer (1961) Excitation and inhibition of single pyramidal cells during hippocampal seizure. Exp. Neurol. *4:*162–179.

Kaplan, M.S., and J.W. Hinds (1977) Neurogenesis in the adult rat: Electron microscopic analysis of light radioautographs. Science *197:*1092–1094.

Konig, N., G. Roch, and R. Marty (1975) The onset of synaptogenesis in rat temporal cortex. Anat. Embryol. *148:*73–87.

Krettek, J.E., and J.L. Price (1978) A description of the amygdaloid complex in the rat and cat with observations on the intra-amygdaloid axonal connections. J. Comp. Neurol. *178:*255–280.

Levitt, P., M.L. Cooper, and P. Rakic (1983) Early divergence and changing proportions of neuronal and glial precursor cells in the primate cerebral ventricular zone. Dev. Biol. *96:*472–484.

Lorente de Nó, R. (1934) Studies on the structure of the cerebral cortex. II. Continuation of the study of the Ammonic system. J. Psychol. Neurol. *46:*113–177.

Marin-Padilla, M. (1970) Prenatal and early postnatal ontogenesis of the human motor cortex: A Golgi study. I. The sequential development of the cortical layers. Brain Res. *23:*167–183.

Marin-Padilla, M. (1972) Prenatal ontogenetic history of the principal neurons of the neocortex of the cat *(Felis domestica).* A Golgi study. II. Developmental differences and their significances. Z. Anat. Entwickl. Gesch., *136:*125–142.

Marin-Padilla, M. (1978) Dual origin of the mammalian neocortex and evolution of the cortical plate. Anat. Embryol. *152:*109–126.

Meibach, R.C., and A. Siegel (1975) The origin of fornix fibers which project to the mammillary bodies in the rat: A horseradish peroxidase study. Brain Res. *88:*518–522.

Molliver, M.E., and H. van der Loos (1970) The ontogenesis of cortical circuitry: The spatial distribution of synapses in somesthetic cortex of newborn dog. Ergeb. Anat. Entwickl. Gesch. *42:*1–54.

Noback, C.R., and D.P. Purpura (1961) Postnatal ontogenesis of neurons in cat neocortex. J. Comp. Neurol. *117:*291–307.

Nowakowski, R.S., and P. Rakic (1981) The site of origin and route and rate of migration of neurons to the hippocampal region of the rhesus monkey. J. Comp. Neurol. *196:*129–154.

Raedler, E., and A. Raedler (1978) Autoradiographic study of early neurogenesis in rat neocortex. Anat. Embryol. *154:*267–284.

Rakic, P., and R.S. Nowakowski (1981) The time of origin of neurons in the hippocampal region of the rhesus monkey. J. Comp. Neurol. *196:*99–128.

Ramón y Cajal, S. (1891) Sur la structure de l'ecorce cerebrale de quelques mammiferes. La Cellule *7:*125–176, plates 1–3.

Ramón y Cajal, S. (1972) Histologie du systeme nerveus de L'Homme et Vertebres, Vol. 2. Madrid: Maloine C S/C, pp. 647–823.

Retzius, G. (1893) Die Cajal'schen Zellen der Grosshirnrinde bei Menschen und bei Sängethieren. Biol. Untersuch. (Stockh.) *V:*1–8, plates I–IV.

Rickmann, M., B.M. Chronwall, and J.R. Wolff (1977) On the development of nonpyramidal neurons and axons outside the cortical plate: The early marginal zone as a pallial anlage. Anat. Embryol. *151:*285–307.

Rosene, D.L., and G.W. van Hoesen (1977) Hippocampal efferents reach widespread areas of cerebral cortex and amygdala in the rhesus monkey. Science *198:*315–317.

Schlessinger, A.R., W.M. Cowan, and D.I. Gottieb (1975) An autoradiographic study of the time of origin and pattern of granule cell migration in the dentate gyrus of the rat. J. Comp. Neurol. *159:*149–176.

Schlessinger, A.R., W.M. Cowan, and L.W. Swanson (1978) The time of origin of neurons in Ammon's horn and the associated retrohippocampal fields. Anat. Embryol. *154:*153–173.

Seifert, W., B. Ranscht, H.J. Fink, F. Förster, B. Beckh, and H.W. Hüller (1983) Development of hippocampal neurons in cell culture: A molecular approach. In W. Seifert (ed): Neurobiology of the Hippocampus. New York: Academic Press, pp. 109–138.

Sidman, R.L., and P. Rakic (1973) Neuronal migration with special reference to developing human brain: A review. Brain Res. *62:*1–35.

Stanfield, B.B., B.R. Nahin, and D.D.M. O'Leary (1987) A transient postmammillary component of the rat fornix during development: Implications for interspecific differences in mature axonal projections. J. Neurosci. *7:*3350–3361.

Steward, O. (1976) Topographic organization of the projections from the entorhinal area to hippocampal formation of the rat. J. Comp. Neurol. *167:*258–314.

Swanson, L.W., and W.M. Cowan (1975) Hippocampo-hypothalamic connections: Origins in the subicular cortex, not Ammon's horn. Science *189:*303–304.

Swanson, L.W., J.M. Wyss, and W.M. Cowan (1978) An autoradiographic study of the organization of intrahippocampal association pathways in the rat. J. Comp. Neurol. *181:*681–716.

van Groen, Th., and M. Wyss (1988) Species differences in hippocampal commissural connections: Studies in rat, guinea pig, rabbit and cat. J. Comp. Neurol. *267:*322–334.

West, J.R., H.O. Nornes, C.L. Barnes, and M. Bronfenbrenner (1979) The cells of origin of the commissural afferents to the area dentata in the mouse. Brain Res. *160:*203–215.

Wyss, J.M. (1981) An autoradiographic study of the efferent connections of the entorhinal cortex in the rat. J. Comp. Neurol. *199:*495–512.

Wyss, J.M., and B. Sripanidkulchai (1985) The development of Ammon's horn and the fascia dentata in the cat. A [³H]thymidine analysis. Dev. Brain Res. *18:*185–198.

Wyss, J.M., B. Sripandkulchai, and T.L. Hickey (1983) An analysis of the time of origin of neurons in the entorhinal and subicular cortices of the cat. J. Comp. Neurol. *221:*341–357.

Zimmer, J. (1971) Ipsilateral afferents to the commissural zone of the fascia dentata, demonstrated in decommissurated rats by silver impregnation. J. Comp. Neurol. *142:*393–416.

The Hippocampus—New Vistas, pages 17–31
© 1989 Alan R. Liss, Inc.

2
Some Implications of Postnatal Maturation of the Hippocampus

LYNN NADEL AND JEFFREY WILLNER

Department of Psychology, University of Arizona, Tucson, Arizona

INTRODUCTION

In most brain systems the generation of nerve cells concludes before birth. The dentate gyrus of the hippocampal formation is one of the few exceptions; postnatal neurogenesis has been documented in this structure in a variety of nonhuman mammals (mouse: Angevine, 1965; rat: Altman and Das, 1965; Bayer, 1980; Schlessinger et al., 1975, 1978; cat: Purpura and Pappas, 1968; Wyss and Sripanidkulchai, 1985; rabbit: Guéneau et al., 1982). Neurogenesis in the dentate gyrus of the rat and rabbit apparently continues well into adulthood, and perhaps throughout life, though at a very low rate (Kaplan and Bell, 1983; Guéneau et al., 1982). It now appears that the same is true for primate development in general and human development in particular. Several recent studies of the development of primate hippocampal formation (Rakic and Nowakowski, 1981; Rakic, 1985; Kretschmann et al., 1986; Brody et al., 1987) indicate that there is also extensive postnatal development in monkeys and humans. Rakic and Nowakowski (1981) showed that although pyramidal cell generation concludes before birth, dentate granule cells continue to be generated for some months postnatally. Kretschmann et al. (1986) concluded from their analysis of 25 male brains from the Yakovlev collection that the maximum rate of growth in hippocampal formation occurs at about 2 months postnatally (the comparable figure for the mouse is 4 days postnatally). Myelination continues considerably beyond this time, reaching adult levels after 3–5 years (Brody et al., 1987); cellular RNA content measures reach adult values in the subiculum only at 9 years (Uemura and Hartmann, 1979). Thus there is every reason to believe that there is in humans, as in rats, a prolonged period of early life during which significant maturation is occurring within the hippocampal region. Though this chapter is most directly concerned with the rat, our assumption is that lessons learned from studies of the rat will prove relevant to humans as well.

IMPLICATIONS

Any consideration of the functional implications of delayed maturation of the hippocampus requires some appreciation of the role of this brain system in behavior. We consider the hippocampus to be a central part of an internal representational system concerned with constructing (and perhaps storing) cognitive/spatial maps of experience (O'Keefe and Nadel, 1978; Nadel et al., 1985). As such, it plays a critical role in the creation of long-lasting memories for episodes and events—what Schacter (1988) has referred to as "explicit" knowledge. O'Keefe discusses some recent evidence for the spatial map hypothesis of hippocampal function (Speakman and O'Keefe, Chapter 27, this volume); we will not expand on the theory here (see O'Keefe and Speakman, 1987). It will be assumed in what follows that the hippocampal formation plays a critical role in only some forms of learning and memory, with an emphasis on memory for places and the events that transpire in those places. Whether or not one accepts this characterization of the role of the hippocampus in learning and memory (cf. O'Keefe and Nadel, 1979), it is clear that hippocampal dysfunction has profoundly disruptive effects on learning and memory in human adults. The classic patient H.M., who suffered extensive hippocampal damage in an operation meant to control epileptic seizures (Scoville and Milner, 1957), describes his condition as something like constantly "waking from a dream."

Given this background, we will consider what consequences might flow from the fact that the hippocampus is not functional during the earliest stages of life. Among the implications that we have explored in recent years is the idea that the absence of the hippocampal memory system at the start of life accounts in part for "infantile amnesia" (Nadel and Zola-Morgan, 1984); the idea that learning that occurs in nonhippocampal systems early in life can be reinstated under stress, thereby creating conditions for the establishment of unusual "fears and phobias" (Jacobs and Nadel, 1985); and, finally, the idea that the late development and maturation of the hippocampus puts it at risk in Down syndrome (Nadel, 1986, 1988).

We will focus on a somewhat different implication of the delayed development and maturation of the hippocampus in this chapter. Here, we will be concerned with the possibility that early experiences could influence the development, and ultimately the functioning, of the hippocampus. The general principle that early experiences can alter emotional and cognitive functioning is well-established. Dogs, for example, display highly aberrant emotional behavior after extensive sensory deprivation during development (Melzack and Thompson, 1956); separation from the mother in early life can induce wide-ranging abnormalities in social, sexual, and parental behavior (Suomi and Harlow, 1971; Levine, 1962); rearing in enriched environments increases various parameters of brain size (Rosenzweig et al., 1972; Greenough, 1984); and extra stimulation in neonates can improve reactions to stress (Meaney et al., 1988).

What has been lacking until now is some understanding of the neurodevelopmental events that were influenced by such early experiences. This situation has begun to change, however, as we will try to show through a discussion of recent work. The picture that emerges from this work is most exciting:

Events occurrring early in life can indeed have a lasting impact on the development of the hippocampal system. Further, depending on the nature (and timing) of these experiences, the functional status of the hippocampus can be altered for better or for worse. Given the importance of the hippocampal system for cognitive function—consider what H.M. is like without a hippocampus—the effects of early experience on hippocampal development and function are of considerable interest.

EARLY EXPERIENCE AND THE MATURATION OF HIPPOCAMPAL FUNCTION

A variety of evidence suggests that the hippocampus of the rat matures at about the end of the third week of postnatal life, just when the pup is ready to be weaned from the mother (for a review of the evidence, see Nadel and Zola-Morgan, 1984). Data from behavioral experiments lead to much the same conclusion; behavioral capacities for which an intact hippocampus is essential do not emerge until this age (cf. Somerville, 1979). This was first observed for spontaneous alternation (Douglas et al., 1973; Frederickson and Frederickson, 1979) and other forms of exploration (Feigley et al., 1972; File, 1978; Williams et al., 1975), and it has most recently been confirmed for development of place learning in the Morris water maze (Rudy et al., 1987).

In our initial studies of early experience and hippocampal development, we examined how extra handling and bouts of overnight isolation from the dam during the first 2 weeks of postnatal life would affect the emergence of exploratory behavior (Kurz et al., 1984). Litters of Long-Evans rats were bred in our laboratory and subjected to a modified handling-isolation procedure.[1] Exploration was then assessed in a large open arena (ca. 6 ft diameter) containing four junk objects that the rats could climb in or on. Rats were lowered into the center of this arena in a closed box, the sides of which opened downwards, giving the rat access to the arena. Mature rats are typically cautious about leaving the safety of this "home base," but they eventually move out and make contact with the objects, which were located at preselected sites midway between the home base and the walls of the arena. The age at which rats first show an interest in these objects was used as a marker for the emergence of exploratory behavior. Rats were tested between 16 and 25 days of age, in one of two ways: with a within-subjects design in which each animal was tested daily for 20 min in the arena or with a between-subjects design in which each animal was tested twice on a single day (10 min per trial).[2] In both cases,

---

[1] All litters were culled to four males and four females on the second day of postnatal life; the day of birth is designated PN1. On postnatal days 5, 6, 7, 8, 10, 12, and 14, rats receiving the handling treatment were removed from the maternal cage, placed in a small cardboard box, and gently shaken from side to side for 5 min. On days 9, 11, and 13, these pups were removed from the maternal cage and maintained as a group on clean shavings in a heated, lit cage for 8 h.

[2] In all the research to be reported here, testing was conducted by researchers who were unaware of which rats had received the early handling-isolation treatment.

interest in the objects (as measured by time spent in the sectors containing objects) emerged sometime between postnatal days 17 and 25 in most rats. What is more, the emergence of exploration in any given rat, as seen in the within-subject study, was quite abrupt. Rats made the transition from spending almost no time in the object sectors to spending the maximum time within a 24-h period (see Fig. 1A). The abrupt emergence of exploration in any individual animal would of course tend to be obscured in group data, giving the misleading impression that it emerged gradually over several days.

What effect did our early experience manipulation have on the normal pattern of development? As shown in Figure 1B, exploration emerged in the control animals between postnatal days 17 and 25, with roughly the same number of rats beginning to explore on each of these days. However, all the rats receiving the early handling-isolation treatment began to explore the objects by postnatal day 21, with both males and females being affected by this treatment. Early handling and isolation speeded up the emergence of exploration, suggesting that this manipulation might be altering the timing of hippocampal development.

SPECIFICITY OF EARLY EXPERIENCE EFFECTS

Although suggestive, the results of our initial studies of exploration are far from definitive. The hippocampus is only one of several brain structures undergoing significant changes during early postnatal life; we cannot simply assume that handling-isolation is exerting its effects on exploration by altering the development of the hippocampal formation. One way to explore the issue of specificity is to determine whether early handling-isolation also affects the development of capacities that do not require the hippocampus. We therefore undertook a study of the effects of early handling-isolation on the emergence of two different forms of learning in the water maze (Willner, Kurz and Nadel, manuscript in preparation). In the *place learning* version of the water maze, rats are trained to find a submerged platform that they cannot see but that is always found in the same location in the tank. Efficient performance on this version of the task requires that the rat learn where the platform is located relative to extramaze cues. As might be expected, lesions of the hippocampus disrupted both the acquisition *and* retention of place learning in the water maze (Morris et al., 1982). In the *cue learning* version of the task, on the other hand, the rat's goal is to find a visible platform whose location in the tank changes from trial to trial. The animal can solve this version of the task by learning to approach a specific cue in the water maze; it does not need to learn about the location of the platform at all. Indeed, efficient performance on the cued version of the water maze task would almost seem to require that the rat learn to ignore the location of the platform in the tank. It should therefore come as no surprise that lesions of the hippocampus have little, if any, impact on the rat's ability to solve this version of the water maze task (Morris et al., 1982). Further, one can see a similar dissociation between place and cue learning during ontogeny. Rudy et al. (1987) observed that rats first displayed a capacity for place learning in the water maze around day 21, whereas the capacity for cue learning in the water maze was present as early as day 17 of

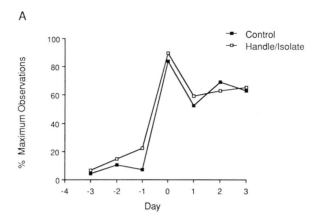

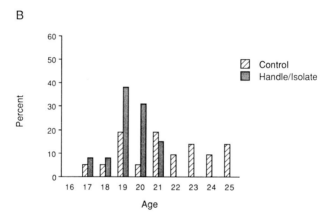

Fig. 1. **A:** Number of observations in object sectors of the arena expressed as a percentage of the maximum number of object-sector observations ever displayed by the animal. Day 0 was defined as the day on which an animal first exceeded 50% of its maximum and represents the day on which an animal began to explore the arena, while the other data points represent the 3 days preceding and following this day. **B:** Percentage of animals beginning to explore on each postnatal day (N = 21 and 13 for control and experimental groups, respectively).

postnatal life. Thus, to the extent that the effects of early handling-isolation on behavior reflect a selective impact on hippocampal development, early handling-isolation should differentially affect place and cue learning in the water maze.

In our study, rats from control and experimental litters received 2 days of training (seven trials per day) on either the cued or place learning versions of the water maze task. Pilot work in our laboratory had confirmed the finding of Rudy et al. (1987) that place and cue learning emerged at different times during ontogeny, so tests of cue learning were conducted with rats 16, 18, 20, or 22 days of age at the start of training, while tests for place learning were conducted with rats 20, 22, 24, or 26 days old at the start of training.[3] Figure 2 shows the course of acquisition for the experimental and control groups on the two tasks. Figure 2A shows the daily mean performance of the controls on the two tasks, and Figure 2B shows the same data for the experimental groups. These data confirm the findings of Rudy et al. (1987) that the capacity for cue learning emerges by day 18 and that rats of a given age perform better on the cue task than do comparable animals tested on the place learning task. Figure 2C,D provides a closer look at the course of cue learning in the two sexes, with Figure 2C showing the data for male animals and Figure 2D showing those for female rats. There are many points that could be made concerning these data, but the major point is that neither sex nor handling-isolation turned out to be an important factor in the ontogeny of cue learning. These data stand in sharp contrast to the results shown in Figure 2E,F, which presents the data on the acquisition of place learning. Here, we observed a clear difference in performance between male and female controls in the acquisition of place learning, with the females showing a greater improvement from day 1 to day 2 of training. This effect was completely absent in the rats subjected to handling-isolation, however; experimental females were no better than control or experimental males and significantly worse than the control females. These data, then, provide initial evidence that there is at least some specificity in the effects of handling-isolation on development. Early handling-isolation had virtually no effects on the ontogeny of cue learning, but did affect the ontogeny of place learning in female rats receiving this treatment, suggesting that this treatment affects the development of the hippocampus.

[3]Groups in the cue learning condition were comprised of 12 rats (six males and six females) from five to six different litters, while place learning groups were comprised of 16 rats (eight males and eight females) from five to eight different litters. As a further safeguard against possible litter effects, the assignment of rats from a given litter to the different conditions of the experiment was counterbalanced as closely as possible for task, sex and age.

The training apparatus was a circular metal tank ≈1.6m in diameter, located in a room containing a number of visual and auditory extramaze cues. The water in the tank was made opaque through the addition of condensed milk and was maintained at a temperature of 25°C throughout training. The platform was 0.015 m below the surface of the water. For animals in the cue learning condition, the location of the platform was marked by a dark rubber ball, 0.05 m in diameter, hung 0.15 m above the top of the platform.

On any given trial, the rats allowed a maximum of 60 s to locate the platform in the tank. Rats who found the platform within the 60 s limit were allowed to remain there for 20 s before being removed to a heated holding cage for a 5 min intertrial interval, while rats who failed to find the platform were gently guided to the platform and allowed to remain there for 20 s before removal from the apparatus.

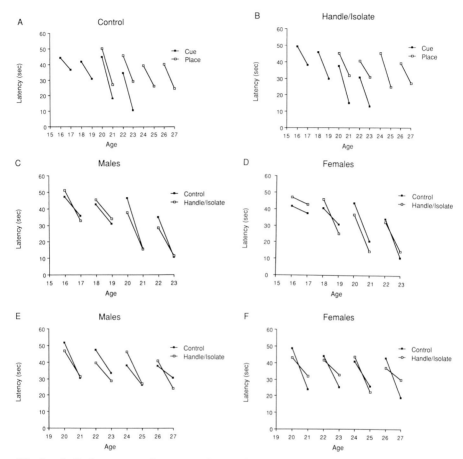

Fig. 2. **A:** Daily mean performance of controls on cue and place versions of the watermaze task. **B:** Daily mean performance of handled-isolated rats on cue and place versions of the watermaze task. **C:** Daily mean performance of control and handled-isolated males on cue version of the watermaze. **D:** Daily mean performance of control and handled-isolated females on cue version of the watermaze. **E:** Daily mean performance of control and handled-isolated males on place version of the watermaze task. **F:** Daily mean performance of control and handled-isolated females on place version of the watermaze.

Somewhat more direct evidence that early handling-isolation alters hippocampal development comes from a study examining the effects of this manipulation on the physiological functioning of the hippocampus (Wilson et al., 1986). We examined long-term potentiation (LTP) in 30–40-day-old control and experimental rats and found that rats receiving the early handling-isolation treatment displayed more LTP than the control rats. This was a surprising finding. On the one hand, our behavioral data suggested that early handling-isolation had detrimental effects on hippocampal development. To the extent that LTP can be viewed as a component of learning processes in the hippocampus, on the other hand, our data seemed to indicate that early handling-isolation was enhancing hippocampal function. A recent study on the ontogeny of LTP suggests a resolution to this apparent contradiction between our behavioral and electrophysiological data. Harris and Teyler (1984) found that LTP, as measured by changes in the population spike, was maximal at an early age (ca. 15 days) and then declined to adult values. Although the functional implications of this pattern of maturation of LTP in the hippocampus still need to be clarified, our results would seem to indicate that early handling-isolation delays the decline in LTP normally seen during development.

LONG-TERM EFFECTS OF EARLY HANDLING-ISOLATION

Our behavioral and physiological data, then, suggest that early handling-isolation alters hippocampal maturation. Do these effects of early handling-isolation have a long-lasting impact on hippocampal function? There are reasons for thinking that this is the case and that the impact is largely a negative one. First, in a follow-up of our original LTP study, we found that early handling-isolation caused long-term changes in hippocampal LTP (Wilson, Willner, Nadel, and Kurz, unpublished data). Unlike the situation in young rats, we observed that rats receiving early handling-isolation showed little or no LTP at 6 months of age. Perhaps the most convincing evidence for a long-term effect of early handling-isolation on hippocampal function, however, comes from behavioral studies we have conducted showing that this manipulation alters spatial problem-solving strategies in the adult rat (Willner, Nadel, and Kurz, manuscript in preparation).

Many of the tasks used to study learning and memory in animals have multiple solutions. When assessing the effects of a given brain manipulation, it is important to determine not only *whether* the animal can solve the task, but also *how* it is doing it. Consider the case of a T-maze discrimination task where the rat is always reinforced with food for choosing the same arm of the maze. One way that the rat could learn to solve this task would be to learn to make a particular response (e.g. "turn right") when it reached the choice point in the maze. Alternatively, the rat could solve the task by learning to go to a particular place on the maze to obtain food independent of the behaviors it must perform to reach that location. Unfortunately, the simple fact that a rat masters the task tells one nothing about how it used the information available to it to solve the task. To do this, one must test the animals with "probe" trials during which the different strategies are pitted against one another. In the case of our T-maze example, one could determine whether a rat was using a place or response "strategy" to solve the task by starting the animal from an arm 180° away from the original start arm. Under these conditions, the rat using a place strategy would make a different response (e.g. "turn left"), but end up in the same location, whereas the rat using a response strategy would make the same response and go to a different location on the maze.

What makes the determination of the strategy that an animal is using to solve a given task so important is the fact that different strategies seem to depend on different neural substrates. The hippocampus, for example, is an essential component of the neural circuitry underlying the use of place strategies in behavior (cf. Black et al., 1977). Even though they acquire a T-maze task like the one we have described as rapidly as normal animals, rats with hippocampal lesions do not use place strategies to solve this task, but rely on response strategies instead (Means and Douglas, 1970). This stands in sharp contrast to what one sees in normal animals, where 75–80% of the animals use a place strategy to solve the task.

We used a T-maze discrimination task to assess the effects of our early handling-isolation manipulation on the adult rat's use of place strategies in problem solving. Control and experimental rats between 6 and 7 months of age were trained on a T-maze discrimination in which the rat was rewarded with food for choosing the arm opposite its initial side preference. Once a rat had reached criterion performance (seven correct in eight consecutive trials), it was given a probe trial with the start arm rotated 180° to the other side of the maze. Although there were no significant between-group differences in the number of trials it took rats to reach criterion, the groups differed in how they tried to solve the discrimination. Figure 3 shows the results of the probe trials for males and females in the control and experimental groups. The first thing to notice in the graph is that more than three-fourths of the animals in the control group used a place strategy to solve the discrimination, an outcome we have replicated on a number of occasions. This situation is reversed in rats receiving the early handling-isolation treatment; almost two-thirds of these rats used a response strategy to solve the task. This latter result closely resembles that obtained with senescent rats (Barnes et al., 1980), who also showed a decreased likelihood of using place strategies when trained on tasks that permit a variety of solutions.

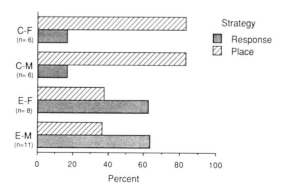

Fig. 3. Percentage of control and handled-isolated rats using place and response strategies on probe trial. C-F, control females; C-M, control males; E-F, experimental females; E-M, experimental males.

The fact that rats given the early handling-isolation manipulation are less likely to use place strategies in problem solving as adults does not mean that they are incapable of using spatial information in a problem-solving setting, however. Although we have found some differences between control rats and rats receiving early handling-isolation on tasks in which they are required to use place strategies (e.g. controls show somewhat better retention from day to day on the place learning version of the water maze), we have not observed any gross impairment of place learning in rats receiving the early handling-isolation treatment. Whether the same thing will be true of these animals as they grow older and spatial ability declines (Barnes, 1979) remains to be determined.

MECHANISMS OF EARLY EXPERIENCE EFFECTS

We are not the only investigators to have observed that early experience can affect the development and function of the hippocampus. It will be useful to consider these other results briefly insofar as they suggest that other types of early experience have somewhat different effects on hippocampal development and because they suggest some possible mechanisms for early experience effects on hippocampus.

One of the lines of evidence suggesting an effect of early experience on hippocampal development is research showing that early handling affects performance on learning tasks that involve the hippocampus. The phenomenon of "latent inhibition" (Lubow, 1973) provides a good example of this. Latent inhibition refers to the observation that animals given nonreinforced exposure to a stimulus are typically retarded in acquiring subsequent conditioning of that stimulus. The hippocampus is regarded as an important structure in mediating the effect, as studies have consistently shown that damage to the hippocampus leads to deficits in latent inhibition. Indeed, a disruption of latent inhibition after hippocampal damage may well be the best-documented effect of hippocampal lesions on classical conditioning (cf. Nadel and Willner, 1980; Nadel et al., 1985; Kaye and Pearce, 1987).

Latent inhibition is also affected by early handling. Weiner et al. (1985, 1987) compared latent inhibition in male and female rats who received either a brief period of handling on each of the first 21 days of life or who were left undisturbed in their home cages during this time. As adults, the rats were trained on two-way active avoidance (Weiner et al., 1985) or conditioned suppression (Weiner et al., 1987), with half of the animals in each group receiving preexposure to the tones that served as conditioned stimuli in these tasks. In both experiments, Weiner and his collegues found that stimulus exposure retarded learning in unhandled females, but not in unhandled males (i.e. no latent inhibition effect in unhandled males). In contrast to this, both males and females who received early handling developed latent inhibition for the pre-exposed stimulus. Early handling, then, made it possible for male rats to develop latent inhibition under conditions in which "normal" males did not display the effect.

The most direct evidence for a beneficial effect of early handling on hippocampus comes from recent studies showing that early handling during the first 3 weeks of life leads to a relatively selective, long-term increase in the concentration of glucocorticoid receptors in rat hippocampus (Meaney et al., 1985). The hippocampus plays an important role in negative feedback regulation of the pituitary-adrenal axis, so one might suspect that altering the concentration of glucocorticoid receptors in hippocampus would influence the rat's capacity to deal with stress, and this does appear to be the case. Meaney et al. (1988) reported that rats receiving early handling secreted less corticosterone in response to stress and exhibited a more rapid recovery of basal corticosterone levels than did rats left unhandled during infancy. They also found that handling attenuated the progressive increase in basal corticosterone levels normally seen in rats as they grow older. Finally, Meaney et al. (1988) found that rats receiving early handling were protected against the cell loss that occurs in the hippocampus with aging and that handled rats did not show the deficits in spatial learning that are characteristic of aged animals.

These data, then, provide evidence that early handling can have beneficial effects on the hippocampus and suggest a role for altered hippocampal regulation of the pituitary-adrenal axis as the basis for these beneficial effects. Whether such an account for the effects of early handling can be extended to explain the negative consequences of our combined early handling-isolation treatment remains to be seen. Recent evidence suggests that isolation has effects that are unlike those produced by early handling. During the second week of postnatal life, extended isolation from the dam (8–24 h) causes an exaggerated release of corticosterone in pups when they are subsequently exposed to novelty stress (Levine, personal communication; Stanton et al., 1987). Given that high levels of corticosterone can have cytotoxic effects on the developing hippocampus (Bohn, 1980; DeKosky et al., 1982), it seems reasonable to think that isolation-enhanced release of corticosterone may play a role in producing the results that we have obtained. We are currently undertaking studies to evaluate this possibility.

CONCLUSIONS

The data we have reviewed indicate that early experience can alter the development and subsequent functioning of the hippocampus. By itself, early handling appears to have beneficial effects on hippocampal development and function, and these benefits become more apparent as the animal ages. The combination of handling and isolation, on the other hand, seems to impair hippocampal functioning, and available evidence suggests that this impairment is not ameliorated with the passage of time.

There are a host of questions that need to be answered before we can expect to have any clear understanding of how early experience affects hippocampal development. Research on this is still in its infancy, and, like the newborn infant, our ignorance far outstrips our knowledge. First, we need a more detailed description of the effects of handling and isolation on hippocampal development. So far, most investigations have been more concerned with showing that these manipulations can affect hippocampal development than with analyzing the nature of the behavioral and neural changes that result from these experiences. We do not know, for example, whether there is a "critical period" for the effects of handling and isolation on hippocampal development. Until we have such knowledge, however, it will not be possible to provide a comprehensive account of how early experience acts to influence the development of the hippocampus, let alone an account of how these effects are manifested across the life span.

We also need more information on what types of early experience can affect hippocampal development. It seems rather unlikely that handling and isolation would be the only types of experience that can affect hippocampal development. Cramer et al. (1988), for example, recently reported that variations in pups' suckling experience led to later differences in performance on the radial-arm maze, a spatial task that is sensitive to hippocampal function. It is only by investigating a broad range of possible experiences that we will be able to determine whether those experiences that affect hippocampal development share common attributes or neural mechanisms.

A final issue that needs to be addressed is whether males and females are differentially sensitive to the effects of early experience on the hippocampus. Although sex differences in response to early experience have been found in a number of studies, there are many studies in which such differences have not been observed. Further, even in those instances in which sex differences have been observed, it is not the case that one sex has always been found to be more reliably affected than the other. Given the potential significance of the issue, however, researchers should give close attention to sex differences in responses to early experience in future work.

Clearly, there is much to be done, and it will undoubtedly be some time before we can hope for closure on any of these issues. Nevertheless, the question of how early experience influences hippocampal development and function is an important one and is well worth the time and effort that will be required to answer it.

ACKNOWLEDGMENTS

We thank Lisa Kurz and Don Wilson for their many cobntributions to the work and ideas discussed in this chapter. We also thank the many students who worked on this seemingly endless project, both at Irvine and Arizona. Lynn Wilson and Diane Amend have made important recent contributions; Sandy Lawrence has spent countless hours analyzing tapes. Gig Levine exchanged ideas and unpublished data during a recent visit to Tucson, for which we are grateful. The research reported here was supported by grants from NINCDS (NS 17712), The March of Dimes Birth Defects Foundation (12-143), The Sloan Foundation (87-2-13), and NIH (BRSG S07 RR07002).

REFERENCES

Altman, J., and G. Das (1965) Autoradiographic and histological evidence of postnatal hippocampal neurogenesis in rats. J. Comp. Neurol. *124*:319–336.

Angevine, J. (1965) Time of neuron origin in the hippocampal region: An autoradiographic study in the mouse. Exp. Neurol. [Suppl.] *13(2)*:1–70.

Barnes, C.A. (1979) Memory deficits associated with senescence: A neurophysiological and behavioral study in the rat. J. Comp. Physiol. Psychol. *93*:74–104.

Barnes, C.A., L. Nadel, and W.K. Honig (1980) Spatial memory deficit in senescent rats. Can. J. Psychol. *34*:29–39.

Bayer, S.A. (1980) Development of the hippocampal region in the rat. I. Neurogenesis examined with ³H-thymidine autoradiography. J. Comp. Neurol. *190*:87–114.

Black, A.H., L. Nadel, and J. O'Keefe (1977) Hippocampal function in avoidance learning and punishment. Psychol. Bull. *84*:1107–1129.

Bohn, M.C. (1980) Granule cell genesis in the hippocampus of rats treated neonatally with hydrocortisone. Neuroscience, *5*:2003–2012.

Brody, B.A., H.C. Kinney, A.S. Kloman, and F.H. Gilles (1987) Sequence of central nervous system myelination in human infancy. I. An autopsy study of myelination. J. Neuropathol. Exp. Neurol. *46*:283–301.

Cramer, C., J.P. Pfister, and K.A. Haig (1988) Experience during suckling alters later spatial learning. Dev. Psychobiol. *21*:1–24.

DeKosky, S.T., A.J. Nonneman and S.W. Scheff (1982) Morphologic and behavioral effects of perinatal glucocorticoid administration. Physiol. Behav. *29*:895–900.

Douglas, R.J., J.J. Peterson, and D.P. Douglas (1973) The ontogeny of a hippocampus-dependent response in two rodent species. Behav. Biol. *8*:27–37.

Feigley, D.A., P.J. Parson, L.W. Hamilton, and N.E. Spear (1972) Development of habituation to novel environments in the rat. J. Comp. Physiol. Psychol. *79*:443–452.

File, S.E. (1978) The ontogeny of exploration in the rat, habituation and effects of handling. Dev. Psychobiol. *11*:321–328.

Frederickson, C.J., and M.H. Frederickson (1979) Emergence of spontaneous alternation in the kitten. Dev. Psychobiol. *12*:615–621.

Greenough, W.T. (1984) Possible structural substrates of plastic neural phenomena. In G. Lynch, J.L. McGaugh and N.M. Weinberger (eds): Neurobiology of Learning and Memory. New York: The Guilford Press, pp. 470–478.

Guéneau, G., A. Privat, J. Drouet, and L. Court (1982) Subgranular zone of the dentate gyrus of young rabbits as a secondary matrix: A high-resolution autoradiographic study. Dev. Neurosci. *5*:345–358.

Harris, K., and T. Teyler (1984) Developmental onset of long-term potentiation in area CA1 of the rat hippocampus. J. Physiol. *346*:27–48.

Jacobs, W.J., and L. Nadel (1985) Stress-induced recovery of fears and phobias. Psychol. Rev. *92*:512–531.

Kaplan, M.S., and D.H. Bell (1983) Neuronal proliferation in the 9-month-old rodent—Radioautographic study of granule cells in the hippocampus. Exp. Brain Res.

Kaplan, M.S., and D.H. Bell (1983) Neuronal proliferation in the 9-month-old rodent—Radioautographic study of granule cells in the hippocampus. Exp. Brain Res. *52*:1–5.

Kaye, H., and J.M. Pearce (1987) Hippocampal lesions attenuate latent inhibition of a CS and of a neutral stimulus. Psychobiology *15*:293–299.

Kretschmann, H.-J., G. Kammradt, I. Krauthausen, B. Sauer, and F. Wingert (1986) Growth of the hippocampal formation in man. Bibl. Anat. *28*:27–52.

Kurz, E.M., B.L. Harkins, and L. Nadel (1984) Ontogeny and plasticity of exploratory behavior and hippocampal development in rats. Poster presented at Second Conference on the Neurobiology of Learning and Memory, University of California, Irvine.

Levine, S. (1962) The effects of infantile experience on adult behavior. In A.J. Bachrach (eds): Experimental Foundations of Clinical Psychology. New York: Basic Books, pp. 139–169.

Lubow, R.E. (1973) Latent inhibition. Psychol. Bull. *79*:398–407.

Meaney, M.J., D.H. Aitken, S.R. Bodnoff, L.J. Iny, J.E. Tatarewicz, and R.M. Sapolsky

(1985) Early postnatal handling alters glucocorticoid receptor concentrations in selected brain regions. Behav. Neurosci. *99:*765–770.

Meaney, M.J., D.H. Aitken, C. van Berkel, S. Bhatnagar, and R.M. Sapolsky (1988) Effect of neonatal handling on age-related impairments associated with the hippocampus. Science *239:*766–768.

Means, L.W., and R.W. Douglas (1970) Effects of hippocampal lesions on cue utilization in spatial discrimination in rats. J. Comp. Physiol. Psychol. *73:*254–260.

Melzack, R., and W.R. Thompson (1956) Effects of early experience on social behavior. Can. J. Psychol. *10:*82–90.

Morris, R.G.M., P. Garrard, J.N.P. Rawlins, and J. O'Keefe (1982) Place navigation impaired in rats with hippocampal lesions. Nature *297:*681–683.

Nadel, L. (1986) Down syndrome in neurobiological perspective. In C.J. Epstein (ed): The Neurobiology of Down Syndrome. New York: The Raven Press, pp. 239–251.

Nadel, L. (1988) The Psychobiology of Down Syndrome. Cambridge, MA: Bradford Books/ MIT Press.

Nadel, L., J. Willner (1980) Context and conditioning: A place for space. Physiol. Psychol. *8:*218–228.

Nadel, L., J. Willner, and E.M. Kurz (1985) Cognitive maps and environmental context. In: P. Balsam and A. Tomie (eds): Context and Learning. Hillsdale, NJ: Lawrence Erlbaum Associates.

Nadel, L., and S. Zola-Morgan (1984) Infantile amnesia: A neurobiological perspective. In M. Moscovitch, (ed): Infant Memory. New York: Plenum Press, pp. 145–172.

O'Keefe, J., and L. Nadel (1978) The Hippocampus as a Cognitive Map. Oxford: The Clarendon Press.

O'Keefe, J., and L. Nadel (1979) Précis of O'Keefe and Nadel's *The Hippocampus as a Cognitive Map*, and author's response to commentaries. Behav. Brain Sci. *2:*487–534.

O'Keefe, J., and A. Speakman (1987) Single unit activity in the rat hippocampus during a spatial memory task. Exp. Brain Res. *68:*1–27.

Purpura, D.P., and G.D. Pappas (1968) Structural characteristics of neurons in the feline hippocampus during postnatal ontogenesis. Exp. Neurol. *22:*379–393.

Rakic, P. (1985) Limits of neurogenesis in primates. Science *227:*1054–1055.

Rakic, P., and R.S. Nowakowski (1981) The time of origin of neurons in the hippocampal region of the rhesus monkey. J. Comp. Neurol. *196:*99–128.

Rosenzweig, M.R., E.L. Bennett M.C. Diamond (1972) Chemical and anatomical plasticity of brain, replications and extensions. In J. Gaito (ed): Macromolecules and Behavior, ed. 2. New York: Appleton-Century-Crofts, pp. 205–277.

Rudy, J.W., S. Stadler-Morris, and P. Albert (1987) Ontogeny of spatial navigation behaviors in the rat: Dissociation of "proximal"- and "distal"-cue based behaviors. Behav. Neurosci. *101:*62–73.

Schacter, D.L. (1989) On the relation between memory and consciousness, dissociable interactions and conscious experience. In H.L. Roediger and F.I.M. Craik (eds): Varieties of Memory and Consciousness: Essays in Honor of Endel Tulving. Hillsdale, N.J.: Erlbaum Associates, pp. 355–389.

Schlessinger, A.R., W.M. Cowan, and D.I. Gottleib (1975) An autoradiographic study of the time of origin and the pattern of granule cell migration in the dentate gyrus of the rat. J. Comp. Neurol. *159:*149–176.

Schlessinger, A.R., W.M. Cowan, and L.W. Swanson (1978) The time of origin of neurons in Ammon's horn and the associated retrohippocampal fields. Anat. Embryol. *154:*153–173.

Scoville, W.B., and B. Milner (1957) Loss of recent memory after bilateral hippocampal lesion. J. Neurol. Neurosurg. Psychiatry *20:*11–21.

Somerville, E. (1979) Postnatal Development of the Hippocampus in the Rat *(Rattus norvegicus):* Correlations Between Hippocampal anatomy, Electroencephalogram and Behavior. Unpublished Ph.D. Thesis, University College, London.

Stanton, M.E., J. Wallstrom, and S. Levine (1987) Maternal contact inhibits pituitary-adrenal stress responses in preweanling rats. Dev. Psychobiol. *20:*131–145.

Suomi, S.J., and H.F. Harlow (1971) Abnormal social behavior in young monkeys. In J. Helmuth (ed): Exceptional Infant: Studies in Abnormality, Vol. 2. New York: Brunner/Mazel, pp. 483–529.

Uemura, E., and H.A. Hartmann (1979) RNA content and volume of nerve cell bodies in human brain. II. Subiculum in aging normal patients. Exp. Neurol. *65:*107–117.

Weiner, I., J. Feldon, D. Ziv-Harris (1987) Early handling and latent inhibition in the conditioned suppression paradigm. Dev. Psychobiol. *20:*233–240.

Weiner, I., I. Schnabel, R.E. Lubow, and J. Feldon (1985) The effects of early handling on latent inhibition in male and female rats. Dev. Psychobiol. *18:*291–297.

Williams, J.M., L.W. Hamilton, and P.L. Carlton (1975) Ontogenetic dissociation of two classes of habituation. J. Comp. Physiol. Psychol. *87:*724–732.

Wilson, D.A., J. Willner, E.M. Kurz, and L. Nadel (1986) Early experience alters brain plasticity. Behav. Brain Res. *21:*223–227.

Wyss, M.J., and B. Sripanidkulchai (1985) The development of Ammon's horn and the fascia dentata in the cat: A [^{3}H]thymidine analysis. Dev. Brain Res. *18:*185–198.

The Hippocampus—New Vistas, pages 33–52

3

Ultrastructure, Development, and Plasticity of Dendritic Spine Synapses in Area CA1 of the Rat Hippocampus: Extending Our Vision With Serial Electron Microscopy and Three-Dimensional Analyses

KRISTEN M. HARRIS, FRANCES E. JENSEN, AND BEATRICE H. TSAO
Neuroscience Department, Children's Hospital, Boston, Massachusetts

INTRODUCTION

In area CA1 of the rat hippocampus, the overwhelming majority of excitatory synapses occur on protrusions from pyramidal cell dendrites referred to as "dendritic spines." Considerable attention has been focused on dendritic spines because changes in their dimensions could modulate synaptic efficacy (Chang, 1952; Rall, 1970, 1974; Harris and Stevens, 1988a; and Brown et al., 1987 for review). Complete anatomical measurements are required to interpret whether changes in spine or synaptic morphology are sufficient to mediate functional plasticity. To date, the only method available to obtain these complete measurements is three dimensional reconstructions from serial electron microscopy. In this chapter, we describe the morphology of CA1 spiny dendrites with Golgi impregnations, freeze-fracture preparations, and thin section electron microscopy. We present the rationale for studying dendritic spines through serial electron microscopy and propose some methods for overcoming the major shortcoming of serial EM—i.e. small sample sizes. Finally, we present some results that illustrate how these complete reconstructions can be used to determine whether changes in spine and synapse morphology could be involved in the ontogeny of hippocampal longterm potentiation.

CA1 Spiny Pyramidal Cell Dendrites: Qualitative Description of Spine and Synaptic Morphology

With light microscopy, it is possible to discern the tiny spines that protrude from CA1 pyramidal cell dendrites, but impossible to obtain accurate measurements of their dimensions (Fig. 1a,b). Viewed with electron microscopy, some fortunate freeze-fracture planes reveal the enormous diversity of spine morphology among near neighbors on a single dendritic shaft (Fig. 2). This diversity of spine morphology is associated with varied synaptic morphology

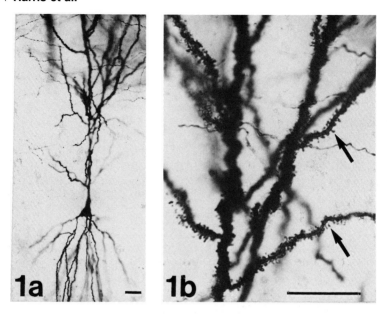

Fig. 1. **a:** A Golgi impregnation of a hippocampal CA1 pyramidal cell with apical den-drites extending up into s. radiatum. **b:** At higher magnification, dendritic spines (arrows) can be seen to stud the surface of these dendrites. Bars = 10 μm. (Reproduced from Harris et al., 1980, with permission of the publisher.)

(Fig. 3). Spines have been qualitatively classified to have stubby, mushroom, and thin shapes (criteria for making these distinctions are described in the Results section). Small dendritic spines have asymmetric synapses with a small continuous postsynaptic density (PSD), which is macular in appearance when viewed through serial thin sections. Large mushroom-shaped dendritic spines usually have perforated asymmetric postsynaptic densities. The presynaptic axonal varicosity associated with each of these PSD morphologies contains round, clear vesicles. The organization of the particles in the fractured synaptic membrane also differs on small and large dendritic spines. The smaller, thinner spines tend to have small, continuous aggregates of particles (Fig. 4), and the larger mushroom-shaped spines have aggregates of particles that are perforated by particle-free regions (Fig. 5). While the identity of these particles is not yet known, they are associated with synapses that have characteristics of excitatory synapses, suggesting that they might be freeze-fracture representations of pro-teins involved in excitatory synaptic transmissions (Harris and Landis, 1986).

Plasticity of Hippocampal Spine Synapses: Single Section Analyses

Following tetanic stimulation, several afferent pathways to hippocampal cells show long-term potentiation (LTP). LTP is a long-lasting enhancement of the postsynaptic response, which can be expressed extracellularly as an

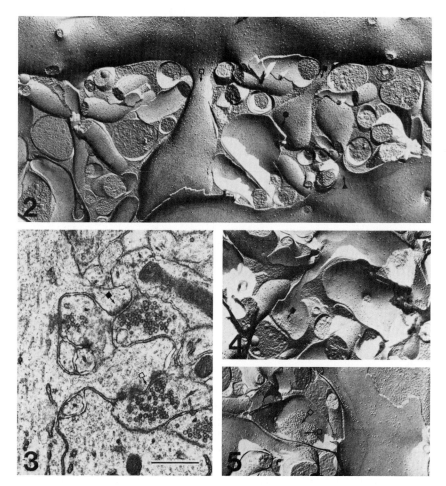

Figs. 2–5. Figure 2 shows cytoplasmic surface of a CA1 pyramidal cell dendrite revealed in profile in a freeze-fracture preparation. Very large mushroom spines (open square) are often located near smaller spines (closed square at neck, closed circle at synaptic cleft) of the same dendritic segment and on different dendritic segments (closed triangle). Figure 3 shows thin section of small dendritic spine with a macular postsynaptic density (closed square), adjacent to a large dendritic spine with a perforated postsynatic density (open square). Figure 4 shows extracellular half of the membrane of a postsynaptic density on a thin spine revealing a particle aggregate (closed square) at the synaptic junction. Figure 5 shows particle aggregate on the extracellular half of a larger dendritic spine with particle-free zones (open squares). Bar = 1 μm in Figure 3 for all of Figures 2–5. (Reproduced from Harris and Landis, 1986, with permission of the publisher.)

increased field excitatory postsynaptic potential (EPSP) and population spike or intracellularly as an increased EPSP, increased probability of cell firing, or decreased latency of cell firing. The conditions for inducing LTP have been well worked out. When sufficient depolarization of the postsynaptic cells occurs in the presence of glutamate, a magnesium block is released and channels associated with the N-Methyl-D-Aspartate receptor are opened. These open channels permit a significant influx of calcium to the postsynaptic cell and thus possibly activates several second messenger-mediated events (for review, see Smith, 1987).

LTP lasts for hours, days, or weeks, depending on the exact stimulation conditions (e.g. Bliss and Lomo, 1970, 1973; Bliss and Gardner-Medwin, 1973; Alger and Teyler, 1976; Barnes, 1979). This endurance of LTP has often lead to the suggestion that LTP results in some permanent or semipermanent change in synaptic number or structure (Crick, 1982; Gray, 1982). As summarized in Figure 6, four hippocampal circuits have been studied for anatomical correlates of this physiological plasticity, including 1) afferents from the entorhinal cortex, perforant pathway (PP), to area dentata granule cells (PP–dentate circuit); 2) afferents from dentate granule cells, the mossy fibers (MF), to proximal regions of the CA3 pyramidal cell dendrites (MF–CA3 circuit); 3) afferents from the septum to distal regions of the CA3 pyramidal cell dendrites (septal–CA3 circuit); and 4) afferents from CA3 pyramidal cells, the Schaffer collaterals and commissural fibers, to CA1 pyramidal cell dendrites (CA3–CA1 circuit). In each of these circuits, a variety of morphological changes have been observed after LTP.

In the potentiated PP–dentate circuit, the spine heads appear to be larger and the spine necks shorter (van Harreveld and Fifkova, 1975; Fifkova and Van Harreveld, 1977; Fifkova and Anderson, 1981; Fifkova et al., 1982). Analyses of the PSD suggest an increase in size and a shift in shape from convex to concave; and the number of presynaptic vesicles adjacent to the synaptic cleft increases (Desmond and Levy, 1983, 1986a,b, 1987).

Analyses of the potentiated MF–CA3 circuit suggest that spines swell, spine necks widen (Moshkov et al., 1977, 1980), and PSDs lengthen, similarly to the PP–dentate circuit (Petukov and Popov, 1986). In contrast to the PP–dentate circuit, vesicle number has been observed to decrease following LTP in parallel with an increase in Smooth Endoplasmic Reticulum (SER) in the axonal varicosity (Petukov and Popov, 1986).

Like the PP–dentate and MF–CA3 circuits, results from the potentiated septal–CA3 circuit suggest spine swelling, though there are no data on the neck dimensions. In contrast to the PP–dentate circuit, the potentiated septal–CA3 circuit appears to have a decrease in both length and thickness of the PSD and a decrease in the number of presynaptic vesicles (Wenzel et al., 1985).

The CA3–CA1 circuit contrasts with all three of the other circuits in that no overt spine swelling or neck widening has been observed with potentiation, though a decrease in the variability of spine perimeters has been interpreted to result from spine "rounding" (Lee et al., 1980; Chang and Greenough, 1984).

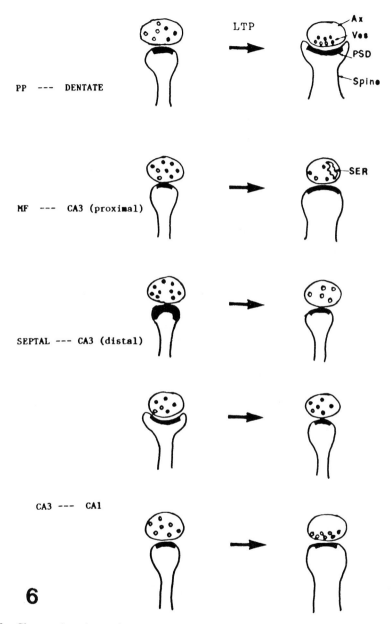

Fig. 6. Changes in spine and synaptic morphologies that have been associated with hippocampal long-term potentiation. See text for description and terminology.

Other studies suggest that spine swelling might occur in the potentiated CA3–CA1 circuit (Applegate et al., 1987). In contrast to the PP–dentate circuit, results from these studies in area CA1 suggest a decrease in PSD length and an interconversion of the PSD shape from concave to convex (Chang and Greenough, 1984). One report suggests no change in vesicle number (Chang and Greenough, 1984), while another suggests that vesicles migrate, producing a higher density at the synaptic cleft in the potentiated CA3–CA1 circuit (Applegate et al., 1987).

All of these results strongly suggest that dramatic changes in spine and synaptic morphology can be associated with hippocampal long-term potentiation. The opposite changes in spine and synaptic morphology that appear to occur in different circuits might be related to differences in receptor types, second-messenger systems, tissue preparation, or other factors.

Several questions remain. How large are the actual anatomical changes in spine or synapse morphology? Are existing synapses growing and changing their shapes, or are new synapses forming to support LTP? Are changes occurring only in a subpopulation of stimulated spines and synapses, or do all the affected spines and synapses show the same shifts in their morphology? Are the changes in spine morphology sufficient to modify the transfer of charge from the synapse through the spine neck to the parent dendrite?

To answer these questions, complete descriptions of spine and synaptic morphologies are required. A serial section analysis allows for a complete description of each spine and its associated synapse, including 1) measurement of the whole spine and synapse, 2) unambiguous identification of each structural element, and 3) three-dimensional reconstructions for quantitative shape analyses. This approach has several advantages over the random-section analyses that have been used thus far to observe changes in dendritic spines and synapses. Relationships between changes in the shape of individual spines and their synapses can be easily discerned. Accurate measurements of individual spine characteristics, such as head diameter, neck diameter, and neck length, can be used to model charge transfer through spines and discern whether measured anatomical changes are sufficient to modify charge transfer (e.g. Wilson et al., 1983; Wilson, 1984; Harris and Stevens, 1988b, 1989). Spine neck and head volumes can be measured and used in theoretical models to determine how changes in shape might alter diffusion properties in the dendritic spine (e.g. Shepherd, 1979; Gamble and Koch, 1987; Brown et al., 1977; Harris and Stevens, 1988b, 1989).

These advantages might be tempered by the time required to obtain a large sample of complete reconstructions from dendritic spines and synapses. However, this must be weighed against the strong advantage of having accurate measurements and identity. Fewer total numbers need be analyzed to reveal dramatic differences in morphology. We present here a strategy we have used to optimize these advantages for analysis of developing hippocampal dendritic spines (Harris et al., 1987; Harris et al., manuscript in preparation) and the possible relationship of developmental changes in their shapes to the ontogeny of LTP (Harris and Teyler, 1984).

DEVELOPMENT AND PLASTICITY OF HIPPOCAMPAL SPINE SYNAPSES:
SERIAL EM ANALYSES

Detailed methods for tissue preparation and serial electron microscopy have been described elsewhere (Stevens et al., 1980; Stevens, 1980; Stevens and Trogadis, 1984; Harris and Landis, 1986; Harris and Stevens, 1988a,b). Here we will describe procedures that have been developed to sample the neuropil to obtain good estimates of the frequency of different spine and synaptic morphologies and accurate measurements of synaptic areas.

To locate sample fields, the photographic screen of the electron microscope was calibrated at the desired magnification (usually 6.6 K on a JEOL 100B) with a calibration grid. Then the calibrated screen was used to measure a distance from the pyramidal cell body layer out to 250 μm in stratum radiatum. This procedure requires a rotation stage so that one can move perpendicularly from the pyramidal cell layer into s. radiatum. Using the calibrated screen, a strip located in s. radiatum measuring about 25 μm wide and running perpendicular to the pyramidal cell bodies was divided into eight to ten equal fields, each about 500 μm^2 (Fig. 7). A random number table was consulted to determine which of these fields to photograph through adjacent serial sections. The "sample" field of 200 μm^2 is located on the middle section of the series. The reason for making the sample field smaller than the photographic field is to allow for slight shifts in the alignment from section to section, which could result in loss of sample structures at the edge of the micrograph if all 500 μm^2 were sampled.

Adjacent sample fields in s. radiatum often have very different structural components occupying the neuropil. In Figure 8, the neuropil is filled with small dendrites, spine heads, and axons. Most of this neuropil contains structures that are part of the synaptic complex. In contrast, large, longitudinally sectioned dendrites fill much of the neuropil of the field in Figure 9. It is impossible for synapses to form in the central cytoplasm of these dendrites; therefore, the sample areas of these two adjacent fields are not equivalent for calculating synaptic densities.

A method was devised to determine which processes should be subtracted from the total sample area to give a corrected sample area with homogeneity of variance among the size of dendritic processes in it. Five randomly selected fields, including these two fields, were photographed. If a blood vessel was in the field, the photographic screen was moved laterally to exclude the vessel. Then the enclosed area of every dendritic process in the field was measured. Spines, unmyelinated axons, and axonal varicosities are smaller than these processes and were excluded from this analysis. The frequencies of dendritic process areas for each field are plotted in Figure 10. The mean process area and variance were computed for each field (Table I, "before correction"). Then the two fields with the most disparate variance (Nos. 2 and 5) were compared for homogeneity of variance among dendritic process areas. All process areas greater than 2 μm^2 were excluded from the sample to achieve homogeneity of variance across the five fields (Table I, "after correction"). The corrected

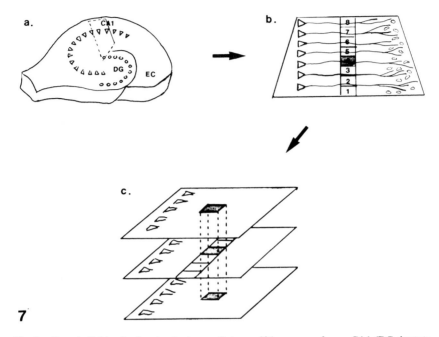

Fig. 7. Sample field selection in stratum radiatum of hippocampal area CA1 (DG-dentate gyrus; EC-entorhinal cortex). **a:** The trapezoid is trimmed to contain the CA1 pyramidal cell bodies and the entire apical dendritic field (full length approximately equalling 0.8 mm). **b:** A sample field located about 250 μm from the outer edge of the pyramidal cell layer is randomly selected from the eight to ten possible fields across the width of the section (approx. 0.2 mm). **c:** The sample field is then photographed through 40 adjacent serial thin sections.

neuropil area (NA) = Total sample area − (glia area − myelinated axon area − dendritic cytoplasm of processes > 2 μm^2).

Every synapse with a portion located on the sample field of the central section was completely reconstructed through adjacent serial sections. For cross-sectioned synapses, the area of the PSD was determined by measuring its length through adjacent sections, multiplying the lengths by section thickness, and then adding across sections. Section thickness was determined empirically as described by Harris and Stevens (1988a,b). For obliquely or tangentially sectioned PSDs, the enclosed area was measured on each section on which it appeared.

Figs. 8, 9. Adjacent sample fields within s. radiatum. These figures contain about 50 μm^2 of the sample fields. They illustrate the extreme inhomogeneity in structural composition of the neuropil where small dendritic processes fill Figure 8 and large dendritic processes occupy much of the field in Figure 9. Bar = 1 μm.

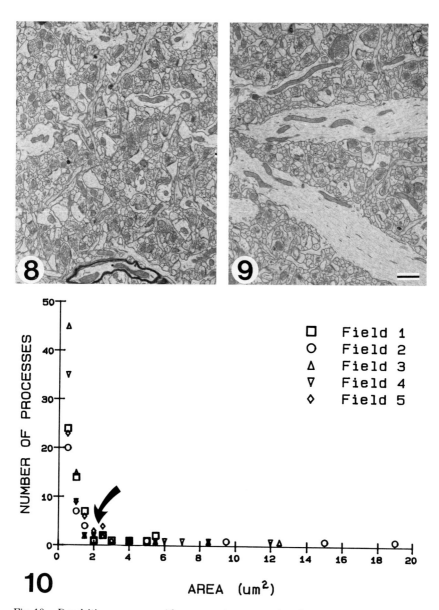

Fig. 10. Dendritic processes with measured cross-sectional areas on the sample fields. To obtain homogeneity of variance in process sectioned areas across these five fields, all processes with areas greater than 2 μm^2 (curved arrow) were excluded from the sample area. See also Table I.

TABLE I. Effect of Excluding Large Dendritic Processes From Sample Fields on the Mean and Variance of the Process Areas Occupying These Fields*

Field	n	Before correction		n'	After correction	
		Mean	Variance		Mean	Variance
1	53	0.98	1.60	46	0.57	0.47
2	38	1.80	15.76	32	0.51	0.46
3	69	0.80	3.38	64	0.39	0.38
4	54	1.15	5.06	48	0.43	0.40
5	47	0.83	0.71	41	0.57	0.48

*Mean is expressed as μm^2; n is number of processes measured in each field, and n' is number of processes remaining after excluding those with areas >2.0 μm^2.

We recognized that the probability of observing part of a synapse on the sample field was proportional to the number of sections that the synapse actually occupied through serial sections. If a synaptic type changed size, shape, or orientation to change significantly the probability of viewing them on the sample field, then the number of sections on which they appeared would change proportionately. For example, if an elliptical synapse was sectioned at 0.07 μm thickness, perpendicular to a short axis with a diameter of 0.21 μm, three sections of the synapse would be obtained. In a nine-section series, with random placement of this synapse in the series, the probability of viewing the synapse on any one of the nine sections is 3/9 or 1/3. If the same synapse were sectioned parallel to a long axis with a diameter of 0.42 μm, six sections of the synapse would be obtained. Random placement in the nine-section series would give a probability of viewing the same synapse in any one section of 6/9 or 2/3— a 100% increase in the probability of viewing that synapse on the sample section.

For each synapse appearing on the sample section, we counted the number of serial sections on which it appeared. Then, when grouping the synapses by type, we computed the average number of sections for each type. If there was a significant difference in the number of sections occupied by a particular synaptic type that occur at one age from another, then the %difference in section number was calculated. Then the following formulae were used to correct the relative synaptic densities (corrSYNdens):

$$uncorrSYNdens = \text{No. of synapses/NA}$$

$$corrSYNdens = uncorrSYNdens - [(\%\text{difference in section No.}) \cdot (uncorrSYNdens)]$$

The postsynaptic element associated with each synapse was identified by viewing it through adjacent serial sections. Dendritic spines were first classified into three shape categories of stubby, mushroom, and thin according to the criteria listed in Figure 11. Then a randomly selected subpopulation of these spines was reconstructed to confirm the shape assignments. The reconstruc-

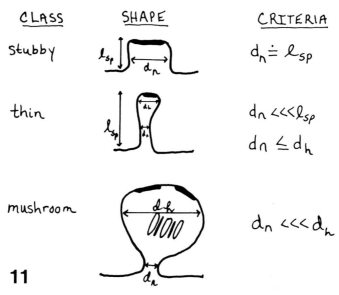

Fig. 11. Classification of dendritic spines by shape as viewed through serial thin sections. The criterion for a stubby dendritic spine was that the diameter of the neck (d_n) be greater than or equal to the spine length (l_{sp}). The criteria for a thin spine were that the neck diameter be much less than the total length and that the diameter of the head (d_h) be not much greater than the neck diameter. A spine was classified as a mushroom shape if the diameter of the neck was very much less than the head diameter. These mushroom spines frequently had perforated synapses and well-developed spine apparatuses in adult hippocampus.

tions were obtained using a reconstruction system that includes a Gould Image Processing System interfaced to a VAX 780 and a Cohu monochromatic camera mounted on a copy stand. Electron micrographs were positioned under the video camera, images captured with the Gould system, and traces superimposed on the EM image viewed on the Gould monitor. Quantitative analyses of the reconstructions were obtained with the PANDORA software (Pearlstein et al., 1986).

RESULTS

Development of Synapses in Stratum Radiatum: Sample Field Analyses

We have used the methods described above to evaluate synaptic morphology in the developing hippocampus at three postnatal ages: P7, P15, and adult. These ages were chosen because it was shown in an earlier study that the ontogeny of LTP begins postnatally in hippocampal area CA1 (Harris and Teyler, 1984). Before P5, tetanic stimulation (100 Hz for 1 s) does not induce long-lasting changes in the population response; by P5, half of the animals showed potentiation of the population spike amplitude; and by P7 all of the animals showed robust LTP. At P15, the magnitude of LTP was three times greater than that observed in adult animals (see Fig. 3 in Harris and Teyler, 1984). Our preliminary anatomical analyses reveal striking differences in the frequencies of the different classes of synaptic and spine morphologies across these ages (a detailed description and quantitative analysis is being prepared by Harris et al.).

Thus far, 232 synaptic PSD areas have been measured through complete reconstructions. Five categories of postsynaptic elements were identified with these synapses by viewing them through serial thin sections, including unclassified, shaft, stubby spine, mushroom spine, or thin spine.

At P7 (LTP onset), four sample fields (100–150 μm^2 each) were analyzed. In these fields, seven synapses could not be unambiguously identified by class. These unclassified P7 synapses were of the same average area as synapses occurring on dendritic shafts (N = 18), stubby spines (N = 5), and a mushroom spine (N = 1; Fig. 12). There are no postsynaptic elements that could be identified as thin spines at P7.

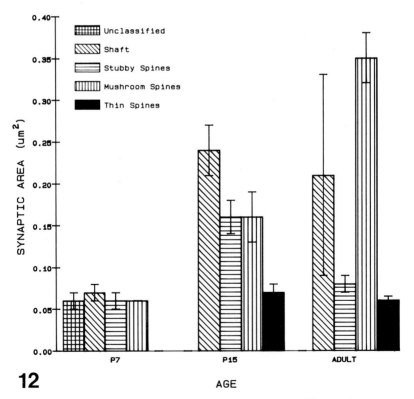

Fig. 12. Synaptic area, measured through serial sections, at different classes of postsynaptic structures (mean ± S.E.M.) at postnatal days 7 (P7), 15 (P15), and adult.

At P15 (LTP peak), two sample fields (NA = 171.06 and 183.76 μm²) were analyzed. All of the postsynaptic elements were readily identified, and all classes of synapses (shaft, N = 13; stubby, N = 21; mushroom, N = 15; and thin, N = 16) were larger than at P7, suggesting growth in synaptic area between these two ages (Fig. 12).

In the adult (LTP decline), analysis of two sample fields (NA = 128.5 and 170.64 μm²) revealed no further significant increase in the size of synapses on dendritic shafts (N = 5). The size of synapses of stubby spines (N = 5) decreased significantly from the P15 value ($P < 0.003$). The size of synapses on mushroom spines (N = 44) increased significantly from the P15 value ($P < 0.0001$). The slight decrease in average synaptic area on thin spines from the P15 to the adult value (N = 87) was not significant (Fig. 12).

The relative densities of these different synaptic classes were computed from each of these sample fields, and the mean values are presented in Figure 13. To obtain an estimate of synaptic densities in each class at each age we first computed the number of synapses per corrected neuropil area as described

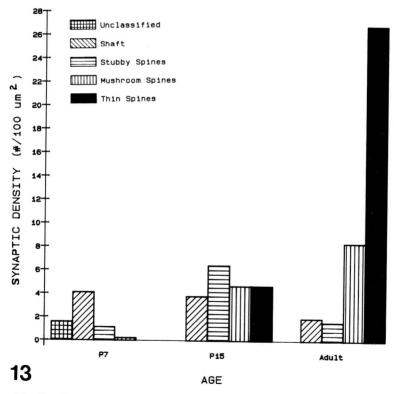

13

Fig. 13.   Density of different classes of postsynaptic structures at each age.

above. We used P15 as the age of comparison for %difference in section number to correct further the relative synaptic densities (as described above for corrSYNdens). Only the mushroom spines showed a significant difference in the number of sections their synaptic PSD occupied, which increased between P15 and P60.

At P7, most synapses were associated with unclassified dendritic shafts or with stubby dendritic spines. Occasionally a mushroom spine was observed. At P15, synapses were distributed relatively evenly between all four classes of postsynaptic elements. In the adult, many fewer shaft and stubby spines are present than at P15. The density of mushroom spines doubles, even when corrected for the increase in the probability of observing them on the sample field because of the significant increase in PSD area. There is a dramatic fourfold increase in the density of synapses located on thin dendritic spines between P15 and adulthood.

Development of Spine Morphology: Three-Dimensional Reconstructions To Confirm Visual Identity

Two P15, stubby dendritic spines are illustrated in Figure 14. These stubby spines had large, well-developed synaptic complexes, complete with a thickened PSD, a widened cleft, and a presynaptic axonal varicosity filled with round, clear vesicles. This spine morphology was rare in the adults, in which thin spines prevailed. To test spine classification as identified by viewing them through serial sections, 12 dendritic spines (two in each spine class from the sample fields at P15 and adult) have been completely reconstructed. Six of these spines are illustrated in Figure 15. Of these 12 spines, 11 were correctly identified. One P15 mushroom spine was misidentified as a thin spine. It had a relatively small head for the mushroom category, but the head diameter was clearly larger than the neck diameter when completely reconstructed. More of these reconstructions are being completed to be tested in biophysical models of charge transfer through the necks and to discern whether they occur in quantitatively discrete shape categories at each age or if there are perhaps more "transitional" shapes at younger ages (e.g. shapes that are halfway between stubby and mushroom or between mushroom and thin).

DISCUSSION: PROPOSED SEQUENCE OF SPINE DEVELOPMENT IN HIPPOCAMPAL AREA CA1—IMPLICATIONS FOR THE ONTOGENY OF LTP

A sequence for spine development in area CA1 is proposed in Figure 16. These anatomical observations would be consistent with the view that hippocampal stubby spines develop from shaft synapses, because more shaft than spine synapses are present at P7. The stubby spine might be a precursor of mushroom spines or of long, thin spines, because more stubby spines are present at P15 than in the adult. It is unlikely that long, thin spines form first and then contract to become stubby spines, because many stubby spines are present at P7 and P15 while very few stubby spines are present in the adult. Alternatively, thin spines might be remodeled from mushroom spines. This second

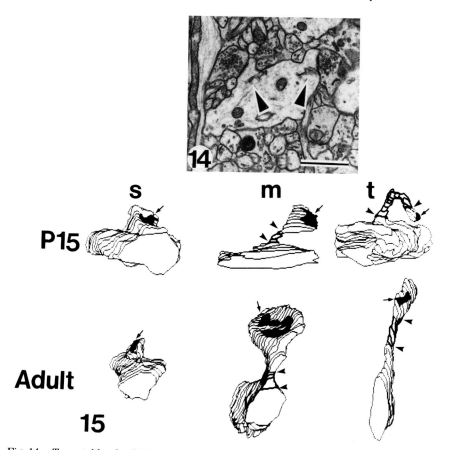

Fig. 14. Two stubby dendritic spines (arrow heads) from P15 hippocampal area CA1. Bar = 1 μm for Figures 14 and 15.

Fig. 15. Three-dimensional reconstructions of dendritic spines at P15 and adult ages to illustrate spine shape categories of stubby (s), mushroom (m), and thin (t). Synaptic areas (arrows) are filled in on the spine heads (thin lines). Spine necks are divided from spine heads for mushroom and thin spines (bold lines between arrowheads). A portion of the dendritic shaft that each spine was connected to is also illustrated. See Figure 14 for scale bar.

view is supported by the relative abundance of stubby and mushroom spines and the relative absence of thin spines at P7 and P15, suggesting that the stubby and mushroom shapes might precede the thin spine shape. Analyses are in progress to determine whether stubby, mushroom, and thin spines occur in discrete categories with quantitative distinctions separating them (e.g. the ratio of head volume to neck diameter) or represent a continuum in shape dimensions across development.

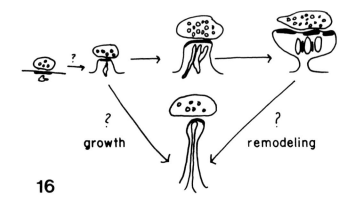

Fig. 16.   Proposed sequence of spine development that is consistent with the preliminary anatomical findings reported here.

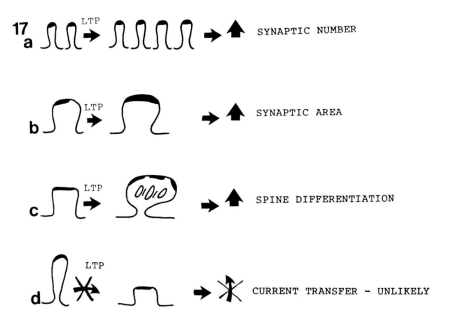

Fig. 17.   Possibilities for changes in spine or synaptic morphology of hippocampal CA1 pyramidal cells that could be associated with LTP at ages P7 and P15. See text for further description.

Since more synapses are present in adult animals than at P15, the peak and decline in LTP around P15 is not directly related to the absolute number of synapses present. Our hypothesis has been that a larger percentage of synapses can produce LTP at P15 than in adult animals (Harris and Teyler, 1984). We proposed that synapses are removed from a pool of "plastic" synapses as they are "used" to process experiences, thus explaining how a peak and decline in LTP production might be related to synaptogenesis (see Fig. 11 in Harris and Teyler, 1984).

The anatomical observations presented here suggest several changes in spine and synaptic morphology that could occur with LTP at P15 (Fig. 17). At P15, tetanic stimulation could induce more synapses (e.g. more thin spines with synapses) to form (Fig. 17a). Synaptic area could grow to produce LTP and might do so at a greater extent during robust synaptogenesis (P15) than in adults (Fig. 17b). Undifferentiated stubby or mushroom spines might be induced to undergo a change in P15 hippocampus more readily than in adult hippocampus (Fig. 17c).

It seems *unlikely* that the peak in LTP magnitude is mediated by a large population of long, thin spines, which shorten and widen to facilitate charge transfer to the parent dendrite (Fig. 17d). If this were so, we would expect the magnitude of LTP observed in adult animals to be larger than at P15, because many more thin spines are available for "contraction" in the adult than at P15. In addition, it seems unlikely that long, thin spines are necessary for LTP induction, because few, if any, are present at P7, an age when LTP is robust.

It could be that spine differentiation from stubby to mushroom or thin spines with constricted spine necks facilitates partitioning of synapses onto relatively isolated compartments, i.e. the spine head (Harris and Stevens, 1988b, 1989). This partitioning of dendritic spines could prevent diffusion of second messengers, phosphorylated proteins, or other postsynaptic products of LTP away from the activated synapses, thereby restricting LTP to those synapses that are potentiated. This restriction might serve to prevent heterosynaptic potentiation. The relative absence of constricted spine necks at P15 might result in nonspecific heterosynaptic potentiation, leading to a larger response magnitude because neighboring "unpotentiated" synapses were also "potentiated" by diffusing substances (see Harris and Stevens, 1988b, 1989; Brown et al., 1987). If this were so, the peak in LTP magnitude observed at P15 could be an immaturity of response specificity, a possibility that will be tested physiologically in subsequent experiments. In conjunction with the serial EM approach described here, it should be possible to discern whether changes in spine shape are sufficient to contribute to the peak and decline in LTP magnitude observed during development.

SUMMARY

The goal of this chapter was to illustrate our strategy for optimizing the use of complete reconstructions from serial EM to obtain accurate measurement and identification of dendritic spines and their associated synapses. We have observed a dramatic shift from stubby and mushroom-shaped dendritic spines at P7 (LTP onset) and P15 (LTP peak) to a predominance of long, thin spines in adult (LTP decline) hippocampal area CA1. We propose a sequence for the genesis of dendritic spines from short stubby protrusions to either mushroom-shaped spines or long, thin spines. Hypotheses concerning the role(s) of dendritic spines in the ontogeny of hippocampal LTP were considered in light of these preliminary anatomical findings.

ACKNOWLEDGMENTS

We thank Gene Zilberstein and Nariman Shambayati of the Image Graphics Laboratory at Children's Hospital for implementing software used for the reconstructions, editing, and displays in these studies. We thank Dr. John Stevens and Judy Trogadis of the University of Toronto for teaching K.M.H. many of the principles of serial EM and for use of their reconstruction system during earlier phases of this work; Dr. D. Max Snodderly and Dr. Thomas Brown for helpful discussions of the results; and Greg Belmont and Dr. Robert Baughman for improving an earlier version of this manuscript. This work is supported by NIH-NINCDS grant NS21184 and The Alfred P. Sloan Foundation (K.M.H.), NIH-NICHD grant HD00807 (F.E.J.), a Radcliffe Summer Project Grant (B.H.T.), NIH grant NS20820 (R.L. Sidman, P.I.), and MRC grants MT-7345 and MA-8304 (J.K. Stevens, P.I.).

REFERENCES

Alger, B.E., and T.J. Teyler (1976) Long-term and short-term plasticity in CA1, CA3, and dentate regions of rat hippocampal slice. Brain Res. *110:*463–480.

Applegate, M.D., D.S. Kerr, and P. Landfield (1987) Redistribution of synaptic vesicles during hippocampal long term potentiation. Brain Res. *401:*401–406.

Barnes, C.A. (1979) Memory deficits associated with senescence: A neurophysiological and behavioral study in the rat. J. Comp. Physiol. Psychol. *93:*74–104.

Bliss, T.V.P., and A.R. Gardner-Medwin (1973) Long-lasting potentiation of synaptic transmission in the dentate area of the unanaesthetized rabbit following stimulation of the perforant path. J. Physiol. *232:*357–374.

Bliss, T.V.P., and T. Lomo (1970) Plasticity in a monosynaptic cortical pathway. J. Physiol. *207:*61P.

Bliss, T.V.P., and T. Lomo (1973) Long-lasting potentiation of synaptic transmission in the dentate area of the anaesthetized rabbit following stimulation of the perforant path. J. Physiol. *232:*331–356.

Brown, T.H., V.C. Chang, A.H. Ganong, C.L. Keenan, and S.R. Kelso (1987) Biophysical properties of dendrites and spines that may control the induction and expression of long-term synaptic potentiation. In P.W. Landfield and S.A. Deadwyler (eds): Long-Term Potentiation: From Biophysics to Behavior. New York: Alan R. Liss, Inc., pp. 201–264.

Chang, H.T. (1952) Cortical neurons with particular reference to the apical dendrites. Cold Spring Harbor Symp. Quant. Biol. *17:*189–202.

Chang, F.L.F., and W.T. Greenough (1984) Transient and enduring morphological correlates of synaptic activity and efficacy in the rat hippocampal slice. Brain Res. *309:*35–46.

Crick, F. (1982) Do dendritic spines twitch? Trends Neurosci. *5:*44–46.

Desmond, N.L., and W.B. Levy (1983) Synaptic correlates of associative potentiation/depression: An ultrastructural study in the hippocampus. Brain Res. *265*:21–30.

Desmond, N.L., and W.B. Levy (1986a) Changes in the numerical density of synaptic contacts with long-term potentiation in the hippocampal dentate gyrus. J. Comp. Neurol. *253*:466–475.

Desmond, N.L., and W.B. Levy (1986b) Changes in the postsynaptic density with long-term potentiation in the dentate gyrus. J. Comp. Neurol. *253*:476–482.

Desmond, N.L., and W.B. Levy (1987) Anatomy of associative long-term synaptic modification. In P.W. Landfield and S.A. Deadwyler (eds): Long-Term Potentiation: From Biophysics to Behavior. New York: Alan R. Liss, pp. 265–305.

Fifkova, E., and C.L. Anderson (1981) Stimulation-induced changes in dimensions of stalks of dendritic spines in the dentate molecular layer. Exp. Neurol. *74*:621–627.

Fifkova, E., C.L. Anderson, S.J. Young, and A. van Harreveld (1982) Effect of anisomyosin on stimulation-induced changes in dendritic spines of the dentate granule cells. J. Neurocytol. *11*:183–210.

Fifkova, E. and A. Van Harreveld (1977) Long-lasting morphological changes in dendritic spines of dentate granular cells following stimulation of the entorhinal area. J. Neurocytol. *6*:211–230.

Gamble, E., and C. Koch (1987) The dynamics of free calcium in dendritic spines in response to repetitive synaptic input. Science *236*:1311–1315.

Gray, E.G. (1982) Rehabilitating the dendritic spine. Trends Neurosci. *5*:5–6.

Harris, K.M., W.L.R. Cruce, W.T. Greenough, and T.J. Teyler (1980) A Golgi impregnation technique for thin brain slices maintained in vitro. J. Neurosci. Methods *2*:363–371.

Harris, K.M., F.E. Jensen, and B. Tsao (1987) Development of hippocampal LTP, synapses, and spines. Soc. Neurosci. Abs. Vol. *13*:394.12.

Harris, K.M., and D.M.D. Landis (1986) Synaptic membrane structure in area CA1 of the rat hippocampus. Neuroscience *19*:857–872.

Harris, K.M., and J.K. Stevens (1988a) Study of dendritic spines by serial electron microscopy and three-dimensional reconstructions. In R.J. Lasek and M.M. Black (eds): Intrinsic Determinants of Neuronal Form and Function. New York: Alan R. Liss, pp. 179–199.

Harris, K.M., and J.K. Stevens (1988b) Dendritic spines of rat cerebellar Purkinje cells: Serial electron microscopy with reference to their biophysical characteristics. J. Neurosci. *8*:4455–4469.

Harris, K.M. and J.K. Stevens, (1989) Dendritic spines of CA1 pyramidal cells in the rat hippocampus: Serial electron microscopy with reference to their biophysical characteristics. J. Neurosci. (in press).

Harris, K.M., and T.J. Teyler (1984) Developmental onset of long-term potentiation in area CA1 of the rat hippocampus. J. Physiol. *346*:27–48.

Lee, K.S., F. Schottler, M. Oliver, and G. Lynch (1980) Brief bursts of high-frequency stimulation produce two types of structural change in the rat hippocampus. J. Neurophysiol. *44*:247–258.

Moshkov, D.A., L.L. Petrovskaia, and A.G. Bragin (1977) Posttetanic changes in the ultrastructure of the giant spious synapses in hippocampal field CA3. Dokl. Akad. Nauk. USSR *237*:1525–1528.

Moshkov, D.A., L.L. Petrovskaia, and A.G. Bragin (1980) Ultrastructural study of the bases of postsynaptic potentiation in hippocampal sections by the freeze-substitution method. Tsitologiia *22*:20–26.

Pearlstein, R.A., L. Kirschner, J. Simons, S. Machell, W.F. White, and R.L. Sidman, (1986) A multimodel system for reconstruction and quantification of neurologic structures. Anal. Quant. Cytol. Histol. *8:*108–115.

Petukhov, V.V., and V.I. Popov (1986) Quantitative analysis of ultrastructural changes in synapses of the rat hippocampal field CA3 in vitro in different functional states. Neuroscience *18(4):*823–835.

Rall, W. (1970) Cable properties of dendrites and effects of synaptic location. In P. Andersen and J.K.S. Jensen (eds): Excitatory Synaptic Mechanisms. Proceedings of the 5th International Meeting of Neurobiologists. Oslo: Universitets Forlaget, pp. 175–187.

Rall, W. (1974) Dendritic spines, synaptic potency and neuronal plasticity. In C. Woody, K. Brown, T. Crow, and J. Knispel (eds): Cellular Mechanisms Subserving Changes in Neuronal Activity. Los Angeles, CA: Brain Information Service, UCLA.

Shepherd, G.M. (1979) The Synaptic Organization of the Brain. New York: Oxford University Press, p. 364.

Smith, S.J. (1987) Progress in LTP at hippocampal synapses—A post synaptic Ca^{2+} trigger for memory storage. Trends Neurosci. *10:*142–144.

Stevens, J.K. (1980) Reconstructing neuronal microcircuitry: Using computers to assemble three dimensional structures from montages of serial electron microscopy. Bull. Micro. Soc. Can *8:*4–12.

Stevens, J.K., T. Davis, N. Friedman, and P. Sterling (1980) A systematic approach to reconstructing microcircuitry by electron microscopy of serial sections. Brain Res. Rev. *2:*265–293.

Stevens, J.K., and J. Trogadis (1984) Computer assisted reconstruction from serial electron micrographs: A tool for systematic study of neuronal form and function. Annu. Rev. Neurobiol. *5:*341–369.

Van Harreveld, A., and E. Fifkova (1975) Swelling of dendritic spines in the fascia dentata after stimulation of the perforant fibers as a mechanism of post-tetanic potentiation. Exp. Neurol. *49:*736–749.

Wenzel, J., C. Schmidt, G. Duwe, W.G. Skrebitz, and I. Kudrjats (1985) Stimulation-induced changes of the ultrastructure of synapses in hippocampus following posttetanic potentiation. J. Hirnfor. *26(5):*573–583.

Wilson, C.J. (1984) Passive cable properties of dendritic spines and spiny neurons. J. Neurosci. *4:*281–297.

Wilson, C.J., P.M. Goves, S.T. Kitai, and J.C. Linder (1983) Three dimensional structure of dendritic spines in rat striatum. J. Neurosci. *3:*383–398.

The Hippocampus—New Vistas, pages 53–69
© 1989 Alan R. Liss, Inc.

4
Connectivity of the Rat Hippocampus

MENNO P. WITTER
Department of Anatomy, Vrije Universiteit, Amsterdam, The Netherlands

INTRODUCTION

As a result of the interest of anatomists, continuing for almost a century, the architectonics and hodology of the hippocampus are considered to be well known. The functional significance of the hippocampus, however, is still not clear, although recent evidence convincingly points toward a function in memory processes (Scoville and Milner, 1957; Mishkin, 1978; Zola-Morgan and Squire, 1986; Zola-Morgan et al., 1986). This hypothesis gave way to a surge of electrophysiological, behavioral, and pharmacological research of hippocampal processes that may underlie memory. With the development of powerful techniques like in vivo and in vitro intracellular recording, it became possible to study the various properties of single neurons and the hippocampal networks to which they belong (for an overview, see Lopes da Silva et al., 1989). Interesting mechanisms have been put forward, for example, long-term potentiation, that may subserve memory formation (Teyler and Discenna, 1987; McNaughton and Morris, 1987), and elegant models have been proposed that functionally describe the hippocampus (O'Keefe and Nadel, 1978; Teyler and Discenna, 1984; McNaughton and Morris, 1987).

In the past decades, using the "slice preparation," investigators discovered in detail the transverse connectivity within the hippocampus, the so-called trisynaptic circuit. Most of the models of the hippocampal circuitry and of the ways intrahippocampal information processing is thought to take place are based on the idea that the hippocampus is organized in a lamellar fashion. (Andersen et al., 1971; O'Keefe and Nadel, 1978). The available anatomical techniques, however, did not permit analyses of the intrinsic circuitry at the same level of precision. As a result, detailed anatomical data on the "trisynaptic circuit" are relatively sparse, and connections between different lamellae, i.e. the longitudinal association fibers (Lorente de Nó, 1934; Fricke and Cowan, 1978; Swanson et al., 1978), have not been documented in detail.

Abbreviations: CA1,2,3, subfields of Ammon's horn; DG, dentate gyrus; LEA, lateral subdivision of the entorhinal cortex; MEA, medial subdivision of the entorhinal cortex; PHA-L, *Phaseolus vulgaris*-leucoagglutinin.

With the recent introduction of the anterograde tracer *Phaseolus vulgaris-leucoagglutinin* (PHA-L), a new powerful anatomical technique became available (for detailed descriptions of this method, see Gerfen and Sawchenko, 1984; Groenewegen et al., 1987). With the use of PHA-L, more detailed data on the intrinsic and extrinsic connections of the hippocampus have emerged. In the present chapter, attempts will be made to describe some of these new findings and to indicate their implications for the functional organization of the hippocampus.

NOMENCLATURE AND ARCHITECTONICS

In the rat the hippocampus extends almost from the septum dorsally to the caudal part of the amygdala ventrally, resembling the shape of a cashew nut. For descriptive purposes, the hippocampus will be divided into a dorsal or septal part and a ventral or temporal part. In between the septal and temporal parts, an intermediate part is distinguished. The longitudinal axis is curved and runs from the septal pole to the temporal pole of the hippocampus. The transverse axis of the hippocampus is defined as the axis in a plane perpendicular to the longitudinal axis (Fig. 1).

The hippocampus consists of Ammon's horn, the dentate gyrus, and the subiculum. In the rat, as in all mammals, the hippocampus consists of two C-shaped, interlocking principal cell layers: the granular cell layer of the dentate gyrus (DG) and the pyramidal cell layer of Ammon's horn (Figs. 1, 2). Various nomenclatures have been used to describe the subdivions of the hippocampus. Based largely on Golgi preparations, Ramón y Cajal (1911) subdivided Ammon's horn into an area of large pyramidal cells (regio inferior) and a region of more densely packed smaller pyramidal cells (regio superior). Another widely used terminology was introduced by Lorente de Nó (1934). Also using the Golgi technique, Lorente de Nó divided Ammon's horn into four subfields: CA (cornu Ammonis) 1 to CA4. Area CA4 corresponds to the polymorphic zone of the DG as described by Ramón y Cajal. More recent evidence strongly support Ramón y Cajal's point of view that these cells belong to the DG and not to the CA (Blackstad, 1956; Amaral, 1978; Gaarskjaer, 1981). Areas CA2 and CA3 together correspond to the regio inferior and area CA1 to the regio superior.

The basic architecture of the hippocampal subfields is very similar (Fig. 2) in that they all consist of one single lamina of neurons of which the apical dendrites extend into a cell-poor zone, the stratum moleculare in the DG and the subiculum and the stratum lacunosum-moleculare and stratum radiatum in Ammon's horn. For convenience, the stratum lacunosum-moleculare will be called the *stratum-moleculare.* Underneath the cell layer lies the polymorphic layer, which in turn is bordered by a fiber zone. For a more extensive description of the basic anatomical features of the hippocampus, reference is given to the original publications, many of which have been comprehensively summarized in several recent reviews (Witter, 1986; Swanson et al., 1987).

The DG consists of a densely packed single cell layer, with granule cells as the major cell type. Because of its (strong) curvature, it encloses the so-called hilar area (Fig. 2). The hilar area contains the polymorphic or infragranular layer of the DG and the proximal part of the pyramidal cell layer of CA3. The granule cell layer of the DG can be subdivided in relation to its location to the pyramidal cells of CA3 into a *suprapyramidal* and an *infrapyramidal* blade, which merge at the *crest* of the DG (Fig. 2). In following the pyramidal cell layer of Ammon's horn along its transverse axis from proximal to distal, i.e. from the dentate gyrus toward the subiculum, the following sequence can be distinguished. The CA3 field merges distally with the CA2 field. Although CA2, as CA3, mainly contains large pyramidal neurons, it has been claimed that CA2 in contrast to CA3 does not receive mossy fiber input from the DG (Lorente de Nó, 1934). The proximal part of CA1 adjoins CA2, and the distal part of CA1 borders the subiculum. The subiculum is distally replaced by the pre- and parasubiculum and the adjacent entorhinal cortex ventrally and the retrosplenial cortex dorsally.

Using cytoarchitectonic criteria, the entorhinal cortex of the rat can be subdivided into various subfields. In general, a lateral (LEA) and medial (MEA) entorhinal area are recognized (Blackstad, 1956; Steward, 1976; Wyss, 1981; Krettek and Price, 1977). Within the entorhinal cortex six cortical layers are distinguished that generally are described as constituting superficial (layers I–III) and deep (IV–VI) layers.

OUTLINE OF THE "LAMELLAR" ORGANIZATION

Anatomical (Blackstad et al., 1970; Hjorth-Simonsen and Jeune, 1972) and even more so electrophysiological data (Andersen et al., 1971) have indicated that the hippocampus is organized in a lamellar fashion. Each lamella, which is oriented more or less perpendicular to the longitudinal axis of the hippocampus, contains a sequence of almost completely unidirectional connections from the DG to the subiculum, via CA3 and CA1 (Fig. 2; see also Fig. 5A). The DG represents the major input structure of the hippocampus, with major cortical afferents arising from the entorhinal cortex. The subiculum is considered to give rise to most of the hippocampal efferents to widespread subcortical and cortical areas, including the entorhinal cortex, although CA1 also contributes to many of these efferent systems (see Witter, 1986; Swanson et al., 1987).

CONNECTIONS BETWEEN THE ENTORHINAL CORTEX AND THE HIPPOCAMPUS

The entorhinal cortex gives rise to a massive projection to the hippocampus, the perforant pathway, that has been reported to terminate predominantly in the DG. Projections to Ammon's horn also have been described (Steward, 1976; Wyss, 1981), but in general they have not been incorporated into models of hippocampal circuitry. It appears well established that the projections to the DG and CA3 arise predominantly from cells in layer II, whereas neurons in layer III give rise to the projections to CA1 (Steward and Scoville, 1976). Minor contributions may originate in the deeper layers of the entorhinal cortex (Köhler, 1985a).

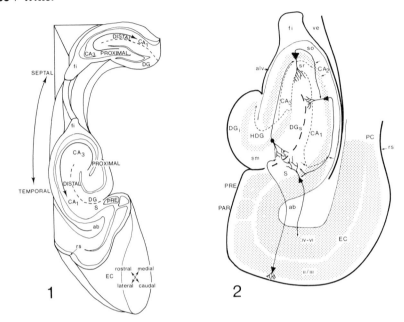

Abbreviations for Figures

II–VI	cortical layers
ab	angular bundle
alv	alveus
CA1,2,3	subfields of Ammon's horn
DG	dentate gyrus
DG$_i$	infrapyramidal blade of the dentate gyrus
DG$_s$	suprapyramidal blade of the dentate gyrus
EC	entorhinal cortex
fi	fimbria
HDG	hilus of the dentate gyrus
hf	hippocampal fissure
PAR	parasubiculum
PC	perirhinal cortex
PRE	presubiculum
rs	rhinal sulcus
S	subiculum
sm	molecular layer
so	stratum oriens
sr	stratum radiatum
ve	lateral ventrical

Fig. 1. Artist's representation of the hippocampus and entorhinal cortex of the rat. The longitudinal or septotemporal axis, which runs from the septal pole to the temporal pole, is indicated. In the two transverse sections at the temporal and septal extreme the proximodistal axis of Ammon's horn and the subiculum is illustrated. This axis runs from the hilus of the dentate gyrus toward the subiculum.

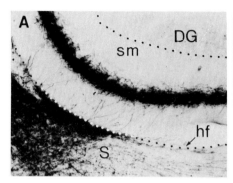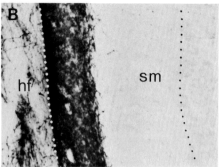

Fig. 3. Photomicrographs of part of the dentate gyrus and adjacent subiculum, showing the terminal distribution of entorhinal fibers in the molecular layer (sm) of the dentate gyrus (DG) following an injection in the MEA **(A)** and the LEA **(B)**. The borders of the molecular layer are indicated by stippling. The injection in the MEA results in a terminal field in approximately one-fifth of the molecular layer, whereas following the LEA injection, the terminal labeling occupies the entire outer one-third. Note in A the fibers that penetrate the hippocampal fissure (hf) on their way to the DG.

Perforant pathway fibers have been observed to leave layers II and III of the entorhinal cortex and enter the underlying white matter and the angular bundle. From here they traverse the pyramidal cell layer of the subiculum proper, although some fibers cross the presubiculum or the distal part of CA1. According to the traditional descriptions (Blackstad, 1956; Hjorth-Simonsen and Jeune, 1972), the majority of the fibers of the perforant pathway traverse the molecular layers of the subiculum and CA1 and subsequently cross the hippocampal fissure to reach the molecular layer of the DG, where they terminate. Using PHA-L we observed that the number of fibers that follow this pathway is not very large (Fig. 3A). In contrast, many of the entorhinal fibers travel in the molecular layer of Ammon's horn along its transverse axis. In CA3, these fibers show en passant varicosities. Subsequently, they enter the suprapyramidal tip of the molecular layer of the DG, where they terminate along its transverse extent. Although confirmation using, for example, intra-cellular EM tracing is needed, these observations imply that next to entorhinal

Fig. 2. Schematic representation of a transverse section, i.e. a section taken perpendicular to the longitudinal axis, through the hippocampus of the rat. The different subfields (dentate gyrus, CA3–CA1, and the subiculum) and their various layers are indicated. Note the input and output relations of the hippocampus with the entorhinal cortex and the trisynaptic circuit: The dentate gyrus gives rise to mossy fibers that course in the stratum lucidum to the dendrites of the CA3 pyramidal cells, where they terminate. CA3 cells distribute the Schaffer collaterals to CA1 cells, which in turn send their axons to the subiculum (see also Fig. 5).

fibers that reach the DG directly, there are fibers that first interact with cells in CA3 before reaching the dentate granule cells.

As is illustrated in Figure 4, the entorhinal cortex projects not only to the DG and CA3 but also very densely to CA1 and the subiculum. The density of the projections to CA1 appears to be related to their site of origin in the entorhinal cortex. A rostrolateral part of the LEA projects preferentially to CA1, almost without projecting to the DG, whereas more medial and caudal parts of the LEA give rise to denser projections to the DG (Witter et al., 1988). Although an entorhinal projection to the subiculum has been previously suggested, the anatomical techniques then available made it very difficult to discriminate actual termination within the subiculum from the many fibers that are passing through. With the use of PHA-L we clearly observed that the entire entorhinal cortex gives rise to fibers that terminate in the outer two-thirds of the molecular layer of the subiculum.

The subiculum and CA1 project back to the entorhinal cortex, in particular to the deep layers of the MEA (Swanson et al., 1978; Köhler, 1985b), although the subiculum also projects to the superficial layers of caudal parts of the MEA (Groenewegen and Witter, unpublished observations). From the data presented above, it is concluded that the traditional circuitry of the hippocampus needs to be revised. Nested within the connectional sequence from the entorhinal cortex to the subiculum via the DG, CA3, and CA1 (Fig. 5A), reciprocal connections of the entorhinal cortex with CA1 and with the subiculum are present. Since the entorhinal cortex also projects to CA3, it appears that within the entorhinal–hippocampal system several parallel but strongly interconnected routes are present (Fig. 5B).

TOPOGRAPHICAL ORGANIZATION OF THE ENTORHINAL–
HIPPOCAMPAL SYSTEM
Afferent Connections of the Entorhinal Cortex

In the cat and the monkey the entorhinal cortex, in particular its lateral part, receives a prominent input from the perirhinal cortex. This pathway was suggested to mediate multimodal sensory information, although other, more direct pathways to the entorhinal cortex are also present (van Hoesen, 1982; Witter et al., 1986; Insausti et al., 1987). In the rat, it was recently suggested that the perirhinal cortex projects to the entorhinal cortex (Köhler, 1986). Our own observations confirmed this and showed that the perirhinal fibers predominantly terminate in lateral portions of the LEA and lateral and caudal parts of the MEA. Similar to the situation in the cat and the monkey, in the rat the perirhinal cortex receives input from widespread sensory-related parts of the cortical surface (Deacon et al., 1983). Electrophysiological data in the

---

Fig. 4.   Photomicrographs of labeling in the hippocampus following injections of PHA-L laterally into the LEA **(A)** and laterally into the MEA **(B)**. Following transcardial perfusion, the hippocampus and adjacent cortices were taken out of the brain and flattened prior to sectioning. This provides the possibility of cutting transverse sections along almost the entire longitudinal extent of the hippocampus and the rostrocaudal extent of the entorhinal cortex. The sections are represented from septal to temporal

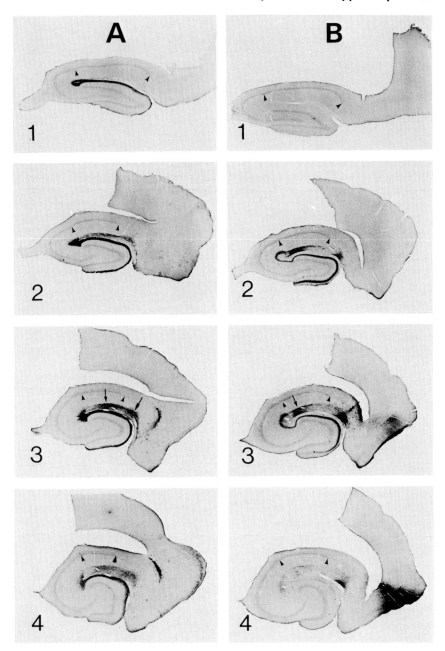

(A 1–4 and B 1–4, respectively). The borders of field CA1 are indicated by arrowheads. Note the dense terminal fields in the subiculum (double-headed arrows) and CA1 (single-headed arrows) and the different localization in CA1 following the LEA and MEA injections (A-3 and B-3).

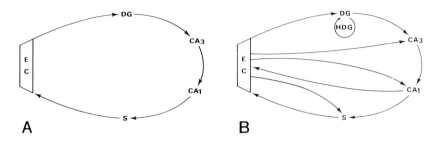

Fig. 5. **A:** Schematic representation of the "traditional" entorhinal–hippocampal circuitry. The entorhinal cortex, in particular the superficial layers, feed into the trisynaptic circuit, and the subiculum projects back to the entorhinal cortex, in particular to its deep layers. Note that the different layers within the entorhinal cortex are not indicated. **B:** Schematic representation of the entorhinal–hippocampal circuitry derived from the results of the PHA-L experiments described in the text. Nested within the traditional circuit (compare with A) parallel circuits are indicated between the entorhinal cortex on the one hand and CA1 and the subiculum on the other. The circuit between the dentate granule cells and the hilus is also indicated (see text for further details).

rat indicate that in superficial layers of lateral parts of the entorhinal cortex sensory convergence takes place (Vaysettes-Courchay and Sessler, 1983). Not much is known in detail with respect to the afferents of more medial parts of the entorhinal cortex. As suggested in the cat and the monkey (Witter et al., 1986, 1989), the medial parts of the entorhinal cortex most probably receive information different from that received by the lateral parts.

The Perforant Pathway

In previous anterograde studies it was reported that the perforant pathway distributes topographically along the entire longitudinal axis of the hippocampus such that the septotemporal axis of the hippocampus is related to a similarly oriented axis in the entorhinal cortex (Hjorth-Simonsen, 1972; Wyss, 1981). In contrast to this, and in line with a recently published retrograde tracer study (Ruth et al., 1982; see also Witter, 1986), we observed that a somewhat obliquely oriented mediolateral axis in the entorhinal cortex corresponds to the septotemporal hippocampal axis. Lateral parts of both the LEA and MEA, as well as the most caudal extreme of the MEA, project preferentially to septal parts of the hippocampus, whereas more medial parts of both subdivisions project to more temporal parts of the hippocampus. This septotemporal organization is most impressive in the entorhinal–dentate projections (cf. Witter and Groenewegen, 1984; Witter et al., 1989). The topographical organization of the perforant pathway is in register with the topographical distribution within the entorhinal cortex of some of its afferents as outlined before. Lateral parts of the entorhinal cortex may thus transmit sensory-related information to the septal part of the hippocampus. We also observed that the reciprocal projections from the subiculum to the entorhinal cortex show a similar topography (Groenewegen and Witter, unpublished observations).

In contrast to the previously described organization, the perforant pathway also shows a topological organization that is related to the cytoarchitectonic organization of the entorhinal cortex. Anterograde studies (Hjorth-Simonsen, 1972; Hjorth-Simonsen and Jeune, 1972; Steward, 1976; Wyss, 1981) showed that fibers that originate in the MEA distribute preferentially to the middle one-third of the molecular layer of the DG and CA3 and to more proximal parts of field CA1 —close to the CA1–CA3 border. Fibers from the LEA project to the outer one-third of the molecular layer of the DG and CA3 and to more distal portions of CA1 —close to the CA1–subicular border. From these data it was concluded that within the perforant pathway a medial and lateral component can be distinguished. According to some investigators, however, the organization of the perforant pathway is a more gradual phenomenon. Therefore, they described a third, intermediate component (Steward, 1976; Wyss, 1981).

The results of our PHA-L experiments (N = 34) indicate that the terminal distribution of the perforant pathway in the molecular layers of the DG and CA3 can be classified into either the outer or middle one-third. Interestingly, injections that resulted in labeling in the middle one-third in most cases did not label the entire width of this terminal zone (Fig. 3A). In these cases, the width of the zone of termination appears to be related not to the size of the injection but to its location along the lateral-to-medial axis in the entorhinal cortex. Lateral parts of the MEA project to the outer part of the middle one-third of the molecular layer, and more medial locations in the MEA distribute fibers to more inner parts of the middle one-third. In contrast, in all cases in which labeling in the outer one-third was observed, the labeling occupied the entire width of this zone (Fig. 3B). Our data confirmed previously published data that indicated that the perforant pathway is organized mainly along the transverse axis of CA1. The lateral perforant pathway distributes to the distal part of CA1 (Fig. 4A-3), whereas the medial perforant pathway projects to the more proximal portion of CA1 (Fig. 4B-3). Within the subiculum both of the components of the perforant pathway appear to distribute homogeneously within the outer two-thirds of the molecular layer (Fig. 4). Our data confirm previous observations that fibers from the LEA show a more extensive distribution along the longitudinal axis of the hippocampus than do fibers that originate in the MEA (compare Fig. 4A and 4B).

It can be concluded that the perforant pathway can be subdivided into two components, which arise from different parts of the entorhinal cortex and which differ with respect to their distribution in the hippocampus. The lateral perforant pathway is organized such that a small part of LEA can interact not only with a relatively large part of the hippocampus along its longitudinal extent but also with a large segment (one-third) of the apical dendrites of the cells of the DG and CA3. The medial component of the perforant pathway exhibits a more restricted distribution. This difference in organization of the two components of the perforant pathway, the lateral somewhat more diffuse and the medial more restricted, suggests that each of the two components may exert a different effect on the same target neurons in the DG and CA3. In contrast, both components may interact with different cell populations of CA1. In the subiculum they may influence the same cells in the same way, although both the lateral and medial components differ with respect to their neuroactive substances and electrophysiological characteristics (McNaughton, 1980; Fredens et al., 1984).

It has been reported that the lateral perforant pathway distributes preferentially to the suprapyramidal blade and that the medial component either does not show a preference or prefers the infrapyramidal blade (Wyss, 1981). From experiments using PHA-L, this description can be refined. Lateral parts of the LEA project predominantly to the suprapyramidal blade, whereas more medial parts of the LEA do not show a clear preference, or in some cases project slightly denser to the infrapyramidal blade. Rostral and caudal parts of the MEA show a preference for the suprapyramidal blade, whereas the remaining parts of the MEA appear to project evenly dense to both blades of the DG, although in a few cases with extremely medially placed injections a slight preference for the infrapyramidal blade is observed. It should be noted, however, that the organization is even more complex, since the terminal densities in the two blades vary along the longitudinal axis of the DG (compare Fig. 4B-2 and 4B-3).

Using the terminal pattern of entorhinal fibers in the molecular layer of the DG as a defining characteristic of the lateral and medial components of the perforant pathway, the origin of both components in the entorhinal cortex can be charted. This chart can subsequently be superimposed on the septotemporal topography of the perforant pathway. The resulting map of the origin and distribution of entorhinal-dentate fibers is schematically illustrated in Figure 6. All parts of the hippocampus along its longitudinal axis are reached by both the lateral and medial components of the perforant pathway. However, their respective sites of origin in the entorhinal cortex and the terminal fields show a very complex spatial relation. For example, septal parts of the DG are reached by the lateral perforant pathway originating laterally in the LEA and by the medial perforant pathway arising from the most caudolateral part of the MEA. In contrast, the more intermediate parts of the DG are reached by the two components both originating at approximately the same rostrocaudal level in the LEA and MEA.

The topographical organization of the entorhinal–dentate projections together with that of the afferents of the entorhinal cortex indicate that the lateral and caudal parts of the entorhinal cortex, which mediate sensory-related information, project densest to septal and intermediate parts of the DG, in particular to the suprapyramidal blade. More medial parts of the entorhinal cortex project preferentially to more temporal levels of the DG and show a slight preference for the infrapyramidal blade. As indicated before, it is to be expected that more medial parts of the entorhinal cortex differ with respect to their afferents from the lateral part (cf. Witter et al., 1986, 1989). Therefore, different subsets of dentate granular cells will most likely mediate different types of information.

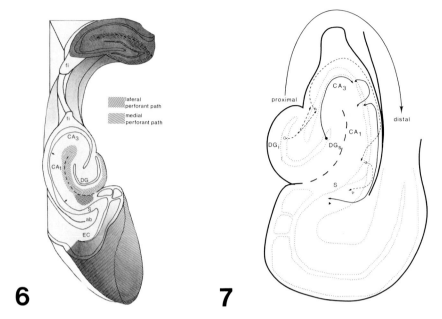

6   **7**

Fig. 6. Artist's representation of the organization of the perforant pathway in the rat (compare with Fig. 1). The septotemporal topography is indicated by corresponding grey levels in the entorhinal cortex and the hippocampus. The origin and distribution of the lateral and medial components of the perforant pathway are illustrated using different hatchings. Note that both components reach the entire septotemporal extent of the hippocampus.

Fig. 7. Summary diagram illustrating the intrinsic circuitry of the hippocampus as described in the text. Two hypothetical circuits are represented, one starting from the infrapyramidal blade of the dentate gyrus (open circles and triangles) and reaching the proximal part of the subiculum. The other (closed circles and triangles) connects the suprapyramidal blade of the dentate gyrus with the distal part of the subiculum. Note that the connections of the hilus and the circuitry of the interneurons are not included.

INTRINSIC HIPPOCAMPAL CIRCUITRY
Detailed Organization of the Trisynaptic Circuit

The dentate granule cells distribute their mossy fibers to the entire transverse or proximodistal extent of CA3. Using intracellular injection of dentate granule cells and small extracellular injections with horseradish peroxidase (HRP) in hippocampal slices, Claiborne et al. (1986) confirmed earlier descriptions (Ramón y Cajal, 1911; Lorente de Nó, 1934; Blackstad et al., 1970; Swanson et al., 1978) and, in addition, showed that the mossy fiber system in the rat exhibits a complicated topology. They observed that the proximal portions of CA3 are preferentially reached by fibers that originate in the infrapyramidal blade, the crest, and adjacent portion of the suprapyramidal blade. Cells in the tip of the suprapyramidal blade interact with more distal portions of the CA3 field (Fig.

7). The mossy fibers that terminate on the basal dendrites of the more prox-imally located CA3 pyramidal cells arise mainly from the infrapyramidal blade of the DG. Therefore, Claiborne and her collaborators (1986) concluded that "the influence of different populations of granule cells upon the cells in field CA3 is a function of their location within the granule cell layer."

The pyramidal cells in field CA3 give rise to the Schaffer collaterals that distribute to the CA1 region. In general, the Schaffer collaterals synapse in the stratum radiatum and stratum oriens with the dendrites of CA1 pyramidal cells. The CA1 pyramidal cells, in turn, give rise to powerful projections to the sub-iculum that terminate in the deep half of the molecular layer and in the py-ramidal cell layer (Fig. 2). The results of recent intracellular and extracellular tracing studies with HRP and PHA-L, respectively, indicate that the connections between CA3 and CA1 and those from CA1 to the subiculum show a columnar organization perpendicular to the cell layer. Both intrinsic systems exhibit the same gradual topology: Neurons in CA3 and CA1 form axonal columns in CA1 and the subiculum, respectively, with a reversed order. Proximal parts of CA3 and CA1 distribute fibers to distal parts of CA1 and the subiculum, respectively, and more distal parts of CA3 and CA1 interact with more proximal parts of CA1 and the subiculum, respectively (Fig. 7) (Tamamaki et al., 1987; unpublished observations; Ishizuka et al., 1988; Amaral, personal communication). In a recent electrophysiological study it was reported that within CA1 an intrinsic inhibitory system is present that also reflects a columnar organization (Dingledine et al., 1987).

Longitudinal Connectivity

The intrinsic connections between the various subfields of the hippocampus also show a longitudinal organization (Ishizuka et al., 1988; Amaral, personal communication; our own unpublished results). Within all fields of the hippo-campus a large number of interneurons is present. These interneurons are known to give rise to widespread axonal arborizations along not only the transverse axis but also the longitudinal axis of the hippocampus (Struble et al., 1978). Therefore, they may interact with many hippocampal principal neu-rons along both the transverse and longitudinal axes of the hippocampus (Buz-sáki, 1984; Swanson et al., 1987). These data thus confirm the existence within the hippocampus of a longitudinal association system that interconnects various lamellae (cf. Lorente de Nó, 1934; Swanson et al., 1978; Fricke and Cowan, 1978).

Connectivity of the Hilus

The dentate granular cells not only give rise to mossy fibers that terminate in CA3 but in addition distribute many axon collaterals within a relatively nar-row lamella of the hilus of the dentate gyrus (Claiborne et al., 1986; Fricke and Cowan, 1978; Swanson et al., 1978). Most of the associational and com-missural input to the dentate gyrus, which terminates in the inner one-third of its molecular layer, arises from hilar cells. The hilar region receives a number of extrinsic afferents, predominantly from the brain stem and the septal area. These afferents include a prominent noradrenergic input from the locus coeruleus, a serotonergic input from the median and dorsal raphe, a cholinergic input from the medial septal nucleus, and a histaminergic input from the supramammillary region. These afferents also reach some of the other subfields of the hippocampus, but, in general, their terminal field in the hilus of the DG is the densest (see Swanson et al., 1987 for a detailed overview and relevant references). It is well established that information flow through the hippocampus is influenced by modulation of one or more of these systems (for review, see Lopes da Silva et al., 1988). Since the dendritic trees of hilar cells have been observed to reach the molecular layer of the DG (Amaral, 1978), they may also be influenced directly by the major cortical inputs to the DG. Thus, it seems appropriate to consider the hilus as a functionally different unit of the hippocampus that may participate in regulatory circuits of the dentate gyrus (Fig. 5B) and thus may enhance or inhibit information flow in the dentate gyrus.

EFFERENT PROJECTIONS OF THE HIPPOCAMPUS

The hippocampus projects to various cortical and subcortical structures, including the entorhinal cortex (see above), the septum, the nucleus accumbens, the amygdaloid complex, and the hypothalamus. Although the subiculum appears to be the major source of most of these extrinsic projections, Ammon's horn, in particular CA1, also contributes to these projections (cf. Swanson et al., 1987). Recently, we reported that the subiculum is heterogeneous with respect to the origin of at least one of its projections. The projection to the nucleus accumbens that arises from the entire longitudinal extent of the subiculum was observed to originate only in cells that are located close to the subicular–CA1 border, i.e. the proximal part. The distal part of the subiculum does not contribute fibers to this efferent pathway (Groenewegen et al., 1987). Preliminary data of both anterograde and retrograde experiments indicate that in the dorsal subiculum the more distally located population of neurons projects to the retrosplenial and perirhinal cortices. These findings indicate that in the subiculum at least two populations of cells are present that interact with different targets in the brain. This does not imply that all targets are reached by fibers that originate in differently located subicular cell populations. For example, it has been reported that subicular projections to the septum and to the entorhinal cortex arise from the same neuronal population, in some cases even as collaterals (Swanson et al., 1981).

SUMMARY OF HIPPOCAMPAL CONNECTIVITY

In summarizing the overall patterns of connectivity of the hippocampus, the following "flow chart" can be constructed (see Fig. 7). Cells in the suprapyramidal blade of the DG, in particular the region near the tip, that receive a more or less well-defined input from sensory-related parts of the entorhinal cortex project densest to distal parts of CA3. Cells closer to the dentate crest or in the infrapyramidal blade project to the more proximal parts of CA3. Subsequently, distal parts of CA3 project to proximal parts of CA1, which in turn project to distal parts of the subiculum. Accordingly, the more proximal parts of the subiculum appear to be indirectly connected with the crest and the infrapyramidal blade of the DG. Within the subiculum, proximal and distal parts give rise to different projections outside the hippocampus.

CONCLUDING REMARKS

It is important to emphasize that not all of the described circuits are documented to the same precision and that some may even be considered speculative. However, the anatomical data presented should lead to changes in concepts of how the hippocampus is organized. First, it seems valid to conclude that the "lamellar hypothesis," which emphasises the transverse connectivity within the hippocampus, only in part reflects the intrinsic organization. The longitudinal intrinsic connectivity should be added to this organization. The observation that the perforant pathway is not organized in a lamellar fashion further stresses the need for models in which the hippocampus is described as a matrix (see, e.g. Teyler and Discenna, 1984; McNaughton and Morris, 1987).

Second, models must incorporate the parallel circuitry that exists within the entorhinal–hippocampal system. The presented data suggest that entorhinal activity is transmitted to not only the DG but also the CA3. This system is organized in such a way that CA3 neurons may be "prepared" by incoming entorhinal activity before they are reached by the dentate-transformed activity. The other parallel circuits, between the entorhinal cortex on the one hand and the CA1 and the subiculum on the other, arise from different cells in the entorhinal cortex than the entorhinal–dentate/CA3 projections. This suggests that within the various circuits different types of information are processed. As a further complicating factor, all hippocampal subfields are reached by the lateral and medial component of the perforant pathway. With the exception of the subiculum, these two components distribute differentially within each field of the hippocampus. As outlined before, in the DG and CA3, these components may interact differently with the same target neurons. In contrast, within CA1 they probably interact with different sets of neurons in a similar way, whereas both components may influence the same set of subicular neurons in the same way.

Third, the intrinsic pathways of the hippocampus show a clear columnar organization that is in accordance with the topography of the perforant pathway and with the origin in the subiculum of hippocampal efferents. Different columns are interconnected in such a way that channels can be distinguished that may process different types of information.

Finally, it is indicated that the hilus of the DG should be incorporated into hippocampal circuits as a functionally different component that may influence the sensitivity of the dentate granule cells to incoming stimuli.

ACKNOWLEDGMENTS

I thank Dr. D.G. Amaral for the many hours of stimulating discussion that preceded the preparation of this manuscript. The critical reading of earlier versions of the manuscript by Drs. P.V.J.M. Hoogland and F.G. Wouterlood, and their valuable suggestions, are greatfully acknowledged. I also thank Mr. D. de Jong for photographic support.

REFERENCES

Amaral, D.G. (1978) A Golgi study of cell types in the hilar region of the hippocampus in the rat. J. Comp. Neurol. *182*:851–914.

Andersen, P., T.V.P. Bliss, and K.K. Skrede (1971) Lamellar organization of hippocampal excitatory pathways. Exp. Brain Res. *13*:222–238.

Blackstad, T.W. (1956) Commissural connections of the hippocampal region in the rat, with special reference to their mode of termination. J. Comp. Neurol. *105*:417–537.

Blackstad, T.W., K. Brink, J. Hem, and B. Jeune (1970) Distribution of hippocampal mossy fibers in the rat. An experimental study with silver impregnation methods. J. Comp. Neurol. *138*:433–450.

Buzsáki, G. (1984) Feed-forward inhibition in the hippocampal formation. Prog. Neurobiol. *22*:131–153.

Claiborne, B.J., D.G. Amaral, and W.M. Cowan (1986) A light and electron microscopic analysis of the mossy fibers of the rat dentate gyrus. J. Comp. Neurol. *246*:453–458.

Deacon, T.W., H. Eichenbaum, P. Rosenberg, and K.W. Eckman (1983) Afferent connections of the perirhinal cortex in the rat. J. Comp. Neurol. *220*:168–190.

Dingledine, R., A.A. Roth, and G.L. King (1987) Synaptic control of pyramidal cell activation in the hippocampal slice preparation in the rat. Neuroscience *22*:553–561.

Fredens, K., K. Stengaard-Pedersen, and L.I. Larsson (1984) Localization of enkephalin and cholecystokinin immunoreactivities in the perforant pathway terminal fields of the rat hippocampal formation. Brain Res. *304*:255–263.

Fricke, R., and W.M. Cowan (1978) Autoradiographic study of the commissural and ipsilateral hippocampal-dentate projections in the adult rat. J. Comp. Neurol. *181*:253–269.

Gaarskjaer, F.B. (1981) The hippocampal mossy fiber system of the rat studied with retrograde tracing techniques. Correlation between topographic organization and neurogetic gradients. J. Comp. Neurol. *203*:717–735.

Gerfen, C.R., and P.E. Sawchenko (1984) An anterograde neuroanatomical tracing method that shows the detailed morphology of neurons, their axons and terminals: Immunohistochemical localization of an axonally transported plant lectin, *Phaseolus vulgaris*-leucoagglutinin. Brain Res. *209*:283–303.

Groenewegen, H.J., E. Vermeulen-van Der Zee, A. te Kortschot, and M.P. Witter (1987) Organization of the projections from the subiculum to the ventral striatum in the rat. A study using anterograde transport of *Phaseolus vulgaris* leucoagglutinin. Neuroscience *23*:103–120.

Hjorth-Simonsen, A. (1972) Projection of the lateral part of the entorhinal area to the hippocampus and fascia dentata. J. Comp. Neurol. *147*:219–232.

Hjorth-Simonsen, A., and B. Jeune (1972) Origin and termination of the hippocampal perforant path in the rat studied by silver impregnation. J. Comp. Neurol. *144*:215–232.

Insausti, R., D.G. Amaral, and W.M. Cowan (1987) The entorhinal cortex of the monkey: II. Cortical afferents. J. Comp. Neurol. *264*:356–395.

Ishizuka, N., J. Weber, and D.G. Amaral (1989) Organization of intrahippocampal projections originating from CA3 pyramidal cells in the rat. J. Comp. Neurol. (manuscript submitted).

Köhler, C. (1985a) A projection from the deep layers of the entorhinal area to the hippocampal formation in the rat brain. Neurosci. Lett. *56*:13–19.

Köhler, C. (1985b) Intrinsic projections of the retrohippocampal region in the rat brain. I. The subicular complex. J. Comp. Neurol. *236*:504–522.

Köhler, C. (1986) Intrinsic connections of the retrohippocampal region in the rat brain. II. The medial entorhinal area. J. Comp. Neurol. *246*:149–169.

Krettek, J.E., and J.L. Price (1977) Projections from the amygdaloid complex and adjacent olfactory structures to the entorhinal cortex and to the subiculum in the rat and cat. J. Comp. Neurol. *172:*723–752.

Lopes da Silva, F.H., M.P. Witter, P.H. Boeijinga, and A.H.M. Lohman (1989) Anatomical organization and physiology of the limbic cortex. Physiol. Rev. (in press).

Lorente de Nó, R. (1934) Studies on the structure of the cerebral cortex. II. Continuation of the study of the ammonic system. J. Psychol. Neurol. *46:*113–177.

McNaughton, B.L. (1980) Evidence for two physiologically distinct perforant pathways to the fascia dentata. Brain Res. *199:*1–19.

McNaughton, B.L., and R.G.M. Morris (1987) Hippocampal synaptic enhancement and information storage within a distributed memory system. TINS *10:*408–415.

Mishkin, M. (1978) Memory in monkeys severely impaired by combined but not separate removal of amygdala and hippocampus. Nature *273:*297–298.

O'Keefe, J., and L. Nadel (1978) The Hippocampus as a Cognitive Map. Oxford: Clarendon Press.

Ramón y Cajal, S. (1911) Histologie du Système Nerveux de l'Homme et des Vertebres. Paris: Norbert Maloine.

Ruth, R.E., T.J. Collier, and R. Routtenberg (1982) Topography between the entorhinal cortex and the dentate septotemporal axis in rats: I. Medial and intermediate entorhinal projecting cells. J. Comp. Neurol. *209:*69–78.

Scoville, W.B., and B. Milner (1957) Loss of recent memory after bilateral hippocampal lesions. J. Neurol. Neurosurg. Psychiatry *20:*11–21.

Steward, O. (1976) Topographic organization of the projections from the entorhinal area to the hippocampal formation in the rat. J. Comp. Neurol. *167:*285–314.

Steward, O., and S.A. Scoville (1976) Cells of origin of entorhinal cortical afferents to the hippocampus and fascia dentata of the rat. J. Comp. Neurol. *169:*347–370.

Struble, R.G., N.L. Desmond, and W.B. Levy (1978) Anatomical evidence for interlamellar inhibition in the fascia dentata. Brain Res. *152:*580–585.

Swanson, L.W., C. Köhler, and A. Björklund (1987) The limbic region. I: The septohippocampal system. In A. Björklund, T. Hökfelt, and L.W. Swanson (eds): Handbook of Chemical Neuroanatomy, Vol. 5: Integrated Systems of the CNS, part 1. Amsterdam: Elsevier Science Publishers B.V., pp. 125–277.

Swanson, L.W., P.E. Sawchenko, and W.M. Cowan (1981) Evidence for collateral projections by neurons in Ammon's horn, the dentate gyrus and the subiculum. A multiple retrograde labeling study in the rat. J. Neurosci. *1:*548–559.

Swanson, L.W., J.M. Wyss, and W.M. Cowan (1978) An autoradiographic study of the organization of intrahippocampal association pathways in the rat. J. Comp. Neurol. *181:*681–716.

Tamamaki, N., K. Abe, and Y. Nojyo (1987) Columnar organization in the subiculum formed by axon branches originating from single CA1 pyramidal neurons in the rat hippocampus. Brain Res. *412:*156–160.

Teyler, T.J., and P. Discenna (1984) The topological anatomy of the hippocampus: A clue to its function. Brain Res. Bull. *12:*711–719.

Teyler, T.J., and P. Discenna (1987) Long-term potentiation. Annu. Rev. Neurosci. *10:*131–161.

Van Hoesen, G.W. (1982) The parahippocampal gyrus. New observations regarding its cortical connections in the monkey. TINS *5:*345–350.

Vaysettes-Courchay, C., and F.M. Sessler (1983) Neurophysiologie. Mise en evidence de convergences sensorielles dans le cortex entorhinal du rat. C.R. Acad. Sci. (Paris) *296:*877–879.

Witter, M.P. (1986) A survey of the anatomy of the hippocampal formation, with emphasis on the septotemporal organization of its intrinsic and extrinsic connections. Adv. Exp. Med. Biol. *23:*67–82.

Witter, M.P., A.W. Griffioen, B. Jorritsma-Byham, and J.L.M. Krijnen (1988) Entorhinal projections to the hippocampal CA1 region in the rat: An underestimated pathway. Neurosci. Lett. *85:*193–198.

Witter, M.P., and H.J. Groenewegen (1984) Laminar origin and septotemporal distribution of entorhinal and perirhinal projections to the hippocampus in the cat. J. Comp. Neurol. *224:*371–385.

Witter, M.P., P. Room, H.J. Groenewegen, and A.H.M. Lohman (1986) The connections of the parahippocampal cortex in the cat. V. Intrinsic connections: Comments on input/output connections with the hippocampus. J. Comp. Neurol. *252:*78–94.

Witter, M.P., G.W. van Hoesen, and D.G. Amaral (1989) Topographical organization of the entorhinal projection to the dentate gyrus of the monkey. J. Neurosci. *9:*216–228.

Wyss, J.M. (1981) An autoradiographic study of the efferent connections of the entorhinal cortex in the rat. J. Comp. Neurol. *199:*495–512.

Zola-Morgan, S., and L.R. Squire (1986) Memory impairment in monkeys following lesions limited to the hippocampus. Behav. Neurosci. *100:*155–160.

Zola-Morgan, S., L.R. Squire, and D.G. Amaral (1986) Human amnesia and the medial temporal region: Enduring memory impairment following a bilateral lesion limited to field CA1 of the hippocampus. J. Neurosci. *6:*2950–2967.

The Hippocampus—New Vistas, pages 71–83
© 1989 Alan R. Liss, Inc.

5
New Anatomical Approaches To Reveal Afferent and Efferent Hippocampal Circuitry

EBERHARD H. BUHL, WALTER K. SCHWERDTFEGER, AND
PETER GERMROTH

*Max-Planck-Institut für Hirnforschung, Frankfurt, Federal Republic of
Germany*

INTRODUCTION

The recently introduced intracellular Lucifer yellow (LY) staining in fixed tissue is a powerful neuroanatomical technique (Tauchi and Masland, 1984). This technique was subsequently combined with retrograde fluorescent tracing to reveal the morphology of projection neurons (Buhl and Peichl, 1986; Schwerdtfeger and Buhl, 1986). Because of visually guided penetration of pre-labeled cells, the method offers high selectivity and, in addition, yields large samples of stained neurons (Buhl and Lübke, 1989). Although LY itself possesses no significant electron density, a relatively simple photo-oxidation procedure can transform the dye into an electron-opaque reaction product, enabling ultrastructural analysis of filled neurons (Maranto, 1982; Buhl and Schlote, 1987).

The present study involves a novel combination of retrograde tracing, intracellular staining in fixed tissue, and electron microscopy (EM). This combination was used to determine the morphology and ultrastructure of neurons constituting the perforant path, a fiber tract originating in the ipsilateral entorhinal cortex and terminating in the molecular layers of the dentate gyrus and Ammon's horn (Hjorth-Simonsen, 1972; Hjorth-Simonsen and Jeune, 1972). Here, entorhinal afferents establish asymmetric synaptic contacts with dendritic spines of dentate granule cells or pyramidal cells, respectively (Matthews et al., 1976). These synapses show activity-dependent modifications after tetanic stimulation of the afferents (Bliss and Lømo, 1973). The phenomenon of long-term potentiation at entorhinodentate synapses is considered to be a model for activity-dependent central nervous system plasticity (Desmond and Levy, 1987).

As for the sources of hippocampal afferents, only limited anatomical data about the neuronal composition of nonpyramidal hippocampofugal projections are available (Chronister and DeFrance, 1979; Alonso and Köhler, 1982; Seress and Ribak, 1983; Seroogy et al., 1983; Totterdell and Hayes, 1987). Because of insufficient filling, results of tract-tracing studies rarely provide detailed information with respect to the identity of labeled neurons other than pyramidal cells. Therefore, commissurally and septally projecting hippocampal neurons were retrogradely labeled with a fluorescent tracer, and their detailed morphology was revealed by LY injection.

MATERIALS AND METHODS

For the first set of experiments adult rats were anesthetized with an intraperitoneal injection of a 4% aqueous chloral hydrate solution (1 ml/100 gm body weight). After positioning the animal in a stereotaxic frame, a craniotomy was performed at the coordinates AP 2.7–3.2 mm and ML 2.5 mm (after Paxinos and Watson, 1982). An injection cannula was advanced vertically with a stereotaxic microdrive for 2.5–3 mm under the pial surface. Small amounts (about 0.25 μl) of a 2% aqueous solution of the fluorescent tracer Fast Blue (FB) were pressure injected into the presumed dentate area.

Following a 3 day survival period, the rats to be used for fluorescence microscopy were deeply reanesthetized and perfused transcardially with a mixture of physiological saline and 0.1% heparin, followed by 500 ml 4% paraformaldehyde in 0.1 M phosphate buffer (PB; pH 7.4). When subsequent EM was required the fixative contained an additional 0.5% glutaraldehyde.

Fixed brains were immediately removed from the skull, trimmed, and serially cut at 100 μm with a vibratome. All sections from the ipsilateral entorhinal cortex were stored in 0.1 M PB at 4°C. Inspection of the injection sites with the fluorescence microscope revealed that the tracer deposit was contained within the ipsilateral dentate area and the CA3 region of Ammon's horn.

For dye filling, entorhinal slices were immersed in an injection chamber containing 0.1 M PB. The chamber was transferred onto a Zeiss fixed stage microscope equipped with epifluorescence illumination and Zeiss UD long-distance objectives (working distance ca. 8 mm). Micropipettes were pulled from omega dot glass capillaries (1.0 mm o.d. × 0.86 mm i.d.) and filled with a 3–8% aqueous solution of LY. A platinum-iridium or silver wire was inserted into the pipettes, which had a DC resistance (measured in 0.1 M PB) ranging between 90 and 300 MΩ. The electrodes were attached to a motor-driven mechanical micromanipulator and moved toward the tissue at an angle of 30–40° from the vertical. Retrogradely labeled entorhinal neurons were identified with the filter combination (Zeiss BP 400-440, FT 460, LP 470) in which both FB and LY can be visualized simultaneously. Under visual control the brightly fluorescent micropipette was advanced toward a labeled cell body. The soma's membrane was penetrated with a brief current pulse or mechanical impulse. Because of the absence of physiological criteria a successful impalement was monitored by applying a negative current pulse, which led to rapid intracellular diffusion of LY. Dye injection was then continued with a negative constant current of 1–3 nA for up to 15 min until all fine dendritic branches appeared

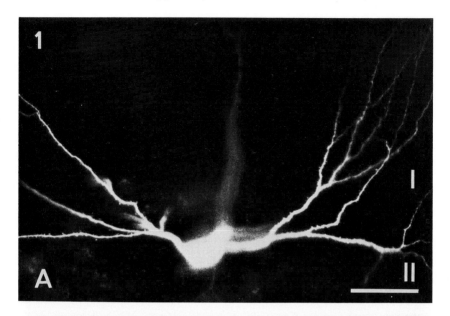

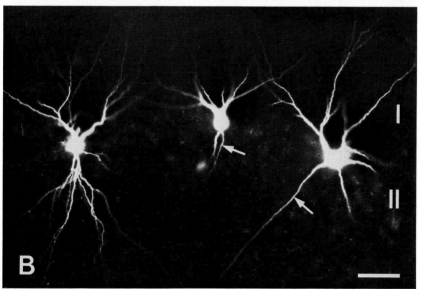

Fig. 1. Stellate cells in layer II of rat lateral entorhinal cortex. After retrogradely pre-labeling the neurons with FB from the ipsilateral hippocampus, we intracellularly injected the cells with LY. At high magnification **(A)** dendritic spines were discernible. When adjacent hippocampally projecting cells were filled **(B)**, their morphological diversity became apparent. Cortical layers are denoted by roman numerals. Axons are labeled by white arrows. Bars = 50 μm.

brightly fluorescent (Fig. 1A). When several neurons had been injected (Fig. 1B) the slice was mounted on a slide and coverslipped with glycerol.

For EM purposes glutaraldehyde-fixed material was used. Slices containing one extensively filled cell were immersed for 5–10 min in a petri dish with 0.1 M PB (pH 7.4) containing 1 mg diaminobenzidine (DAB)/ml (Buhl and Schlote, 1987). Following preincubation, injected neurons were irradiated with the LY excitation wavelength until all visible fluorescence had faded (20–25 min), resulting in the intracellular formation of a homogeneously distributed brown reaction product. Immediately after photoconversion slices were rinsed in three changes of 0.1 M PB (10 min each). Postfixation for 10 min with 0.5% osmium tetroxide in 0.1 M PB was followed by a further three rinses in 0.1 M PB. Then the slices were dehydrated and flat-embedded in Durcupan (Fluka). After serial photography (Fig. 2) and camera lucida reconstruction, photo-oxidized cells were serially cut for EM purposes. Finally, ultrathin sections were contrasted with lead citrate (Fig. 3).

For the second part of the study rats received stereotaxic injections of FB into either the contralateral hippocampus or ipsilateral septum, involving both the medial and lateral septal nuclei. After a 5 day survival period retrogradely labeled hippocampal neurons were intracellularly filled with LY to determine their morphology. Apart from small modifications, the injection protocol was essentially the same as described above (for details, see Schwerdtfeger and Buhl, 1986).

RESULTS
Morphology of Entorhinal Neurons, Which Contribute to the Perforant Path

In lateral entorhinal cortex 54 neurons were extensively filled throughout their dendritic arbor (Fig. 1A). Frequently the axon (Figs. 1B,2) and, at higher magnification, axonal collaterals were traced for considerable distances until these processes left the plane of section. A morphological variety of neuronal types was encountered (Fig. 1B). Pyramidal cells, mainly located in layer III, were identified by the presence of an apical dendrite whose length varied with the laminar position of the cell body. Spiny stellate cells (Fig. 1), the most frequent cell class, were further subdivided into three morphological subtypes with respect to the laminar distribution and branching pattern of dendrites (Fig. 1B). In contrast to pyramidal cells their somata were predominantly located in layer II.

In addition to densely spined entorhinohippocampal neurons, two populations of sparsely spinous cells were identified. As distinguishing criteria, several morphological features were considered, such as the mode of origin and laminar distribution of dendrites. Accordingly two subtypes, sparsely spinous horizontal and multipolar neurons, were discriminated. Despite their morphological heterogeneity, all neurons constituting the perforant path shared one distinct property, namely, a rather elaborate dendritic plexus within layer I, known to receive a variety of entorhinal afferents (for review, see Swanson et al. 1987).

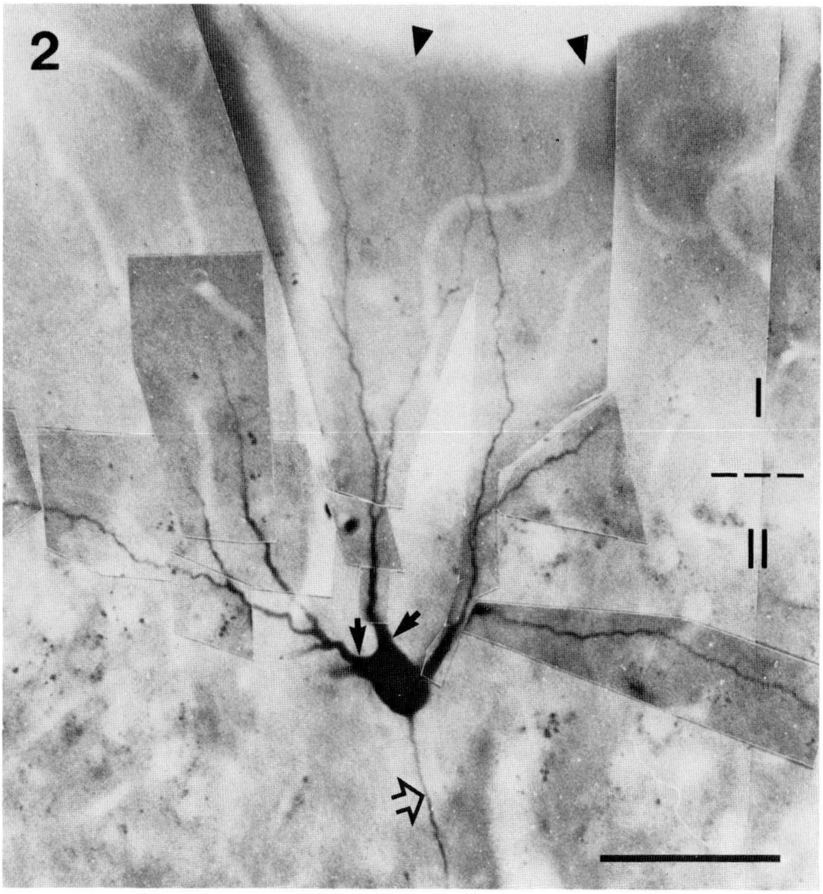

Fig. 2.   Golgi-like, light microscopical appearance of flat-embedded layer II spiny stellate cell after LY-filling and photo-oxidation. Two of its primary dendrites (arrows) and the axon initial segment (open arrow) were identified on the EM micrograph in Figure 3. Cell bodies with endogenous peroxidase activity and capillaries provide an inhomogeneous background pattern. Roman numerals indicate cortical laminae. Pial surface (arrowheads) is at the top. Bar = 50 μm.

Correlated Electron Microscopy

The morphology of photo-oxidized neurons was determined after flat-embedding, as exemplified by a layer II spiny stellate neuron with apically ascending dendrites (Fig. 2). Dark brown diaminobenzidine (DAB) reaction product filled the entire dendritic arbor and main axon, thus providing a Golgi-like image. Three primary dendrites originated from the soma in a polar ori-

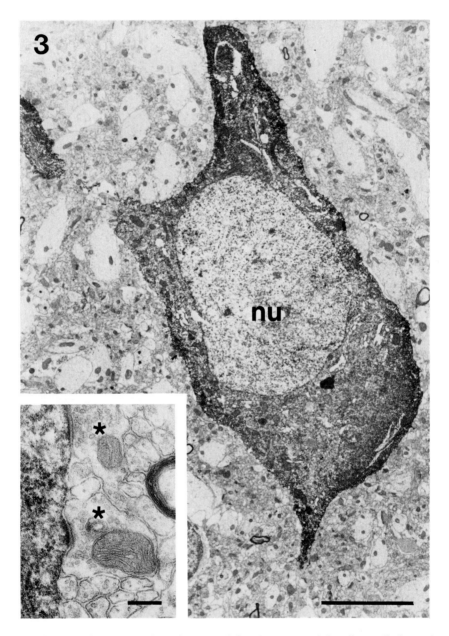

Fig. 3. Ultrathin section through soma of the photoconverted stellate cell shown in Figure 2. Because of the content of fine, electron-opaque precipitate, the cell is darkly contrasted and therefore readily identified in the EM micrograph. Both cell shape and origin of processes correlate well at the light and EM levels. The neuron's oval, pale nucleus (nu) was surrounded by a broad rim of cytoplasm. At higher magnification (insert) boutons (asterisks) containing mitochondria and pleomorphic synaptic vesicles were found to have established axosomatic contacts. Bar = 5 μm; insert, bar = 0.2 μm.

entation. They dichotomously branched into a small number of vertically oriented secondary and tertiary dendrites.

Ultrastructurally, the intracellularly injected spiny stellate cell appeared darkly contrasted because of its content of electron-opaque reaction product (Fig. 3). Since the fine, granular precipitate was distributed rather homogeneously throughout the cell's karyo- and cytoplasm, many cytological details were discernible. The ovoid pale nucleus was surrounded by a broad rim of cytoplasm containing numerous mitochondria and stacks of endoplasmatic reticulum. Two of the primary dendrites (Fig. 2, black arrows) and the axon initial segment (Fig. 2, open arrow) were recognized in the EM micrograph (Fig. 3).

At higher magnification (Fig. 3, insert) it was apparent that a number of terminal boutons, containing pleomorphic vesicles established synaptic contacts with the soma. A varying degree of electron-dense precipitate in apposition to the postsynaptic membrane (Fig. 3, insert) was potentially misleading with regard to the question of whether synapses established symmetrical or asymmetrical contacts with photoconverted entorhinal neurons. Nevertheless, by comparing a larger sample, the majority of axosomatic synapses were tentatively classified as symmetrical. When the shafts of labeled dendrites and the axon initial segment were traced in consecutive sections further symmetrical synaptic contacts were discovered. Conversely, spine heads received asymmetrical synaptic input.

Nonpyramidal Neurons as a Source of Hippocampal Efferents

In agreement with previous reports (Berger et al., 1980; Seroogy et al., 1983) most of the neurons labeled from the contralateral hippocampus in the present study were located in the hilus of the dentate area (Fig. 4A,B) or the pyramidal layer of subfield CA3c (Fig. 4C). In CA3c most of the retrogradely labeled neurons injected with LY were classified as pyramidal cells. However, as well as inverted fusiform cells at the lucidum/pyramidal border, some multipolar neurons (Fig. 4C), resembling Amaral's "giant aspiny stellate cells" (1978) were observed.

Approximately one-half of the contralaterally projecting hilar neurons possessed densely spined dendrites. Some of them may correspond to Amaral's class of "unaligned pyramidal cells," whereas others, located in the tip of the hilus, were identified as "mossy cells" (Fig. 4B). The remainder of injected hilar cells, usually close to the granular cell layer, was classified as sparsely spinous. In addition to "stellate cells of the dentate/hilar border" (Amaral, 1978) and multipolar cells, some fusiform cells (Fig. 4A) with bipolarly arranged dendritic tufts were identified.

Stereotaxic injections involving the ipsilateral septal nuclei led predominantly to retrograde labeling of neurons in Ammon's horn and, to a lesser extent, in the hilus. In the latter region "stellate cells at the dentate/hilus border" (Amaral, 1978) and "aspiny stellate cells" (Fig. 4G) were injected. In subfields CA1 and CA3 of Ammon's horn, pyramidal basket cells (Fig. 4D) constituted the most frequent nonpyramidal cell type. Some of their axonal collaterals

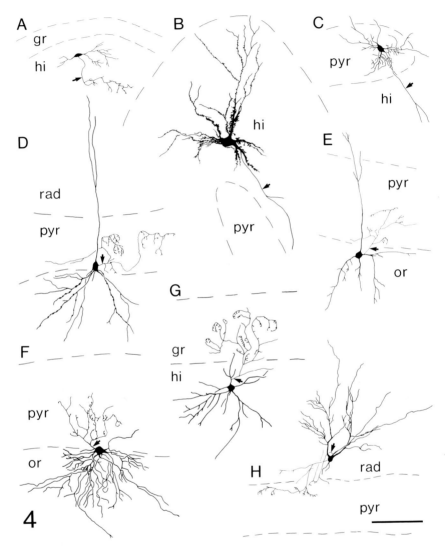

Fig. 4. Graphic reconstructions of LY-filled nonpyramidal hippocampal neurons that projected to either contralateral hippocampus (A–C) or ipsilateral septal nuclei (D–H). **A:** Fusiform cell in the hilus (hi) of the area dentata. **B:** Mossy cell in dentate hilus. **C:** Giant aspiny stellate cell in the pyramidal layer (pyr) of subfield CA3c. **D:** Pyramidal basket cell. **E:** Polygonal basket cell in stratum oriens (or). **F:** Horizontal basket cell. **G:** Aspiny stellate cell in the dentate hilus. **H:** Stellate stratum radiatum (rad) cell in Ammon's horn. gr, granule cell layer. Axons are indicated by arrows. Bar = 100 μm.

established a basket-like plexus around adjacent pyramidal cell bodies. The somata of polygonal (Fig. 4E) and horizontal basket cells (Fig. 4F) were located in the stratum oriens of CA1 and CA3. Axon collaterals of both cell types ramified within the pyramidal layer. Further nonpyramidal cells were filled in the stratum radiatum of CA1. Among them was a stellate cell (Fig. 4H), which had a local axon plexus in the pyramidal layer.

DISCUSSION
Neurons Constituting the Perforant Path: Comparative Aspects

In agreement with published data (Hjorth-Simonsen and Jeune, 1972; Steward and Scoville, 1976; Schwartz and Coleman, 1981) the present results indicate that the perforant path originates predominantly from layers II and III of the entorhinal cortex. Stereotaxic injections of FB into the septal hippocampus labeled neurons confined to the lateral entorhinal cortex. The finding confirms the reported lateromedial to septotemporal topography of the perforant path (Hjorth-Simonsen and Jeune, 1972).

Recently the retrograde transport of horseradish peroxidase was employed to determine the neuronal composition of the entorhinohippocampal projection (Schwartz and Coleman, 1981). Although dendritic labeling appeared incomplete, morphological similarities to LY-filled entorhinal neurons can be readily discerned. Structural correlates of injected entorhinal cells were also identified in published Golgi material (Lorente de Nó, 1933). Interestingly, in the latter study various impregnated neurons were assessed as having a "short axis cylinder," i.e. presumed to be local-circuit neurons. Data presented above, however, indicate that a number of them, e.g. layer III sparsely spinous multipolar cells, project to the ipsilateral hippocampus.

Neurons Constituting the Perforant Path: Functional Implications

The present study provided further evidence that the perforant path originates to a large extent from entorhinal layer II spiny stellate cells (Steward and Scoville, 1976). Their dendritic architecture should be considered a crucial determinant for the direct "availability" of laminar specific input to the entorhinal cortex. Since the majority of the relay cell's dendrites were confined to layers I–III, they are less likely to be directly contacted by terminations in deeper laminae. Indeed, the ipsilateral projection from the subiculum and region CA1 terminates predominantly in the deeper entorhinal layers (Hjorth-Simonsen, 1971), whereas afferents to the upper entorhinal layers arise from a multitude of sources, as diverse as olfactory bulb, olfactory cortex, amygdala, septum, basal forebrain, thalamus, and brain stem (for review, see Swanson et al., 1987).

Recently, synapses of olfactory (mitral cell) axons with dendrites of layers II and III neurons of the entorhinal cortex have been demonstrated (Wouterlood and Nederlof, 1983). In addition, our preliminary findings (Schwerdtfeger et al., 1988) suggest that olfactory input is monosynaptically relayed to the hippocampus. However, a number of olfactory axons also contact local-circuit neurons containing the inhibitory neurotransmitter γ-aminobutyric acid

(GABA), thus providing a model for feed-forward inhibition of entorhinal relay cells (Wouterlood et al., 1985). Indeed, GABAergic axon terminals are most densely distributed in layer II, where they establish symmetric axodendritic and axosomatic contacts with GABA-negative neurons (Köhler et al., 1985). In conjunction with the latter findings, our demonstration of similar, symmetrical synapses on injected *relay cells* (Fig. 3) provides further evidence for GABA-ergic inhibition of neurons constituting the perforant path.

The Concept of Hippocampal Local-Circuit and Projection Neurons

Prior to the introduction of sensitive tracing techniques long-range projections of nonpyramidal neurons were largely unknown, leading to the classical subdivision into projection and local-circuit neurons. This concept is, however, challenged by findings indicating that nonpyramidal neurons project to distant targets, such as the contralateral hippocampus (Seress and Ribak, 1983; Seroogy et al., 1983), septum (Chronister and DeFrance, 1979; Alonso and Köhler, 1982), and nucleus accumbens (Totterdell and Hayes, 1987). Recently, the morphology of hippocampal projection neurons was revealed with a combination of retrograde tracing and intracellular injection, enabling the identification of various nonpyramidal cell types previously classified as interneurons (Schwerdtfeger and Buhl, 1986) (see Fig. 4). However, the *dual* nature of these neurons is revealed by the simultaneous presence of a local axon collateral system with putative contacts on adjacent somata. Indeed, double-labeling studies employing two fluorescent tracers already indicated that both commissural and associational fibers may originate from an individual neuron in either the dentate area or Ammon's horn (Swanson et al., 1981).

The morphological properties of injected hippocampofugal nonpyramidal cells indicate their GABAergic nature, and the presence of GABA was demonstrated in hippocampal neurons with commissural or septal projections (Seress and Ribak, 1983; Shinoda et al., 1987). Abundant physiological and anatomical evidence suggests that excitatory commissural and septal afferents may terminate on hippocampal interneurons, thus providing a basis for feed-forward inhibition (Buzsáki, 1984; Frotscher et al., 1984; Seress and Ribak, 1984; Schwerdtfeger, 1986). However, the existence of GABAergic long-range projection neurons (Seress and Ribak, 1983; Shinoda et al., 1987) suggests that this may not be the sole mechanism for relaying inhibition to intra- and extrahippocampal targets.

Intracellular Staining in Fixed Slices: New Vistas?

A novel approach has been taken to investigate hippocampal afferent and efferent neurons by successively combining retrograde tracing, intracellular staining, and EM. Using three different anatomical techniques in the same tissue rendered information about projection targets, dendritic morphology, ultrastructure, and synaptic input of individual neurons. In principle, tract tracing with either horesradish peroxidase or fluorescent markers combined with the Golgi technique (Freund and Somogyi, 1983; Catsicas et al., 1986) may provide similar results. However, for most studies the selective staining of individual, preselected neurons is preferable to the randomness of Golgi impregnations. In addition, the latter technique, when applied for EM purposes (Fairén et al., 1977), is technically rather difficult and requires considerably more steps than the relatively simple LY EM protocol.

For the future of hippocampal neuroanatomy it appears realistic to predict more sophisticated combinations of intracellular staining with other techniques, such as anterograde tracing, autoradiography, and immunocytochemistry. Hence more complicated experimental paradigms may provide new answers to old questions.

SUMMARY

Retrograde fluorescent tracing was combined with intracellular Lucifer yellow staining in fixed tissue to determine the neuronal composition of hippocampal afferent and efferent neurons. Simple photo-oxidation of injected neurons led to the intracellular formation of an electron-dense precipitate. Subsequently photoconverted neurons were analyzed ultrastructurally. The latter methodological approach was tested in two experimental paradigms.

Neurons in the upper layers of lateral entorhinal cortex were retrogradely labeled from the ipsilateral hippocampus. Intracellular injections predominantly revealed spiny neurons, such as spiny stellate and pyramidal cells. However, sparsely spinous horizontal and multipolar cells also contributed to the entorhinohippocampal projection. These findings provide evidence for an unrecognized complexity of the neuronal sources that constitute the perforant path.

In addition, a variety of hippocampal nonpyramidal cell types provide afferent input to the septum and contralateral hippocampus. However, a number of hippocampofugal neurons also had a local axon plexus, and their morphology corresponded to previously described types of interneurons. Therefore, hippocampal neurons may possess the properties of both local-circuit and projection neurons.

ACKNOWLEDGMENTS

We are indebted to Dr. L. Peichl, Prof. W. Singer, and Prof. H. Wässle for providing the facilities. We are grateful to W. Hofer, R. Krauss, and G.-S. Nam for valuable technical assistance. Sincere thanks are extended to Drs. J.F. Dann and C.M. Müller for critically commenting on the manuscript.

REFERENCES

Alonso, A., and C. Köhler (1982) Evidence for separate projections of hippocampal pyramidal and non-pyramidal neurons to different parts of the septum in the rat brain. Neurosci. Lett. *31:*209–214.

Amaral, D.G. (1978) A Golgi study of cell types in the hilar region of the hippocampus in the rat. J. Comp. Neurol. *182:*851–914.

Berger, T.W., S. Semple-Rowland, and J.L. Basset (1980) Hippocampal polymorph neurons are the cells of origin for ipsilateral association and commissural afferents to the dentate gyrus. Brain Res. *215:*329–336.

Bliss, T.V.P., and T. Lømo (1973) Long-lasting potentiation of synaptic transmission in the dentate area of the anaesthetized rabbit following stimulation of the perforant path. J. Physiol. (Lond.) *232*:331–356.

Buhl, E.H., and J. Lübke (1989) Intracellular Lucifer yellow injection in fixed brain slices combined with retrograde tracing, light and electron microscopy. Neuroscience *28:* 3–16.

Buhl, E.H., and L. Peichl (1986) Morphology of rabbit retinal ganglion cells projecting to the medial terminal nucleus of the accessory optic system. J. Comp. Neurol. *253:*163–174.

Buhl, E.H., and W. Schlote (1987) Intracellular Lucifer yellow staining and electron microscopy of neurones in slices of fixed epitumourous human cortical tissue. Acta Neuropathol. *75:*140–146.

Buzsáki, G. (1984) Feed-forward inhibition in the hippocampal formation. Prog. Neurobiol. *22:*131–153.

Catsicas, S., P.J. Berbel, and G.M. Innocenti (1986) A combination of Golgi impregnation and fluorescent retrograde labeling. J. Neurosci. Methods *18:*325–332.

Chronister, R.B., and J.F. DeFrance (1979) Organization of projection neurons of the hippocampus. Exp. Neurol. *66:*509–523.

Desmond, N.L., and W.B. Levy (1987) Anatomy of associative long-term synaptic modification. In P.W. Landfield and S.A. Deadwyler (eds): Long-Term Potentiation: From Biophysics to Behavior. New York: Alan R. Liss, pp. 265–305.

Fairén, A., A. Peters, and J. Saldanha (1977) A new procedure for examining Golgi impregnated neurons by light and electron microscopy. J. Neurocytol. *6:*311–337.

Freund, T.F., and P. Somogyi (1983) The section-Golgi impregnation procedure. 1. Description of the method and its combination with histochemistry after intracellular iontophoresis or retrograde transport of horseradish peroxidase. Neuroscience *9:*463–474.

Frotscher, M., C. Léránth, K. Lübbers, and W.H. Oertel (1984) Commissural afferents innervate glutamate decarboxylase immunoreactive non-pyramidal neurons in the guinea pig hippocampus. Neurosci. Lett. *46:*137–143.

Hjorth-Simonsen, A. (1971) Hippocampal efferents to the ipsilateral entorhinal area: An experimental study in the rat. J. Comp. Neurol. *142:*417–438.

Hjorth-Simonsen, A. (1972) Projection of the lateral part of the entorhinal area to the hippocampus and fascia dentata. J. Comp. Neurol. *146:*219–232.

Hjorth-Simonsen, A., and B. Jeune (1972) Origin and termination of the hippocampal perforant path in the rat studied by silver impregnation. J. Comp. Neurol. *144:*215–232.

Köhler, C., J.-Y. Wu, and V. Chan-Palay (1985) Neurons and terminals in the retrohippocampal region in the rat's brain identified by anti-γ-aminobutyric acid and anti-glutamic acid decarboxylase immunocytochemistry. Anat. Embryol. *173:*35–44.

Lorente de Nó, R. (1933) Studies on the structure of the cerebral cortex. I. The area entorhinalis. J. Psychol. Neurol. *45:*381–438.

Maranto, A.R. (1982) Neuronal mapping: A photooxidation reaction makes Lucifer yellow useful for electron microscopy. Science *217:*953–955.

Matthews, D.A., C. Cotman, and G. Lynch (1976) An electron microscopic study of lesion-induced synaptogenesis in the dentate gyrus of the adult rat. I. Magnitude and time course of degeneration. Brain Res. *115:*1–21.

Paxinos, G., and C. Watson (1982) The Rat Brain in Stereotaxic Coordinates. London: Academic Press.

Schwartz, S.P., and P.D. Coleman (1981) Neurons of origin of the perforant path. Exp. Neurol. *74:*305–312.

Schwerdtfeger, W.K. (1986) Afferent fibers from the septum terminate on gamma-aminobutyric acid (GABA-) interneurons and granule cells in the area dentata of the rat. Experientia *42*:392–394.

Schwerdtfeger, W.K., and E. Buhl (1986) Various types of non-pyramidal hippocampal neurons project to the septum and contralateral hippocampus. Brain Res. *386*:146–154.

Schwerdtfeger, W.K., E.H. Buhl, and P. Germroth (1988) Fine structure of identified entorhinal cortical neurons projecting to the hippocampus. A study combining retrograde tracing, intracellular injection and electron microscopy. In N. Elsner and F.G. Barth (eds): Sense Organs—Interfaces Between Environment and Behaviour. Stuttgart: Thieme, p. 332.

Seress, L., and C.E. Ribak (1983) GABAergic cells in the dentate gyrus appear to be local circuit and projection neurons. Exp. Brain Res. *50*:173–182.

Seress, L., and C.E. Ribak (1984) Direct commissural connections to the basket cells of the hippocampal dentate gyrus: Anatomical evidence for feed-forward inhibition. J. Neurocytol. *13*:215–225.

Seroogy, K.B., L. Seress, and C.E. Ribak (1983) Ultrastructure of commissural neurons of the hilar region in the hippocampal dentate gyrus. Exp. Neurol. *82*:594–608.

Shinoda, K., M. Tohyama, and Y. Shiotani (1987) Hippocampofugal γ-aminobutyric acid (GABA)-containing neuron system in the rat: A study using a double-labeling method that combines retrograde tracing and immunocytochemistry. Brain Res. *409*:181–186.

Steward, O., and S.A. Scoville (1976) Cells of origin of entorhinal cortical afferents to the hippocampus and fascia dentata of the rat. J. Comp. Neurol. *169*:347–370.

Swanson, L.W., C. Köhler, and A. Björklund (1987) The limbic region. I: The septohippocampal system. In A. Björklund, T. Hökfelt, and L.W. Swanson (eds): Handbook of Chemical Neuroanatomy, Vol. 5. Amsterdam: Elsevier, pp. 125–277.

Swanson, L.W., P.E. Sawchenko, and M.W. Cowan (1981) Evidence for collateral projections by neurons in Ammon's horn, the dentate gyrus, and the subiculum: A multiple retrograde labeling study in the rat. J. Neurosci. *1*:548–559.

Tauchi, M., and R.H. Masland (1984) The shape and arrangement of the cholinergic neurons in the rabbit retina. Proc. R. Soc. Lond. (Biol.) *223*:101–119.

Totterdell, S., and L. Hayes (1987) Non-pyramidal projection neurons: A light and electron microscopic study. J. Neurocytol. *16*:477–485.

Wouterlood, F.G., E. Mugnaini, and J. Nederlof (1985) Projection of olfactory bulb efferents to layer I GABAergic neurons in the entorhinal area. Combination of anterograde degeneration and immunoelectron microscopy in rat. Brain Res. *343*:283–296.

Wouterlood, F.G., and J. Nederlof (1983) Terminations of olfactory afferents on layer II and III neurons in the entorhinal area: Degeneration-Golgi-electron microscopic study in the rat. Neurosci. Lett. *36*:105–110.

The Hippocampus—New Vistas, pages 85–96
© 1989 Alan R. Liss, Inc.

6

Cholinergic Innervation of Identified Neurons in the Hippocampus: Electron Microscopic Double Labeling Studies

MICHAEL FROTSCHER, ROBERT NITSCH, AND CSABA LERÁNTH

Institute of Anatomy, Johann Wolfgang Goethe University, Frankfurt am Main, Federal Republic of Germany (M.F., R.N.); Section of Neuroanatomy, Yale University School of Medicine, New Haven, Connecticut (C.L.)

INTRODUCTION

A description of the cholinergic innervation of the hippocampus comprises two sets of neurons, i.e. the cells of origin of the cholinergic terminals and the various types of target cells in the hippocampal formation. It is well documented that large neurons in the medial septum–diagonal band complex (MSDB) give rise to a cholinergic projection to hippocampal and dentate neurons (e.g. Lewis and Shute, 1967; Lewis et al., 1967; Baisden et al., 1984; Woolf et al., 1984; Amaral and Kurz, 1985). Using antibodies against choline acetyltransferase (ChAT), the acetylcholine-synthesizing enzyme, and immunocytochemical techniques, Houser et al. (1983) were the first to describe an additional population of cholinergic neurons, small nonpyramidal cells in the hippocampus and fascia dentata (see also Levey et al., 1984; Frotscher et al., 1986; Matthews et al., 1987), as a possible source of hippocampal cholinergic innervation. However, recent studies did not provide evidence that these neurons contribute much to the cholinergic innervation of the hippocampus. One month after unilateral complete transection of the fimbria-fornix, which disconnects the hippocampus from its cholinergic septal input, an almost complete lack of cholinergic terminals persists in the hippocampus and fascia dentata ipsilateral to the lesion (Frotscher, 1988). The ChAT-immunoreactive hippocampal neurons, however, were not affected and were found as usual in all hippocampal layers. This clearly indicates that medial septal neurons but not ChAT-positive cells in the hippocampus play a major role in hippocampal cholinergic innervation. Moreover, it also demonstrates that ChAT-immunoreactive hippocampal neurons are not capable of compensating for the loss of septal cholinergic afferents by sprouting.

A light microscopic analysis of ChAT-immunostained sections of hippo-campus and fascia dentata suggests that the principal cells, pyramidal neurons and granule cells, receive a dense cholinergic innervation. The septohippo-campal cholinergic fibers form a pericellular plexus around their cell bodies. In fact, electron microscopic analysis revealed symmetric synaptic contacts on the cell bodies of both types of neuron (Clarke, 1985; Frotscher and Leránth, 1985, 1986). Moreover, in these cases identification of the target cells was rel-atively easy, because perikarya of both pyramidal and granule cells exhibit some fine structural characteristics that differ from those of nonpyramidal neurons (Ribak and Anderson, 1980; Ribak and Seress, 1983; Schlander and Frotscher, 1986).

Fine varicose ChAT-immunoreactive fibers as observed in the vicinity of the cell layers were also found in other layers, i.e. in stratum oriens and stratum radiatum of the hippocampus proper and in the molecular layer of the fascia dentata. Here, they formed contacts on dendritic shafts and spines. Identifi-cation of the type of target neuron was again easy in the case of contacts on spines, because spines are numerous on pyramidal and granule cell dendrites but are absent on dendrites of nonpyramidal cells, at least in the rodent hip-pocampus (Schlander and Frotscher, 1986). As a rule, identification of target neurons was not possible in the case of synaptic contacts of cholinergic ter-minals on dendritic shafts. Here the target cells could include pyramidal cells as well as GABAergic or peptidergic nonpyramidal neurons, and identification would require double labeling procedures.

In the present study we analyzed identified pyramidal neurons and GABAergic nonpyramidal cells in the hippocampus proper for synaptic contacts with cholinergic terminals. The cholinergic terminals were labeled by immu-nocytochemistry using a monoclonal antibody against ChAT and the peroxidase-antiperoxidase (PAP) technique. Immunostaining with an antibody against glu-tamate decarboxylase (GAD), the GABA-synthesizing enzyme, and ferritin as a second electron-dense marker allowed us to identify GABAergic elements. A combination of ChAT immunocytochemistry and Golgi impregnation (gold-toning; cf. Fairén et al., 1977) was used to study the cholinergic innervation of identified pyramidal neurons. In this sense, the present study is a continuation of our previous work on the fascia dentata, which has demonstrated a cho-linergic innervation of Golgi-impregnated granule cells (Frotscher and Leránth, 1986) and GABAergic and peptidergic neurons in the hilar region (Leránth and Frotscher, 1987).

MATERIALS AND METHODS
Tissue Fixation

Adult male Sprague Dawley rats (200–250 gm body weight) kept under stan-dard laboratory conditions were used for the present study. Under ether anes-thesia the animals were transcardially perfused with 70 ml of oxygenated iso-tonic saline followed by a solution of 4% paraformaldehyde, 0.08%

glutaraldehyde, and 15% saturated picric acid in 0.1 M phosphate buffer (Somogyi and Takagi, 1982). The brains were removed from the skull, and the hippocampi were dissected out and divided perpendicular to the longitudinal (septotemporal) axis into about 3-mm-thick tissue blocks from the septal (dorsal), middle, and temporal (ventral) regions. These blocks were stored for 3 h in a glutaraldehyde-free fixative solution. Then Vibratome sections (40 μm) perpendicular to the longitudinal axis of the hippocampus were cut and washed in several changes of phosphate buffer prior to immunostaining.

Immunostaining for ChAT

Sections to be double immunostained for ChAT and GAD were briefly incubated in 10% sucrose and rapidly frozen in liquid nitrogen (Frotscher and Leránth, 1985) to allow for a better penetration of antibodies. Immunostaining for ChAT was performed with a monoclonal antibody from rat-mouse hybridoma (type I, Boehringer Mannheim GmbH, Mannheim, FRG) (see Eckenstein and Thoenen, 1982) as described in more detail elsewhere (Frotscher and Leránth, 1985, 1986). Incubation times and dilutions were as follows: anti-ChAT (diluted 1:9) for 48 h at 4°C; rabbit antirat IgG (1:40) for 1.5 h at 20°C; rat PAP complex (1:40) for 2 h at 20°C. The sections were washed between each incubation step in several changes of phosphate buffer. The tissue-bound peroxidase was finally visualized by incubating the sections with 3,3'-diaminobenzidine (DAB, 0.07%) and H_2O_2 in Tris buffer (0.1 M, pH 7.6) for 5–10 min. In parallel control experiments the sections were treated in the same way except that the primary antiserum was omitted.

Combined ChAT Immunocytochemistry and Golgi Impregnation

ChAT immunostaining was performed as described except that the sections were not frozen in liquid nitrogen because this was found to interfere with subsequent Golgi impregnation (Frotscher and Leránth, 1986). For Golgi impregnation of the immunostained Vibratome sections a modification of the section Golgi procedure (Freund and Somogyi, 1983) was applied, which has been described in detail elsewhere (Frotscher and Leránth, 1986; Frotscher and Zimmer, 1986). Briefly, the sections were placed onto pieces of Parafilm and kept moist with phosphate buffer. Then the sections, with intervening Parafilm, were piled on top of each other and were covered with agar to form a "tissue block" of rejoined sections that was Golgi impregnated. Thereafter, the sections were again separated by cutting away the covering agar and then examined in the light microscope. Sections containing well-impregnated pyramidal neurons were further processed according to the gold-toning procedure (Fairén et al., 1977), described in detail elsewhere (Frotscher et al., 1981). The sections were dehydrated (block stained with uranyl acetate in 70% ethanol) and embedded flat in Araldite between foils of aluminium and transparent plastic. After hardening, selected pyramidal neurons were photographed and drawn using a microscope drawing tube and re-embedded in plastic capsules for thin sectioning. During sectioning drawings of the remaining nonsectioned parts of the cells were repeatedly made on transparent paper to help in identifying single processes of the gold-toned cells in the electron microscope. The sections were stained with lead nitrate and studied in a Siemens Elmiskop 101.

Double Immunolabeling for ChAT and GAD

The double immunostaining procedure applied in the present experiments has been described in previous studies (e.g. Leránth and Frotscher, 1987). The principle of the method is to demonstrate the second antigen, i.e. GAD in the present experiments, with ferritin by using Ferritin-Avidin D (Vector Labs, Burlingame, CA 94010) and a biotinylated secondary antibody. Avidin is known to have a high affinity to biotin.

In the electron microscope, the ferritin grains are easily differentiated from the diffuse DAB reaction product, which was used to label ChAT immunoreactivity. Incubation times and dilutions were performed as follows. After immunostaining for ChAT, which was performed as described above, the Vibratome sections were incubated in sheep antiserum S3 against GAD (Oertel et al., 1982), diluted 1:2,000, for 48 h at 4°C. This was followed by incubation in biotinylated rabbit antigoat IgG (1:250) for 2 h at 20°C and in Ferritin-Avidin D (1:60) for 12 h at 4°C. After completion of the immunostainings, the Vibratome sections were rinsed in phosphate buffer, osmicated for 1 h in 1% osmium tetroxide, dehydrated (stained with 1% uranyl acetate in 70% ethanol), and flat-embedded as described above for the ChAT-immunostained and Golgi-impregnated sections. However, for better visualization of immunoreactive structures, we omitted staining the ultrathin sections with lead nitrate.

In control experiments the specificity of double immunostainings was tested by omission of one of the secondary antibodies. Only single immunolabeling was found under these experimental conditions.

RESULTS

The present study was aimed at identifying the postsynaptic elements of septohippocampal cholinergic terminals in the hippocampus of the rat. For a more general description of ChAT immunoreactivity in the hippocampus and fascia dentata as seen under the light microscope, the reader is referred to the works of Houser et al. (1983), Clarke (1985), Frotscher and Leránth (1985, 1986), Frotscher et al. (1986), and Matthews et al. (1987). It should be sufficient here to summarize these studies by mentioning that ChAT-immunoreactive fibers were observed in all layers of the hippocampus and fascia dentata, with a somewhat higher concentration in the vicinity of the cell layers. Occasionally small ChAT-immunoreactive cell bodies were found, mainly in stratum lacunosum-moleculare of CA1. In the present electron microscopic study we focused on the CA1 region of the hippocampus, and we studied Golgi-impregnated identified pyramidal neurons and GAD-immunoreactive, supposedly GABAergic nonpyramidal cells for synaptic contacts with cholinergic terminals.

Cholinergic Innervation of Identified Pyramidal Cells

Thin sections revealed numerous varicose unmyelinated ChAT-immuno-reactive fibers and vesicle-filled terminal boutons that formed synaptic contacts. The contacts on cell bodies and dendritic shafts were mainly symmetric, whereas asymmetric synaptic contacts occurred on dendritic spines. As mentioned, these latter contacts strongly suggest a cholinergic innervation of pyramidal cells, since nonpyramidal neurons in the rodent hippocampus lack dendritic spines. Figure 1a shows an asymmetric contact on a spine in the stratum radiatum of CA1.

Although the Vibratome sections were not frozen in these experiments, the penetration of the ChAT antibody was good enough to expect some immunoreactive terminals to be in the same plane of the section as the cell bodies and dendrites of Golgi-impregnated pyramidal cells. As can be seen in Figures 1b,c and 2, the gold-toned pyramidal cells were easily identified by the gold particles in the cytoplasm. However, often the gold grains were concentrated along the surface membrane, which made the identification of synaptic contacts difficult (Fig. 1b,c). Nevertheless, in some cases parts of the synaptic membrane specializations were visible, or electron-dense cleft material suggested a synaptic contact. We mainly looked for contacts on pyramidal cell dendritic shafts (Figs. 1c, 2b) because these contacts in particular require identification of the postsynaptic neuron (see above). Contacts on gold-toned spines and cell bodies (Fig. 2a) of identified pyramidal cells were similarly observed. We can conclude that septohippocampal cholinergic fibers terminate on spines, dendritic shafts, and cell bodies of pyramidal cells in the CA1 region.

Cholinergic Innervation of GABAergic Neurons

Immunolabeling with ferritin is not detectable under the light microscope. For a light microscopic control of the second immunolabeling (immunostaining for GAD), some sections were separated after the incubation in the biotinylated antigoat antibody, and instead of being incubated in avidinated ferritin, they were incubated in the Vectastain ABC complex, and the "second" tissue-bound peroxidase was detected using a DAB reaction. With this procedure, we observed the characteristic DAB immunostaining of cell bodies and proximal dendrites of GABAergic neurons and numerous terminal-like puncta surrounding immunonegative pyramidal cells (cf. Ribak et al., 1978).

Electron microscopy of sections labeled with ferritin for GAD and with DAB for ChAT similarly demonstrated ferritin grains in some cell bodies, thick proximal dendrites, and axon terminals, the latter forming symmetric synaptic contacts with immunonegative cell bodies in the pyramidal layer. A few DAB-labeled ChAT-positive terminals were observed that formed symmetric synaptic contacts with ferritin-labeled cell bodies (Fig. 3a) and dendritic shafts of GABAergic neurons (Fig. 3b,c). It should be mentioned that the number of cholinergic synapses on GABAergic neurons is certainly underestimated in the present experiments. Only proximal dendritic segments were labeled with fer-

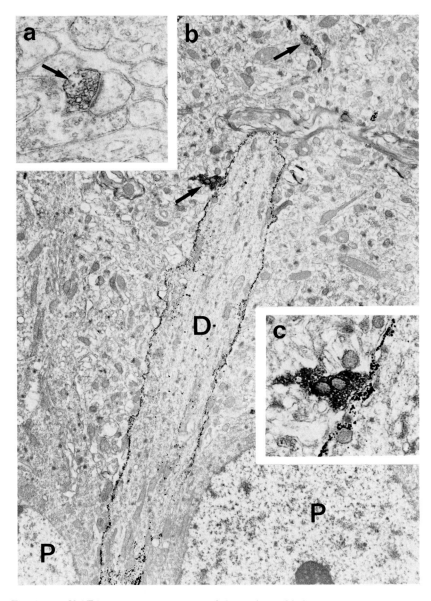

Fig. 1. **a:** ChAT-immunoreactive terminal (arrow) establishing asymmetric synaptic contact on a spine in the stratum radiatum of CA1. ×34,000.   **b:** Two ChAT-positive terminals (arrows), one of them impinging on the gold-toned apical dendrite (D) of an identified CA1 pyramidal cell. Dendrite running through the inner part of the stratum radiatum in CA1. Cell bodies of two pyramidal neurons (P) indicate outer border of pyramidal layer. ×5,700.   **c:** Higher magnification of the ChAT-immunoreactive bouton shown in b. Parts of the putative synaptic contact zone are masked by gold particles. ×18,000.

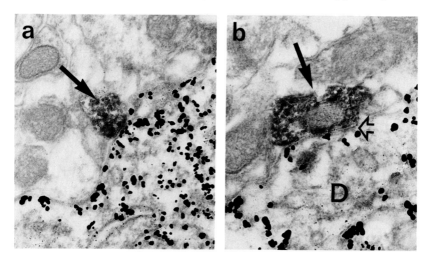

Fig. 2. **a:** ChAT-positive terminal (arrow) contacting the gold-toned cell body of an identified pyramidal cell in CA1. Electron-dense cleft material suggests a synaptic contact. **b:** ChAT-positive terminal (black arrow) in synaptic contact with proximal dendrite (D) of a gold-toned CA1 pyramidal cell. Open arrow indicates zone of synaptic contact. ×42,000.

ritin, but it is likely that peripheral dendrites of GABAergic cells also receive a cholinergic input. In fact, many ChAT-immunoreactive terminals formed synaptic contacts on thin (unlabeled) dendritic branches.

DISCUSSION

The results of the present study demonstrate that two major cell types in the CA1 region of the rat hippocampus, i.e. pyramidal neurons and GABAergic nonpyramidal cells, establish synaptic contacts with septohippocampal cholinergic afferents. One and the same ChAT-immunoreactive terminal may form a symmetric synaptic contact on the cell body of a GABAergic neuron and an asymmetric contact on an immunonegative spine, most likely arising from a pyramidal cell dendrite (Fig. 3a). This observation does not support previous speculations that the two different types of contact, i.e. symmetric and asymmetric ones, are formed by cholinergic fibers of different origin (cf. Frotscher and Leránth, 1986). Moreover, recent experiments with medial septal lesions or unilateral fimbria-fornix transections have provided strong evidence that the overwhelming majority of cholinergic fibers in the hippocampus and fascia dentata arise from neurons in the medial septum (Matthews et al., 1987; Frotscher, 1988) (see the Introduction). The question remains as to the role of intrahippocampal ChAT-positive neurons.

The present findings confirm and extend our previous studies on the fascia dentata, which have similarly shown that the main cell types there, granule

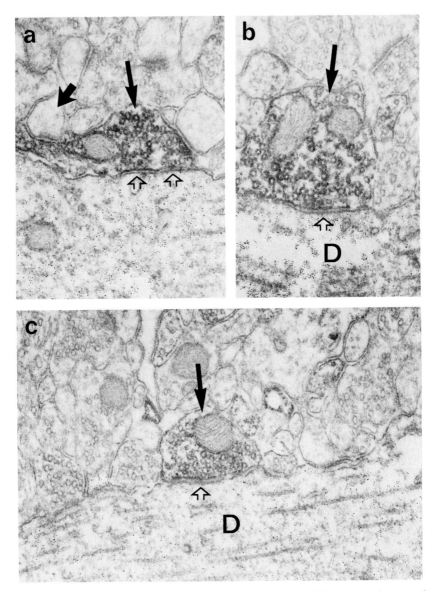

Fig. 3. **a:** ChAT-immunoreactive terminal (long black arrow) in symmetric synaptic contact (open arrows) with GAD-positive cell body labeled by small ferritin grains (stratum oriens of CA1). Note that the terminal also forms an asymmetric contact on a spine (short black arrow). ×42,000. **b,c:** ChAT-positive terminals (black arrows) establishing symmetric synaptic contacts (open arrows) on ferritin-labeled thick proximal dendrites (D) of GAD-immunoreactive neurons (stratum radiatum of CA1). ×42,000.

cells and GABAergic and peptidergic hilar neurons, receive a cholinergic innervation (Frotscher and Leránth, 1986; Leránth and Frotscher, 1987). Obviously the cholinergic afferents do not select between different types of target cells. This is consonant with previous studies on other fiber systems that were also found to terminate on both pyramidal neurons and nonpyramidal cells. Thus, commissural fibers from the contralateral hippocampus, labeled by anterograde degeneration caused by contralateral fimbria-fornix transection, established synaptic contacts with spines of identified (Golgi-impregnated) pyramidal neurons (Blackstad, 1970; Frotscher, 1983) and varicose dendritic shafts of GABAergic and peptidergic nonpyramidal cells (Frotscher and Zimmer, 1983; Leránth and Frotscher, 1983; Frotscher et al., 1984). The same holds true for a well-characterized ipsilateral fiber system, the mossy fiber projection from the fascia dentata. The giant mossy fiber boutons form synaptic contacts on large spines (excrescences) of pyramidal neurons in CA3 but also on smooth dendrites of basket cells (Frotscher, 1985). GABAergic basket cells in turn do not only form the characteristic basket plexus around the cell bodies of pyramidal neurons and granule cells but also contact GABAergic neurons in the hippocampus proper and fascia dentata (Frotscher et al., 1984; Misgeld and Frotscher, 1986). Recent double immunolabeling experiments with antibodies against tyrosine hydroxylase and GAD provided evidence that catecholaminergic brain stem afferents are no exception: Tyrosine hydroxylase-immunoreactive terminals were found to establish asymmetric synaptic contacts on spines of pyramidal cells and symmetric contacts on dendritic shafts and cell bodies of GABAergic neurons (Frotscher and Leránth, 1988). The manifold connections of GABAergic cells with extrinsic and intrinsic fibers suggest that these inhibitory neurons are involved in feed-forward inhibition, recurrent inhibition, and disinhibition of pyramidal neurons and granule cells. GABAergic synapses on GABAergic neurons in particular indicate inhibition of inhibitory neurons resulting in a disinhibitory effect on pyramidal cells.

The physiological effect of acetylcholine on pyramidal neurons and granule cells is a slow depolarization of these neurons associated with an enhancement of their excitability (e.g. Dodd et al., 1981; Benardo and Prince, 1982; Cole and Nicoll, 1984; Müller and Misgeld, 1986). The action of acetylcholine on GABAergic nonpyramidal cells is controversial, but it is now possible to record intracellularly from nonpyramidal cells in the hippocampus and fascia dentata and to identify these cells by intracellular staining (Schwartzkroin and Mathers, 1978; Schwartzkroin and Kunkel, 1985; Misgeld and Frotscher, 1986). One can envisage studies on the physiological effects of acetylcholine on identified (intracellularly recorded and intracellularly stained) nonpyramidal neurons in the near future.

ACKNOWLEDGMENTS

The authors thank Dr. W.H. Oertel for providing the GAD antiserum and E. Thielen for excellent technical assistance. This study was supported by the Deutsche Forschungsgemeinschaft (Fr 620/1-3 and SFB 45).

REFERENCES

Amaral, D.G., and J. Kurz (1985) An analysis of the origins of the cholinergic and non-cholinergic septal projections of the hippocampal formation of the rat. J. Comp. Neurol. *240*:37–59.

Baisden, R.H., M.L. Woodruff, and D.B. Hoover (1984) Cholinergic and noncholinergic septo-hippocampal projections: A double-label horseradish peroxidase-acetylcholinesterase study in the rabbit. Brain Res. *290*:146–151.

Benardo, L.S., and D.A. Prince (1982) Cholinergic excitation of mammalian hippocampal pyramidal cells. Brain Res. *249*:315–331.

Blackstad, T.W. (1970) Electron microscopy of Golgi preparations for the study of neuronal relations. In W.J.H. Nauta and S.O.E. Ebbesson (eds): Contemporary Research Methods in Neuroanatomy. New York: Springer Verlag, pp. 186–216.

Clarke, D.J. (1985) Cholinergic innervation of the rat dentate gyrus: An immunocytochemical and electron microscopical study. Brain Res. *360*:349–354.

Cole, A.E., and R.A. Nicoll (1984) The pharmacology of cholinergic excitatory responses in the hippocampal pyramidal cells. Brain Res. *305*:283–290.

Dodd, J., R. Dingeldine, and J.S. Kelly (1981) The excitatory action of acetylcholine on hippocampal neurons of the guinea-pig and rat maintained in vitro. Brain Res. *207*:109–127.

Eckenstein, F., and H. Thoenen (1982) Production of specific antisera and monoclonal antibodies to choline-acetyltransferase: Characterization and use for identification of cholinergic neurons. EMBO J. *1*:363–368.

Fairén, A., A. Peters, and J. Saldanha (1977) A new procedure for examining Golgi impregnated neurons by light and electron microscopy. J. Neurocytol. *6*:311–337.

Freund, T., and P. Somogyi (1983) The section-Golgi impregnation procedure. I. Description of the method and its combination with histochemistry after intracellular iontophoresis or retrograde transport of horseradish peroxidase. Neuroscience *9*:463–474.

Frotscher, M. (1983) Dendritic plasticity in response to partial deafferentation. In W. Seifert (ed): Neurobiology of the Hippocampus. New York: Academic Press, pp. 65–80.

Frotscher, M. (1985) Mossy fibres form synapses with identified pyramidal basket cells in the CA3 region of the guinea pig hippocampus: A combined Golgi-electron microscope study. J. Neurocytol. *14*:245–259.

Frotscher, M. (1988) Cholinergic neurons in the rat hippocampus do not compensate for the loss of septohippocampal cholinergic fibers. Neurosci. Lett. *87:* 18–22.

Frotscher, M., and C. Leránth (1985) Cholinergic innervation of the rat hippocampus as revealed by choline acetyltransferase immunocytochemistry: A combined light and electron microscopic study. J. Comp. Neurol. *239*:237–246.

Frotscher, M., and C. Leránth (1986) The cholinergic innervation of the rat fascia dentata: Identification of target structures on granule cells by combining choline acetyltransferase immunocytochemistry and Golgi impregnation. J. Comp. Neurol. *243*:58–70.

Frotscher, M., and C. Leránth (1988) Catecholaminergic innervation of pyramidal and GABAergic nonpyramidal neurons in the rat hippocampus. Double label immunostaining with antibodies against tyrosine hydroxylase and glutamate decarboxylase. Histochemistry *88*:313–319.

Frotscher, M., C. Leránth, K. Lübbers, and W.H. Oertel (1984) Commissural afferents innervate glutamate decarboxylase immunoreactive non-pyramidal neurons in the guinea pig hippocampus. Neurosci. Lett. *46*:137–143.

Frotscher, M., U. Rinne, R. Hassler, and A. Wagner (1981) Termination of cortical afferents on identified neurons in the caudate nucleus of the cat: A combined Golgi/EM degeneration study. Exp. Brain Res. *41*:329–337.

Frotscher, M., M. Schlander, and C. Leranth (1986) Cholinergic neurons in the hippocampus: A combined light and electron microscopic immunocytochemical study in the rat. Cell Tissue Res. *246*:293–301.

Frotscher, M., and J. Zimmer (1983) Commissural fibers terminate on nonpyramidal neurons in the guinea pig hippocampus—a combined Golgi/EM degeneration study. Brain Res. *265*:289–293.

Frotscher, M., and J. Zimmer (1986) Intracerebral transplants of the rat fascia dentata: A Golgi/electron microscope study of dentate granule cells. J. Comp. Neurol. *246*:181–190.

Houser, C.R., G.D. Crawford, R.P. Barber, P.M. Salvaterra, J.E. Vaughn, (1983) Organization and morphological characteristics of cholinergic neurons: An immunocytochemical study with a monoclonal antibody to choline acetyltransferase. Brain Res. *266*:97–119.

Leránth, C., and M. Frotscher (1983) Commissural afferents to the rat hippocampus terminate on vasoactive intestinal polypeptide-like immunoreactive non-pyramidal neurons. Brain Res. *276*:357–361.

Leránth, C., and M. Frotscher (1987) Cholinergic innervation of hippocampal GAD- and somatostatin-immunoreactive commissural neurons. J. Comp. Neurol. *261*:33–47.

Levey, A.I., B.H. Wainer, D.B. Rye, E.J. Mufson, and M.M. Mesulam (1984) Choline-acetyltransferase-immunoreactive neurons intrinsic to rodent cortex and distinction from acetylcholinesterase-positive neurons. Neuroscience *13*:341–353.

Lewis, P.R., and C.C.D. Shute (1967) The cholinergic limbic system: Projections to hippocampal formation, medial cortex, nuclei of the ascending cholinergic reticular system and the subfornical organ and supra-optic crest. Brain *90*:521–537.

Lewis, P.R., C.C.D. Shute, and A. Silver (1967) Confirmation from choline acetylase analyses of a massive cholinergic innervation to the rat hippocampus. J. Physiol. *191*:215–224.

Matthews, D.A., P.M. Salvaterra, G.D. Crawford, C.R. Houser, and J.E. Vaughn (1987) An immunocytochemical study of choline-acetyltransferase-containing neurons and axon terminals in normal and partially deafferented hippocampal formation. Brain Res. *402*:30–43.

Misgeld, U., and M. Frotscher (1986) Postsynaptic GABAergic inhibition of non-pyramidal neurons in the guinea-pig hippocampus. Neuroscience *19*:193–206.

Müller, W., and U. Misgeld (1986) Slow cholinergic excitation of guinea pig hippocampal neurons is mediated by two muscarinic receptor subtypes. Neurosci. Lett. *67*:107–112.

Oertel, W.H., D.E. Schmechel, E. Mugnaini, M.L. Tappaz, and I.J. Kopin (1982) Immunocytochemical localization of glutamate decarboxylase in the rat cerebellum with a new antiserum. Neuroscience *6*:2715–2735.

Ribak, C.E., and C.L. Anderson (1980) Ultrastructure of the pyramidal basket cells in the dentate gyrus of the rat. J. Comp. Neurol. *192*:903–916.

Ribak, C.E., and L. Seress (1983) Five types of basket cell in the hippocampal dentate gyrus: A combined Golgi and electron microscopic study. J. Neurocytol. *12*:577–597.

Ribak, C.E., J.E. Vaughn, and K Saito (1978) Immunocytochemical localization of glutamic acid decarboxylase in neuronal somata following colchicine inhibition of axonal transport. Brain Res. *140*:315–332.

Schlander, M., and M. Frotscher (1986) Non-pyramidal neurons in the guinea pig hippocampus. A combined Golgi-electron microscope study. Anat. Embryol. *174*:35–47.

Schwartzkroin, P.A., and D.D. Kunkel (1985) Morphology of identified interneurons in the CA1 regions of guinea-pig hippocampus. J. Comp. Neurol. *232*:205–218.

Schwartzkroin, P.A., and L.H. Mathers (1978) Physiological and morphological identification of a nonpyramidal hippocampal cell type. Brain Res. *157*:1–10.

Somogyi, P., and H. Takagi (1982) A note on the use of picric acid-paraformaldehyde-glutaraldehyde fixative for correlated light and electron microscopic immunocytochemistry. Neuroscience *7*:1779–1784.

Woolf, N.J., F. Eckenstein, and L.L. Butcher (1984) Cholinergic systems in the rat brain: I. Projection to the limbic telencephalon. Brain Res. Bull. *13*:751–784.

The Hippocampus—New Vistas, pages 97–117
© 1989 Alan R. Liss, Inc.

7
Excitatory and Inhibitory Amino Acids in the Hippocampus

O.P. OTTERSEN AND J. STORM-MATHISEN
Anatomical Institute, University of Oslo, Oslo, Norway

INTRODUCTION

The hippocampus is a widely used model system for exploring the cellular mechanisms underlying important neurobiological phenomena such as long-term potentiation, epilepsy, and seizure-related and ischemic cell damage (see e.g. symposium proceedings by Schwarcz and Ben-Ari [1986] and review by Mayer and Westbrook [1987]). The neuroactive amino acids, most notably glutamate, aspartate, and γ-aminobutyric acid (GABA), are thought to be critically involved in all of these phenomena, and it must therefore be considered a task of major importance to identify the hippocampal fiber systems that use these amino acids as neurotransmitters. The aim of the present review is to show how far this work has come, with emphasis on recent neurochemical and immunocytochemical data. The older literature has been discussed previously (Storm-Mathisen, 1977a; Cotman and Nadler, 1981; Storm-Mathisen and Ottersen, 1984; Walaas, 1984).

EXCITATORY AMINO ACIDS
Release and Uptake Studies

Figure 1 shows the main excitatory pathways in the hippocampal formation. The major excitatory input is by way of the perforant path fibers, which originate in the entorhinal cortex and terminate in the outer two-thirds of the dentate molecular layer in synaptic contact with dendrites of granule cells. The latter cells give rise to mossy fibres, which interact synaptically with CA3 pyramidal cell dendrites in the stratum lucidum. The third link in the polysynaptic excitatory pathway through the hippocampus is provided by CA3 pyramidal cell axons (Schaffer collaterals) terminating on the dendrites of CA1 pyramidal cells, whose axons in turn project to the subiculum and entorhinal cortex. CA3 pyramidal cells emit additional excitatory collaterals to the lateral septum and to the contralateral hippocampus and intrinsic collaterals that run longitudinally to more septal or temporal parts of CA3. A further (mixed) com-

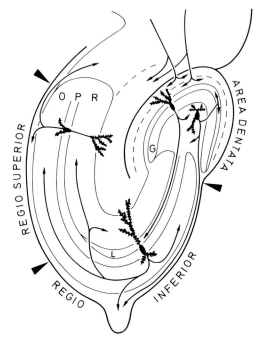

Abbreviations in figures

DLEA	dorsal subdivision of the lateral entorhinal cortex
E	endothelial cell
F	second reflected blade
G	stratum granulosum
IP	inner plexiform layer of the guinea pig hilus
L	stratum lucidum
LM	stratum lacunosum-moleculare
LU	stratum lucidum
M	dentate molecular layer
Mi	inner zone of the dentate molecular layer
Mo	outer zone of the dentate molecular layer
O	stratum oriens
OP	outer plexiform layer of the guinea pig hilus
P	stratum pyramidale
R	stratum radiatum
SUB	subiculum
T	mossy fiber terminal
V	vessel lumen
VLEA	ventral subdivision of the lateral entorhinal cortex

Fig. 1. Putative glutamate or aspartate connections of the hippocampal formation (see text for explanation). (Reproduced from Storm-Mathisen and Ottersen, 1988, with permission of the publisher.)

missural and ipsilateral system, formed by hilar cell projections to the inner one-third of the contralateral and ipsilateral dentate molecular layer, is also excitatory in nature (although a minor subpopulation of the fibers may be inhibitory; see below). As will be discussed, there is today substantial evidence that glutamate and/or aspartate are transmitters in all of the excitatory pathways described above.

Among the first experiments to implicate glutamate and aspartate as transmitters in hippocampal excitatory projections were those of Nadler et al. (1976, 1978), who recorded a decrease in calcium-dependent, potassium-stimulated efflux of endogenous excitatory amino acids in superfused hippocampal slices after removal of the entorhinal cortex or contralateral hippocampus. The entorhinal lesion selectively depressed glutamate release in the dentate gyrus, whereas the commissurotomy was followed by a decreased release of aspartate as well as glutamate in regio superior and a selective decrease in aspartate release in the dentate gyrus. Evidence has also been obtained concerning excitatory amino acid release from the CA3 pyramidal cell projections to the ipsilateral CA1, contralateral hippocampus, and lateral septum after electrical stimulation of the respective pathways in vitro (Malthe-Sørenssen et al., 1979, 1980; Skrede and Malthe-Sørenssen, 1981; Spencer et al., 1981).

Terminals that are thought to release glutamate or aspartate as transmitter are endowed with high-affinity uptake pumps that accept either of these amino acids (Davies and Johnston, 1976). Autoradiographic studies have revealed uptake of radiolabeled glutamate or aspartate in the termination areas of all of the excitatory pathways depicted in Figure 1 (Fig. 2A) (Taxt and Storm-Mathisen, 1984), although the intensity of labeling varies among the different pathways. This is particularly evident in the dentate molecular layer, where the uptake is much lower in the intermediate and outer zones than in the inner zone (Fig. 2A). It remains to be resolved whether this pattern reflects differences in the density of the excitatory terminals or different uptake capacities in the individual terminals.

Electron microscopic studies have confirmed that the major fraction of the accumulated label resides in nerve terminals (Storm-Mathisen and Iversen, 1979). In agreement, interruptions of the perforant path, the dentate commissural/ipsilateral projection, or the bilateral CA3 projections to the hippocampus or lateral septum lead to a substantial decrease in autoradiographically recorded D-[^{3}H]aspartate uptake in the respective termination areas (Taxt and Storm-Mathisen, 1984). All of these pathways plus the mossy fiber system have also been shown to take up and axonally transport D-[^{3}H]aspartate in vivo (Fig. 3; Storm-Mathisen, 1982; Fischer et al., 1986, 1989). The autoradiographic data are fully consistent with the biochemical analyses of changes in D-[^{3}H]aspartate and L-[^{3}H]glutamate uptake after lesions (Nadler et al., 1976, 1978; Storm-Mathisen, 1977b, 1982; Fonnum and Walaas, 1978; Storm-Mathisen and Woxen Opsahl, 1978; Taxt and Storm-Mathisen, 1984). Studies based on uptake also implicate glutamate or aspartate as transmitters in projections from CA1 and subiculum to the amygdala (Ottersen et al., 1986) and from subiculum to nucleus accumbens, nucleus interstitialis striae terminalis, corpus mammillare, and

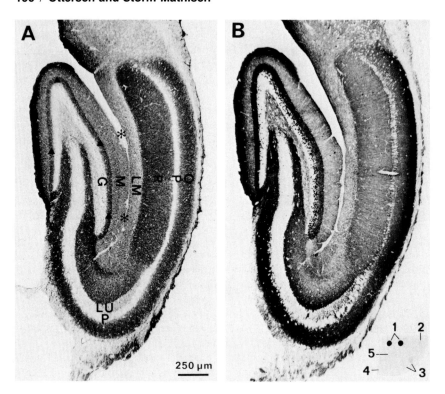

Fig. 2. Autoradiographic localization of D-[³H]aspartate uptake sites **(A)** and immunocytochemical localization of glutamate-like immunoreactivity **(B)** in adjacent sections of a rat hippocampal slice. The slice (300 μm) was incubated in Krebs' solution containing 2 μM D-[³H]aspartate for 10 min at 19°C, rinsed, fixed in 5% glutaraldehyde, frozen in sucrose, and resectioned at 20 μm. The two labeling patterns are very similar. Asterisks, fissura hippocampi; triangles, strong labeling of the inner zone of the dentate molecular layer (target zone of hilar associational/commissural projection). Inset: Nitrocellulose test filter incubated together with the section. The spots contain conjugates made by reacting rat brain protein with an amino acid (1, glutamate; 2, glycine; 3, GABA; 4, L-aspartate; and 5, none) in the presence of glutaraldehyde. Note selective staining of glutamate spots. Conjugates prepared from other amino acids such as glutamine and D-aspartate were also unstained (data not shown). Bar = 250 μm.

mediobasal hypothalamus (Storm-Mathisen and Woxen Opsahl, 1978; Walaas and Fonnum, 1979, 1980; Walaas, 1981).

Transmitter-Synthesizing Enzymes

The distributions in hippocampus of the glutamate- and aspartate-synthesizing enzymes phosphate-activated glutaminase (PAG) and aspartate aminotransferase (AAT) have been subjected to both immunocytochemical and his-

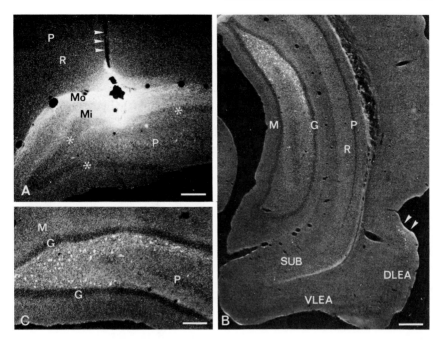

Fig. 3. Dark-field photomicrographs of autoradiograms showing retrogradely labeled neurons in the dorsal subdivision of the lateral entorhinal cortex **(B)** and in the hilus **(B,C)** after an implantation of D-[³H]aspartate containing gel beads in the molecular layer of rat fascia dentata **(A)**. Arrowheads indicate micropipette track (A) and labeled neurons in DLEA (B). Asterisks, granular layer. Section in B (part of which is enlarged in C) is 1,600 μm caudal to the implantation site shown in A. A,C, bars = 250 μm; B, bar = 0.5 mm. (Reproduced from Fischer et al., 1986, with permission of the publisher.)

tochemical investigations. PAG-like immunoreactivity was reported to be concentrated in the stratum lucidum (Altschuler et al., 1985), although results obtained with another antiserum suggested a rather uniform distribution in all hippocampal zones (Svenneby and Storm-Mathisen, 1983). AAT has been demonstrated histochemically in several excitatory fiber systems in the hippocampus (Schmidt and Wolf, 1987), but was not detected immunocytochemically (Altschuler et al., 1985). The results on the glutamate- and aspartate-synthesizing enzymes are difficult to interpret in terms of transmitter action of the amino acids, since these enzymes are also responsible for the formation of the metabolic pools of glutamate and aspartate.

Endogenous Contents of Excitatory Amino Acids

The biochemically recorded glutamate concentration shows little variation among the different layers and subfields of the hippocampal formation (Berger et al., 1977; Nitsch and Okada, 1979). Interruptions of excitatory pathways either have failed to produce any changes in glutamate contents in the deafferented areas (e.g. the commissural projection; Nadler et al., 1976, 1978) or have produced only modest effects (mossy fiber pathway, Nadler et al., 1978; commissural projection, Nitsch et al., 1979; perforant pathway, Nadler and Smith, 1981; commissural and Schaffer collaterals, Storm-Mathisen, 1978). These results can readily be explained by the prevalence of "metabolic" glutamate (Fonnum, 1984), a substantial amount of which will remain in neuronal cell bodies, dendrites, and glial cells in the deafferented areas. The metabolic pool might even increase following lesions.

Amino Acid Immunocytochemistry

The development of antisera to glutamate and aspartate (Storm-Mathisen et al., 1983; Ottersen and Storm-Mathisen, 1984a,b, 1985) has made it possible to study the distribution of the respective amino acids at a resolution exceeding by far that provided by biochemical techniques. By means of immunocytochemistry we should be able to determine whether glutamate or aspartate are concentrated in the terminals of the excitatory fiber systems in the hippocampus. Our initial immunocytochemical preparations of perfusion-fixed tissue did not resolve this issue because of inappropriate labeling of nerve terminals (Fig. 4B) (Ottersen and Storm-Mathisen 1984b, 1985). This technical difficulty was considered to reflect inadequate access of the antibodies to the transmitter pools and an obscuring effect of the metabolic pools (Storm-Mathisen and Ottersen, 1988). We reasoned that these problems might be alleviated if the antisera were applied to ultrathin plastic-embedded sections rather than to the Vibratome or frozen sections routinely used. The former procedure, besides providing a much higher resolution, detects only antigenic epitopes exposed at the surface of the section and therefore avoids penetration problems. The use of colloidal gold particles as an immunocytochemical marker permitted us to quantify the immunolabeling (Somogyi et al., 1986; Ottersen, 1987). Following incubation with a glutamate antiserum, the terminals of the major excitatory fiber systems (mossy fiber terminals and terminals establishing asymmetric synapses with dendritic spines in strata radiatum, oriens, and dentate molecular layer) displayed two- to fivefold higher gold particle densities than the postsynaptic elements (mostly dendrites of putative glutamatergic pyramidal cells) and presumed inhibitory nerve terminals (terminals with pleomorphic vesicles establishing symmetric contacts with dendritic stems or neuronal perikarya) (Fig. 5A). The excitatory nerve terminals appeared to be enriched in glutamate-like immunoreactivity relative to their parent cell bodies, whereas this was not the case with the inhibitory fiber systems (Ottersen and Bramham, 1988). Comparisons between the different fiber systems further suggested that the Schaffer collateral/commissural terminals in CA1 stratum radiatum contain a significantly higher level of glutamate-like immunoreactivity than mossy fiber terminals. Comparable data are not yet available for aspartate.

What do these differences in gold particle densities correspond to in terms of absolute glutamate concentrations? This question was addressed by incu-

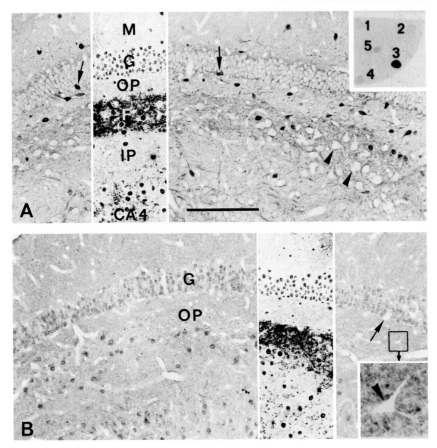

Fig. 4. Photomicrographs showing closely spaced sections of guinea pig area dentata stained with an antiserum against GABA **(A)** or glutamate **(B).** From perfusion-fixed material. The staining patterns are almost complementary: Basket cells (arrows) and cells in the outer plexiform layer are stained for GABA, but unstained for glutamate, whereas the converse is true for the majority of the large neurons (arrowheads in A) in the second reflected blade. A glutamate immunonegative neuron in OP has been enlarged in B (arrowhead). Although cell body staining for glutamate is not restricted to glutamatergic or aspartatergic neurons (see Discussion in Ottersen and Storm-Math-isen, 1985) it is noteworthy that the population of large glutamate-like immunoreactive cell bodies in F probably includes the mossy cells, which are thought to give rise to the majority of the excitatory fibers in the dentate commissural/associational projection (see text). Note that the pattern of glutamate-like immunoreactivity differs considerably from that seen in immersion-fixed material, where terminals are preferentially stained (Fig. 2B). Inset in A shows test filter prepared as in Figure 2 and processed together with the section: 1, aspartate; 2, glutamate; 3, GABA; 4, taurine; 5, none. (The glutamate antiserum is equally selective; see Fig. 2.) Vertical strips show parts of section treated according to the Timm/Haug procedure and used for orientation; note intense staining of mossy fiber terminals in F. Bar = 200 μm.

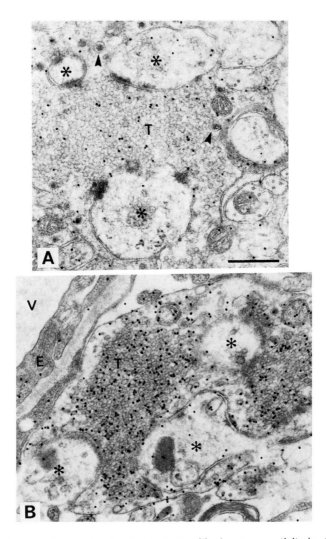

Fig. 5. Electron micrographs showing glutamate-like immunoreactivity in stratum lucidum of perfusion-fixed **(A)** and immersion-fixed **(B)** rat hippocampus. Postembedding immunogold technique. The contrast in immunolabeling between mossy fiber terminals (T) and dendritic spines (asterisks) is very much enhanced in the immersion-fixed material (same incubation procedure as in Fig. 2B). Not all mossy fiber terminals are equally intensely labeled (see Fig. 2B). It should be emphasized that the *absolute* gold particle densities in A and B are not comparable, since the two figures were from different experiments. Arrowheads, dense core vesicles. B was obtained from material prepared in collaboration with W. Schmidt. Bar = 0.5 μm.

bating a series of glutamate conjugates, each made from a different glutamate concentration, together with the tissue sections (Ottersen, 1989). A preliminary analysis suggests that the average glutamate concentration in the excitatory nerve terminals is of the order of 20 mM, which is only about twice the biochemically measured average tissue concentration (Berger et al., 1977). This estimate may be too low, since it does not take into account the possibility that the nerve terminals lose a disproportionately large fraction of their glutamate contents during fixation. However, it is compatible with the modest decreases in endogenous glutamate levels after deafferentation (see above).

The relatively small differences in immunolabeling intensity between profiles presumed to contain transmitter glutamate and those believed to contain only metabolic glutamate necessitate a statistical evaluation of the gold particle densities. This is a time-consuming procedure, since it requires the analysis of a large number of profiles. The identification of putative glutamatergic terminals would therefore be greatly facilitated if ways were found to depress selectively the metabolic pool of glutamate. This can apparently be achieved by incubating fresh hippocampal slices in artificial cerebrospinal fluid before immersion fixation with glutaraldehyde (Storm-Mathisen et al., 1986a,b). Under certain conditions, such slices display an almost complete loss of glutamate-like immunoreactivity (as well as aspartate-like immunoreactivity) from cell bodies and dendrites, the remaining immunoreactivity being restricted to nerve terminals considered to be glutamatergic or aspartatergic on other grounds (compare Fig. 2B with Fig. 4B and Fig. 5A with Fig. 5B). The nerve terminal labeling can be abolished in a calcium-dependent manner by exposing the slice to high concentrations of potassium or to veratridine for prolonged periods (Storm-Mathisen et al., 1986a,b). The loss of nerve terminal staining is associated with a greatly increased glial staining, suggesting that part of the released glutamate is taken up into glia. Further studies based on the use of enzyme inhibitors or on manipulation of the precursor levels have shown that the nerve terminal pools of glutamate and aspartate behave as expected of transmitter pools (Storm-Mathisen et al., 1986a,b; Storm-Mathisen and Ottersen, 1988).

The mechanisms underlying the loss of metabolic glutamate under the in vitro conditions have not been elucidated. One possibility is that there is a general efflux of glutamate and that high levels of glutamate are only maintained at sites of rapid glutamate synthesis and turnover, i.e. in the transmitter pools. Interestingly, a pattern of immunostaining similar to that observed in slices was produced in brain tissue that had been perfusion fixed after prolonged perfusion with buffer alone (Yoshida et al., 1987)

Receptor Distribution and Function

Autoradiographic studies have demonstrated the presence of glutamate binding sites in the termination zones of all of the main excitatory amino acid pathways in the hippocampus (for reviews, see Cotman et al., 1987; Cotman and Monaghan, 1987). The three classes of glutamate receptors appear to be heterogeneously distributed. N-methyl-D-aspartate (NMDA) displaceable glutamate binding is prevalent in stratum radiatum and stratum oriens, particularly in CA1, whereas kainic acid displaceable binding is concentrated in the mossy fiber zone. The distribution of quisqualate sites resembles that of the NMDA sites, although the former type predominates over the latter in the pyramidal cell layer.

A number of electrophysiological studies suggest that classical, fast excitatory synaptic transmission mainly involves quisqualate and kainic acid receptors (Collingridge et al., 1983a; Crunelli et al., 1983; Ganong et al., 1986) and that the NMDA receptor rather engages in slower modulatory events such as long-term potentiation (Collingridge et al., 1983b; Collingridge and Bliss, 1987) and kindling (Mody and Heinemann, 1987). However, monosynaptic NMDA responses can be evoked by a single volley if Mg^{2+} is removed from the bathing medium, as shown in CA1 (Wigström et al., 1985; Coan and Collingridge, 1985). This is consistent with the idea that the NMDA sensitive ion channel is subject to a voltage-dependent block by Mg^{2+} (for reviews, see Ascher and Nowak, 1987; Mayer and Westbrook, 1987). Hablitz and Langmoen (1986) suggest that the NMDA receptor mediates a minor part of the monosynaptic excitatory postsynaptic potential (EPSP) in CA1 even in the presence of 2 mM Mg^{2+}. Hippocampal receptors for excitatory amino acids may also act through second messenger systems (Nicoletti et al., 1986).

Transmitter Identity

The finding that the reversal potential for glutamate is similar to that for the natural transmitter in the Schaffer collateral system (Hablitz and Langmoen, 1982) as well as in the perforant path (Crunelli et al., 1984) adds to the large amount of data favoring glutamate as an important transmitter in hippocampal excitatory pathways. Furthermore, it should be clear from the evidence reviewed above that aspartate must be regarded as a likely transmitter candidate in addition to glutamate, particularly in the dentate commissural projection. The possible involvement of yet other excitatory amino acids should be explored. A particularly interesting compound in this respect is homocysteic acid, which has recently been claimed to be a more likely transmitter candidate than glutamate in excitatory synapses in layer III of neocortex (Zeise et al., 1988).

It must also be emphasized that most of the excitatory pathways appear to contain one or several neuroactive substances in addition to the excitatory amino acids(s). *The dentate associational/commissural pathway* displays four different transmitter candidates. The mossy cells give rise to the majority of the fibers in this pathway (Ribak et al., 1985) and are likely to use glutamate or aspartate as transmitter (Nadler et al., 1976, 1978; Fischer et al., 1986). A smaller, presumed inhibitory component consists of fibers that originate from cells different from the mossy cells; these fibers contain glutamic acid decarboxylase (GAD) and establish symmetric junctions in the inner zone of the molecular layer (Ribak et al., 1986). Still another population of hilar neurons (which may overlap with the GAD-containing one) emits somatostatin-immunoreactive fibers to the outer zone of the dentate molecular layer (Bakst et al., 1986). Finally, cholecystokinin is present in the dentate commissural system, at least in mice (Gall et al., 1986). *The lateral and medial perforant paths* contain enkephalin and cholecystokinin, respectively (Fredens et al., 1984), whereas the *mossy fiber zone* is enriched in enkephalin and dynorphin (Fitzpatrick and Johnson, 1981; Stengaard-Pedersen et al., 1981) as well as cholecystokinin (Stengaard-Pedersen et al., 1983; Gall et al., 1986). The distribution of some of the above peptides appears to vary considerably among different species. An important question that remains to be resolved is whether these peptides coexist with glutamate or aspartate or occur in separate fibers.

INHIBITORY AMINO ACIDS

GABA appears to be the major inhibitory transmitter candidate in the hippocampus. Its inhibitory effect on hippocampal neurons was reported by Biscoe and Straughan (1966), and it was later shown that bicuculline blocks the effect of microiontophoretically applied GABA on hippocampal neurons, as well as the synaptically evoked inhibitory potentials (Curtis et al., 1970, 1971). The reversal potential for GABA is similar to that of the inhibitory postsynaptic potential (Andersen et al., 1980; Ben-Ari et al., 1981).

Identification of Putative GABAergic Neurons

A large body of evidence suggests that the GABAergic inhibition in the hippocampus is mediated by nonprincipal cells (Andersen et al. 1964; Andersen, 1975; Storm-Mathisen, 1977a; Ribak et al., 1978). Unlike the pyramidal and granule cells, nonprincipal cells are found in all layers of the hippocampus and can be subdivided into numerous subpopulations based on their morphology and location (Lorente de Nó, 1934; Amaral, 1978; Ribak and Seress, 1983). Judged from immunocytochemical studies of GAD (Ribak et al., 1978) or GABA (Ottersen and Storm-Mathisen, 1984a; Somogyi et al., 1984; Gamrani et al., 1986) a large majority of the nonprincipal neurons are likely to use GABA as transmitter. The exact proportion is difficult to determine with immunocytochemical techniques because of the possible occurrence of false-negative staining. With this caveat in mind, results obtained by Kosaka et al. (1985) point to the existence of a GAD-immunonegative subpopulation of vasoactive intestinal polypeptide (VIP)-containing interneurons. The question whether these or other nonprincipal neurons in the hippocampus are indeed incapable of GABA synthesis will probably soon be resolved by the use of in situ hybridization techniques for the detection of GAD mRNA.

Detailed immunocytochemical studies have localized GAD to basket neurons in the pyramidal cell layer and to different types of neurons in strata oriens, radiatum, and lacunosum-moleculare (Ribak et al., 1978; Somogyi et al., 1983b). A particular type of GAD and GABA-immunopositive neuron has been described that exclusively contacts the initial axon segment of pyramidal cell neurons (the axoaxonic cell; Somogyi et al., 1983a,b, 1985). The fascia dentata contains a variety of GABA-immunopositive (Fig. 4A) and GAD-immunopositive cells, including five different types of basket cells (Seress and Ribak, 1983).

The distribution of GABA-like immunoreactivity in the hippocampus (Ottersen and Storm-Mathisen, 1984a; Gamrani et al., 1986) is strikingly similar to that of GAD. Direct evidence that GABA and GAD generally coexist in the same cell bodies was provided by Somogyi et al. (1984), using postembedding immunolabeling of consecutive semithin sections. A slight discrepancy may exist in the hilus of rats, where GABA antisera appear to label fewer neurons than do the antisera against GAD (cf. Sloviter and Nilaver, 1987; Seress and Ribak, 1983). Most of the neurons that contain GAD-like immunoreactivity, but no demonstrable GABA-like immunoreactivity, are situated in the deep hilar region and may include the cells that give rise to the GABAergic component of the associational/commissural projection. This would fit with observations from other brain regions suggesting that GABAergic projection neurons are generally more difficult to stain for GABA than are local interneurons (see, e.g. Ottersen and Storm-Mathisen, 1984b).

Studies based on immunocytochemistry of GABA or GAD (see above) or on autoradiography of GABA uptake (Taxt and Storm-Mathisen, 1984) have shown that although GABA terminals are distributed in all layers of the hippocampus, they are particularly concentrated in the pyramidal and granule cell layers. In these layers the GABA terminals establish axosomatic synapses and densely innervate the initial axon segments (Ribak et al., 1978; Somogyi et al., 1983b; Gamrani et al., 1986). In the dendritic layers the GABA terminals contact the dendritic stems, as opposed to the dendritic spines, which are the targets of the excitatory input. With very few exceptions (Kosaka et al., 1984) the GABA terminals form symmetric contacts.

Biochemical analyses of the GAD level after deafferentation suggest that the majority of the GABAergic fibers in the hippocampus originate from intrinsic neurons (Storm-Mathisen, 1972). Some of these neurons may project their axons for rather long distances within the hippocampal region, e.g. from CA3 to CA1, subiculum, and medial entorhinal area (Köhler and Chan-Palay, 1983). Two sources of extrinsic GABAergic inputs have been demonstrated. First, Ribak et al. (1986) showed that GAD immunopositive neurons in the hilus could be retrogradely labeled by axonal transport of tracer from the contralateral fascia dentata and also provided evidence of a minor GABAergic component in the CA3–CA3 commissural pathway. Second, using a similar approach, Köhler et al. (1984) demonstrated that the septohippocampal projection is not exclusively cholinergic but probably includes GABAergic fibers as well. The latter projection appears to be reciprocated by a minor GABA-containing pathway originating predominantly from nonprincipal neurons in strata oriens, radiatum, and pyramidale of CA1 (Shinoda et al., 1987). Nonprincipal neurons in the same locations also project to nucleus accumbens (Totterdell and Hayes, 1987). Obviously, the term *interneuron* is no longer generally applicable to the GABA neurons in the hippocampus.

GABA/Peptide Colocalization

Most, if not all, of the GABA neurons in the hippocampus also contain one or several neuroactive peptides. Somogyi et al. (1984) demonstrated that all of the cholecystokinin-positive neurons and most of the somatostatin-positive neurons in cat hippocampus were GAD immunoreactive and that the two peptides occurred in separate neurons. Colocalization of VIP and GAD has been described in the hippocampus of rat (Kosaka et al., 1985), although a majority of the VIP-positive cells were GAD immunonegative. A small number of neurons appear to contain GAD, VIP, and cholecystokinin (Kosaka et al., 1985; Sloviter and Nilaver, 1987). Other compounds that have been immunocytochemically localized to nonprincipal neurons in the hippocampus include parvalbumin (Kosaka et al., 1987), enkephalin (Gall et al., 1981), and choline acetyltransferase (Frotscher et al., 1986).

Little is known about the functional significance of GABA/peptide coexistence in the hippocampus. From other systems it is known that peptides may serve to modulate the neuronal signalling mediated by the cocontained "classical" transmitter (Hökfelt, 1986). The most imminent question is whether the peptides are actually released and, if so, under what conditions. Recent studies suggest that somatostatin enhances a voltage-dependent outward K^+ current in hippocampal neurons that tends to clamp the membrane potential at resting level (Moore et al., 1988). The effect of cholecystokinin on hippocampal cells is still an issue of controversy (see MacVicar et al., 1987).

Feedback Vs. Feed-Forward Inhibition

GABA is thought to mediate classical recurrent inhibition in the hippocampus. This function has traditionally been ascribed to the basket cells (Andersen, 1975), but the axoaxonic cell described by Somogyi et al. (1983a,b; 1985) appears equally well suited to control the output of pyramidal neurons by virtue of their dense innervation of the axon initial segments.

It has become increasingly clear that the principal cells are also strongly influenced by a GABAergic inhibition of feed-forward type. Indeed, most of the excitatory input pathways to the hippocampus may directly excite both principal cells and interneurons (for review, Buzsáki, 1984). There is evidence that the same nonprincipal interneurons can mediate feed-forward as well as feedback inhibition (Schwartzkroin and Kunkel, 1985), but the existence of neuronal subpopulations specifically devoted to one or the other type of inhibition cannot be ruled out.

The presence of feed-forward inhibitory mechanisms receives support from anatomical studies that have demonstrated that commissural axons establish synapses with GAD-immunopositive neurons in CA1 (Frotscher et al., 1984) and with Golgi-impregnated nonpyramidal neurons in the dentate gyrus (Seress and Ribak, 1984). Furthermore, choline acetyltransferase-containing axons have been shown to contact GAD-immunopositive neurons in the fascia dentata (Leránth and Frotscher, 1987). Immunocytochemical and electrophysiological data also indicate that inhibitory neurons are contacted by GABAergic terminals (Misgeld and Frotscher, 1986), suggesting that disinhibition may be an important feature of information processing in the hippocampus. Acetylcholine (Krnjević et al., 1988) and norepinephrine (Madison and Nicoll, 1988) have also been reported to cause disinhibition.

Receptor Distribution and Function

The hyperpolarizing effect of GABA in the hippocampus can be mediated through two different sets of receptors. The GABA$_A$ receptor is the "classical"

GABA receptor; it is bicuculline sensitive, coupled to a chloride channel, and responsible for the "fast" inhibitory postsynaptic potential (IPSP). The $GABA_B$ receptor is insensitive to bicuculline and activated by baclofen; it is connected to a G protein and produces a "slow" IPSP by increasing the membrane conductance for K^+ (Newberry and Nicoll, 1984, 1985). This functional role of the $GABA_B$ receptor has recently been corroborated by the use of phaclofen, a selective $GABA_B$ antagonist (Dutar and Nicoll, 1988). The $GABA_B$ receptors are activated only by strong afferent inputs, which may reflect their rather low affinity to GABA compared with the $GABA_A$ receptor (Newberry and Nicoll, 1985; Dutar and Nicoll, 1988). Interestingly, other transmitter candidates, such as serotonin and noradrenaline, may exert their effect on the same second-messenger systems as the $GABA_B$ receptor, allowing for an interaction at the cellular level between the different transmitter systems (e.g. Andrade et al., 1986). In addition to the postsynaptic $GABA_B$ receptors referred to above, some $GABA_B$ receptors appear to be localized presynaptically and may serve to regulate transmitter release. Thus the selective $GABA_B$ agonist baclofen has been found to block synaptic transmission in the mossy fibers and Schaffer collaterals (Lanthorn and Cotman, 1981; Olpe et al., 1982).

Autoradiographic studies have revealed slightly different distributions of $GABA_A$ and $GABA_B$ binding sites. Notably, the former binding site predominates over the latter in the cellular layers (Bowery et al., 1987; also see Chan-Palay, 1978). This observation fits with electrophysiological evidence suggesting that the $GABA_A$ receptor mediates basket cell recurrent inhibition (Curtis et al., 1970) and that the $GABA_B$ response is much weaker in the cellular than in the dendritic layers (Newberry and Nicoll, 1984). However, it should be noted that recent results obtained with antibodies against the $GABA_A$ receptor disagree with the binding data in suggesting a very low receptor density in the cellular layers (Richards et al., 1987; de Blas et al., 1988). The reason for this discrepancy is unclear.

Although the action of GABA is usually associated with hyperpolarization, a depolarizing effect has also been described (Andersen et al., 1980). This effect, which is only seen in the dendritic layers, is due to an increased membrane conductance and serves to short-circuit the postsynaptic potentials produced by the excitatory input (Alger and Nicoll, 1982).

SUMMARY

Our understanding of the amino acid transmitter systems in the hippocampus has greatly improved during the last few years. There is now strong evidence that excitatory amino acids (probably glutamate and possibly also aspartate) are the predominant transmitters in the main excitatory pathways in the hippocampus and that the inhibitory amino acid GABA is the major transmitter of the nonprincipal neurons. However, much remains to be learned about how the amino acid transmitter systems interact anatomically and physiologically with other transmitter systems and, in the case of colocalization, how the amino acid interacts with the cocontained peptide. Another important task for future research is to advance further our knowledge about the physiological characteristics of the individual amino acid-using synapses, particularly in regard to their plastic properties.

ACKNOWLEDGMENTS

This work was supported by the Norwegian Research Council for Science and the Humanities, the Norwegian Council on Cardiovascular Disease, the Norwegian Society for Fighting Cancer, and the Royal Norwegian Academy of Sciences.

REFERENCES

Alger, B.E., and R.A. Nicoll (1982) Pharmacological evidence for two kinds of GABA receptor on rat hippocampal pyramidal cells studied in vitro. J. Physiol. (Lond.) *328*:125–141.

Altschuler, R.A., D.T. Monaghan, W.G. Haser, R.J. Wenthold, N.P. Curthoys, C.W. Cotman (1985) Immunocytochemical localization of glutaminase-like and aspartate amino-transferase-like immunoreactivities in the rat and guinea pig hippocampus. Brain Res. *330*:225–233.

Amaral, D.G. (1978) A Golgi study of cell types in the hilar region of the hippocampus in the rat. J. Comp. Neurol. *182*:851–914.

Andersen, P. (1975) Organization of hippocampal neurons and their interconnections. In R.L. Isaacson, K.H. Pribram (eds): The Hippocampus, Vol. 1. New York: Plenum Press, pp. 155–175.

Andersen, P., R. Dingledine, L. Gjerstad, I.A. Langmoen, and A. Mosfeldt Laursen (1980) Two different responses of hippocampal pyramidal cells to application of gamma-amino butyric acid. J. Physiol. (Lond.) *305*:279–296.

Andersen, P., J.C. Eccles, and Y. Løyning (1964) Pathway of postsynaptic inhibition in the hippocampus. J. Neurophysiol. *27*:608–619.

Andrade, R. R.C. Malenka, and R.A. Nicoll (1986) A G protein couples serotonin and GABA$_B$ receptors to the same channels in hippocampus. Science *234*:1261–1265.

Ascher, P., and L. Nowak (1987) Electrophysiological studies of NMDA receptors. Trends Neurosci. *10:* 284–288.

Bakst, I., C. Avendano, J.H. Morrison, and D.G. Amaral (1986) An experimental analysis of the origins of somatostatin-like immunoreactivity in the dentate gyrus of the rat. J. Neurosci. *6*:1452–1462.

Ben-Ari, Y., K. Krnjević, R.J. Reiffenstein, and W. Reinhardt (1981) Inhibitory conductance changes and action of γ-aminobutyrate in rat hippocampus. Neuroscience *6*:2445–2463.

Berger, S.J., J.G. Carter, and O.H. Lowry (1977) The distribution of glycine, GABA, glutamate and aspartate in rabbit spinal cord, cerebellum and hippocampus. J. Neurochem. *28*:149–158.

Biscoe, T.J., and D.W. Straughan (1966) Micro-electrophoretic studies of neurones in the cat hippocampus. J. Physiol. (Lond.) *183*:341–359.

Bowery, N.G., A.L. Hudson, and G.W. Price (1987) GABA$_A$ and GABA$_B$ receptor site distribution in the rat central nervous system. Neuroscience *20*:365–383.

Buzsáki, G. (1984) Feed-forward inhibition in the hippocampal formation. Prog. Neurobiol. *22*:131–153.

Chan-Palay, V. (1978) Quantitative visualization of γ-aminobutyric acid receptors in hippocampus and area dentata demonstrated by [^{3}H]muscimol autoradiography. Proc. Natl. Acad. Sci. U.S.A. *75*:2516–2520.

Coan, E.J., and G.L. Collingridge (1985) Magnesium ions block an N-methyl-D-aspartate receptor-mediated component of synaptic transmission in rat hippocampus. Neurosci. Lett. *53*:21–26.

Collingridge, G.L., and T.V.P. Bliss (1987) NMDA receptors—Their role in long-term potentiation. Trends Neurosci. *10*:288–293.

Collingridge, G.L., S.J. Kehl, and H. McLennan (1983a) The antagonism of amino acid-induced excitations of rat hippocampal CA1 neurones in vitro. J. Physiol. (Lond.) *334*:19–31.

Collingridge, G.L., S.J. Kehl, and H. McLennan (1983b) Excitatory amino acids in synaptic transmission in the Schaffer collateral–commissural pathway of the rat hippocampus. J. Physiol. (Lond.) *334*:33–46.

Cotman, C.W., and D.T. Monaghan (1987) Chemistry and anatomy of excitatory amino acid systems. In H.Y. Meltzer (ed): "Psychopharmacology: The Third Generation of Progress." New York: Raven Press, pp. 197–210.

Cotman, C.W., D.T. Monaghan, O.P. Ottersen, and J. Storm-Mathisen (1987) Anatomical organization of excitatory amino acid receptors and their pathways. Trends Neurosci. *10*:273–280.

Cotman, C.W., and J.V. Nadler (1981) Glutamate and aspartate as hippocampal transmitters: Biochemical and pharmacological evidence. In P.J. Roberts, J. Storm-Mathisen, and G.A.R Johnston (eds): "Glutamate: Transmitter in the Central Nervous System." Chichester: John Wiley & Sons, pp. 117–154.

Crunelli, V., S. Forda, and J.S. Kelly (1983) Blockade of amino acid-induced depolarizations and inhibition of excitatory postsynaptic potentials in rat dentate gyrus. J. Physiol (Lond.) *341*:627–640.

Crunelli, V., S. Forda, and J.S. Kelly (1984) The reversal potential of excitatory amino acid action on granule cells of the rat dentate gyrus. J. Physiol. (Lond.) *351*:327–342.

Curtis, D.R., A.W. Duggan, D. Felix, G.A.R. Johnston, and H. McLennan (1971) Antagonism between bicuculline and GABA in the cat brain. Brain Res. *33*:57–73.

Curtis, D.R., D. Felix, and H. McLennan (1970) GABA and hippocampal inhibition. Br. J. Pharmacol. *40:* 881–883.

Davies, L.P., and G.A.R. Johnston (1976) Uptake and release of D- and L-aspartate by rat brain slices. J. Neurochem. *26*:1007–1014.

de Blas, A.L., J. Vitorica, and P. Friedrich (1988) Localization of the $GABA_A$ receptor in the rat brain with a monoclonal antibody to the 57,000 M_r peptide of the $GABA_A$ receptor/benzodiazepine receptor/Cl^- channel complex J. Neurosci. *8*:602–614.

Dutar, P., R.A. Nicoll (1988) A physiological role for $GABA_B$ receptors in the central nervous system. Nature *332:*156–158.

Fischer, B.O., O.P. Ottersen, and J. Storm-Mathisen (1986) Implantation of D-[^{3}H]aspartate loaded gel particles permits restricted uptake sites for transmitter selective axonal transport. Exp. Brain Res. *63*:620–626.

Fischer, B.O., O.P. Ottersen, and J. Storm-Mathisen (1989) In vivo axonal transport of D-[^{3}H]aspartate in intrinsic and afferent fibre connections of the rat and guinea pig hippocampus. Manuscript submitted.

Fitzpatrick, D., and R.P. Johnson (1981) Enkephalin-like immunoreactivity in the mossy fiber pathway of the hippocampal formation of the tree shrew *(Tupaia glis)*. Neuroscience *6*:2485–2494.

Fonnum, F. (1984) Glutamate: A neurotransmitter in mammalian brain. J. Neurochem. *42*:1–11.

Fonnum, F., and I. Walaas (1978) The effect of intrahippocampal kainic acid injections and surgical lesions on neurotransmitters in hippocampus and septum. J. Neurochem. *31*:1173–1181.

Fredens, K., K. Stengaard-Pedersen, and L.-I. Larsson (1984) Localization of enkephalin and cholecystokinin immunoreactivities in the perforant path terminal fields of the rat hippocampal formation. Brain Res. *304:*255–263.

Frotscher, M., C. Leránth, K. Lübbers, and W.H. Oertel (1984) Commissural afferents innervate glutamate decarboxylase immunoreactive non-pyramidal neurons in the guinea pig hippocampus. Neurosci. Lett. *46:*137–143.

Frotscher, M., M. Schlander, and C. Leránth (1986) Cholinergic neurons in the hippocampus: A combined light and electron microscopic immunocytochemical study in the rat. Cell Tissue Res. *246:*293–301.

Gall, C., L.M. Berry, and L.A. Hodgson (1986) Cholecystokinin in the mouse hippocampus: Localization in the mossy fiber and dentate commissural systems. Exp. Brain Res. *62:*431–437.

Gall, C., N. Brecha, H.J. Karten, and K.J. Chang (1981) Localization of enkephalin-like immunoreactivity to identified axonal and neuronal populations of the rat hippocampus. J. Comp. Neurol. *198:*335–350.

Gamrani, H., B. Onteniente, P. Seguela, M. Geffard, and A. Calas (1986) Gamma-aminobutyric acid-immunoreactivity in the rat hippocampus. A light and electron microscopic study with anti-GABA antibodies. Brain Res. *364:*30–38.

Ganong, A.H., A.W. Jones, J.C. Watkins, and C.W. Cotman (1986) Parallel antagonism of synaptic transmission and kainate/quisqualate responses in the hippocampus by piperazine-2,3-dicarboxylic acid analogs. J. Neurosci. *6:*930–937.

Hablitz, J.J., and I.A. Langmoen (1982) Excitation of hippocampal pyramidal cells by glutamate in the guinea-pig and rat. J. Physiol. *325:*317–331.

Hablitz, J.J., and I.A. Langmoen (1986) N-methyl-D-aspartate receptor antagonists reduce synaptic excitation in the hippocampus. J. Neurosci. *6:*102–106.

Hökfelt, T. (1986) Chemical neurotransmission as seen from the histochemical side. In P. Panula, H. Päivärinta, and S. Soinila (eds): Neurohistochemistry: Modern Methods and Applications. New York: Alan R. Liss pp. 331–353.

Köhler, C., and V. Chan-Palay (1983) Gamma-aminobutyric acid interneurons in the rat hippocampal region studied by retrograde transport of glutamic acid decarboxylase antibody after in vivo injections. Anat. Embryol. *166:*53–66.

Köhler, C., V. Chan-Palay, and J.-Y. Wu (1984) Septal neurons containing glutamic acid decarboxylase immunoreactivity project to the hippocampal region in the rat brain. Anat. Embryol. *169:*41–44.

Kosaka, T., K. Hama, and J.-Y. Wu (1984) GABAergic synaptic boutons in the granule cell layer of rat dentate gyrus. Brian Res. *293:*353–359.

Kosaka, T., H. Katsumaru, K. Hama, J.-Y. Wu, and C.W. Heizmann (1987) GABAergic neurons containing the Ca^{2+}-binding protein parvalbumin in the rat hippocampus and dentate gyrus. Brain Res. *419:*119–130.

Kosaka, T., K. Kosaka, K. Tateishi, Y. Hamaoka, N. Yanaihara, J.-Y. Wu, and K. Hama (1985) GABAergic neurons containing CCK-8-like and/or VIP-like immunoreactivities in the rat hippocampus and dentate gyrus. J. Comp. Neurol. *239:*420–430.

Krnjević, K., N. Ropert, and J. Casullo (1988) Septohippocampal disinhibition. Brain Res. *438:*182–192.

Lanthorn, T.H., and C.W. Cotman (1981) Baclofen selectively inhibits excitatory synaptic transmission in the hippocampus. Brain Res. *225:*171–178.

Leránth, C., and M. Frotscher (1987) Cholinergic innervation of hippocampal GAD- and somatostatin-immunoreactive commissural neurons. J. Comp. Neurol. *261:*33–47.

Lorente de Nó, R. (1934) Studies on the structure of the cerebral cortex. II. Continuation of the study of the ammonic system. J. Physiol. Neurol. (Lpz.) *46:*113–177.

MacVicar, B.A., J.P. Kerrin, and J.S. Davison (1987) Inhibition of synaptic transmission in the hippocampus by cholecystokinin (CCK) and its antagonism by a CCK analog (CCK$_{27-33}$). Brain Res. *406*:130–135.

Madison, D.V., and R.A. Nicoll (1988) Norepinephrine decreases synaptic inhibition in the rat hippocampus. Brain Res. *442*:131–138.

Malthe-Sørenssen, D., K.K. Skrede, and F. Fonnum (1979) Calcium-dependent release of D-[^{3}H]aspartate evoked by selective electrical stimulation of excitatory afferent fibers to hippocampal pyramidal cells in vitro. Neuroscience *4*:1255–1263.

Malthe-Sørenssen, D., K.K. Skrede, and F. Fonnum (1980) Release of D-[^{3}H]aspartate from the dorsolateral septum after electrical stimulation of the fimbria in vitro. Neuroscience *5*:127–133.

Mayer, M.L., and G.L. Westbrook (1987) The physiology of excitatory amino acids in the vertebrate central nervous system. Prog. Neurobiol. *28*:197–276.

Misgeld, U., and M. Frotscher (1986) Postsynaptic-GABAergic inhibition of non-pyramidal neurons in the guinea pig hippocampus. Neuroscience *19*:193–206.

Mody, I., and U. Heinemann (1987) NMDA receptors of dentate gyrus granule cells participate in synaptic transmission following kindling. Nature *326*:701–704.

Moore, S.D., S.G. Madamba, M. Joëls, and G.R. Siggins (1988) Somatostatin augments the M-current in hippocampal neurons. Science *239*:278–280.

Nadler, J.V., and E.M. Smith (1981) Perforant path lesion depletes glutamate content of fascia dentata synaptosomes. Neurosci. Lett. *25*:275–280.

Nadler, J.V., K.W. Vaca, W.F. White, G.S. Lynch, and C.W. Cotman (1976) Aspartate and glutamate as possible transmitters of excitatory hippocampal afferents. Nature (Lond.) *260*:538–540.

Nadler, J.V., W.F. White, K.W. Vaca, B.W. Perry, and C.W. Cotman (1978) Biochemical correlates of transmission mediated by glutamate and aspartate. J. Neurochem. *31*:147–155.

Newberry, N.R., and R.A. Nicoll (1984) Direct hyperpolarizing action of baclofen on hippocampal pyramidal cells. Nature *308*:450–452.

Newberry, N.R., and R.A. Nicoll (1985) Comparison of the action of baclofen with γ-aminobutyric acid on rat hippocampal pyramidal cells in vitro. J. Physiol. *360*:161–185.

Nicoletti, F., J.L. Meek, M.J. Idarola, D.M. Chuang, B.L. Roth and E. Costa (1986) Coupling of inositol phospholipid metabolism with excitatory amino acid recognition sites in rat hippocampus. J. Neurochem. *46*:40–46.

Nitsch, C., J.-K. Kim, C. Shimada, and Y. Okada (1979) Effect of hippocampus extirpation in the rat on glutamate levels in target structures of hippocampal efferents. Neurosci. Lett. *11*:295–299.

Nitsch, C., and Y. Okada (1979) Distribution of glutamate in layers of the rabbit hippocampal fields CA1, CA3, and the dentate area. J. Neurosci. Res. *4*:161–167.

Olpe, H.-R., M. Baudry, L. Fagni, and G. Lynch (1982) The blocking action of baclofen on excitatory transmission in the rat hippocampal slice. J. Neurosci. *2*:698–703.

Ottersen, O.P. (1987) Postembedding light and electron microscopic immunocytochemistry of amino acids: Description of a new model system allowing identical conditions for specificity testing and tissue processing. Exp. Brain Res. *69*:167–174.

Ottersen, O.P. (1989) Postembedding immunogold labelling of fixed glutamate: an electron microscopic analysis of the relationship between gold particle density and antigen concentration. J. Chem. Neuroanat. (in press)

Ottersen, O.P., and C.R. Bramham (1988) Quantitative electron microscopic immunocytochemistry of excitatory amino acids. In E.A. Cavalheiro, J. Lehmann, and L. Turski (eds): Frontiers in excitatory amino acid research. New York: Alan R. Liss, pp. 93–100.

Ottersen, O.P., B.O. Fischer, E. Rinvik, and J. Storm-Mathisen (1986) Putative amino acid transmitters in the amygdala. In R. Schwarcz and Y. Ben-Ari (eds): Excitatory Amino Acids and Epilepsy. New York: Plenum, pp. 53–66.

Ottersen, O.P., and J. Storm-Mathisen (1984a) Neurons containing or accumulating transmitter amino acids. In A. Björklund, T. Hökfelt, and M.J. Kuhar (eds): Handbook of Chemical Neuroanatomy, Vol. 3. Amsterdam: Elsevier/North Holland, pp. 141–246.

Ottersen, O.P. and J. Storm-Mathisen (1984b) Glutamate- and GABA-containing neurons in the mouse and rat brain, as demonstrated with a new immunocytochemical technique. J. Comp. Neurol. 229:374–392.

Ottersen, O.P., and J. Storm-Mathisen (1985) Different neuronal localization of aspartate-like and glutamate-like immunoreactivities in the hippocampus of rat, guinea-pig and senegalese baboon *(Papio papio)* with a note on the distribution of γ-aminobutyrate. Neuroscience 16:589–606.

Ribak, C.E., and L. Seress (1983) Five types of basket cells in the hippocampal dentate gyrus. A combined Golgi and electron microscopic study. J. Neurocytol. 12:577–597.

Ribak, C.E., L. Seress, and D.G. Amaral (1985) The development, ultrastructure and synaptic connections of the mossy cells of the dentate gyrus. J. Neurocytol. 14:835–857.

Ribak, C.E., L. Seress, G.M. Peterson, K.B. Seroogy, J.H. Fallon, and L.C. Schmued (1986) A GABAergic inhibitory component within the hippocampal commissural pathway. J. Neurosci. 6:3492–3498.

Ribak, C.E., J.E. Vaughn, and K. Saito (1978) Immunocytochemical localization of glutamic acid decarboxylase in neuronal somata following colchicine inhibition of axonal transport. Brain Res. 140:315–332.

Richards, J.G., P. Schoch, P. Häring, B. Takacs, and H. Möhler (1987) Resolving GABA$_A$/benzodiazepine receptors: Cellular and subcellular localization in the CNS with monoclonal antibodies. J. Neurosci. 7:1866–1886.

Schmidt, W., and G. Wolf (1987) Activity of aspartate aminotransferase in hippocampal formation of the rat during post-natal development and after lesion of the hippocampal Schaffer's collaterals: A quantitative histochemical study. Neurochem. Int. 11:39–47.

Schwarcz, R., and Y. Ben-Ari (1986) Excitatory Amino Acids and Epilepsy. New York: Plenum, 735 pp.

Schwartzkroin, P.A., and D.D. Kunkel (1985) Morphology of identified interneurons in the CA1 regions of guinea pig hippocampus. J. Comp. Neurol. 232:205–218.

Seress, L., and C.E. Ribak (1983) GABAergic cells in the dentate gyrus appear to be local circuit and projection neurons. Exp Brain Res. 50:173–182.

Seress, L., and C.E. Ribak (1984) Direct commissural connections to the basket cells of the hippocampal dentate gyrus: Anatomical evidence for feed-forward inhibition. J. Neurocytol. 13:215–225.

Shinoda, K., M. Tohyama, and Y. Shiotani (1987) Hippocampofugal γ-aminobutyric acid (GABA)-containing neuron system in the rat: A study using a double-labeling method that combines retrograde tracing and immunocytochemistry. Brain Res. 409:181–186.

Skrede, K.K., and D. Malthe-Sørenssen (1981) Differential release of D-[^{3}H]aspartate and [^{14}C]γ-aminobutyric acid following activation of commissural fibres in a longitudinal slice preparation of guinea pig hippocampus. Neurosci. Lett. 21:71–76.

Sloviter, R.S., G. Nilaver (1987) Immunocytochemical localization of GABA-, cholecystokinin-, vasoactive intestinal polypeptide-, and somatostatin-like immunoreactivity in the area dentata and hippocampus of the rat. J. Comp. Neurol. 256:42–60.

Somogyi, P., T.F. Freund, A.J. Hodgson, J. Somogyi, D. Beroukas, and I.W. Chubb (1985) Identified axo-axonic cells are immunoreactive for GABA in the hippocampus and visual cortex of the cat. Brain Res. 332:143–149.

Somogyi, P., K. Halasy, J. Somogyi, J. Storm-Mathisen, and O.P. Ottersen (1986) Quantification of immunogold labelling reveals enrichment of glutamate in mossy and parallel fibre terminals in cat cerebellum. Neuroscience *19:*1045–1050.

Somogyi, P., A.J. Hodgson, A.D. Smith, M.G. Nunzi, A. Gorio, and J.-Y. Wu (1984) Different populations of GABAergic neurons in the visual cortex and hippocampus of cat contain somatostatin- or cholecystokinin-immunoreactive material. J. Neurosci. *4:*2590–2603.

Somogyi, P., M.G. Nunzi, A. Gorio, and A.D. Smith (1983a) A new type of specific interneuron in the monkey hippocampus forming synapses exclusively with the axon initial segments of pyramidal cells. Brain Res. *259:*137–142.

Somogyi, P., A.D. Smith, M.G. Nunzi, A. Gorio, H. Takagi, and J.-Y. Wu (1983b) Glutamate decarboxylase immunoreactivity in the hippocampus of the cat: Distribution of immunoreactive synaptic terminals with special reference to the axon initial segment of pyramidal neurons. J. Neurosci. *3:*1450–1468.

Spencer, H.J., G. Tominez, and B. Halpern (1981) Mass spectrographic analysis of stimulated release of endogenous amino acids from rat hippocampal slices. Brain Res. *212:*194–197.

Stengaard-Pedersen, K., K. Fredens, and L.-I. Larsson (1981) Enkephalin and zinc in the hippocampal mossy fiber system. Brain Res. *212:*230–233.

Stengaard-Pedersen, K., K. Fredens, and L.-I. Larsson (1983) Comparative localization of enkephalin and cholecystokinin immunoreactivities and heavy metals in the hippocampus. Brain Res. *273:*81–96.

Storm-Mathisen, J. (1972) Glutamate decarboxylase in the rat hippocampal region after lesions of the afferent fibre system. Evidence that the enzyme is localized in intrinsic neurones. Brain Res. *40:*215–235.

Storm-Mathisen, J. (1977a) Localization of transmitter candidates in the brain: The hippocampal formation as a model. Prog. Neurobiol. *8:*119–181.

Storm-Mathisen, J. (1977b) Glutamic acid and excitatory nerve endings: Reduction of glutamic acid uptake after axotomy. Brain Res. *120:*379–386.

Storm-Mathisen, J. (1978) Localization of putative transmitters in the hippocampal formation with a note on the connection to septum and hypothalamus. In K. Elliott and J. Whelan (eds): Functions of the Septohippocampal System, Ciba Foundation symposium 58 (New Series). Amsterdam: Elsevier/Excerpta Medica/North Holland, pp. 49–86.

Storm-Mathisen, J. (1982) Amino acid compartments in hippocampus: An autoradiographic approach. In H.F. Bradford (ed): Neurotransmitter Interaction and Compartmentation. New York: Plenum, pp. 395–409.

Storm-Mathisen, J., and L.L. Iversen (1979) Uptake of [^{3}H]glutamic acid in excitatory nerve endings: Light and electron microscopic observations in the hippocampal formation of the rat. Neuroscience *4:*1237–1253.

Storm-Mathisen, J., A.K. Leknes, A.T. Bore, J.L. Vaaland, P. Edminson, F.-M.S. Haug, and O.P. Ottersen (1983) First visualization of glutamate and GABA in neurones by immunocytochemistry. Nature (Lond.) *301:*517–520.

Storm-Mathisen, J., and O.P. Ottersen (1984) Neurotransmitters in the hippocampal formation. In F. Reinoso-Suárez, and C. Ajmone-Marsan (eds): Cortical Integration. New York: Raven Press, pp. 105–130.

Storm-Mathisen, J., and O.P. Ottersen (1988) Localization of excitatory amino acid transmitters. In D. Lodge (ed): Excitatory Amino Acids in Health and Disease. Sussex, England: John Wiley & Sons, Ltd., pp. 107–141.

Storm-Mathisen, J., O.P. Ottersen, and T. Fu-Long (1986a) Antibodies for the localization of excitatory amino acids. In P.J. Roberts, J. Storm-Mathisen, and H.F. Bradford (eds): Excitatory Amino Acids. London: Macmillan, pp. 101–116.

Storm-Mathisen, J., O.P. Ottersen, T. Fu-Long, V. Gundersen, J.H. Laake, and G. Nordbø (1986b) Metabolism and transport of amino acids studied by immunocytochemistry. Med. Biol. 64:127–132.

Storm-Mathisen, J., and M. Woxen Opsahl (1978) Aspartate and/or glutamate may be transmitters in hippocampal efferents to septum and hypothalamus. Neurosci. Lett. 9:65–70.

Svenneby, G., and J. Storm-Mathisen (1983) Immunological studies on phosphate activated glutaminase. In L. Hertz E. Kvamme, E.G. McGeer, and A. Schousboe (eds): Glutamine, Glutamate, and GABA in the Central Nervous System. New York: Alan R. Liss, pp. 69–76.

Taxt, T., and J. Storm-Mathisen (1984) Uptake of D-aspartate and L-glutamate in excitatory axon terminals in hippocampus: Autoradiographic and biochemical comparison with γ-aminobutyrate and other amino acids in normal rats and in rats with lesions. Neuroscience 11:79–100.

Totterdell, S., and L. Hayes (1987) Non-pyramidal hippocampal projection neurons: A light and electron microscopic study. J. Neurocytol. 16:477–485.

Walaas, I. (1981) Biochemical evidence for overlapping neocortical and allocortical glutamate projections to the nucleus accumbens and rostral caudatoputamen in the rat brain. Neuroscience 6:399–405.

Walaas, I. (1984) The hippocampus. In P.C. Emson (ed): Chemical Neuroanatomy. New York: Raven Press, pp. 337–358.

Walaas, I., and F. Fonnum (1979) The effect of surgical and chemical lesions on neurotransmitter candidates in the nucleus accumbens of the rat. Neuroscience 4:209–216.

Walaas, I., and F. Fonnum (1980) Biochemical evidence for glutamate as a transmitter in hippocampal efferents to the basal forebrain and hypothalamus in the rat brain. Neuroscience 5:1691–1698.

Wigström, H., B. Gustafsson, and Y.Y. Huang (1985) A synaptic potential following single volleys in the hippocampal CA1 region possibly involved in the induction of long-lasting potentiation. Acta Physiol. Scand. 124:175–178.

Yoshida, M., M. Teramura, M. Sakai, N. Karasawa, T. Nagatsu, and I. Nagatsu (1987) Immunohistochemical visualization of glutamate- and aspartate-containing nerve terminal pools in the rat limbic structures. Brain Res. 410:169–173.

Zeise, M.L., T. Knöpfel, and W. Zieglgänsberger (1988) (±)-β-Parachlorophenylglutamate selectively enhances the depolarizing response to L-homocysteic acid in neocortical neurons of the rat: Evidence for a specific uptake system. Brain Res. 443:373–376.

The Hippocampus—New Vistas, pages 119–130
© 1989 Alan R. Liss, Inc.

8
Localization of Transmitter-Metabolizing Enzymes by Enzyme Histochemistry in the Rat Hippocampus

PETER KUGLER

Department of Anatomy, University of Würzburg, Würzburg, Federal Republic of Germany

INTRODUCTION

In contrast to immunocytochemistry, enzyme histochemistry utilizes the catalytic activity of enzymes to demonstrate the local metabolic activity of enzymes, while the enzymes, unlike in biochemical reactions in test tubes, are present in the structural matrix of tissue (Kugler, 1988b). This chapter deals with histochemical results for enzymes of the amino acid transmitter metabolism in the rat hippocampus using catalytic enzyme histochemistry (Kugler, 1988a–c). Concerning amino acids with transmitter functions, there is strong evidence that, in the hippocampus of rats, glutamate (Glu) or aspartate (Asp) is used as an excitatory transmitter (Storm-Mathisen, 1977; White et al., 1977; Taxt and Storm-Mathisen, 1979; Fonnum et al., 1979; Storm-Mathisen and Iversen, 1979; Crunelli et al., 1983; Fonnum, 1984; Cotman et al., 1986).

Because of improved techniques of catalytic enzyme histochemistry it is now possible to demonstrate Glu/Asp-metabolizing enzymes in the rat hippocampus in their laminar and sometimes cellular localization (see below) (Kugler, 1988a). However, in the demonstration of such enzymes one should bear in mind that these amino acids not only serve as transmitters but also occupy a central position in the general metabolism and that it is difficult to separate metabolic Glu from transmitter Glu (Fonnum et al., 1979). Furthermore, the biochemical processes that serve to replenish and regulate the neurotransmitter pool of Glu have not been established (Shank and Campbell, 1982). It is therefore important to gather more information about the topographic distribution and activities of enzymes metabolizing these amino acids by enzyme

Abbreviations: Asp, aspartate; AT, aspartate aminotransferase; CA, cornu Ammonis; cAT, cytoplasmic aspartate aminotransferase; GABA, γ-amino butyric acid; GFAP, glial fibrillary acidic protein; Gldh, glutamate dehydrogenase; Glu, glutamate; mAT, mitochondrial aspartate aminotransferase; OT, ornithine aminotransferase; PAG, phosphate-activated glutaminase; PAP, peroxidase-antiperoxidase.

histochemical means and to find out whether there is a match with glutamatergic or aspartatergic pathways in the hippocampus.

Another important respect in which the amino acid transmitters differ from other neurotransmitters (e.g. acetylcholine and monoamines) is the metabolic relationship between neuron and glia in the turnover and metabolism of amino acid transmitters (Schousboe and Hertz, 1983). Particular attention is also given in this chapter to this complex compartmentation of the Glu/Asp metabolism in situ.

ENZYMES FOR GLUTAMATE SYNTHESIS

All of the major intrinsic pathways of the hippocampus, e.g. the dentate granular cell axons (mossy fibers), which run in the lucidum layer of the cornu Ammonis (CA) 3 and terminate on the proximal dendrites of the CA3 pyramidal cells, the projections of the CA3 pyramidal cells to the strata radiatum and oriens layers of CA1 and to the inner zone of the dentate gyrus molecular layer (Schaffer collaterals) and its major input, and the perforant pathway from the area entorhinalis terminating in the outer two-thirds of the dentate gyrus molecular layer and its commissural fibers to the contralateral hippocampus, have been proposed to be glutamatergic or aspartatergic (White et al., 1977; Taxt and Storm-Mathisen, 1979; Fonnum et al., 1979; Storm-Mathisen and Iversen, 1979; Crunelli et al., 1983; Cotman et al., 1986). The main methods used to reveal these putative Glu/Asp- using pathways are Glu/Asp uptake and release techniques combined with lesion and electrophysiological techniques, but quantitative autoradiographic methods to determine Glu receptors (Halpain et al., 1984; Zilles, 1988) and histochemical methods to study enzymes (Altschuler et al., 1985; Kugler, 1988a) and Glu itself (Storm-Mathisen et al., 1983) are becoming more promising.

The more important Glu-synthesizing or -degrading enzymes are the enzymes aspartate aminotransferase (AT), glutamate dehydrogenase (Gldh), phosphate-activated glutaminase (Salganicoff and de Robertis, 1965), and perhaps other aminotransferases, e.g. ornithine aminotransferase (OT). These enzymes are thought to be not specifically associated with neurotransmitter synthesis because no clear distinction can be made between the participation of these enzymes in the metabolism of the transmitter-related pool and the nontransmitter-related pool of Glu (Schousboe and Hertz, 1983). However, Altschuler et al. (1982) and Kugler (1988a) have recently suggested that a presynaptic enrichment of AT is associated with glutamatergic and aspartatergic neurotransmitter functions.

Aspartate Aminotransferase

AT catalyses the reversible reactions of Asp to oxaloacetate and α-ketoglutarate to Glu. Biochemical studies reveal that two isoenzymes of AT are present in brain; one is associated with the cytoplasm (cAT) and the other with mitochondria (mAT; Salganicoff and de Robertis, 1965).

Together with a lead salt procedure, histochemical studies at the light microscopic level reveal a layered reaction pattern of AT in the rat hippocampus

(Fig. 1) (Schmidt and Wolf, 1987; Kugler, 1988a). Pronounced activities are observed in the radiatum and oriens layers of CA1, in the lucidum and lacunosum-moleculare layers of CA3, and in the middle zone of the dentate gyrus molecular layer. Lower activities are demonstrated in the other hippocampal regions. AT is also demonstrable in the perikarya of most granule cells and by a further improvement of the demonstration procedure (unpublished results) in some perikarya scattered throughout the hippocampus. However, very low activities are shown in the perikarya and proximal dendrites of pyramidal cells (Fig. 2).

Because cAT could have special importance for the production of releasable Glu (see below), in preliminary experiments (unpublished results) we tried to differientiate between the two isoenzymes by heating the sections (70°C for 15 min) before incubation. This heating procedure destroys more than 98% of the mAT activity without affecting cAT activity (Parli et al., 1985). From this procedure resulted almost the same AT reaction pattern, but the demonstrable activities were significantly lower in most hippocampal regions and in the pyramidal cell layer. The smallest changes were observed in the lucidum layer. This might indicate that the pyramidal cell perikarya contain almost exclusively mAT and the mossy fiber system of the lucidum layer preferentially cAT, whereas in other regions of the hippocampus both isoenzymes seem to display the same localization pattern with variable proportions. These results and their interpretation are in agreement with the findings concerning the ultrastructural distribution of AT.

At the electron microscopic level (Kugler, 1988c) AT is localized at two sites corresponding to biochemical data (see above), i.e. in the cytoplasm (cAT) and in mitochondria (mAT). cAT together with mAT is demonstrated in a large number of boutons in all regions of the hippocampus, frequently side to side with negatively reacting boutons. Also, most of the mossy fibers and their giant boutons (Fig. 3) and numerous unmyelinated and myelinated fibers as well as the perikarya of a large number of granule cells react positively for cAT and mAT. An exclusive mAT reaction (without cytoplasmic staining) is shown in a small number of granule cells and in the perikarya of most pyramidal cells. Astrocytes have a negative reaction. It is suggested that AT activities are either below the demonstration limit or the enzyme is really not expressed in astrocytes. Moreover, kinetic studies indicate that the enzyme is associated more closely with neuronal than glial structures (Berl and Clarke, 1978).

The different distribution of the AT isoenzymes might indicate that cAT is associated with the neurotransmitter metabolism whereas mAT is involved in more general metabolic pathways (Salganicoff and de Robertis, 1965). This suggestion is supported by the finding that cAT is preferentially localized in boutons, the best example being the giant boutons of the mossy fibers, which are thought to be glutamatergic or aspartatergic (Cotman et al., 1986). A cAT enrichment is also found by immunocytochemistry in presumed glutamatergic terminals in the retina and the cochlear nucleus (Altschuler et al., 1982).

Any relationship between AT and neurotransmission is not a straight forward one, since AT is also involved in aspects of energy metabolism. However, it

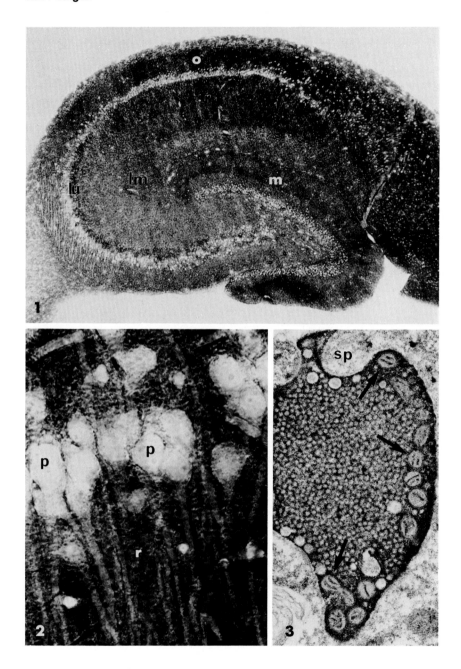

can be suggested that glutamatergic or aspartatergic neurons might use Glu and Asp in energy metabolism to a greater extent than neurons that do not use these amino acids as transmitters (Ross and Godfrey, 1987). Finally, it is remarkable that the AT reaction pattern in the hippocampus shows a conspicuously good correlation with the distribution of glutamate receptors demonstrated by quantitative autoradiography (Halpain et al., 1984; Zilles, 1988), supporting the view that AT is involved in the metabolism of Glu as neurotransmitter.

Glutamate Dehydrogenase

Gldh is principally a mitochondrial matrix enzyme, but other cellular localizations in the brain are also discussed (for references, see Kugler, 1988b). It is involved in the interconversion of Glu and α-ketoglutarate provided by the tricarboxylic acid cycle (Dennis and Clark, 1977).

Recently, in an immunocytochemical study, it was shown that Gldh exhibits low-intensity, uniform immunoreactivity in neurons and intense heterogeneous labeling of glial cells of rat brain, which have been identified as astrocytes (Aoki et al., 1987). Almost at the same time we demonstrated Gldh by enzyme histochemical means in glial cells of the rat hippocampus, and, on the basis of their shape and localization, we proposed that those positively reacting were astrocytes, whereas in neurons Gldh was almost not demonstrable (Kugler, 1988a).

We have now established a double labeling method in which Gldh is demonstrated by enzyme histochemistry and glial fibrillary acidic protein (GFAP), a marker protein of astrocytes (Bignami et al., 1972) by immunohistochemistry (PAP technique) sequentially in the same section (unpublished results). This procedure confirmed that the Gldh-positive glial cells were astrocytes (Fig. 4, inset).

The most important finding in our single and double labeling studies was the heterogeneous Gldh reaction of astrocytes in the rat hippocampus, which was also demonstrated but in less detail by Aoki et al. (1987) using immu-

---

Fig. 1. Demonstration of aspartate aminotransferase (AT) in a 5-μm-thick glutaraldehyde-fixed cryostat section. AT reaction product is demonstrable in all regions of the hippocampus, preferentially in the radiatum (r) and oriens (o) layers of CA1, the lucidum (lu) and lacunosum-moleculare (lm) layers of CA3, and the molecular (m) layer of the fascia dentata. × 40.

Fig. 2. Demonstration of AT in a Vibratome section of a perfusion-fixed hippocampus (Kugler, 1988c). AT reaction product is barely detectable in the perikarya and mainstem dendrites of pyramidal cells (p) of the CA1, whereas the space between the dendrites contain reaction product. r, radiatum layer. × 400.

Fig. 3. Ultracytochemical demonstration of AT (Kugler, 1988c) in a mossy fiber bouton. AT reaction product is detected in the bouton cytoplasm and in the cristae of mitochondria (arrows), whereas synaptic vesicles and a dendritic spine (sp) contain no reaction product. × 33,000.

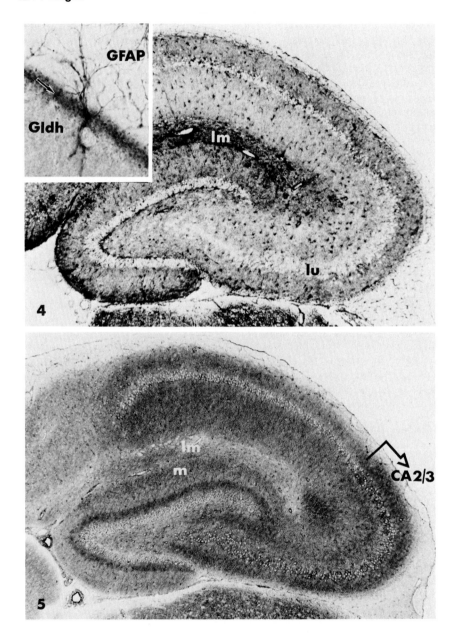

nocytochemistry. Astrocytes labeled by GFAP antiserum were distributed throughout the hippocampus, showing a high density of profiles in the lacunosum-moleculare layer of the hippocampus proper, in the alveus, and in the hilus of the fascia dentata. Gldh-positive astrocytic profiles of different densities were also detected throughout the hippocampus (Fig. 4). The highest density was found in the lacunosum-moleculare layer of the hippocampus proper, which is in agreement with the GFAP immunocytochemistry, and low density in the hilus of fascia dentata and lucidum layer of the CA3, which does not match the distribution of astrocytes labeled by the GFAP antiserum.

It is also worth noting that Gldh-stained fine processes were significantly more numerous throughout the hippocampus than were those processes labeled by the GFAP antiserum. This implies that Gldh might be distributed in the fine ramifications of astrocytic processes that contain no glial filaments (Kosaka and Hama, 1986). Double labeling was observed in most astrocytic perikarya (with the exception of the hilus and the lucidum layer) and their proximal thick processes.

This astrocytic Gldh reaction pattern might provide an indication that local Glu uptake and Glu metabolism depend on glutamatergic pathways (Aoki et al., 1987; Kugler, 1988a) and supports the importance of neuron–glia interactions in the Glu metabolism (Schousboe and Hertz, 1983). The high density of Gldh-positive astrocytic profiles in the lacunosum-moleculare layer of the hippocampus proper and the molecular layer of the fascia dentata corresponds with the high density of glutamatergic terminals in these layers. However, the lucidum layer, which is also presumed to be a glutamatergic (or aspartatergic) termination field (see Aspartate Aminotransferase, above) did not exhibit a pronounced astrocytic reaction pattern. A possible explanation could be that in certain regions neuronal reuptake mechanisms are of more importance than glia–neuron interactions in the Glu metabolism or the metabolic processing of Glu taken up in astrocytes is established preferentially by other enzymes. This also leads to the suggestion that the astrocytic Gldh reaction pattern is not firmly associated with glutamatergic pathways, a finding substantiated by observations in other brain regions (Aoki et al., 1987).

Fig. 4. Demonstration of glutamate dehydrogenase (Gldh) in a 10-μm-thick cryostat section. Gldh is demonstrable almost only in astrocytic profiles forming fibers and puncta. The highest density of profiles is demonstrable in the lacunosum-moleculare layer (lm) of the hippocampus proper and very low density in the lucidum layer (lu). $\times$ 40. Inset: An astrocyte that is stained for Gldh in its perikaryon and labeled with GFAP antiserum in its processes. The dark zone (arrow) marks the front of the Gldh incubation medium. $\times$ 600.

Fig. 5. Demonstration of phosphate-activated glutaminase (PAG) in a 10-μm-thick cryostat section. PAG is observed in all regions of the hippocampus. A strong reaction is detected in the layers of CA2/3 (with the exception of the region of mossy fiber boutons) and in the inner one-third of the molecular layer (m) of the fascia dentata and a preferentially weak reaction in the lacunosum-moleculare layer (lm) of CA1. $\times$ 40.

Furthermore, it should be mentioned that astrocytic Gldh could be involved in the metabolism not only of neuronally released Glu as neurotransmitter but also of Glu produced in the degradation of GABA. It is well established that astrocytic GABA uptake is of pysiological significance for the inactivation of GABA (for references, see Schousboe and Hertz, 1983). By the action of astrocytic GABA transaminase GABA is metabolized to succinic semialdehyde and Glu, which can be converted by Gldh. It is noteworthy that the overall reaction pattern of GABA transaminase in the hippocampus (Kugler, 1988a) matches partly the Gldh reaction pattern.

Phosphate-Activated Glutaminase

PAG, the major glutamine-degrading enzyme in the brain, is localized in mitochondria and leads to Glu formation (Kvamme, 1984). Glutamine is a precursor of the transmitter Glu as well as of GABA (for references, see Shank and Campbell, 1982; Schousboe and Hertz, 1983; Fonnum, 1984). PAG has been detected in neurons and astrocytes and appears to be associated with GABAergic nerve terminals rather than with glutamatergic terminals (for references, see Schousboe and Hertz, 1983).

In a recent enzyme histochemical study different levels of PAG were shown to be present in all regions of the rat hippocampus (Fig. 5) (Kugler, 1988a). With the exception of the lucidum layer, a strong reaction is observed in the layers of the regio inferior and in the inner one-third of the dentate gyrus molecular layer. Lower activities have been detected in the other hippocampal regions, especially in the lacunosum-moleculare layer of CA1 and in the localization of mossy fiber boutons. PAG is also present in astrocytes (Kugler, 1988a).

With respect to the production of releasable Glu, cAT (see above) seems to be a more likely candidate than PAG regarding the topochemistry of both enzymes. However, the contribution of these enzymes to the amino acid transmitter pool in the hippocampus should be investigated by studying the loss of enzyme activities following lesion of glutamatergic and aspartatergic pathways.

Ornithine Aminotransferase

OT catalyzes the transfer of the amino group of ornithine to α-ketoglutarate, producing Glu and glutamic semialdehyde. Recently, we adapted an enzyme histochemical procedure (unpublished results) that allows the demonstration of OT. On the whole, the demonstrable activities in the hippocampus were low. However, some regions of the hippocampus showed elevated activities, i.e. the dentate gyrus molecular layer (particularly the inner and outer one-thirds) and the lacunosum-moleculare layer of the hippocampus proper (Fig. 6). Using various incubation conditions, we have shown that OT is localized in both neuronal structures and astrocytes.

Uptake and metabolic studies (Shank and Campbell, 1984) on cellular fractions of mouse cerebellum have shown that ornithine may serve as a metabolic precursor of the transmitter pool of Glu and possibly GABA (see also Yoneda

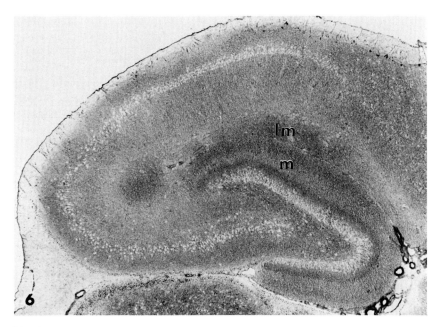

Fig. 6.   Demonstration of ornithine aminotransferase (OT) in a 10-μm-thick section. Low OT activities are detected in most regions of the hippocampus. Higher activities are demonstrable preferentially in the lacunosum-moleculare layer (lm) of CA1/3 and in the molecular layer (m) of the fascia dentata. × 40.

et al., 1982). However, the slow conversion, at least in cellular fractions of mouse cerebellum, indicates that Glu is synthesized de novo in terminals more readily from α-ketoglutarate and glutamine than from ornithine (Shank and Campbell, 1984). From our topochemical view OT could be one of the enzymes in the rat hippocampus producing neurotransmitter Glu in glutamatergic regions, but probably with low activities. Using the histochemical procedure for the demonstration of OT we have also shown other amino acid aminotransferase (unpublished results); of these, tyrosine and leucine aminotransferases should be mentioned, which displayed almost the same hippocampal reaction pattern as OT, but with somewhat lower activities.

It is important to note that the brain has an efficient uptake system for many of the circulating amino acids (for references, see Cooper and Meister, 1985). It has been shown that, following an intravenous injection of [^{14}C]leucine, label in rat brain is rapidly converted to a number of metabolites, most notably Glu (for references, see Cooper and Meister, 1985). Therefore, the sum of activities of different aminotransferases could contribute to the replenishment of the Glu transmitter pool.

CONCLUSIONS

Catalytic enzyme histochemistry together with improved detection methods could be a valuable tool for studying the enzymes of amino acid metabolism in situ and showing the precise topography of Glu- or Asp-metabolizing enzymes in presumed glutamatergic or aspartatergic regions of the hippocampus. These topochemical results might provide evidence for the participation of specific enzymes in the production of releasable Glu/Asp and in the glial or neuronal metabolism of these amino acids. Concerning the topochemistry of Glu/Asp-metabolizing enzymes, there are some indications that cAT plays an important role in the production of releasable Glu, whereas other aminotransferases (e.g. OT) are of minor importance. The contribution of these enzymes and of PAG to the amino acid transmitter pool in the hippocampus should be investigated by quantitative histochemical methods, studying the loss of enzyme activities following lesions of glutamatergic and aspartatergic pathways.

From the described topochemistry, it is apparent that astrocytes play an active role in the control of the neurotransmission process mediated by glutamate and GABA (cf. Schousboe and Hertz, 1983). With the exception of AT, all other Glu-metabolizing enzymes (i.e. PAG, ornithine, leucine, and tyrosine transaminases) can be demonstrated not only in neuronal structures but also differentially in astrocytes, whereas Gldh is almost exclusively found in astrocytes. Especially Gldh, which is heterogeneously distributed in astrocyes, should be included in further studies to show its functional significance in the metabolism of neuronally released Glu and the Glu produced by the degradation of GABA and also its possible role for Glu synthesis, which has been suggested by pharmacohistochemical experiments with gabaculine (Kugler, 1988a).

ACKNOWLEDGMENTS

This study was supported by the Deutsche Forschungsgemeinschaft (Ku 541/2-1).

REFERENCES

Altschuler, R.A., D.T. Monaghan, W.G. Haser, R.J. Wenthold, N.P. Curthoys, and W.C. Cotman (1985) Immunocytochemical localization of glutaminase-like and aspartate aminotransferase-like immunoreactivities in the rat and guinea pig hippocampus. Brain Res. 330:225–233.

Altschuler, R.A., J.L. Mosinger, G.G. Harmison, M.H. Parakkal, and R.J. Wenthold (1982) Aspartate aminotransferase-like immunoreactivity as a marker for aspartate/glutamate in guinea pig photoreceptors. Nature 298:657–659.

Aoki, C., T.A. Milner, K.-T.R. Sheu, J.P. Blass, and V.M. Pickel (1987) Regional distribution of astrocytes with intense immunoreactivity for glutamate dehydrogenase in rat brain: Implications for neuron–glia interactions in glutamate transmission. J. Neurosci. 7:2214–2231.

Berl, S., and D.D. Clarke (1978) Metabolic compartmentation of the glutamate–glutamine system. Glial contribution. In F. Fonnum (ed): Amino Acids as Chemical Transmitters. New York: Plenum Press, pp. 691–708.

Bignami, A., L.F. Eng, D. Dahl, and C.T. Uyeda (1972) Localization of the glial fibrillary acidic protein in astrocytes by immunofluorescence. Brain Res. 43:429–435.

Cooper, A.J.L., and A. Meister (1985) Metabolic significance of transamination. In P. Christen and D.E. Metzler (eds): Transaminases. Biochemistry, Vol. 2. New York: John Wiley & Sons, pp. 534–586.

Cotman, C.W., J.A. Flatman, A.H. Ganong, and M.N. Perkins (1986) Effects of excitatory amino acid antagonists on evoked and spontaneous excitatory potentials in guinea-pig hippocampus. J. Physiol. [Lond.] 378:403–415.

Crunelli, V., S. Forda, and J.S. Kelly (1983) Blockade of amino acid-induced depolarizations and inhibition of excitatory postsynaptic potentials in rat dentate gyrus. J. Physiol. [Lond.] 341:627–640.

Dennis, S.C., and J.B. Clark (1977) The pathway of glutamate metabolism in rat brain mitochondria. Biochem. J. 168:521–527.

Fonnum, F. (1984) Glutamate: A neurotransmitter in mammalian brain. J. Neurochem. 42:1–11.

Fonnum, F., R. Lund-Karlsen, D. Malthe-Sørensen, K.K. Skrede, and I. Walaas (1979) Localization of neurotransmitters, particularly glutamate, in hippocampus, septum, nucleus accumbens and superior colliculus. Prog. Brain Res. 51:167–191.

Halpain, S., C.M. Wieczorek, and T.C. Rainbow, (1984) Localization of L-glutamate receptors in rat brain by quantitative autoradiography. J. Neurosci. 4:2247–2258.

Kosaka, T., and K. Hama (1986) Three-dimensional structure of astrocytes in the rat dentate gyrus. J. Comp. Neurol. 249:242–260.

Kugler, P. (1988a) Enzyme histochemistry of the neurotransmitter metabolism. In M. Frotscher, P. Kugler, U. Misgeld, and K. Zilles (eds): Neurotransmission in the hippocampus. Adv. Anat. Embryol. Cell Biol. 111:40–60.

Kugler, P. (1988b) Quantitative enzyme histochemistry in the brain. Histochemistry 90:99–107.

Kugler, P. (1988c) Cytochemical demonstration of aspartate aminotransferase in the mossy-fibre system of the rat hippocampus. Histochemistry 87:623–625.

Kvamme, E. (1984) Enzymes of cerebral glutamine metabolism. In D. Häusinger and H. Sies (eds): Glutamine metabolism in mammalian tissues. Berlin: Springer, pp. 32–48.

Parli, J.A., D.A. Godfrey, and C.D. Ross (1985) Separate enzymatic assays for cytosolic and mitochondrial aspartate aminotransferase activities. Soc. Neurosci. Abstr. 11:107.

Ross, C.D., and D.A. Godfrey (1987) Distribution of activities of aspartate aminotransferase isoenzymes and malate dehydrogenase in guinea pig retinal layers. J. Histochem. Cytochem. 35:669–674.

Salganicoff, L., and E. de Robertis (1965) Subcellular distribution of the enzymes of the glutamic acid, glutamine and γ-amino-butyric acid cycles in rat brain. J. Neurochem. 12:287–309.

Schmidt, W., and G. Wolf (1987) Activity of aspartate aminotransferase in the hippocampal formation of the rat during post-natal development and after lesion of the hippocampal Schaffer's collaterals: A quantitative histochemical study. Neurochem. Int. 11:39–147.

Schousboe, A., and L. Hertz (1983) Regulation of glutamatergic and GABAergic neuronal activity by astroglial cells. In N.N. Osborne (eds): Dale's Principle and Communication Between Neurons. Oxford: Pergamon Press, pp. 113–141.

Shank, R.P., and G.L.M. Campbell (1982) Glutamine and alpha-ketoglutarate uptake and metabolism by nerve terminal enriched material from mouse cerebellum. Neurochem. Res. 7:601–616.

Shank, R.P., and G.L.M. Campbell (1984) Amino acid uptake, content, and metabolism by neuronal and glial enriched cellular fractions from mouse cerebellum. J. Neurosci. 4:58–69.

Storm-Mathisen, J. (1977) Glutamic acid and excitatory nerve endings: Reduction of glutamic acid uptake after axotomy. Brain Res. *120*:379–386.

Storm-Mathisen, J., and L.L. Iversen (1979) Uptake of [^{3}H]glutamic acid in excitatory nerve endings: Light and electron-microscopic observations in the hippocampal formation of the rat. Neuroscience *4*:1237–1253.

Storm-Mathisen, J., A.K. Leknes, A.T. Bore, J.L. Vaaland, F., Edminson, F.-M.S. Haug, and O.P. Otterson (1983) First visualization of glutamate and GABA in neurons by immunocytochemistry. Nature *301*:517–519.

Taxt, T., and J. Storm-Mathisen (1979) Tentative localization of glutamergic and aspartergic nerve endings in brain. J. Physiol. [Paris] *75*:677–684.

White, W.F., J.V. Nadler, A. Hamberger, C.W. Cotman, and J.T. Cummins (1977) Glutamate as transmitter of hippocampal perforant path. Nature *270*:356–357.

Yoneda, Y., E. Roberts, and G.W. Dietz (1982) A new synaptosomal biosynthetic pathway of glutamate and GABA from ornithine and its negative feedback inhibition by GABA. J. Neurochem. *38*:1686–1694.

Zilles, K. (1988) Receptor autoradiography in the hippocampus of man and rat. In M. Frotscher, P. Kugler, U. Misgeld, and K. Zilles (eds): Neurotransmission in the hippocampus. Adv. Anat. Embryol. Cell Biol. 111:61–80.

The Hippocampus—New Vistas, pages 131–144
© 1989 Alan R. Liss, Inc.

9

Ontogenetic Variance of Substance P in the Human Hippocampus

MARINA DEL FIACCO AND MARINA QUARTU

Dipartimento di Citomorfologia, University of Cagliari, Cagliari, Italy

INTRODUCTION

Since the seminal work of Shute and Lewis using acetylcholinesterase histochemistry and choline acetyltransferase analysis (Shute and Lewis, 1961; Lewis and Shute, 1967; Lewis et al., 1967), great strides have been taken in recent years in the knowledge of the neurochemistry of hippocampal formation. Thus, both "classical" neurotransmitters and/or their metabolizing enzymes and a continuously growing list of more recently discovered neuroactive substances have been localized in this region in several animal species, including man. No attempt is made here to cover the extensive literature in this field. The reader is referred to Storm-Mathisen (1978) and Walaas (1983) and to appropriate chapters of this volume.

Immunohistochemical techniques, since their first introduction by Geffen and coworkers (1969), have proved powerful tools for the detection of chemically identified neurons (Cuello, 1978; Hökfelt et al., 1984; Roberts and Allen, 1986; Gibson and Polak, 1986). Their use in combination with a variety of experimental procedures, such as mechanic, electrolytic, or neurotoxic lesions, tracers and axonal flow blockers injection, and autoradiography (see Chan-Palay, 1983; Cuello et al., 1983; Skirboll and Hökfelt, 1983), abutted on the identification of transmitter-specific neurons and, in several cases, of their projection pathways and fields. Unfortunately, the inaccessibility of the human central nervous system to most of the experimental manipulations that can be carried out in laboratory animals represents a major hindrance to the achievement of a close representation of the dynamic in vivo processes. It is well known that in the adult tissue immunoreactivity for the neurotransmitters and their markers is restricted in most cases to preterminal and terminal networks and that blockers of the axonal transport are needed to produce accumulations of the antigen in the cell bodies up to levels detectable by immunocytochemistry (Dahlström, 1968; Hökfelt and Dahlström, 1971; Ljungdahl et al., 1978; Del Fiacco and Cuello, 1980: Del Fiacco et al., 1982). On the other hand, at the juvenile and particularly at the perinatal stages of ontogenesis, neuronal perikarya are often readily stained by the immunoreaction (Ljungdahl et al., 1978; Inagaki et al., 1982; Sakanaka et al., 1982; Gall et al., 1984). Moreover, areas populated by nerve fibers and terminals may show a different density of immunoreactive material with age; finally, neuronal perikarya are detectable in some regions only in the adult tissue (Del Fiacco et al., 1984, 1988). These findings suggest that the immunocytochemical analyses performed on human material from subjects at different ontogenetic stages may be complementary to each other.

A few years ago we started to study the immunohistochemical localization of substance P in the human nervous system. The undecapeptide substance P, discovered by von Euler and Gaddum (1931), is widely and unevenly distributed in both the central and peripheral nervous systems (Cuello and Kanazawa, 1978; Ljungdahl et al., 1978; Schultzberg, 1983). Its presence in different neuronal systems suggests its involvement in a variety of nervous functions (Nicoll et al., 1980). Abnormalities in the distribution of this peptide have been demonstrated in several neurological disorders (Kanazawa et al., 1977; Gale et al., 1978; Emson et al., 1980; Spokes, 1981; Pearson et al., 1982; Crystal and Davies, 1982; Mauborgue et al., 1983; Yates et al., 1983). In this chapter we will present the results obtained from studies on the localization of substance P-like immunoreactivity in the hippocampal formation and parahippocampal gyrus of human subjects at different ontogenetic stages. Autoptic specimens (30 h maximum postmortem delay) were examined by the indirect immunofluorescence technique of Coons and Kaplan (1950).

RESULTS
Fetus

The specimen at the earliest stage of ontogenetic development we could examine belonged to a fetus at the 4th month of gestation. It was at the beginning of the third stage as defined by Macchi (1951), when the subiculum-ammonic portion of the hippocampus and the fascia dentata are clearly delineated. In this specimen (Fig. 1), whereas numerous substance P-like immunoreactive structures were present in several diencephalic areas, only rare intensely immunoreactive beaded fibers in the entorhinal region (Fig. 2) and even more sporadic in the hippocampus proper were detectable.

Premature Newborn

In one premature newborn at the 25th week of gestation, two types of immunoreactive elements were present: neuronal perikarya and beaded fibers. The immunoreactivity present within positive cell bodies appeared in the form of tiny granules dispersed in the cytoplasm. Their density varied among the detectable cells so that a wide range in the intensity of labeling was appreciable at this stage. Immunoreactive perikarya were reliably found in the stratum oriens of the hippocampus proper, being somewhat more numerous in the CA1 sector, and in the hilus of the fascia dentata. While in the stratum oriens several immunoreactive perikarya showed an intense staining (Fig. 3), most of the positive cell bodies in the hilus of the fascia dentata were only weakly labeled (Fig. 4). The principal field of distribution of the beaded positive fibers was the stratum lacunosum-moleculare of the hippocampus proper. Such fibers, parallel to the long axis of the hippocampus, were abundant in sectors CA3 and CA2 (Fig. 5) and were rarely found in CA1. Extremely sporadic short tracts of beaded fibers were present in the molecular layer of the subiculum, in the alveus, and in the hilus of the fascia dentata, whereas no immunoreactive elements were detectable in the entorhinal cortex or in the granular and molecular layers of the fascia dentata.

Full-Term Newborn

In six specimens from full-term newborn subjects aged 2 to 11 days, the presence of immunoreactive perikarya was the most impressive feature. They were diffusely disseminated in the stratum oriens of the hippocampus proper, being somewhat more numerous in the CA1 sector (Figs. 6, 7). Toward the boundary between the CA1 and the subiculum, the layer populated by positive neurons became gradually wider. Many of the perikarya appeared spindle-shaped, with proximal branches filled with immunoreactive material and parallel to the fibers of the alveus. Irregularly shaped, triangular, or multipolar neurons were also frequently found. Several of them seemed to merge into the pyramidal layer. In this layer, scattered positive cell bodies were occasionally detectable, particularly in the dorsal CA1 and in the CA2 and CA3 sectors. Sector CA4, within the hilus of the fascia dentata, was densely populated by substance P-containing neurons (Fig. 8). Oval, pear-shaped, fusiform triangular, or multipolar perikarya could be easily identified. Although distributed throughout the polymorphic layer, they appeared to be somewhat more frequently located in its peripheral part, facing the stratum granulare of the fascia dentata. Very occasionally, labeled cell bodies were detected in other layers of the hippocampal formation, such as strata radiatum and moleculare of the hippocampus proper and stratum moleculare of the fascia dentata.

Although less numerous than in the hippocampal formation, immunoreactive perikarya were also frequently found in the parahippocampal gyrus. The population of positive cell bodies present in the stratum oriens of the CA1 sector extended to the deep cortical layers of the subicular complex. Scattered neurons were also labeled in the superficial layers of the subiculum. In the entorhinal area positive cell bodies were sparse in the deep cortical layers and even more deeply in the field of the white matter.

Beaded fibers and tubule-like and dot-like elements were present at these perinatal stages. In the hippocampus proper, the alveus showed only sporadic beaded fibers at its boundary with the stratum oriens. A scanty punctate fluorescence was homogeneously distributed in the stratum pyramidale (Fig. 9). Short tracts of intensely immunoreactive neuronal processes were abundant in sector CA4. Strata radiatum, lacunosum, and moleculare showed a dot-like immunoreaction of progressively increasing density. As observed in the new-

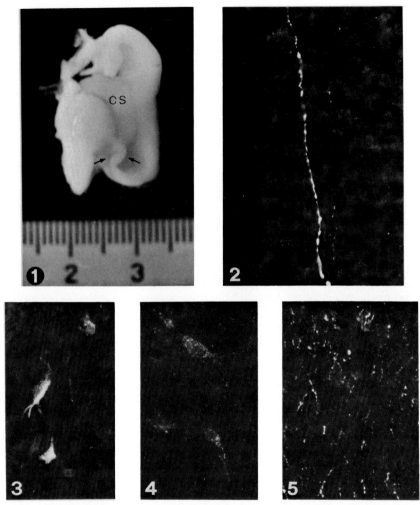

Fig. 1. Fetus, 4th month of gestation. Posterior view of frontal section of the right half of the brain. CS, corpus striatum. Arrows indicate the hippocampal formation.

Fig. 2. Fetus, 4th month of gestation. Strongly immunofluorescent beaded fiber in the entorhinal cortex. ×260.

Fig. 3. Premature newborn, 25 weeks of gestation. Immunoreactive cell bodies in the stratum oriens of the CA1 sector of the hippocampus proper. ×220.

Fig. 4. Premature newborn, 25 weeks of gestation. Weak immunofluorescence in the form of sparse granules in the neuronal perikarya of the hilus of the fascia dentata. ×350.

Fig. 5. Premature newborn, 25 weeks of gestation. Strongly immunofluorescent beaded fibers in the stratum lacunosum-moleculare of the CA2 sector of the hippocampus proper. ×220.

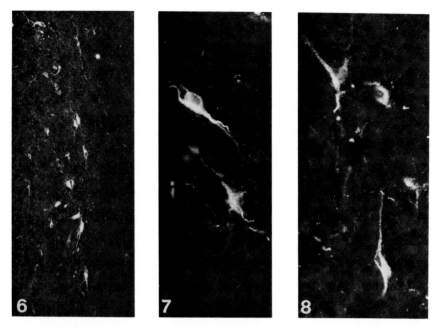

Fig. 6.   Full-term 5-day-old newborn. Numerous immunoreactive perikarya in the stratum oriens of the CA1 sector of the hippocampus proper. ×85.

Fig. 7.   Full-term 5-day-old newborn. Two intensely immunofluorescent cell bodies and their proximal branches in the stratum oriens of the CA1 sector of the hippocampus proper. ×220.

Fig. 8.   Full-term 3-day-old newborn. Immunoreactive perikarya in the hilus of the fascia dentata. ×200.

born at the 25th week of gestation, strongly fluorescent beaded fibers parallel to the long axis of the hippocampus were present in the stratum moleculare, with decreasing density from CA3 toward CA1. The stratum granulare of the fascia dentata was negative to the immunoreaction. The stratum moleculare, on the contrary, showed a homogeneously dispersed, finely dot-like fluorescence, rare long beaded fibers, and thicker tubular neuronal processes (Fig. 10). Extremely sporadic varicose fibers were seen in the fimbria. A scanty dot-like immunoreaction and scattered tracts of fibers were distributed over the parahippocampal cortical layers.

In one specimen from a 45-day-old newborn, the overall pattern of distribution of the immunoreactivity was similar to that described above. However, two main differences must be pointed out: 1) although present in the fields previously indicated, the immunoreactive perikarya were detected in smaller number; and 2) a dot-like immunoreactivity of low density was present over the stratum granulare of the fascia dentata.

Adult

The adult specimens examined were obtained from eight subjects aged 27 to 72 years. Compared with the distribution pattern of the substance P-like immunoreactive material observed in the newborn tissue, in the adult hippocampal formation and parahippocampal gyrus the immunoreactive cell bodies were by far less numerous, whereas positive nerve fibers and terminals appeared more precisely organized and, in some fields, more densely packed.

In the hippocampus proper, substance P-containing perikarya were present in the stratum oriens, being again more numerous in sector CA1; rare immunoreactive neurons were detected in sectors CA1, CA2, and CA3 of the stratum pyramidale, more frequently located among the deep rows of pyramidal cells facing the stratum oriens. Numerous cell bodies of various sizes and shapes were labeled in the hilus of the fascia dentata. Many of them showed a peripheral location close to the stratum granulare. Several immunoreactive neurons were seen in the multiform layer of the parahippocampal cortex.

Alveus, stratum oriens, and strata radiatum, lacunosum, and moleculare of the adult hippocampus proper showed a distribution pattern of dot- and fiber-like specific fluorescence not dissimilar to that seen in the newborn tissue. On the contrary, remarkable differences existed at the level of the stratum pyramidale and stratum moleculare of the fascia dentata. The stratum pyramidale showed a finely punctate immunoreaction scantily dispersed in the CA1 sector. The density of the specific reaction increased abruptly in the CA2 sector, where a plexus of intensely fluorescent fibers with large varicosities appeared interspersed among the neuronal cell bodies (Fig. 11). Such fibers were also present in CA3 and CA4 sectors, although their density decreased progressively toward the hilus of the fascia dentata.

In the fascia dentata a punctate immunoreactivity was densely packed in the superficial three-fourths of the stratum moleculare (Fig. 12). The deeper one-fourth of this layer was poorly immunoreactive. Varicose fluorescent fibers could be followed radially crossing this part of the layer. In the specimens from elderly subjects, the superficial edge of the stratum granulare was bordered by a rich plexus of substance P-positive nerve fibers and terminals, whereas the rest of the layer was negative. However, in two specimens from subjects aged 27 and 35 years, dot- and fiber-like elements were present in the full depth of the layer. A light punctate immunoreactivity was localized over the molecular layer of the parahippocampal cortex.

The results of this study, schematically represented in Figure 13, show the presence of numerous perikarya in the human hippocampal formation and parahippocampal cortex. Substance P-containing neuronal structures begin to appear in the human hippocampal formation during fetal life. A few intensely immunoreactive perikarya are already evident at the 25th week of gestation (Fig. 13A). Moreover, the dispersed granular immunoreactive material within numerous weakly fuorescent cell bodies indicates that, although perhaps in quantity just sufficient to allow detection by the technique adopted, the antigen is being produced in them. However, besides the strongly immunoreactive long

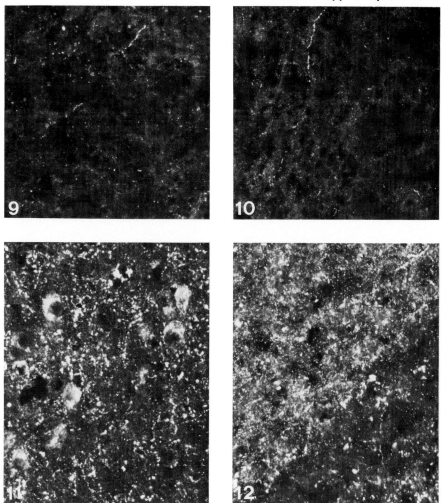

Fig. 9.   Full-term 5-day-old newborn. Scanty punctate immunoreactivity and sporadic beaded fibers in the pyramidal layer of CA2 sector of the hippocampus proper. × 225.

Fig. 10.   Full-term 5-day-old newborn. Scanty dot-like immunoreactivity and rare beaded fibers in the stratum moleculare of the fascia dentata. × 220.

Fig. 11.   Sample from a 63-year-old adult. Dense plexus of strongly immunoreactive beaded fibers and punctate elements in the pyramidal layer of the CA2 sector of the hippocampus proper. The fluorescence over the cell bodies is nonspecific. × 220.

Fig. 12.   Sample from a 63-year-old adult. Dense punctate immunoreactivity in the superficial part and poor immunoreactivity in the deep one-fourth of the stratum moleculare of the fascia dentata. × 220.

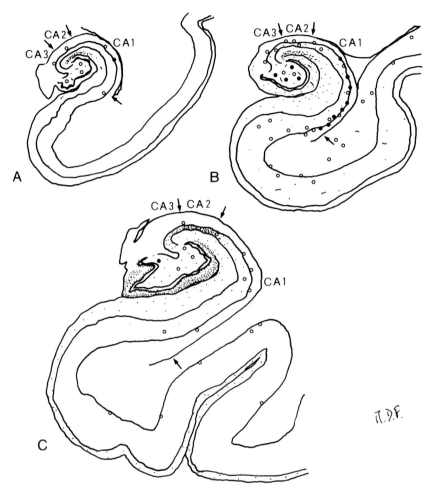

Fig. 13.   Distribution of substance P-like immunoreactivity in the human hippocampal formation and parahippocampal gyrus. Schematic diagrams were obtained from cresyl violet coronal sections. **A:** Premature newborn, 25 weeks of gestation; **B:** full-term newborn; **C:** adult. Dots and short lines indicate immunoreactive nerve fibers and terminals; open circles represent one to three perikarya; solid circles represent 4 to 15 perikarya. Arrows indicate boundaries between subiculum and subfields CA1, CA2, and CA3 of Ammon's horn. ×5.

varicose fibers well confined to the hippocampal superficial layers, all other fields are almost completely devoid of immunoreactive material at this stage. The numbers and morphological varieties of immunoreactive structures increase successively. Among the ontogenetic stages we could examine, the number of substance P-containing perikarya reaches a peak during the first days after birth (Fig. 13B). In this period positive cell bodies are present also in the parahippocampal gyrus. Thin filamentous and punctate elements, probably representing preterminal and terminal nerve processes (Ljungdahl et al., 1978), also appear at this stage. However, they seem lightly and homogeneously dispersed and, when compared with the distribution pattern observed at later stages, poorly organized. A remarkable decrease in the number of labeled cell bodies occurs at successive stages. This phenomenon is already evident in the specimen at postnatal day 45, although such a statement derived from a single observation requires confirmation from a greater number of cases. The number of immunoreactive neurons is by far smaller in the adult (Fig. 13C) than in the newborn tissue. Only in the former, on the other hand, do densely packed varicose fibers and dot-like structures characterize a few well-defined fields of the hippocampal formation (cf. Figs. 9 and 11 and Figs. 10 and 12).

DISCUSSION

Numerous ontogenetic studies point out the existence of differences in the distribution of a variety of neuroactive substances at different stages in both the experimental animals (Olson and Seiger, 1972; Emson et al., 1979; Pátey et al., 1980; McGregor et al., 1982; Senba et al., 1982; Inagaki et al., 1982; Sakanaka et al., 1982; Gall et al., 1984; Hayashi and Oshima, 1986) and man (Chayvialle et al., 1980; Charnay et al., 1983, 1985; Del Fiacco et al., 1984, 1987, 1988; Paulin et al., 1986), often suggesting that such a variance might reflect changes in their functional roles. The early ontogenetic presence in conspicuous amounts of some neuropeptides suggests their involvement in brain development (McGregor et al., 1982; Zagon et al., 1985). Substance P, in particular, has been demonstrated to possess neurotrophic and growth-stimulatory effects (Narumi and Fujita, 1978; Nakai and Kasamatsu, 1984) and to prevent the 6-hydroxy-dopamine-induced degeneration of developing noradrenergic neurons (Jonsson and Hallman, 1982). Moreover, Black et al. (1984) have shown that neurotransmitter expression and metabolism may vary not only during development but also through adulthood.

Morphological and biochemical studies on human postmortem brain tissue have shown that alterations in neurotransmitters and their metabolizing enzymes occur in a number of neurological or psychiatric diseases (see Vinken and Bruyn, 1977; Spokes, 1981; Coyle et al., 1983; Nemeroff et al., 1983; Sagar et al., 1984; Martin and Barchas, 1986; Chan-Palay et al., 1985, 1986), thus stressing the importance of a detailed knowledge of the distribution and cellular localization of the neuroactive substances in the human brain. The hippocampus appears in many diseases of the nervous system as a region of selective vulnerability for degenerative phenomena. A cell loss caused by anoxic damage in the so-called Sommer's sector is common in brains from epileptic patients (Meyer, 1957). Degenerative changes in senile dementia and Alzheimer's disease (Hyman et al., 1984) also occur in this region. Indeed, recent studies have shown a severe loss of somatostatin and neuropeptide Y in the human hippocampus in cases of Alzheimer-type dementia (Chan-Palay et al., 1986; Chan-Palay, 1987). Moreover, infant pathology demonstrates that the immature brain differs significantly from the adult one with respect to the reactivity against the action of various noxious agents. This fact emphasizes the need for chemoarchitectonic studies of the hippocampal region during morphological and functional development of the brain. Immunocytochemical studies of neurotransmitter-specific neuronal systems during ontogenesis, combined with analysis of cell proliferation and differentiation, synaptogenesis, regulation of neurotransmitter production by in situ hybridization, and specific receptors appearance, might elucidate their role in development and shed light on their physiological significance at different ontogenetic stages.

SUMMARY

The distribution of substance P-like immunoreactive structures was studied in specimens of the hippocampal formation and parahippocampal gyrus from fetal, newborn and adult human brains. By indirect immunofluorescence, the presence of the antigen was revealed within neuronal perikarya, beaded fibers, and punctate nerve terminals. Such elements show a different distribution and density at different ontogenetic stages. They are already present during fetal life. However, neuronal perikarya are particularly abundant during the perinatal stages and decrease in number successively. On the contrary, nerve fibers and terminals appear more precisely organized and, in some areas, more densely packed in the adult brain. Such variance might reflect differences in the functional role of the peptide. Ontogenetic analysis of the appearance, presence, and cellular distribution of the neuropeptide is helpful in drawing a map of the neuropeptide's localization and might shed light on its functional significance at different stages.

ACKNOWLEDGMENTS

This work was supported by grants from the Ministero della Pubblica Istruzione and the Consiglio Nazionale delle Ricerche.

REFERENCES

Black, I.B., J.E. Adler, C.F. Dreyfus, G.M. Jonakait, D.M. Katz, E.F. LaGamma, and K.M. Markey (1984) Neurotransmitter plasticity at the molecular level. Science *225:*1266–1270.

Chan-Palay, V. (1983) Combined immunohistochemistry and autoradiography. In A.C. Cuello (eds): Immunohistochemistry. New York: John Wiley & Sons, pp. 449–464.

Chan-Palay, V. (1987) Somatostatin immunoreactive neurons in the human hippocampus and cortex shown by immunogold/silver on Vibratome sections: Coexistence with neuropeptide Y neurons and effects in Alzheimer-type dementia. J. Comp. Neurol. *260:*201–223.

Chan-Palay, V., W. Lang, V. Haesler, C. Köhler, and G. Ysargil (1986) Distribution of hippocampal neurons and axons immunoreactive with antisera against neuropeptide Y in Alzheimer's-type dementia. J. Comp. Neurol. *248:* 376–394.

Chan-Palay, V., W. Lang, Y.S. Allen, U. Haesler, and J.M. Polak (1985) Cortical neurons immunoreactive with antisera against neuropeptide Y are altered in Alzheimer's type dementia. J. Comp. Neurol. *238:*390–400.

Charnay, Y., J.-A. Chayvialle, S.I. Said, and P.M. Dubois (1985) Localization of vasoactive intestinal peptide immunoreactivity in human foetus and newborn infant spinal cord. Neuroscience 14:195–205.

Charnay, Y., C. Paulin, J.A. Chayvialle, and P.M. Dubois (1983) Distribution of substance P-like immunoreactivity in the spinal cord and dorsal root ganglia of the human foetus and infant. Neuroscience 10:41–55.

Chayvialle, J.A., C. Paulin, P.M. Dubois, F. Descos, and M.P. Dubois (1980) Ontogeny of somatostatin in the human gastrointestinal tract, endocrine pancreas and hypothalamus. Acta Endocrinol. [Kbhn] 94:1–10.

Coons, A.H., and M.H. Kaplan (1950) Localization of antigens in tissue cells. II. Improvements in a method for the detection of antigen by means of fluorescent antibody. J. Exp. Med. 91:1–9.

Coyle, J.T., D.L. Price, and M.R. DeLong (1983) Alzheimer's disease: A disorder of cortical cholinergic innervation. Science 219:1184–1190.

Crystal, H.A., and P. Davies (1982) Cortical substance P-like immunoreactivity in cases of Alzheimer's disease and senile dementia of the Alzheimer type. J. Neurochem. 38: 1781–1784.

Cuello, A.C. (1978) Immunocytochemical studies of the distribution of neurotransmitters and related substances in CNS. In L.L. Iversen, S.D. Iversen, and S.H. Snyder (eds): Handbook of Psychopharmacology, Vol. 9. New York: Plenum Press, pp. 69–137.

Cuello, A.C., M. Del Fiacco-Lampis, and G. Paxinos (1983) Combined immunohistochemistry with stereotaxic lesions. In A.C. Cuello (ed): Immunohistochemistry. New York: John Wiley & Sons, pp. 477–496.

Cuello, A.C., and I. Kanazawa (1978) The distribution of substance P immunoreactive fibers in the rat central nervous system. J. Comp. Neurol. 178:129–156.

Dahlström, A. (1968) Effect of colchicine on transport of amine storage granules in sympathetic nerves of rat. Eur. J. Pharmacol. 5:111–112.

Del Fiacco, M., and A.C. Cuello (1980) Substance P- and enkephalin-containing neurones in the rat trigeminal system. Neuroscience 5:803–815.

Del Fiacco, M., M.L. Dessi, and M.C. Levanti (1984) Topographical localization of substance P in the human post-mortem brainstem. An immunohistochemical study in the newborn and adult tissue. Neuroscience 12:591–611.

Del Fiacco, M., G. Paxinos, and A.C. Cuello (1982) Neostriatal enkephalin-immunoreactive neurones project to the globus pallidus. Brain Res. 231:1–17.

Del Fiacco, M., M.T. Perra, M. Quartu, M.D. Rosa, G. Zucca, and M.C. Levanti (1988) Evidence for the presence of substance P-like immunoreactivity in the human cerebellum. Brain Res. 446:173–177.

Emson, P.C., A. Arregui, V. Clement-Jones, B.E.B. Sandberg, and M. Rossor (1980) Regional distribution of methionine-enkephalin- and substance P-like immunoreactivity in normal human brain and in Huntington's disease. Brain Res. 119: 147–160.

Emson, P.C., R.T.F. Gilbert, I. Loren, J. Fahrenkrug, F. Sundler, and O.B. Schaffalitzky de Muckadell (1979) Development of vasoactive intestinal polypeptide (VIP) containing neurones in the rat brain. Brain Res. 177:437–444.

Gale, J.S., E.D. Bird, E.G. Spokes, L.L. Iversen, and T. Jessell (1978) Human brain substance P: Distribution in controls and Huntington's chorea. J. Neurochem. 30:633–634.

Gall, C., N. Brecha, K.-J. Chang, and H.J. Karten (1984) Ontogeny of enkephalin-like immunoreactivity in the rat hippocampus. Neuroscience 11:359–380.

Geffen, L.B., B.G. Livett, and R.A. Rush (1969) Immunohistochemical localization of protein components of catecholamine storage vesicles. J. Physiol. [Lond.] 204:593–605.

Gibson, S.J., and J.M. Polak (1986) Neurochemistry of the spinal cord. In J.M. Polak and S. van Noorden (eds): Immunocytochemistry Modern Methods and Applications. Bristol: John Wright & Sons Ltd, pp. 360–389.

Hayashi, M., and K. Oşhima (1986) Neuropeptides in cerebral cortex of macaque monkey *(Macaca fuscata fuscata):* Regional distribution and ontogeny. Brain Res. *364:* 360–368.

Hökfelt, T., and A. Dahlström (1971) Effect of two mitosis inhibitors (colchicine and vinblastine) on the distribution and axonal transport of noradrenaline storage particles, studied by fluorescence and electron microscopy. Z. Zellforsch. Mikrosk. Anat. *119:*460–482.

Hökfelt, T., O. Johansson, and M. Goldstein (1984) Chemical anatomy of the brain. Science *225:*1326–1334.

Hyman, B.T., G.W. van Hoesen, A.R. Damasio, and C.L. Barnes (1984) Alzheimer's disease: Cell-specific pathology isolates the hippocampal formation. Science *225:* 1168–1170.

Inagaki, S., M. Sakanaka, S. Shiosaka, E. Senba, K. Takatsuki, H. Takagi, Y. Kawai, H. Minigawa, and M. Tohyama (1982) Ontogeny of substance P-containing neuron system of the rat: Immunohistochemical analysis. I. Forebrain and upper brain stem. Neuroscience *7:*251–277.

Jonsson, G., and H. Hallman (1982) Substance P modifies the 6-hydroxydopamine induced alteration of postnatal development of central noradrenaline neurons. Neuroscience *7:* 2909–2918.

Kanazawa, I., E. Bird, R. O'Connell, and D. Powell (1977) Evidence for a decrease in substance P content of substantia nigra in Huntington's chorea. Brain Res. *120:*387–392.

Lewis, P.R., and C.C.D. Shute (1967) The cholinergic limbic system: Projection to the hippocampal formation, medial cortex, nuclei of the ascending cholinergic reticular system, and the subfornical organ and supraoptic crest. Brain *90:*521–540.

Lewis, P.R., C.C.D. Shute, and A. Silver (1967) Confirmation of choline acetylase analyses of a massive cholinergic innervation to the rat hippocampus. J. Physiol. [Lond.] *191:*215–224.

Ljungdhal, Å., T. Hökfelt, and G. Nilsson (1978) Distribution of substance P-like immunoreactivity in the central nervous system of the rat. I. Cell bodies and nerve terminals. Neuroscience *3:*861–943.

Macchi, G. (1951) The ontogenetic development of the telencephalon in man. J. Comp. Neurol. *95:*245–305.

Martin, J.B., and J.D. Barchas (eds) (1986) Neuropeptides in Neurologic and Psychiatric Disease. New York: Raven Press.

Mauborgue, A., F. Javoy-Agid, J.C. Legrand, Y. Agid, and F. Cesselin (1983) Decrease of substance P immunoreactivity in the substantia nigra and pallidum of parkinsonian brains. Brain Res. *268:*167–170.

McGregor, G.P., P.L. Woodhams, D.J. O'Shaughnessy, M.A. Ghatei, J.M. Polak, and S.R. Bloom (1982) Developmental changes in bombesin, substance P, somatostatin and vasoactive intestinal polypeptide in the rat brain. Neurosci. Lett. *28:* 21–27.

Meyer, A. (1957) Hippocampal lesions in epilepsy. In D. Williams (ed): Modern Trends in Neurology. London: Butterworths, pp. 301–306.

Nakai, K., and T. Kasamatsu (1984) Accelerated regeneration of central catecholamine fibres in cat occipital cortex: Effects of substance P. Brain Res. *323:*374–379.

Narumi, S., and T. Fujita (1978) Stimulatory effects of substance P and nerve growth factor (NGF) on neurite outgrowth in embryonic chick dorsal root ganglia. Neuropharmacology *17*:73–76.

Nemeroff, C.B., W.W. Youngblood, P.J. Manberg, A.J. Prange, and J.S. Kizer (1983) Regional brain concentrations of neuropeptides in Huntington's chorea and schizophrenia. Science *221*:972–975.

Nicoll, R.A., C. Schenker, and S.E. Leeman (1980) Substance P as a transmitter candidate. Annu. Rev. Neurosci. *3*:227–268.

Nieuwenhuys, R. (1985) Chemoarchitecture of the Brain. Berlin: Springer-Verlag.

Olson, L., and A. Seiger (1972) Early ontogeny of central monoamine neurons in the rat: Fluorescence histochemical observations. Z. Anat. EntwGesch. *137*:301–316.

Pátey, G., S. de la Baume, C. Gros, and J.C. Schwartz (1980) Ontogenesis of enkephalinergic systems in rat brain: Postnatal changes in enkephalin levels, receptors and degrading enzyme activities. Life Sci. *27*:245–252.

Paulin, C., Y. Charnay, J.A. Chayvialle, S. Danière and P.M. Dubois (1986) Ontogeny of substance P in the digestive tract, spinal cord and hypothalamus of the human foetus. Regul. Pept. *14*:145–153.

Pearson, J., L. Brandeis, and A.C. Cuello (1982) Depletion of substance P-containing axons in substantia gelatinosa of patients with diminished pain sensitivity. Nature *295*:61–63.

Roberts, G.W., and Y.S. Allen (1986) Immunocytochemistry of brain neuropeptides. In J.M. Polak and S. van Noorden (eds): Immunocytochemistry: Modern Methods and Applications. Bristol: John Wright & Sons Ltd, pp. 349–359.

Sagar, S.M., M.F. Beal, P.E. Marshall, D.M. Landis, and J.B. Martin (1984) Implication of neuropeptides in neurological diseases. Peptides [Suppl. 1] *5*:255–262.

Sakanaka, M., S. Inagaki, S. Shiosaka, E. Senba, H. Takagi, K. Takatsuki, Y. Kawai, H. Iida, Y. Hara, and M. Tohyama (1982) Ontogeny of substance P-containing neuron system of the rat: Immunohistochemical analysis. II. Lower brain stem. Neuroscience *7*:1097–1126.

Schultzberg, M. (1983) The peripheral nervous system. In P.C. Emson (ed): Chemical Neuroanatomy. New York: Raven Press, pp. 1–51.

Senba, E., S. Shiosaka, Y. Hara, S. Inagaki, M. Sakanaka, K. Takatsuki, Y. Kawai, and M. Tohyama (1982) Ontogeny of the peptidergic system in the rat spinal cord: Immunohistochemical analysis. J. Comp. Neurol. *208*:54–66.

Shute, C.C.D., and P.R. Lewis (1961) The use of cholinesterase techniques combined with operative procedures to follow nervous pathways in the brain. In: Histochemistry of cholinesterase: Symposium, Basel 1960. Bibl. Anat. *2*:34–49.

Skirboll, L., and T. Hökfelt (1983) Transmitter specific mapping of neuronal pathways by immunohistochemistry combined with fluorescent dyes. In A.C. Cuello (ed): Immunohistochemistry. New York: John Wiley & Sons, pp. 465–476.

Spokes, E.G.S. (1981) The neurochemistry of Huntington's chorea. TINS *4*:115–118.

Storm-Mathisen, J. (1978) Localization of putative transmitters in the hippocampal formation. With a note on the connections to septum and hypothalamus. In: Functions of the Septo-Hippocampal System. Ciba Foundation Symposium 58 (New Series). Amsterdam: Elsevier Excerpta Medica, pp. 49–79.

Vinken, P.J., and G.E. Bruyn (eds) (1977) Metabolic and Deficiency Diseases of the Nervous System. Handbook of Clinical Neurology, Vol. 19. Amsterdam: Elsevier.

von Euler, U.S., and J.H.G. Gaddum (1931) An unidentified depressor substance in certain tissue extracts. J. Physiol. [Lond.] *72*:74–87.

Walaas, I. (1983) The hippocampus. In P.C. Emson (ed): Chemical Neuroanatomy. New York: Raven Press, pp. 337–358.

Yates, C.M., A.J. Harmar, R. Rosie, J. Sheward, G. Sanchez de Levy, J. Simpson, A.F.J. Maloney, A. Gordon, and G. Fink (1983) Thyrotropin-releasing hormone, luteinizing hormone-releasing hormone and substance P-immunoreactivity in post-mortem brain from cases of Alzheimer-type dementia and Down's syndrome. Brain Res. 258:45–52.

Zagon, I.S., R.E. Rhodes, and P.J. McLaughlin (1985) Distribution of enkephalin immunoreactivity in germinative cells of developing rat cerebellum. Science 227:1049–1051.

The Hippocampus—New Vistas, pages 145–151
© 1989 Alan R. Liss, Inc.

10
Simultaneous Demonstrations of Neuropeptide Y Gene Expression and Peptide Storage in Single Hippocampal Neurons of the Human Brain

VICTORIA CHAN-PALAY

Department of Neurology, University Hospital, Zürich, Switzerland

Neuropeptide Y (NPY) is a 36-amino acid peptide (Tatemoto, 1982) that is distributed widely in both the central (Allen et al., 1983; Chan-Palay et al., 1985a, 1986a) and the peripheral nervous systems (Terenghi et al., 1983; Sundler et al., 1983). Morphological studies on the human brain have shown NPY immunoreactivity in numerous cortical interneuronal cell bodies and in a rich plexus of cortical nerve fibers (Chan-Palay et al., 1985a, 1986a). The function of these NPY-containing neurons is under investigation, as they exhibit numerical and morphological changes in certain neurological diseases (Chan-Palay et al., 1985b, 1986b). The regulation of NPY may include alterations in the levels of mRNA encoding for the peptide or its precursors. Steady-state levels of mRNA in single neurons can be assessed by the in situ hybridization method. Through complementary base-pairing, radiolabeled polynucleotides anneal to the specific sequences of the polynucleotides in the mRNA for NPY, and the neurons containing these hybrids are detected by autoradiography.

The structure of the precursor for human NPY has been deduced by analysis of the cDNA sequence. The NPY cDNA was directionally cloned behind the bacteriophage SP6 promotor. A specific single-stranded cRNA probe complementary to NPY mRNA was then synthesized with SP6 polymerase. This probe was used to analyze total RNA from pheochromocytomas, adrenal medullas, and other tissues (Minth et al., 1984). With this probe to human NPY, we recently demonstrated the NPY transcription sites in human cerebral cortical neurons by applying in situ hybridization to samples of human cerebral cortex from surgical biopsy samples and from brains obtained at autopsy after brief post-mortem delays (Terenghi et al., 1987) and described techniques for the simultaneous demonstration of NPY gene expression by in situ hybridization and of peptide storage by immunocytochemistry with antibodies against NPY in individual human brain cortical neurons (see Fig. 1 in Chan-Palay et al.,

1988).This goal required technical innovation because of the limitations imposed by the relatively poor visual sensitivity of the in situ hybridization methods, the difficulties of dealing with human tissue, and the necessity for maintaining sufficient cellular immunoreactivity for successful antigen–antibody reactions. We attempted to enhance the reliability and sensitivity of the in situ hybridization method to demonstrate mRNA encoding while maintaining a sufficient level of immunoreactivity to allow visualization of the peptide. Neuropeptides exist in relatively low quantities in brain neurons compared with that in cells containing peptide hormones, for example in the pituitary or in the enteric nervous system. Since the steady-state level of mRNA copes per neuron coding for NPY is also relatively low, the sensitivities of both detection methods must be very high to ensure some success.

The nonpostmortem tissues used in this study consisted of specimens of neocortex collected from temporal or hippocampal areas from patients who underwent surgery primarily for large brain tumors or for intractable temporal lobe epilepsy. Cortical specimens varying in thickness from 2 to 4 mm were removed together with the tumor as an integral part of the neurosurgical procedure necessitated by the disease. The areas immediately adjacent to the tissue used for immunocytochemistry were checked in stained sections by macroscopic and microscopic examination to eliminate the possibility of tumor or alterations caused by tumor invasion. (The protocol guiding the collection of neurosurgical specimens was accepted by the Internal Ethics Committee of the University Hospital, Zürich, and conforms to the guidelines established by the U.S. National Institute of Health for the use of human tissues.) The samples were either fixed immediately by immersion in a variety of fixatives or quick-frozen in liquid nitrogen and fixed after cryostat sectioning. In addition to the biopsies, postmortem samples of temporal cortex from four patients with no clinical manifestations of neurological disease, confirmed by gross and microscopic neuropathological examination at autopsy, were also used. The areas immediately adjacent to those used here were checked in Nissl sections to confirm the absence of pathologic changes. All postmortem brains, between 1.5 and 4.5 h after death, were perfused through the vascular system with 4% paraformaldehyde. Cryostat sections (10 μm) of the frozen material were mounted onto poly(L-lysine)-coated slides (Huang et al., 1983) and dried overnight at 37°C. Vibratome sections 20 μm thick were cut from the prefixed material and processed similarly. Sections were processed for in situ hybridization followed by immunocytochemistry and normal histology as explained below.

The preparation of the cRNA probe from the 600 base cDNA insert of pNPY 3–75, the prehybridization treatment of the sections, and the hybridization procedure and blot analyses have been described in detail elsewhere (Terenghi et al., 1987; Maniatis et al., 1982). Hybridization was carried out with 3 ng of [^{32}p]labeled probe per section (5×10^5 cpm per section) diluted in a buffer containing 50% formamide, 10% dextran sulfates, 0.30 M sodium chloride, 0.30 M sodium citrate, 0.25% bovine serum albumin, 0.25% Ficoll 400, 0.25% polyvinylpyrrolidone 360, 250 mM Tris/HCl (pH 7.5), 0.5% sodium pyrophosphate,

0.5% NaDodSO$_4$ (sodium dodecyl sulphate), and 250 μg of denatured salmon sperm DNA per milliliter.

Hybridization for double labeling studies was conducted as above with the omission of dextran sulfate from the buffer to increase the signal to noise ratio of the subsequent antigen–antibody reaction. After hybridization, nonspecifically bound single-stranded probe was removed by treatment with a solution containing 20 μg of RNase A per milliliter, 0.5 M sodium chloride, 10 mM Tris/HCl (pH 8), and 1 mM EDTA for 30 min at 37°C. Thereafter, the same sections were immediately prepared for immunocytochemistry without further dehydration. Sections were incubated in 0.5% hydrogen peroxide for up to 2 h and in 1.0% Triton for 1 h before antibody incubation. They were then incubated overnight in primary antisera, diluted in 0.5% Triton X-100/1% normal goat serum to a titer of 1:200 and in fresh antibody solution for an additional 3 h. Subsequent processing followed the peroxidase-antiperoxidase (PAP) method (Sternberger, 1979) or the procedures for immunofluorescence or immunogold silver (IGSS) visualization (Chan-Palay, 1987). The following parameters were used for the PAP technique: goat antirabbit antibody (1:200, Miles) in 0.5% Triton and 1% normal goat serum in phosphate-buffered saline, followed by PAP reagent (1:400, Arnel), then visualization by diaminobenzidine (Chan-Palay et al., 1985a). The immunofluorescence technique utilized goat antirabbit second antibody linked to Texas red (1:20, Miles) in 1% normal goat serum: The sections were washed extensively prior to visualization. The IGSS method was performed as previously described (Chan-Palay, 1987), with a goat-antirabbit-gold antibody enhanced for visualization with silver development (Janssen Pharma).

Anti-NPY was raised in rabbits against unconjugated porcine NPY (1086). The antibody showed negligible cross reactivity with neuropeptide PYY and avian pancreatic polypeptide and no cross reactivity with other peptides such as somatostatin and substance P. Incubation of tissue sections with antiserum preabsorbed with synthetic NPY completely blocked staining of neuronal processes in the hippocampus (Allen et al., 1983). Control sections were incubated with primary antiserum or with primary antiserum preabsorbed with synthetic NPY antigen (0.1 nmol/ml of diluted antiserum; Bachem, Torrance, CA).

Thereafter, sections that had been hybridized and those with double labeling (hydridization and immunocytochemistry) were dipped in Kodak NTB-2 emulsion (1:1 dilution in distilled water) and exposed for 5–7 days at 4°C before being developed in D19 developer Kodak. The in situ hybridization autoradiograms were then dehydrated with graded ethanol solutions and coverslipped.

In each sequence of experiments, four sets of sections were prepared from each specimen under examination. They were respectively 1) for Nissl preparations stained by cresyl violet for morphological confirmation of the location of labeled cells in the laminae of the cortex, 2) for in situ hybridization alone as a control without double labeling with immunocytochemistry, 3) for in situ hybridization and immunocytochemistry together, and 4) for immunocytochemistry alone without in situ hybridization as a control.

For controls, a separate set of sections was treated with RNase (20 μg/ml, 1 h at 37°C) before hybridization. A further control was carried out by omitting the probe during hybridization, although all other conditions were maintained constant. Blot analysis using human cortex poly(A)$^+$ mRNA was prepared from postmortem tissue according to standard methods (Feinberg and Vogelstein, 1983) and has been previously described (Terenghi et al., 1987).

A successful solution to the problem of achieving consistent double labeling with in situ hybridization and antibody peptide immunocytochemistry depends on finding an acceptable compromise among the requirements for morphological fixation of the brain tissue, preservation of the specific mRNA despite the high levels of natural RNAase, preservation of the specific immunoreactivity of the peptide, and the simultaneous display of both, in intact neurons. Brief post-mortem delays and perfusion of the brains at autopsy resulted in the well-fixed samples of postmortem temporal cortex used in this study. These are likely to be among the fundamental reasons for the success of the double labeling procedures. A previous study (Terenghi et al., 1987) demonstrated that prefixed human brain tissues hybridized consistently, with the tissues retaining a better morphology than cortical samples rapidly frozen and then postfixed. Although the latter could produce material showing neurons with a strong hybridization signal, the morphology was poor. Several previous studies (Chan-Palay et al., 1986a,b; Shivers et al., 1986) have demonstrated the suitability of brief prefixed material for the demonstration of NPY in human cortical neurons by immunocytochemistry with antigen–antibody reactions. The present study has demonstrated the conditions under which both antibody reactions and hybridization can be successful, particularly in prefixed material.

Successful hybridization, as expressed by the presence of autoradiographic silver grains clustered over neurons, was readily apparent in all the preparations in the small interneurons of the deeper layers of the hippocampal cortex, particularly in CA1. (Terenghi et al., 1987). Successful double labeling was seen most consistently with the conventional PAP method, with diaminobenzidine as chromogen in the antigen–antibody reaction, and the description has been taken from these results. The deep brown/red color resulting from the NPY antigen–antibody reaction after the PAP procedure is present throughout the neuronal somata and in the issuing primary dendrites. Overlying the cell soma, and less over the dendrites, are dense clusters of autoradiographic silver grains because of successful simultaneous hybridization. Neuronal nuclei, when discernible in our preparations, are not labeled by either the antigen–antibody or the mRNA hybridization procedure. The incidence of these double labeled neurons is high in optimal preparations, matching quantitatively our expectations on the basis of the single labeled control preparations made from the adjacent sections in each set of experiments.

This double labeling procedure overcomes a few problems that were encountered when the immunocytochemistry procedure was done before the in situ hybridization. In contrast to two previous reports, one about virus-infected cell cultures (Gendelman et al., 1985) and another about the pituitary (Shivers et al., 1986), our studies show that prior staining resulted in considerable loss of the in situ signal possibly because of the lengthy incubations in the primary and secondary antibodies and subsequent reactions or perhaps because of

RNase activity. The procedures that we have described with in situ hybridization preceding immunocytochemistry allows a strong in situ signal and a relative weakening of the antigen–antibody reaction when results of the double labeled experiments are compared with the single labeled controls of in situ hybridization alone and immunocytochemistry alone. Clearly, double labeling experiments are compromises between successful results obtainable from the simultaneous juxtaposition of more than one difficult technique. However, it remains the only valid way of demonstrating the simultaneous existence of both gene expression and peptide storage in the same cell. Because of the inherent effects that the techniques of in situ hybridization had on the immunocytochemical staining, it is difficult to assess the quantitative aspects of this form of double labeling work. In many preparations all cells with grain clusters from the in situ signal had NPY immunoreactivity. However, several preparations with neurons labeled by in situ *signal* had only weak or no NPY immunoreactivities. Rather than concluding with the possible biological explanation—that some neurons that express the NPY gene do not store the peptide—we refer to conclude that technical difficulties can impair consistent demonstrations of NPY immunoreactivity.

In the control preparations treated with RNase prior to hybridization, no hybridized cells could be found. Similar results were found when the probe was omitted during the hybridization step. RNA blot hybridization analysis with a human NPY cDNA probe detected a single species of approximately 800 bases (Terenghi et al., 1987). These results of blot analysis are consistent with previous ones on several RNA preparations, including those from human pheochromocytoma, a tissue known to contain significant NPY immunoreactivity. RNAs prepared from other tissue sources do not show significant hybridization to the cRNA probe. In control preparations for NPY antibody specificity, incubation of adjacent sections in antibody solutions preadsorbed with NPY demonstrated no reactive neurons or fibers.

Thus the results show that the NPY gene transcript is present in neuronal cells of the human cortex in well-preserved samples of surgical biopsies and perfused postmortem brain with brief postmortem delays, as demonstrated by in situ hybridization with cRNA probes. This type of probe has been shown to produce a more specific and sensitive hybridization than others. The specificity of these results was confirmed by the lack of hybridization signal in control preparations and by blot analysis of electrophoretically fractionated poly(A)$^+$ RNA from human postmortem cortex. The results of blot analysis are consistent with previous ones on several RNA preparations, including those from human pheochromocytoma, a tissue known to contain significant NPY immunoreactivity. RNAs prepared from other tissue sources do not show significant hybridization to the cRNA probe. This suggests that very little, if any, NPY mRNA is present in these samples. It also demonstrates that the NPY cRNA probe does not cross react with other mRNAs. In situ hybridization in this type of tumor has been demonstrated already by using biotinylated probes, and more recently with the same [^{32}p]labeled cDNA probe as used here (unpublished observations).

The distribution of neurons positive for in situ hybridization was consistent with that of NPY-immunoreactive cells. The small numerical difference observed between neurons showing positive hybridization and immunostaining for NPY might be the reflection of different metabolic states of the cells. Indeed, gene transcription might not be a continuous event for all cells, whereas accumulated amounts of mature peptide could be more readily revealed by immunocyto-chemistry. Also, it cannot be excluded that the use of cross-linking fixative, although superior for the retention of morphological details and of peptide antigenicity, might reduce the efficiency of the hybridization.

We have described the methods by which NPY gene transcription and NPY storage can be simultaneously demonstrated in single human cortical neurons by using in situ hybridization with cRNA probes and antigen–antibody im-munocytochemistry. The marriage of those two powerful methods has provided us with the unequivocal demonstration that single human intracortical neurons identified as having the genetic apparatus and transcription capabilities for NPY also store the peptide. This demonstration lays to rest a question often brought against demonstrations of neurons containing peptide immunoreac-tivities with specific antibodies. That is, do peptide neurons have a demonstrable genetic apparatus for the manufacture of the neuroactive peptide in question, or is the presence of the peptide purely incidental? We envision that further applications of the methodological advances will include investigations into the question of genetic transcription of multiple neuroactive substances in single neurons.

There is no doubt that the in situ hybridization technique is a valuable meth-od for investigating protein biosynthesis in the central nervous system. In par-ticular, it could supply useful information on the role of specific neuronal sub-populations in neurological diseases that are associated with quantitative and morphological changes of NPY-immunoreactive neurons and with reductions of RNA levels for other peptides. Moreover, approaches combining in situ hy-bridization methods and other neuropeptide tracer methods such as immu-nocytochemistry could lead to a better understanding of the regulation and control of synthesis of multiple neuroactive substances in neurons in which more than one active neuromediator or neurotransmitter coexist.

ACKNOWLEDGMENTS

This work was supported by US AFOSR grant 86-0176. I thank U. Haesler and M. Höchli for technical assistance.

REFERENCES

Allen, Y.S., J.E. Adrian, J.M. Allen, K. Tatemoto, T.J. Crow, S.P. Bloom, and J.M. Polak (1983) Neuropeptide Y distribution in the rat brain. Science 221:877–879.

Chan-Palay, V. (1987) Somatostatin immunoreactive neurons in the human hippocampus and cortex shown by immunogold silver intensification on Vibratome setions: Co-existence with neuropeptide Y neurons. J. Comp. Neurol. 257:208–215.

Chan-Palay, V., Y.S. Allen, W. Lang, U. Haesler, and J.M. Polak (1985a) Cytology and distribution in normal human cerebral cortex of neurons immunoreactive with anti-sera against neuropeptide Y. J. Comp. Neurol. 238:382–389.

Chan-Palay, V., C. Köhler, U. Haesler, W. Lang, and G. Yasargil (1986a) Distribution of neurons and axons immunoreactive with antisera neuropeptide Y in the normal human hippocampus. J. Comp. Neurol. *248*:360–375.

Chan-Palay, V., W. Lang, Y.S. Allen, U. Haesler, and J.M. Polak (1985b) Cortical neurons immunoreactive with antisera against neuropeptide Y are altered in Alzheimer's type dementia. J. Comp. Neurol. *238*:390–400.

Chan-Palay, V., W. Lang, U. Haesler, C. Köhler, and G. Yasargil (1986b) Distribution of altered hippocampal neurons and axons immunoreactive with antisera against neuropeptide Y are altered in Alzheimer's type dementia. J. Comp. Neurol. *248*:376–394.

Chan-Palay, V., G. Yasargil, O. Hamid, J.M. Polak and S.L. Palay (1988) Simultaneous demonstrations of neuropeptide Y gene expression and peptide storage in single neurons of the human brain. Proc. Natl. Acad. Sci. U.S.A. *85*:3213–3215.

Feinberg, A.P., and B. Vogelstein (1983) A technique for radiolabelling DNA restriction endonuclease fragments to high specific activity. Anal. Biochem. *132*:6–13.

Gendelman, H.E., T.R. Moench, O. Narayan, D.E. Griffin, and J.E. Clements (1985) A double labeling technique for performing immunocytochemistry and in situ hybridization in virus infected cell cultures and tissues. J. Virol. Methods *11*:93–103.

Huang, W.M., S.J. Gibson, P. Facer, J. Gu, and J.M. Polak (1983) Improved section adhesion for immunocytochemistry using high molecular weight polymers of L-lysine as a slide coating. Histochemistry *77*:275–279.

Maniatis, T., E.F. Fritsch, and J. Sambrook (1982) Molecular Cloning: A Laboratory Manual. Cold Spring Harbor, NY: Gold Spring Harbor Laboratory, pp. 196–203.

Minth, C.D., S.R. Bloom, J.M. Polak, and J.E. Dixon (1984) Cloning characterization and DNA sequence of a human cDNA encoding neuropeptide tyrosine. Proc. Natl. Acad. Sci. U.S.A. *81*:4577–4581.

Shivers, B.D., R.E. Harlan, D.W. Pfaff, and B.S. Schacter (1986) In situ hybridization for the study of gene expression in the brain. J. Histochem. Cytochem. *34*:39–43.

Sternberger, L.A. (1979) Immunocytochemistry, ed 2. NY: John Wiley & Son, pp. 104–169.

Sundler, F., E. Moghimradeh, R. Hakanson, M. Ekelund, and P. Emson (1983) Nerve fibers in the rat displaying neuropeptide-Y-immunoreactivity. Intrinsic and extrinsic origin. Cell Tissue Res. *230*:487–493.

Tatemoto, K. (1982) Neuropeptide Y: Complete amino acid sequence of the brain peptide. Proc. Natl. Acad. Sci. U.S.A. *75*:5485–5489.

Terenghi, G., J.M. Polak, J.M. Allen, S.O. Zhang, W.G. Unger, and S.R. Bloom (1983) Neuropeptide Y-immunoreactive nerves in the uvea of guinea pig and rat. Neurosci. Lett. *42*:33–38.

Terenghi, G., J.M. Polak, O. Hamid, E. O'Brien, P. Denny, S. Legon, J. Dixon, C.D. Minth, S.L. Palay, G. Yasargil, and V. Chan-Palay (1987) Localization of neuropeptide Y in neurons of human cerebral cortex by means of in situ hybridization with a complementary RNA probe. Proc. Natl. Acad. Sci. U.S.A. *84*:7315–7318.

The Hippocampus—New Vistas, pages 153–170

11
Studies on the Expression of Opioid Peptides and Their Respective mRNAs in Hippocampal Seizure

CHRISTINE GALL AND JEFFREY WHITE

Department of Anatomy and Neurobiology, University of California at Irvine, Irvine, California (C.G.); Division of Endocrinology, Department of Medicine, State University of New York, Stony Book, New York (J.W.)

INTRODUCTION

One of the more recent and intriguing advances in our understanding of the plastic capacities of mature CNS neurons is the appreciation that their synthetic activities are to some extent regulated by extrinsic influences. The synthesis and/or resting levels of messenger molecules in particular have been demonstrated to be differentially responsive to such diverse manipulations as adrenalectomy (Davis et al., 1986; Sawchenko, 1987), deafferentation (Baker et al., 1983; Young et al., 1986), pharmacological antagonism of specific neurotransmitter receptors (Hong et al., 1979b; Romano et al., 1987), experimentally induced arthritis (Millan et al., 1986; Iadarola et al., 1986a), and changes in physiological activity (vide infra). These results have attracted a great deal of interest in part because they provide a potential mechanism for "information storage" in the brain (Black et al., 1987) whereby relatively brief physiological events might have a lasting influence on intercellular communication.

Some of the best evidence that the regulation of neuroactive substances is influenced by physiological activity comes from the effects of seizures on the synthesis and resting levels of two opioid peptides, enkephalin and dynorphin, within neurons of the hippocampus. Hong et al. first noted that seizure activity leads to dramatic but transient increases in enkephalin immunoreactivity in whole brain (1979a) and hippocampus (1980) as measured by radioimmunoassay (RIA). Since that time, a number of experimental paradigms that induce recurrent limbic seizures have been found to alter the amounts of both enkephalin and dynorphin in hippocampus, in some instances in dramatically different ways. Our own work has focused on the effects of recurrent limbic seizures, induced by electrolytic lesion of the dentate gyrus hilus (Gall et al., 1981), on neuropeptides contained within the hippocampal mossy fiber system. These studies indicate that the expression of opioid peptides is surprisingly plastic and suggest that the rate of synthesis at any given time is a function of recent physiological activity.

These results suggest one route through which trophic influences between hippocampal neurons might be achieved. They also may be of clinical significance. Enkephalin has epileptogenic properties when applied to hippocampus (Frenk et al., 1978) and hippocampal region CA3, the area in which the enkephalin-containing mossy fibers terminate, has one of the lowest thresholds for seizure of any area in the brain. This raises the possibility that seizure-induced increases in enkephalin synthesis contribute to lowered seizure thresholds.

In this chapter, we will first briefly summarize the distribution of certain opioid peptides in hippocampus and describe how these are affected by an episode of recurrent seizures. We will then turn to the mechanisms responsible for the seizure-induced effects and, in particular, their relationship to genomic expression.

DISTRIBUTION AND SEIZURE-INDUCED PLASTICITY OF HIPPOCAMPAL OPIOIDS

The synthetically distinct opioid peptides enkephalin and dynorphin are both localized within aspects of hippocampal circuitry with the distribution of enkephalin immunoreactivity (ENK-I) being the more complex by far. As described in detail by Gall et al. (1981), ENK-I in rat hippocampus is found within perikarya of varied morphologies that are very sparsely distributed across all laminae of the hippocampus proper and dentate gyrus hilus, as well as within a few dentate gyrus granule cells. In addition, at least three separate axonal systems contain ENK-I: 1) the temporoammonic and perforant pathway afferents from the lateral entorhinal and perirhinal cortices, which are distributed within stratum lacunosum-moleculare and the distal dentate gyrus molecular layer, respectively (Fredens et al., 1984); 2) axons distributed along the interface between stratum lacunosum-moleculare and stratum radiatum of region CA1; and 3) the mossy fiber axons of the dentate gyrus granule cells. The former two systems of immunoreactive axons increase in density along the septotemporal arc of hippocampus. In contrast to enkephalin, immunoreactivity to either dynorphin A (1–8) or dynorphin B (DYN-I, collectively) is restricted to the mossy fiber axonal system and a very few perikarya contained for the most part within the dentate gyrus molecular layer (McGinty et al., 1983; Gall, 1988b). The distributions of ENK-I and DYN-I observed in rat hippocampus are fairly representative of the patterns of immunoreactivity observed in other mammals, although there is variability in the localization of ENK-I within the temporoammonic and perforant pathways (Gall, 1988a).

The first reports of the codistribution of enkephalin and dynorphin immunoreactivities in the mossy fibers raised concerns about the possibility of spurious identification of ENK-I because of cross reactivity of the antileucine enkephalin with dynorphin peptides (Gall et al., 1981; McGinty et al., 1983). However, more recent biochemical (White et al., 1986) and in situ hybridization studies (Gall et al., 1987), to be described below, as well as further immunocytochemical analyses using noncross-reactive antisera (Gall, 1984b; McGinty et al., 1984), have corroborated the original description of enkephalin localization within rat hippocampus. Specifically, it is now certain that the dentate gyrus granule cells synthesize, and the mossy fiber axons contain, synthetically distinct enkephalin and dynorphin, although, in the untreated rat, a much greater proportion of the mossy fiber terminal boutons contain DYN-I than contain ENK-I. Moreover, while ENK-I and DYN-I have not been demonstrated to coexist within individual granule cells (McGinty, 1985) or their mossy fiber boutons, the cellular localization of preproenkephalin A mRNA observed in rats sacrificed following seizure activity discourages the conclusion that there are distinct populations of enkephalin- and dynorphin-synthesizing dentate gyrus granule cells.

As mentioned above, recurrent seizures lead to dramatic changes in the synthesis and amount of the opioid peptides in hippocampus. This is most strikingly evident in the mossy fiber system following seizures induced by electrolytic lesion of the dentate gyrus hilus. Small unilateral hilus lesions, placed with stainless steel electrodes, cause bilateral epileptiform activity within hippocampus and intermittent behavioral seizures of the type that accompanies limbic kindling (Racine, 1972; Gall et al., 1988). In rat, both electrographic and behavioral seizures are first observed from 1.5 to 2 h postlesion and recur for approximately 8–10 h thereafter. The vast majority of full paroxyzmal discharges recorded from hippocampal region CA3 occur between 2 and 5 h postlesion, and no paroxyzmal discharges have been recorded after 12 h postlesion. We have found the hilus lesion (HL) paradigm to be particularly advantageous for studies of the effects of seizure activity on opioid peptide regulation in that HL-induced seizures reliably stimulate extremely large changes in neuropeptide expression (relative to some of the other recurrent seizure paradigms) without the potential involvement of unidentified drug effects and without any apparent cell death or mossy fiber degeneration in hippocampus contralateral to the lesion. For comparison purposes, we have also examined the effects of seizure induced by intracerebroventricular (i.c.v.) injection of kainic acid. Kainic acid induces epileptiform activity within hippocampus, which lasts several hours (Sloviter and Damiano, 1981), but, in contrast to the effects of hilus lesions, this activity is much more continuous and leads to the death of hippocampal neurons most particularly within the rostral stratum pyramidale of region CA3.

Immunocytochemical preparations have demonstrated that at both 6 and 12 h following either a hilus lesion or injection of fairly low convulsant doses of kainic acid (i.c.v.) in rat or mouse, there is a severe depletion to total elimination of immunoreactivities to both methionine-enkephalin and dynorphin (dynorphin A 1–8 and dynorphin B) from the intact mossy fibers of both hippocampi (Gall et al., 1988; White and Gall, 1987a). Following this depletion, ENK-I rapidly returns to the mossy fibers, appears normal by 18 to 20 h postlesion, but continues to increase to well above normal levels by 4–5 days after the seizure episode (Figs. 1, 2). At this postlesion interval there is a tremendous increase in the number of mossy fiber terminal boutons that contain ENK-I, although in HL animals, as in the untreated rat, few of the granule cell bodies

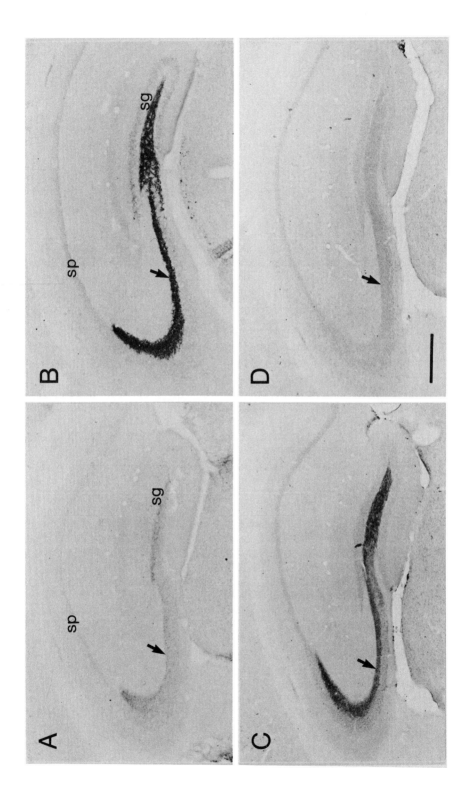

are visibly immunoreactive. While seizure-induced increases in ENK-I are most striking within the mossy fibers of HL animals, fairly large increases in ENK-I are also apparent in entorhinal cortex, the temporoammonic and perforant pathway afferents from entorhinal cortex to hippocampus, the lateral septum, and aspects of the amygdala. At maximal elevation, 4 days following either HL or i.c.v. kainic acid, total hippocampal ENK-I is increased three- to fivefold above normal levels as measured by RIA.

In contrast to the dramatic increase in mossy fiber ENK-I seen after recurrent seizures, DYN-I is reduced within the mossy fibers of rats and mice for several days following either HL or i.c.v. kainic acid (Gall, 1988b) (Fig. 1). In both paradigms, the influence of seizures on mossy fiber DYN-I is much more modest than it is on ENK-I. While ENK-I was consistently elevated in rats or mice sacrificed 4 days after a seizure-producing hilus lesion, mossy fiber DYN-I in the same animals was only partially reduced or, in a few cases, was not clearly different than that seen in paired controls. Interestingly, in mouse, recurrent seizures reliably effect a much more pronounced reduction in immunoreactivity to cholecystokinin octapeptide (CCK-I). CCK is codistributed with enkephalin and dynorphin in the mossy fibers of mouse (Gall et al., 1986), as in guinea pig and monkey (Gall, 1984a, 1988a) but not rat (Greenwood et al., 1981). In mouse, both HL- and kainic acid-induced seizures result in a large bilateral reduction to total elimination of CCK-I from the mossy fibers that persists throughout the full period of enkephalin elevation (Gall, 1988b).

In rat, the effects of recurrent seizures on the opioid peptides in hippocampus are transient. Following a hilus lesion, the level of ENK-I in the mossy fiber system slowly declines to normal levels by about 2 weeks postlesion; mossy fiber DYN-I appears normal by 2 weeks postlesion as well. As such, the duration of increased hippocampal ENK-I is about the same following either HL- or kainic acid-induced seizures (Hong et al., 1980; Gall, unpublished observations). The period of enkephalin elevation is much more variable in mouse hippocampus following the same treatments. Although hippocampal ENK-I appears normal in most mice sacrificed 14 to 20 days following seizure induction by either HL or i.c.v. kainic acid, we observed four cases (two HL and two kainic acid) in which mossy fiber ENK-I was still dramatically elevated (and mossy fiber CCK-I was absent) as late as 2 to 6 months following the initial seizure episode (Gall et al., 1988). These cases suggest the possibility that one episode of extreme recurrent seizures can effect a permanent change in the pattern of neuropeptide expression by the dentate gyrus granule cells. However, the

---

Fig. 1. Low magnification photomicrographs of sections through hippocampus of an untreated mouse **(A,C)** and a mouse sacrificed 4 days following a contralateral hilus lesion **(B,D)** processed for the localization of ENK-I (A,B) and DYN-I (C,D) (peroxidase-antiperoxidase technique). Note the large increase in ENK-I and the decrease in DYN-I in the mossy fibers (arrows) of the HL mouse relative to the paired control. sg, stratum granulosum; sp, stratum pyramidale. Calibration bar: 300μm.

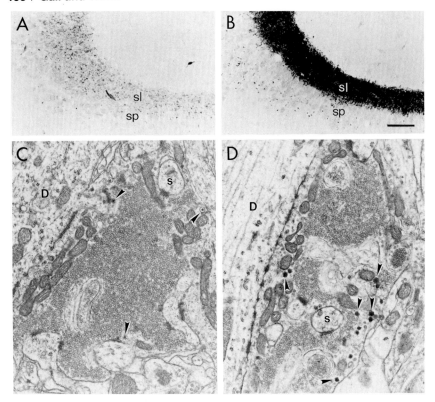

Fig. 2. Light and electron micrographs illustrating the influence of HL-induced seizures on ENK-I in rat mossy fibers and corresponding ultrastructural changes. The upper micrographs show immunostaining for ENK-I in the mossy fibers within the stratum lucidum (sl) of region CA3b in an untreated rat **(A)** and in a paired HL rat sacrificed 4 days after a contralateral lesion **(B)**. The lower electron micrographs each show individual large mossy fiber terminal boutons from region CA3b of an untreated rat **(C)** and a paired HL rat sacrificed 4 days postlesion **(D)**. In both cases, the mossy fiber boutons exhibit the characteristic clusters of agranular vesicles, less numerous dense-cored vesicles (arrowheads), and multiple synaptic contacts with embedded spines (s). However, during the period of elevated mossy fiber ENK-I illustrated in D, there is a dramatic increase in the number of large full-core dense-cored synaptic vesicles. D, dendritic shaft; sp, stratum pyramidale. Bar = 75 μm for A and B. C and D photographed at ×30,000.

possibility that these particular mice experienced further seizures within days of the time of sacrifice cannot be excluded.

Our observations of HL- and kainic acid-induced increases in ENK-I within rodent hippocampus are consistent with the findings of other investigators. In studies using a wide range of experimental paradigms, treatments that stimulate *recurrent* seizures have consistently been found to increase ENK-I in hippocampus and elsewhere. This is not to say that all treatments are equivalent; major differences in the magnitude and regional distribution of changes in ENK-I have been reported. For example, electroconvulsive shock (ECS) has been found to stimulate the largest increases in ENK-I in the hypothalamus (Yoshikawa et al., 1985). In contrast, seizures induced by intrastriatal kainic acid stimulate large increases in ENK-I in hippocampus but do not alter immunoreactivity or preproenkephalin A mRNA in hypothalamus (Kanamatsu et al., 1986b). Within hippocampus, HL- and kainic acid-induced seizures have been found to cause large increases in ENK-I in both the mossy fibers and the perforant pathways, whereas ECS (Kanamatsu et al., 1986a) and amygdaloid kindling (McGinty et al., 1986) reportedly only effect reliable increases in ENK-I in the perforant pathway.

Reports of the effects of seizure activity on dynorphin have been much less consistent. In agreement with our results, repeated ECS (Kanamatsu et al., 1986a) and stimulation-induced limbic kindling (Iadarola et al., 1986b; McGinty et al., 1986) are found to decrease DYN-I in the rat hippocampal mossy fiber system. However, kindling has been reported to increase DYN-I in rabbit hippocampus (Przewlocki et al., 1983), and Kanamatsu et al. (1986b) observed that DYN-I is increased within the hippocampal mossy fibers following seizures induced by intrastriatal kainic acid. Moreover, unlike ENK-I, the direction of the change in DYN-I appears to differ between brain areas in some experimental seizure paradigms; while DYN-I is decreased in hippocampus following ECS, it increases in the substantia nigra, hypothalamus, and ventral pallidum of the same animals (Kanamatsu et al., 1986a).

Before moving to a consideration of the mechanisms through which seizures alter the concentration of opioid peptides in hippocampus, it is appropriate to note that electron microscopic analyses have identified interesting ultrastructural correlates to the seizure-induced changes in enkephalin content within the mossy fibers of rat. The mossy fiber terminal boutons possess a unique morphology in the normal rat in that they are very large (having an estimated mean diameter of 8 μm in region CA3B), are virtually filled with densely packed agranular synaptic vesicles and fewer dense-cored vesicles, envelop and form multiple synaptic contacts with the complex thorny spines of the CA3 pyramidal cells (Amaral and Dent, 1981; Laatsch and Cowan, 1965; Blackstad and Kjaerheim, 1961) (Fig. 2), and contain extremely high concentrations of zinc (Haug, 1967). The significance of the heterogeneity of vesicle type and the presence of zinc are not understood, although it appears that the zinc is present in a releasable pool in that it is depleted from the mossy fibers following stimulation-induced epileptiform activity (Sloviter, 1985).

We have examined the ultrastructure of the mossy fiber boutons 5 h, 11 h, 4 days, and 14 days following contralateral, seizure-producing hilus lesions. As described above, these represent postlesion intervals at which mossy fiber ENK-I is depleted (5 h, 11 h), is elevated far above normal (4 days), and has returned to normal (14 days). At the two early time points, which are placed during and near the termination of seizure activity, there is a dramatic reduction in packing density and bouton area occupied by the agranular vesicles and in the number of dense-cored vesicles. By 4 days, the agranular vesicle population appears normal, but there is a striking and significant increase in the numbers of very large (>80 nm diameter) full-core dense-cored vesicles (Fig. 2). By 14 days, all indices of the synaptic vesicle populations have returned to normal (Pico et al., manuscript in preparation). These data describe a biphasic fluctuation in the number and size of full-core dense-cored vesicles that follows the depletion, elevation, and return to normal levels of ENK-I within the mossy fiber boutons. It is tempting to propose that enkephalin is, in fact, contained within the dense-cored vesicle matrix material, although it is also quite possible that other releasable substances undergo seizure-induced changes that follow the same time course as enkephalin.

The functional consequence of seizure-induced alterations in mossy fiber opioid peptide levels is not understood. This is largely due to the lack of information about what these endogenous opioids contribute to synaptic physiology in hippocampus. Although exogenously applied enkephalin and dynorphin both facilitate the excitation of CA3 and CA1 pyramidal cells in response to stimulation of nonopioid-containing afferents, opioid antagonists have not been found to disrupt synaptic transmission at the mossy fiber synapse (Lynch et al., 1981; Chavkin and Bloom, 1986). The primary neurotransmitter at the mossy fiber synapse is thought to be a glutamate-like acidic amino acid (Alschuler et al., 1985; Crawford and Connor, 1973). As such, one would anticipate that the actions of enkephalin and dynorphin have modulatory functions in this system.

MECHANISMS OF SEIZURE-INDUCED ALTERATIONS IN HIPPOCAMPAL OPIOIDS

All available evidence indicates that the seizure-induced changes in opioid peptides within hippocampus and elsewhere are due to changes in synthesis, with the regulation most likely occurring at the level of transcription. In situ hybridization analyses have demonstrated a decrease in the abundance of preprodynorphin mRNA within the dentate gyrus granule cells following hippocampal kindling and intense local electrical stimulation (Morris et al., 1987, 1988). Northern blot analyses have demonstrated seizure-dependent increases in preproenkephalin A mRNA (mRNA[enk]) within hippocampus following recurrent seizure induction by ECS (Kanamatsu et al., 1986a; Yoshikawa et al., 1985) or by i.c.v. kainic acid (Kanamatsu et al., 1986b) or hilus lesion (White and Gall, 1987a; White et al., 1987). We have found the abundance of mRNA[enk] within rat dentate gyrus to be elevated as soon as 3 h following a contralateral hilus lesion. In this paradigm, messenger RNA levels continue to increase through 18 to 30 h postlesion, are somewhat reduced by 48 h, and have returned to near normal levels by 4 days postlesion. At maximal elevation, mRNA[enk] within the dentate gyrus of HL rats increases to 15- to 30-fold above normal levels. We should note that the dentate samples used in these experiments include pooled mRNA from the dentate gyrus granule cells as well as from neurons within the hilus and the overlying field CA1. Northern blot analysis of entorhinal cortex in rats sacrificed 6, 18, and 30 h after a contralateral hilus lesion indicates a similarly rapid increase in mRNA^{enk} in the region that gives rise to the enkephalin-containing perforant pathway afferents to hippocampus (White and Gall, 1987b). These studies indicate that, within hippocampus, epileptiform activity effects a rapid increase in the transcription of the gene encoding preproenkephalin A, beginning quite early in the recurrent seizure episode, and that the abundance of mRNA^{enk} within hippocampal neurons continues to increase well beyond the period of seizure activity.

Although elevated levels of mRNA^{enk} only suggest increases in the rate of enkephalin synthesis within the affected neurons, increased synthesis has been directly demonstrated for the dentate gyrus granule cells. Using in vivo radiolabeling, we demonstrated elevated enkephalin synthesis by the dentate gyrus granule cells during the period of maximal mRNA^{enk} increase (White et al., 1987). In this study, [^{35}S]methionine was infused into the dentate gyrus of alert rats from 24 to 28 h following a contralateral, seizure-producing hilus lesion. At 30 h postlesion, the incorporation of the label into four proenkephalin A fragments within the mossy fiber terminal field was evaluated. We found a 14-fold increase in incorporation of the label into chromatographically purified Met^5-enkephalin, Met-enkephalin-ArgGlyLeu, Met-enkephalin-ArgPhe, and Bam 18P in HL rats relative to paired controls. Moreover, following seizure there was no change in either the molar ratios of these radiolabeled proenkephalin A products or the proportion of total Met-enkephalin present in larger molecular forms. These data demonstrate that in HL rats there is a large increase in proenkephalin A synthesis within the dentate gyrus granule cells and prompt transport of the newly synthesized opioids to the mossy fiber terminal boutons, but no fundamental change in post-translational processing.

Recently the application of in situ hybridization techniques have advanced our appreciation of the full population of neurons that are capable of enkephalin biosynthesis in hippocampus and have demonstrated that seizure-induced increases in mRNA^{enk} are much more broadly distributed across the forebrain than anticipated on the basis of immunocytochemical observations. Using a 911 base length [^{35}S]cRNA probe (transcribed from the Sac 1–Sma I fragment of rat preproenkephalin cDNA clone pRPE2 (Yoshikawa et al., 1984) and both film and emulsion autoradiographic techniques, we found relatively low levels of hybridization to mRNA^{enk} within hippocampus of the untreated Sprague-Dawley rat. In these animals, the densities of autoradiographic grains overlying the granule cells of the dentate gyrus indicate variability in the abundance of mRNA^{enk} within cells across the population: Generally a few cells, scattered irregularly across the depth and the suprapyramidal-to-infrapyramidal arc of stratum granulosum, are moderately well labeled, whereas the remainder are either lightly labeled or are not labeled above background density (Fig. 3). Moderate to low densities of autoradiographic grains are also seen to overlie a small number of neurons sparsely distributed across all laminae of the hippocampus proper (CA3, CA1) and a few large neurons within the central hilus of the temporal hippocampus. As such, the distribution of [^{35}S]cRNA-labeled neurons is consistent with the reported distribution of neurons containing ENK-I in the untreated rat (Gall et al., 1981).

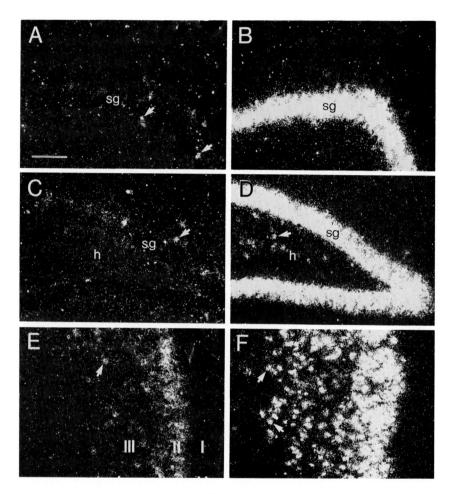

Fig. 3. Dark-field photomicrographs illustrating the in situ hybridization labeling of mRNA^{enk} in tissue sections through the dentate gyrus **(A–D)** and entorhinal cortex **(E,F)** of untreated rats (A,C,E) and paired HL rats sacrificed either 4 h (B) or 24 h (D,F) after contralateral HL placement. Arrows indicate a few of the [^{35}S]labeled neurons. Roman numerals in E indicate cortical layers. Note that only a small number of neurons are labeled in the stratum granulosum (sg) of the untreated rat, whereas what appears to be the full population of neurons in this layer are labeled at both 4 (B) and 24 (D) h postlesion. In each area there is a clear seizure-dependent increase in both the number of labeled neurons and the autoradiographic grain density overlying individual neurons. h, dentate gyrus hilus. Bar = 120 μm for A and B and 150 μm for C–F.

As early as 1.5 h after the onset of HL-induced seizure activity, there is a clear increase in the density of hybridization to mRNA^{enk} within stratum granulosum. By 6 h postlesion, hybridization is elevated within neurons in the entorhinal and piriform cortices in experimental animals relative to paired controls as well. The density of autoradiographic labeling in these areas increases further by 24 h postlesion, at which time virtually all of the dentate gyrus granule cells appear heavily labeled (Fig. 3). In addition, there is a clear increase in hybridization within neurons of the central hilus and the subiculum. As noted above, the former area is lightly labeled in untreated rats, whereas hybridization to mRNA^{enk} is only detectable in a large number of neurons in the subiculum of experimental animals. These changes in hybridization to mRNA^{enk} appear dependent on seizure activity in this paradigm in that equivalent-sized hilus lesions placed with platinum-iridium wire, which do not induce seizure activity (Campbell et al., 1984; Pico and Gall, unpublished observations), do not induce changes in hybridization to mRNA^{enk} within hippocampus or elsewhere.

The increases in hybridization to mRNA^{enk} in stratum granulosum and the entorhinal cortex were anticipated on the basis of the immunocytochemical and Nortern blot studies described above. However, one striking and surprising result of the in situ hybridization analysis was the observation of large increases in mRNA^{enk} throughout the olfactory/limbic forebrain of HL rats, including many areas in which seizure-induced changes in ENK-I were not detected by immunocytochemistry. In the untreated rat, low to moderate levels of hybridization are observed within the granule cell layer of the olfactory bulb, layer II, and, to a lesser extent, layer III of the piriform cortex, the basolateral and posteromedial cortical amygdaloid nuclei, and the medial olfactory tubercle. Twenty-four hours post-HL, large seizure-dependent increases in hybridization are observed in all of these areas (Fig. 4) and involve increases in both the number of neurons labeled with the [^{35}S]cRNA probe and the density of autoradiographic grains overlying individual neurons. These regions all receive input from olfactory cortex (Luskin and Price, 1983) and would be expected to have close association with seizure activity initiating within hippocampus either directly or via intermediate connections with septum or entorhinal cortex. Hybridization densities within other brain areas that would also be expected to be influenced by limbic seizures, but that normally exhibit relatively high levels of mRNA^{enk}, are less affected by HL-induced seizure activity; this is the case for the lateral olfactory tubercle and the ventromedial hypothalamus (Fig. 4). Finally, modest increases in hybridization are seen in some regions outside the olfactory/limbic axis, most notably within neurons of the caudate/putamen.

A major outcome of these in situ hybridization studies is an appreciation of the fact that we are not seeing the full population of hippocampal neurons capable of enkephalin synthesis in the resting state. This is most particularly true in regard to the granule cells of the dentate gyrus. In the normal, untreated rat the localization of moderate densities of mRNA^{enk} within but a few dentate gyrus granule cells is in good agreement with the localization of ENK-I in a small minority of mossy fiber terminal boutons in region CA3. The presence of dense mRNA^{enk} in virtually all of the granule cells 24 h after a recurrent

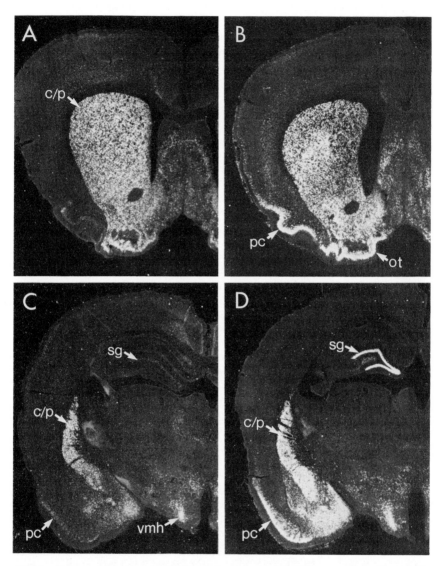

Fig. 4. Low magnification dark-field photomicrographs of tissue sections through the forebrain of an untreated rat **(A,C)** and a paired HL rat sacrificed 24 h after contralateral lesion placement **(B,D)** processed for the in situ hybridization localization of mRNA[enk] using a [35S]cRNA probe and emulsion autoradiography. Note the large seizure-induced increases in mRNA[enk] in the piriform cortex (pc), stratum granulosum (sg), and medial olfactory tubercle (ot) of the HL rat relative to the paired control. c/p, caudate putamen; vmh, ventromedial hypothalamus. (× 7.5)

seizure episode indicates that some aspect of the physiological activity, or its concomitants, experienced during seizure can move the remaining granule cells from an enkephalin-quiescent to an enkephalin-synthesizing mode. Given this capacity for plasticity in enkephalin expression, it is not appropriate to consider there being cells within the population that invariably synthesize enkephalin or dynorphin. It is probably also not appropriate to consider the regulation of dynorphin and enkephalin expression within the granule cells to necessarily be reciprocal: Although an increase in mossy fiber enkephalin is associated with a decrease in dynorphin following HL-induced seizures (Gall, 1988a,b) and intense electrical stimulation (Morris et al., 1988), instances of simultaneously increased ENK-I and DYN-I have also been reported (Kanamatsu et al., 1986a). As such, the expression of the two opioid peptide genes within individual granule cells appears to be independently regulated or at least regulated by different factors. This conclusion is consistent with the large differences observed in the ontogenies of ENK-I and DYN-I within the mossy fiber system. In both rat and mouse, DYN-I is apparent with immunocytochemistry early in the period of mossy fiber outgrowth and synaptogenesis. In contrast, ENK-I is not detected in the mossy fiber terminal boutons until approximately 2 weeks postnatal, well after the establishment of synaptic function (Gall et al., 1984; Gall, 1984b).

We do not, as yet, have a direct indication of the effective stimulus or cellular mechanism through which epileptiform physiological activity influences the synthesis of opioid peptides within hippocampal neurons. In regard to potential regulatory mechanisms, it is noteworthy that HL-induced seizures have been found to stimulate within hippocampus large increases in the activity and abundance of mRNA for the enzyme ornithine decarboxylase (ODC) (Baudry et al., 1986) and in the amount of mRNA for the proto-oncogene *c-fos* (White and Gall, 1987b). As a consequence of its role as the rate-limiting enzyme in polyamine synthesis, ODC has been suggested to be involved as an intracellular mediator of trophic influences and in the initiation or support of RNA transcription (Canellakis et al., 1979). As discussed in another contribution to this volume, the oncogene *c-fos* encodes a nuclear protein (Fos) that has been suggested to play a role in genomic regulation (Morgan et al., 1987). Rapid increases in *c-fos* mRNA and/or Fos immunoreactivity have also been demonstrated in hippocampal neurons following treatment with the convulsant metrazol (Morgan et al., 1987) and in association with hippocampal kindling (Dragunow and Robertson, 1987). Our own recent in situ hybridization studies have demonstrated bilateral increases in *c-fos* mRNA in the dentate gyrus granule cells within 15 min of electrically stimulated seizure initiation, and, following the hilus lesion, there are large increases in hybridization to *c-fos* mRNA within both the dentate gyrus granule cells and the enkephalin-synthesizing cells of the entorhinal cortex. As such, the increase in *c-fos* mRNA is present within (but not limited to) those hippocampal neurons that exhibit increased enkephalin synthesis following seizures and appears to precede increased transcription of preproenkephalin A. The cellular localization and temporal order of these events are compatible with an involvement of *c-fos* induction in the more delayed initiation of accelerated enkephalin synthesis, but there is as yet no direct evidence for a causal relationship.

One of the more interesting questions to arise from this area of research is whether seizure activity is actually necessary to effect changes in opioid peptide expression by hippocampal neurons. It is quite possible that the neurochemical changes observed following these extreme manipulations also appear in response to the natural variation in physiological activity. Bursting activity in hippocampus does not occur only during seizures; studies using chronic recording from behaving animals have shown that some pyramidal cells fire in short, high-frequency bursts and that these episodes can be expected several times a second (Eichenbaum et al., 1987). Moreover, granule cells commonly discharge for prolonged periods (seconds) at high frequency when rats are engaged in locomotor activity (Rose et al., 1983). It is not unreasonable then to speculate that the widespread changes seen after synchronous epileptiform discharges occur in a much smaller percentage of cells, and presumably to a much lesser degree, in certain behavioral circumstances. Of interest in this regard is the observation that patterned bursts of activity designed to mimic physiological activity recorded in behaving rats produce long-term potentiation of hippocampal synapses (Larson and Lynch, 1988) that can persist for weeks (Staubli and Lynch, 1987). Experiments are now in progress to determine if these events are accompanied by the types of changes in genomic expression described in the present review.

SUMMARY

Work with experimental seizure paradigms have demonstrated unexpected plasticity in the expression of the opioid peptides enkephalin and dynorphin by hippocampal neurons. This is particularly evident for the dentate gyrus granule cells and in their mossy fiber axons. In the normal rat, only a few granule cells synthesize and mossy fiber terminal boutons contain the peptide methionine-enkephalin, whereas the great majority of mossy fiber boutons are dynorphin immunoreactive. However, in situ hybridization analysis has demonstrated that within a few hours of the onset of recurrent limbic seizures virtually all of the granule cells contain abundant mRNA for the enkephalin precursor preproenkephalin A. This transient increase in preproenkephalin A mRNA is associated with a more than tenfold increase in enkephalin synthesis by the granule cells and precedes a marked increase in enkephalin immunoreactivity within the mossy fibers that lasts approximately 2 weeks. In striking contrast to these results, dynorphin immunoreactivity within the mossy fibers is reduced in the same seizure paradigm. These experiments have demonstrated that seizure activity differentially alters the expression of the opioids enkephalin and dynorphin within hippocampal neurons, most probably at the level of transcription, and raise questions about the functional consequence of activity-dependent alterations in the expression of neuromodulatory peptides.

REFERENCES

Altschuler, R.A., D.T. Monaghan, W.G. Hasser, R.J. Wenthold, N.P. Curthoys, and C.W. Cotman (1985) Immunocytochemical localization of glutaminase-like and aspartate aminotransferase-like immunoreactivities in the rat and guinea pig hippocampus. Brain Res. *330*:225–223.

Amaral, D., and J. Dent (1981) Development of the mossy fibers of the dentate gyrus. I. A light and electron microscopic study of the mossy fibers and their expansions. J. Comp. Neurol. *195*:51–86.

Baker, H., T. Kawano, F.L. Margolis, and T.H. Joh (1983) Transneuronal regulation of tyrosine hydroxylase expression in olfactory bulb of mouse and rat. J. Neurosci. *3*:69–78.

Baudry, M., G. Lynch, C. Gall (1986) Induction of ornithine decarboxylase as a possible mediator of seizure-induced changes in genomic expression in rat hippocampus. J. Neurosci. *6*:3430–3435.

Black, I.B., J.E. Adler, C.F. Dreyfus, W.F. Friedman, E.F. LaGamma, and A.H. Roach (1987) Biochemistry of information storage in the nervous system. Science *236*:1263–1268.

Blackstad, T.W., and A. Kjaerheim (1961) Special axodendritic synapses in the hippocampal cortex: Electron and light microscopic studies on the layer of mossy fibers. J. Comp. Neurol. *117*:133–159.

Campbell, K.A., B. Bank, and N.W. Milgram (1984) Epileptogenic effects of electrolytic lesions in the hippocampus: Role of iron deposition. Exp. Neurol. *86*:506–514.

Canellakis, E.S., D. Viceps-Madore, D.A. Kyriakidis, and J.S. Heller (1979) The regulation and function of ornithine decarboxylase and of the polyamines. Curr. Top. Cell. Regul. *15*:155–202.

Chavkin, C., and F.E. Bloom (1986) Opiate antagonists do not alter neuronal responses to stimulation of opioid-containing pathways in rat hippocampus. Neuropeptides *7*:19–22.

Crawford, I.L., and J.D. Connor (1973) Localization and release of glutamic acid in relation to the hippocampal mossy fibre pathway. Nature [Lond.] *244*:442–443.

Davis, L.G., R. Arentzen, J.M. Reid, R.W. Manning, B. Wolfson, K.L. Lawrence, and Baldino, R. Jr. (1986) Glucocorticoid sensitivity of vasopressin mRNA levels in the paraventricular nucleus of the rat. Proc. Natl. Acad. Aci. U.S.A. *83:* 1145–1149.

Dragunow, M., and H.A. Robertson (1987) Kindling stimulation induces c-*fos* protein(s) in granule cells of the rat dentate gyrus. Nature *329:*441–442.

Eichenbaum, H., M. Kuperstein, A. Fagan, and J. Nagode (1987) Cue-sampling and goal-approach correlates of hippocampal unit activity in rats performing an odor-discrimination task. J. Neurosci. *7*:716–732.

Fredens, K., K. Stengaard-Pedersen, and L.-T. Larsson (1984) Localization of enkephalin and cholecystokinin immunoreactivities in the perforant path terminal fields of the rat hippocampal formation. Brain Res. 304:255–263.

Frenk, H., R. Motles, Y. Wly, and R. Simantov (1978) Epileptic properties of leucine- and methionine-enkephalin: Comparison with morphine and reversibility by naloxone. Brain Res. *147*:327–337.

Gall, C. (1984a) The distribution of cholecystokinin-like immunoreactivity in the hippocampal formation of the guinea pig: Localization in the mossy fibers. Brain Res. *306*:73–83.

Gall, C. (1984b) Ontogeny of dynorphin-like immunoreactivity in the hippocampal formation of the rat. Brain Res. *307:*327–331.

Gall, C. (1988a) Localization and seizure-induced alterations of opioid peptides and CCK in the hippocampus. In J.F. McGinty (ed): Opioids in the Hippocampus. NIDA Research Monograph 75. Rockville, MD: DHHS Pub. No. (ADM 88-1568), pp. 12–32.

Gall, C. (1988b) Seizures induce dramatic and distinctly different changes in enkephalin, dynorphin, and cholecystokinin immunoreactivities in mouse hippocampal mossy fibers. J. Neurosci. 8:1852–1862.

Gall, C., L. Berry, and L. Hodgson (1986) Cholecystokinin in the mouse hippocampus: Localization in the mossy fiber and dentate commissural system. Exp. Brain Res. 62:431–437.

Gall, C., N. Brecha, K.-J. Chang, and H.J. Karten (1984) Ontogeny of enkephalin-like immunoreactivity in the rat hippocampus. Neuroscience 11:359–380.

Gall, C., N. Brecha, H.J. Karten, and K.-J. Chang (1981) Localization of enkephalin-like immunoreactivity in identified axonal and neuronal populations in the rat hippocampus. J. Comp. Neurol. 198:335–350.

Gall, C., R. Pico, J. Lauterborn (1988) Seizures induce distinct long-lasting changes in mossy fiber peptide immunoreactivity. Peptides 9:79–84.

Gall, C., J.D. White, and J.C. Lauterborn (1987) In situ hybridization analyses of increased preproenkephalin mRNA following seizures. Soc. Neurosci. Abstr. 13:1277.

Greenwood, R.S., S. Godar, T.A. Reaves, Jr., and J. Wayward (1981) Cholecystokinin in hippocampal pathways. J. Comp. Neurol. 203:335–350.

Haug, F.-M.S. (1967) Electron microscopical localization of the zinc in hippocampal mossy fiber synapses by a modified sulphide silver procedure. Histochemie 8:355–368.

Hong, J.S., C. Gillin, H. Yang, and E. Costa (1979a) Repeated electroconvulsive shocks and the brain content of endorphins. Brain Res. 177:273–278.

Hong, J.S., P.L. Wood, J.C. Gillin, H.Y.T. Yang, and E. Costa (1980) Changes of hippocampal Met-enkephalin content after recurrent motor seizures. Nature 285:231–232.

Hong, J.S., H.-Y.T. Yang, J.C. Gillin, W. Fratta, and E. Costa (1979b) Chronic treatment with haloperidol accelerates the biosynthesis of enkephalins in rat striatum. Brain Res. 160:192–195.

Iadarola, M.J., J. Douglass, O. Civelli, and J.R. Naranjo (1986a) Increased spinal cord dynorphin mRNA during peripheral inflammation. In J.W. Holaday, P.-Y. Law, and A. Herz (eds): Progress in Opioid Research. N.I.D.A. Research Monograph 75, pp. 406–409.

Iadarola, M.J., C. Shin, J.O. McNamara, and H.Y.T. Yang (1986b) Changes in dynorphin, enkephalin and cholecystokinin content of hippocampus and substantia nigra after amygdala kindling. Brain Res. 365:181–191.

Kanamatsu, T., J.F. McGinty, C.L. Mitchell, and J.S. Hong (1986a) Dynorphin- and enkephalin-like imunoreactivity is altered in limbic-basal ganglia regions of rat brain after repeated electroconvulsive shock. J. Neurosci 6:644–649.

Kanamatsu, T., J. Obie, L. Grimes, J.F. McGinty, K. Yoshikawa, S. Sabol, and J.S. Hong (1986b) Kainic acid alters the metabolism of Met^5-enkephalin and the level of dynorphin A in the rat hippocampus. J. Neurosci. 6:3094–3102.

Laatsch, R.H., and W.M. Cowan (1965) Electron microscopic studies of the dentate gyrus of the rat. I. Normal structure with special reference to synaptic organization. J. Comp. Neurol. 128: 359–396.

Larson, J. and G. Lynch (1988) Role of N-methyl-D-aspartate receptors in the induction of synaptic potentiation by burst stimulation patterned after the hippocampal theta rhythm. Brain Res. 441:111–118.

Luskin, M.B., and J.L. Price (1983) The topographic organization of associational fibers of the olfactory system in the rat, including centrifugal fibers to the olfactory bulb. J. Comp. Neurol. *216*:264–291.

Lynch, G.S., R.A. Jensen, J.L. McGaugh, K. Davila, and M. Oliver (1981) Effects of enkephalin, morphine, and naloxone on the electrical activity of the in vitro hippocampal slice preparation. Exp. Neurol. *71*:527–540.

McGinty, J.F. (1985) Prodynorphin immunoreactivity is located in different neurons than proenkephalin immunoreactivity in the cerebral cortex of rats. Neuropeptides *5*:465–468.

McGinty, J.F., S.J. Henriksen, A. Goldstein, L. Terenius, and F.E. Bloom (1983) Dynorphin is contained within hippocampal mossy fibers: Immunohistochemical alterations after kainic acid administration and colchicine-induced cytotoxcity. Proc. Natl. Acad. Sci., U.S.A. *80*:589–593.

McGinty, J.F., T. Kanamatsu, J. Obie, R.S. Dyer, C.L. Mitchell, and J.S. Hong (1986) Amygdaloid kindling increases enkephalin-like immunoreactivity but decreases dynorphin A-like immunoreactivity in rat hippocampus. Neurosci. Lett. *71*:31–36.

McGinty, J.F. D. VanDer Kooy, and F.E. Bloom (1984) The distribution of opioid peptide immunoreactive neurons in the cerebral cortex of rats. J. Neurosci. *4*:1104–1117.

Millan, M.J., M.H. Millan, A. Czlonkowski, V. Hollt, W.T. Pilcher, A. Herz, and F.C. Colpaert (1986) A model of chronic pain in the rat: Response of multiple opioid systems to adjuvant-induced arthritis. J. Neurosci. *6*:899–906.

Morgan, J.I., D.R. Cohen, J.L. Hempstead, and T. Curran (1987) Mapping patterns of c-*fos* expression in the central nervous system after seizure. Science *237*:192–197.

Morris, B.J., K.J. Feasley, G. ten Bruggencate, A. Herz, and V. Hollt (1988) Electrical stimulation in vivo increases the expression of proenkephalin mRNA and decreases the expression of prodynorphin mRNA in rat hippocampal granule cells. Proc. Natl. Acad. Sci. U.S.A. *85*:3226–3230.

Morris, B.J., M.E. Moneta, G. ten Bruggencate, and V. Hollt (1987) Levels of prodynorphin mRNA in rat dentate gyrus are decreased during hippocampal kindling. Neurosci. Lett. *80*:298–302.

Przewlocki, R., W. Lason, R. Stach, and D. Kacz (1983) Opioid peptides, particularly dynorphin, after amygdaloid-kindled seizures. Regul Pept. *6*:385–392.

Racine, R. (1972) Modulation of seizure activity by electrical stimulation: II. Motor seizure. Electroencephalogr. Clin. Neurophysiol. **32**:281–294.

Romano, G.J., B.D. Shivers, R.E. Harlan, R.D. Howells, and D.W. Pfaff (1987) Haloperidol increases preproenkephalin mRNA levels in the caudate-putamen of the rat: A quantitative study at the cellular level using in situ hybridization. Mol. Brain Res. *2*:33–41.

Rose, G., D. Diamond, and G. Lynch (1983) Dentate granule cells in the rat hippocampal formation have the behavioral characteristics of theta neurons. Brain Res. *266*:29–37.

Sawchenko, P.E. (1987) Adrenalectomy-induced enhancement of CRF and vasopressin immunoreactivity in parvocellular neurosecretory neurons: Anatomic, peptide and steroid specificity. J. Neurosci. *7*:1093–1106.

Sloviter, R.S. (1985) A selective loss of hippocampal mossy fiber Timm stain accompanies granule cell seizure activity induced by perforant path stimulation. Brain Res. *330*:150–153.

Sloviter, R.S., and B.P. Damiano (1981) On the relationship between kainic acid-induced epileptiform activity and hippocampal neuronal damage. Neuropharmacology *20*:1003–1011.

Staubli, U., and G. Lynch (1987) Stable hippocampal long-term potentiation elicited by "theta" pattern stimulation. Brain Res. *435*:227–234.

White, J.D., and C.M. Gall (1987a) Increased enkephalin gene expression in hippocampus following seizures. In J.W. Holliday, P.Y. Law and A. Herz (eds): Progress in Opioid Research. NIDA Research Monograph, pp. 393–396.

White, J.D., and C.M. Gall (1978b) Differential regulation of neuropeptide and proto-oncogene mRNA content in the hippocampus following recurrent seizures. Mol. Brain Res. *3:*21–29.

White, J.D., C.M. Gall, and J.F. McKelvy (1986) Proenkephalin is processed in a projection specific manner in the rat central nervous system. Proc. Natl. Acad. Sci. U.S.A. *83:*7099–7103.

White, J.D., C.M. Gall and J.F. McKelvy (1987) Enkephalin biosynthesis and enkephalin gene expression are increased in hippocampal mossy fibers following a unilateral lesion of the hilus. J. Neurosci. *7:*753–759.

Yoshikawa, K., J.S. Hong, and S.L. Sabol (1985) Electroconvulsive shock increases pre-proenkephalin messenger RNA abundance in rat hypothalamus. Proc. Natl. Acad. Sci. U.S.A. *82:*589–593.

Yoshikawa, K., C. Williams, and S.L. Sabol (1984) Rat brain preproenkephalin mRNA. J. Biol. Chem. *259:*14301–14308.

Young, S.W., III, T.I. Bonner, and M.R. Brann (1986) Mesencephalic dopamine neurons regulate the expression of neuropeptide mRNAs in the rat forebrain. Proc. Natl. Acad. Sci. U.S.A. *83:*9827–9831.

The Hippocampus—New Vistas, pages 171–187
© 1989 Alan R. Liss, Inc.

12
Neuropeptide Receptors in the Hippocampal Region in the Rat, Monkey, and Human Brain

CHRISTER KÖHLER AND VICTORIA CHAN-PALAY

Astra Research Center, Södertälje, Sweden (C.K.); Neurology Clinic, University Hospital, Zürich, Switzerland (V. C.-P.)

INTRODUCTION

Normal hippocampal function depends on neurotransmission along a chain of association pathways referred to as the *trisynaptic hippocampal circuit*, which interconnects the entorhinal area with the area dentata and, further, the area dentata with subfields CA3 and CA1 of Ammon's horn (Fig. 1). There is a good evidence that one or more excitatory amino acids mediate neurotransmission at several synapses along this intrahippocampal circuit (Cotman et al., 1986; Storm-Mathisen and Iversen, 1979). However, transmission along these pathways is likely to be modulated by afferent projections from cells situated in different cortical and subcortical areas as well as by local interneurons known to be present in all layers of the hippocampal region (see Swanson et al., 1988, and references therein).

In recent years, interest has focused on the chemical identity of hippocampal afferents and interneurons. It is well established that the hippocampus receives serotoninergic, noradrenergic, and dopaminergic inputs from brain stem monoaminergic cell groups (Swanson et al., 1988; Köhler and Steinbusch, 1982; Scatton et al., 1980; Swanson and Hartman, 1975). At more rostral levels, several hypothalamic nuclei have been shown to project to the hippocampus. Thus, histamine, γ-aminobutyric acid (GABA), and galanin producing cells in the tuberomammillary nuclei of the posterior hypothalamus as well as α-melanocyte-stimulating hormone (α-MSH) containing cells in the lateral hypothalamic area and substance P-positive projections from the supramammillary nucleus innervate the hippocampal region (Köhler et al., 1984a,b, 1985b, 1986a; Haglund et al., 1984; Gall and Selawski, 1984) as do cholinergic (Amaral and Kurz, 1985), GABAergic (Köhler et al., 1984a,b), and galanin containing (Melander et al., 1988) neurons situated in the medial septum and the diagonal band of Broca.

Furthermore, histochemical analysis of hippocampal interneurons shows that these constitute a chemically heterogeneous population: whereas the ma-

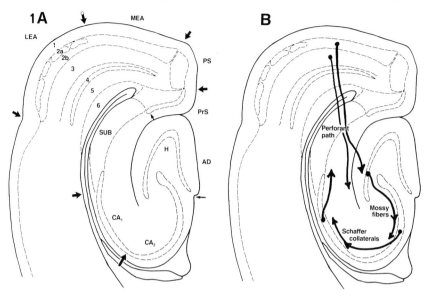

Abbreviations in figures

AD	area dentata
CA1, 3	cornu Ammonis subfields 1 and 3
CCK	cholecystokinin
CCK-ir	cholecystokinin immunoreactive
GAL	galanin
GAL-ir	galanin immunoreactive
H	hilus
LEA	lateral entorhinal area
MEA	medial entorhinal area
NPY	neuropeptide Y
NPY-ir	neuropeptide Y immunoreactive
NT	neurotensin
NT-ir	neurotensin immunoreactive
PrS	presubiculum
PS	parasubiculum
SUB	subiculum

Fig. 1. Line drawings of horizontal sections cut through the midtemporal level of the rat hippocampal region, showing in **A** the major subfields and lamina and in **B** the major components of the intrinsic trisynaptic hippocampal circuit.

jority are GABA containing, recent studies indicated that some neuropeptides are co-stored with GABA in hippocampal interneurons (see Swanson et al., 1988, and references therein). Indeed, the findings of several recent studies imply that neuropeptides are important modulators of hippocampal neurotransmission (Mühlethaler et al., 1984).

Cholecystokinin octapeptide (CCK-8) and neuropeptide tyrosine (NPY) are two peptides that have been located in hippocampal interneurons in the rat and monkey and in postmortem human brain (Chan-Palay et al., 1986; Greenwood et al., 1982; Handelman et al., 1981; Köhler and Chan-Palay, 1982; Lotstra and Vanderhaegen, 1987a,b; Roberts et al., 1984; Sloviter and Nilaver, 1987; Swanson et al., 1988; Köhler et al., 1987b). The morphology of CCK-8 and NPY cells and the laminar distribution of their axons suggest that these two peptides are present in separate groups of interneurons, which implies that they participate in different aspects of hippocampal neurotransmission. For example, while cells containing CCK-8 make frequent axosomatic contacts with hippocampal pyramidal cells, the NPY axons appear to form a more loosely organized network within the hippocampus (see Köhler, 1986; Swanson et al., 1988).

The peptides neurotensin (NT) and galanin have also been identified in cells and terminals within the rodent and primate brain (Hara et al., 1982; Köhler et al., 1986a,b; Melander and Staines, 1986; Melander et al., 1985; Michel et al., 1986; Roberts et al., 1984; Swanson et al., 1988). Unlike CCK-8 and NPY, these peptides are not primarily located in interneurons but are found in cells of the subiculum (neurotensin, Hara et al., 1982; Roberts et al., 1984; Michel et al., 1986) and in afferent projections from the septum/diagonal band complex (galanin, Melander et al., 1985).

While some of the peptidergic afferents have relatively well-defined targets within the hippocampus, others show a more diffusely organized innervation of the structure. It is therefore not always possible to determine in anatomical terms, where the released peptide may exert its primary action. One way of approaching this problem is to supplement information about chemically specified inputs to the hippocampus with maps of receptor localization within this region. The term *receptor* is used here only to denote the existence of a binding site for a drug or a transmitter and does not imply that a functional response has been associated with this binding site. In the present chapter, we review the distribution of receptors for the neuropeptides CCK-8, NPY, neurotensin, and galanin in the rat, monkey, and the postmortem human brain.

MATERIALS AND METHODS

The procedure for in vitro receptor autoradiography was essentially the same as that previously reported by us and by other investigators (Köhler et al., 1987a,b; Kuhar et al., 1986). The ligands used and the conditions of incubations are summarized in Table I. Sections from male Sprague-Dawley rats, male *Cynomologus* monkeys, and postmortem human brains were cut on a cryostat and stored at −70°C until used. The postmortem human brains were collected at autopsy at the University Hospital of Zürich, Switzerland. The postmortem interval until brain tissues were removed and frozen ranged between 3.5 and 23 h. The human brains were from males and females who had no diagnoseable neurological illnesses. After incubations the sections were dried and put in contact with tritium-sensitive film and exposed in darkness for a period of 2 weeks to 2 months at −20°C. The autoradiograms were analyzed by computerized microdensitometry using an IBAS 2000 image-analyzer,

TABLE I. Summary of Ligands and Binding Conditions Used in the Present Study of the Neuropeptide Receptors

Receptor	Ligand	Concentration (nM)	Buffers	Nonspecific (μM)
CCK-8	[^{125}I]CCK-8	0.25	Hepes	CCK-8 (1)
NPY	[^{125}I]NPY	0.20	Krebs-Ringer	NPY (10)
Neurotensin	[^{3}H]NT	7.0	Tris-HCl	NT (1)
Galanin	[^{125}I]Galanin	0.5	Hepes	Galanin (1)

which converted optical densities into molar quantities of bound ligand (for futher discussion of the method, see Palacios and Mengod, Chapter 14, and Zilles, Chapter 13, both this volume).

RESULTS
CCK-8 Receptors

In the three species studied, the highest density of specifically bound [^{125}I]CCK-8 was found in the retrohippocampal region, with moderate to low densities detected in Ammon's horn and the area dentata (Figs. 2–4). In some areas (e.g. pre- and parasubiculum) a similar pattern of binding was found in rat, monkey, and human tissues, while in other subfields differences in the laminar receptor distribution were evident (Fig. 4).

The entorhinal area was found to harbor more CCK-8 receptors than any of the other hippocampal subfields. In the rat, the highest receptor density was present in layers 1 and 3 of the medial entorhinal area, while layers 2, 4, 5, and 6 harbored moderate to low densities of specifically bound [^{125}I]CCK-8. The lateral entorhinal area contained far fewer CCK-8 receptors that did the medial part (Figs. 2A, B, 3), and most of these were located in layer 1 (Fig. 2).

In the monkey hippocampus, the receptor density was lower than, and showed a different pattern of laminar distribution to that, in the rat. Thus, layer 4 was found to be more enriched in CCK-8 receptors than were the other layers. This band of high receptor density in layer 4 could be followed into the lateral entorhinal area.

In the postmortem human brain, the entorhinal area harbored relatively few specific binding sites for [^{125}I]CCK-8, and, in the specimen examined here, little variation in the laminar distribution of specific [^{125}I]CCK-8 binding was noted (Fig. 4). However, the second layer and layers 5 and 6 harbored slightly more binding sites than did the other layers. In all three species, a high density of CCK-8 receptors was found in layer 2 of the presubiculum, while the other fields of the subicular complex showed moderate to low densities of binding.

In the area dentata, which contained a relatively low number of specific binding sites for [^{125}I]CCK-8, some species differences were noted: A moderate density of binding was found in the molecular layer of the monkey and human area dentata, while in the rat the molecular layer appeared to be devoid of

CCK-8 receptors. In all three species, moderate binding densities were found in the hilus of the area dentata.

In the hippocampal region, immunoreactive CCK-8 is present within local interneurons and their processes (Greenwood et al., 1982; Handelman et al., 1981; Köhler and Chan-Palay, 1982; Sloviter and Nilaver, 1987; Roberts et al., 1984; Swanson et al., 1988). Immunohistochemical studies in the rat show that the CCK-8–positive cells innervate primarily layer 2 of the entorhinal area and presubiculum, the pyramidal layer of Ammon's horn, and the hilar and granule cells of the area dentata (Greenwood et al., 1982; Köhler and Chan-Palay, 1982; Sloviter and Nilaver, 1987), where they form axosomatic contacts (Hendry and Jones, 1985; Nunzi et al., 1985). In addition, the lateral entorhinal area of the rat brain is more densely innervated by CCK-8–immunoreactive fibers than is the medial part (Köhler, 1986; Köhler and Chan-Palay, 1982), and in the lateral part all layers receive a dense innervation by CCK-8–positive axons.

The identity and regional distribution of CCK-8–immunoreactive neurons and their processes are less well known in the monkey and human as compared with the rat hippocampus. However, recent studies (Lotstra and Vanderhaegen, 1987a) suggest that the pattern of CCK-8 innervation of the human hippocampus is based on a similar fundamental scheme as that seen in experimental animals.

A comparison between the regional and laminar distributions of CCK-8 receptors and CCK-8–immunoreactive terminals of the hippocampus shows a discrepancy in the sense that the areas richest in CCK-8 receptors were not the ones showing the densest innervation by CCK-8–containing axons. This is not surprising, however, since there must not necessarily exist a perfect relationship, quantitatively speaking, between receptor density and innervation for normal neurotransmission to occur. More disturbing, however, is the finding that the pyramidal layer, which is rich in CCK-8–containing afferent terminals, has among the lowest density of receptors in the entire hippocampal region: little or no specific binding was detected in this layer at the concentration of ligand used here. The reason(s) and biological significance of such a poor concordance are difficult to assess at the moment. Important, however, is the finding that electrophysiological responses can be recorded from hippocampal pyramidal cells after iontophoretic application of CCK-8 (Dodd and Kelly, 1981), and a detailed examination of these effects suggest that the hippocampal CCK-8 receptor is of the so-called central or B type (Böhme et al., 1988).

Neuropeptide Y Receptors

In contrast to CCK-8, the concentration of NPY receptors is highest in Ammon's horn, with moderate to low densities in the area dentata and the retrohippocampal structures (Figs. 2C,D, 4). In the retrohippocampal region, small differences between subfields as well as between individual lamina were discerned. In subfields CA1 through CA3 of Ammon's horn, on the other hand, a high density of binding was found in the strata oriens and radiatum, while strata pyramidale and lacunosum-moleculare were poor in specifically bound peptides in all three species. In the area dentata, the inner part of the molecular layer harbored NPY receptors in the rat, but this was not obvious in monkey

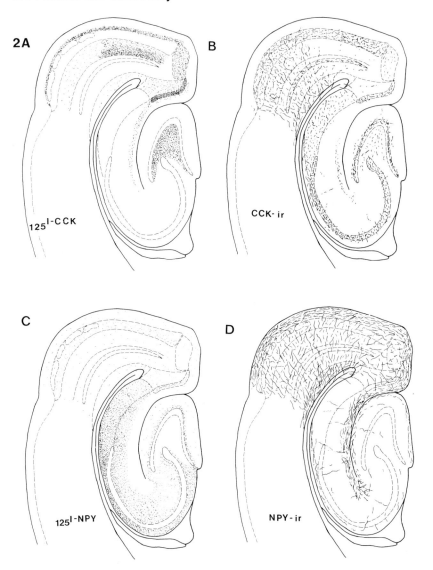

Fig. 2.   Line drawings of horizontal sections through the midtemporal portion of the rat hippocampal region showing the relative density of CCK-8 **(A,B)**, NPY **(C,D)**, NT **(E,F)**, and galanin **(G,H)** receptors (A,C,E,G) and innervation (B,D,F,H).

and human brains. All subfields of the hippocampus contained more NPY receptors in the rat than in the monkey and the postmortem human brain. In general, however, the pattern of NPY receptor distribution was similar in the three species examined.

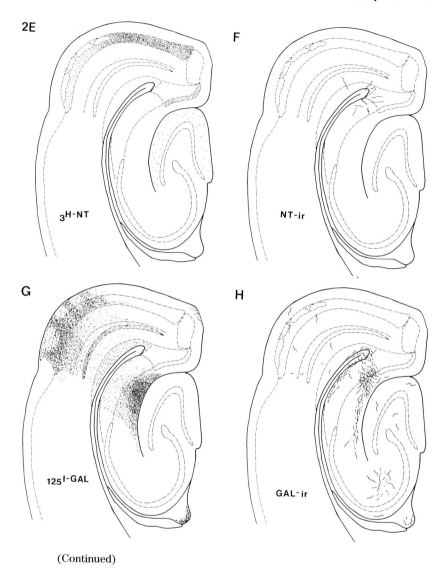

2E 3H-NT

F NT-ir

G 125I-GAL

H GAL-ir

(Continued)

The hippocampal region receives a rich innervation by NPY-positive neurons in the rat (Köhler et al., 1986b), monkey (Köhler et al., 1986b), and postmortem human (Chan-Palay et al., 1986) brain. The pattern of NPY innervation is remarkably similar in the three species: a dense innervation of all layers of the retrohippocampal areas and a more heterogenous innervation of layers in the hippocampal formation. Thus, in Ammon's horn, the majority of the NPY fibers are found in the stratum moleculare, with less prominent innervation of strata

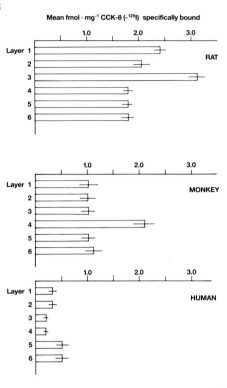

Fig. 3. Histograms showing the laminar distribution of specific [^{125}I]CCK-8 binding sites in rat, monkey, and human entorhinal area as determined by quantitative microdensitometry using an IBAS 2000 image analysis system.

radiatum, pyramidale, and oriens (Köhler et al., 1986b). The NPY receptors are present primarily in those layers of Ammon's horn that contain the basal and apical dendrites, respectively, of the pyramidal cells.

It is obvious from these findings that for NPY, too, there exists a discrepancy between the density of laminar receptor distribution and the density of NPY innervation. Assuming that the receptor distribution reveals the site(s) of action of NPY, the present findings suggest that the dendrites of the hippocampal pyramidal cells or their afferent inputs are the primary targets for neuronally released NPY in all three species. Indeed, several electrophysiological studies have shown that NPY applied onto hippocampal pyramidal cells in vitro causes hyperpolarization of their dendritic membranes, possibly through a presynaptic mechanism that reduces the excitatory input to the pyramidal neurons (Haas et al., 1987; Colmers et al., 1985, 1986).

4

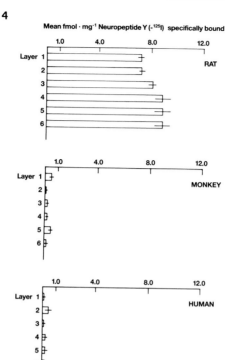

Fig. 4. Histograms showing the laminar distribution of specific [^{125}I]NPY binding sites in the entorhinal area of the rat, monkey, and postmortem human brain.

Neurotensin Receptors

The highest density of specifically bound [^{125}I]neurotensin ([^{125}I]NT) was found in the retrohippocampal region in all three species. Ammon's horn and area dentata contained far less [^{125}I]NT binding sites, but the receptor density tended to increase at more temporal levels of the hippocampal formation.

In the retrohippocampal region, a high density of NT receptors was found in layer 2 of the para- and presubiculum in the rat, monkey, and human brain. The highest receptor density was found in the entorhinal area. In the rat, virtually all of the specifically bound [^{125}I]NT was restricted to layer 2 and the deep part of layer 1 in the medial entorhinal area. At ventral levels, binding was also detected in layer 2b of the lateral entorhinal area. The deep layers, on the other hand, harbored low to undetectable levels of specific [^{125}I]NT binding.

The laminar pattern of entorhinal [^{125}I]NT binding was found to be partly similar in the rat and in the postmortem human brain. In the human brain, too, the outer two layers were enriched in NT receptors, but, in contrast to the situation in the rat, NT receptors were also present in large numbers in the deep layers (Figs. 2E,F, 5). In the monkey brain, the laminar distribution of NT receptors was found to be somewhat different from that in both the rat and human. Thus, the highest receptor density was found in layer 4 of the entorhinal area, while moderate to low binding densities were detected in the other layers.

In all three species the hippocampal formation was found to be poor in NT receptors. In the area dentata, the molecular layer contained a low density of NT receptors in the rat and human brain. In the monkey, a moderate receptor density was found in the hilus, while the molecular layer appeared to be devoid of NT receptors. Ammon's horn apparently contains low densities of NT re-

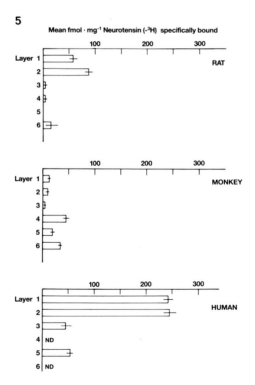

Fig. 5. Histograms showing the laminar distribution of specific [^{125}I]NT binding sites in the entorhinal area of the rat, monkey, and postmortem human brain.

ceptors in rat and human. Low receptor densities could be detected in the stratum radiatum of the monkey hippocampus.

In all three species examined here, the NT receptors appeared to occupy a strategic position within the hippocampus: The high receptor density in layer 2 of the entorhinal area in the rat and human brain suggests that NT may affect cells that give rise to the perforant pathway, the most prominent association pathway of the hippocampal region. In contrast, NT receptors were not associated with these cells in the monkey brains studied here. Instead, layers 4 and 6, which harbor cells that give rise to extrahippocampal projections of the entorhinal area, were enriched in NT receptors.

The exact distribution of NT-immunoreactive (ir) cells and fibers within the hippocampus is still poorly understood. Reports of NT-ir cells in the subiculum of the adult rat (Roberts et al., 1984) has been challenged by failures to detect immunoreactive NT in this region using biochemical methods (Emson et al., 1982). However, immunohistochemical studies have shown NT-ir in subicular cells and in fibers in rat and human fetuses (Hara et al., 1982; Kataoka et al., 1970; Michel et al., 1986). In a study of the human fetus by Michel et al. (1986), NT-ir neurons were found in the subicular complex and NT-ir axons could be traced into the entorhinal area. It is possible that NT receptors are associated with the projections of the subicular complex onto the entorhinal area. The fact that NT immunoreactivity is detected more readily in young animals could indicate a specific role of hippocampal NT during ontogeny.

Galanin Receptors

Specifically bound [^{125}I]galanin could be detected in the rat and to a lesser degree in the monkey and human hippocampi (Figs. 2G,H, 6). In the rat hippocampus, the highest receptor density was found in its ventral part: primarily in the lateral entorhinal area, where all layers harbored galanin receptors, and in the molecular layer of the subiculum (Fig. 2). The dorsal (septal) hippocampus did not contain specific [^{125}I]galanin binding sites.

In the monkey and human hippocampal region, the highest receptor densities were detected in the hilus of area dentata and in the presubiculum. In the entorhinal area low binding densities were detected in rat and human brain. While the distribution was homogeneous in the monkey, the deep (4–6) layers of the human entorhinal cortex were more enriched in [^{125}I]galanin binding sites.

Galanin innervation of the hippocampus has been studied extensively in the rat brain (Melander et al., 1986a,b; Ching et al., 1985; Skofitsch and Jacobiwitz, 1985). The majority of hippocampal galanin-containing axons derive from cells in the diagonal band of Broca, which also costores acetylcholine, and have been shown to project to the ventral but not to the dorsal hippocampal region (Melander et al., 1985). In contrast to several other neurotransmitter candidates, a relatively good correlation appears to exist between receptor distribution and galanin-containing afferent projections. Indeed, a recent study (Fisione et al., 1987) has shown that galanin can inhibit the release of acetylcholine from nerve endings in the ventral but not in the dorsal hippocampus,

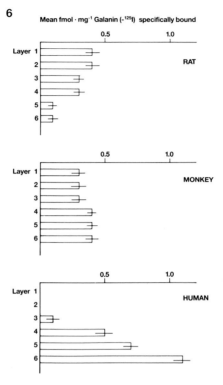

Fig. 6. Histograms showing the laminar distribution of specific [^{125}I]galanin binding sites in different layers of the entorhinal area in the rat, monkey, and postmortem human brain.

presumably through an action on galanin receptors situated on acetylcholine galanin-containing axon terminals. This observation is of fundamental importance, since it implies that a functional heterogeneity of septal cholinergic afferents to the hippocampal region may exist.

The galanin innervation of the monkey and human hippocampi is less well known than in the rat. However, studies in the monkey suggest that in this species, too, the hippocampus receives a galanin-containing projection from cells located in the diagonal band of Broca (Melander and Staines, 1986). The fact that the hippocampus does have galanin receptors suggests that this peptide may play a role in the function of the primate hippocampal region. The lack of detailed information about the terminal distribution of galanin axons in the hippocampus makes a direct comparison with receptor distribution difficult at present.

DISCUSSION

The present chapter has reviewed the laminar distribution of four neuro-peptide receptors (CCK-8, NPY, NT, and galanin) within the hippocampal region of the rat, monkey, and postmortem human brain. These studies partly confirm previous studies in the rat (Köhler et al., 1985a,b; 1987a; Melander et al., 1988) and extend those studies to the primate and to the postmortem normal human brain. With the exception of NT, all other peptide receptors studied were found to be more enriched in the rodent and monkey when compared with the human hippocampus. Whether this represents a true phylogenetic difference in hip-pocampal receptor density is unclear at present. The relatively low receptor numbers noted for CCK-8, NPY, and galanin in the human compared with the rat and the monkey brain may be due to the technical problems presented with tissue handling, including postmortem intervals for the human tissue that may be more detrimental to some peptide receptors (CCK-8, NPY, galanin) than to others (NT).

Previous studies have shown the existence of CCK-8 (Köhler and Chan-Palay, 1982; Sloviter and Nilaver, 1987; Roberts et al., 1984), NPY (Köhler et al., 1987a,b), NT (Michel et al., 1986; Roberts et al., 1984) and galanin (Melander et al., 1986a,b) immunoreactive cells and terminals in the rat and primate brain, which suggests that these peptides may be released at different levels within the hippocampus. Using the receptor autoradiographic technique, presumed receptors for these peptides have been demonstrated in the hippocampus, which further supports the idea that they may participate in hippocampal neu-rotransmission. The exact focus of these receptors may indicate where the neuropeptides excert their primary action(s). Layers 2 and 3 of the entorhinal cortex play important roles in hippocampal neurotransmission, since they give rise to the perforant pathway (Steward, 1976; Steward and Scoville, 1976) as well as to commissural connections with the contralateral entorhinal cortex. More specifically, layer 2 innervates primarily the molecular layer of the area dentata, while layer 3 projects to the molecular layer of Ammon's horn. Both layers 2 and 3 receive input from the pre- and parasubiculum (Köhler et al., 1978; Shipley, 1975), and thus these layers may serve as a gateway for thalamic and cortical inputs to the hippocampus. In the rat brain, the other layers of the entorhinal area are rich in NT (layer 2) and CCK-8 (layer 3) receptors. Although the exact cellular localization of these receptors is unknown at pres-ent, it is reasonable to assume that they participate in the control of neuro-transmission within these layers. This in turn implies that NT and CCK-8 se-lectively affect transmission in different components of the perforant pathway. The layers of the perforant pathway did harbor binding sites for [125I]NPY and [125I]galanin, albeit at far lower densities than in other parts of the hippocampus. Both receptor and immunohistochemical (Köhler et al., 1986a,b; Melander et al., 1986a,b) studies have provided evidence that the activity in layers 2 and 3 of the entorhinal area may be regulated by these two peptides. High densities of galanin receptors were found in all layers of the ventral one-third of the entorhinal area. It is possible that galanin receptors are associated with cholinergic nerve terminals innervating all layers of the entorhinal cortex, thereby affecting the output of both intrinsic (perforant pathway) and extrinsic projections of this area. It is striking that the highest density of NPY receptors was not in the entorhinal area but in Ammon's horn, where they occupied the dendritic zones of regio superior and -inferior. It appears thus that NPY released in Ammon's horn affects a large population of pyramidal cells that have both intrinsic and extrinsic projections.

REFERENCES

Amaral, D.G., and J. Kurz (1985) An analysis of the origins of the cholinergic and noncholinergic septal projections to the hippocampal formation of the rat. J. Comp. Neurol. 1985:37–59.

Böhme, G.-A., J.-M. Stutzman, and J.-C. Blanchard (1988) Excitatory effects of cholecystokinin in rat hippocampus: Pharmacological response compatible with "central" or B-type CCK-8 receptors. Brain Res. 451:309–318.

Chan-Palay, V., C. Köhler, V. Haesler, and W. Lang (1986) Distribution of neurons and axons immunoreactive with antisera against neuropeptide Y in the normal human hippocampus. J. Comp. Neurol. 248:360–375.

Ching, J.L.C., N.D. Christofides, P. Anand, S.J. Gibson, Y.S. Allen, H. Su, U. Tatemoto, F.F.B. Morrison, and J.M. Polak (1985) Distribution of galanin immunoreactivity in the central nervous system and the responses of galanin containing neuronal pathways to injury. Neuroscience 16:343–354.

Colmers, W.F., K. Lujowiak, and Q.J. Pittman (1985) Neuropeptide Y reduces orthodromically evoked population spike in rat hippocampal CA1 by a possibly presynaptic mechanism. Brain Res. 346:404–408.

Colmers, W.F., K. Lukowiak, and Q.J. Pittman (1986) Presynaptic action of neuropeptide Y in area CA1 of the rat hippocampal slice. J. Physiol. [Lond.] (in press).

Cotman, C.W., J.A. Flatman, A.H. Ganong, and M.N. Perkins (1986) Effects of excitatory amino acid antagonists on evoked and spontaneous excitatory potentials in guinea pig hippocampus. J. Physiol. [Lond.] 378:403–415.

Dodd, J., and J.S. Kelly (1981) The actions of cholecystokinin and related peptides on pyramidal neurons in the mammalian hippocampus. Brain Res. 205:337–350.

Emson, C.P., M. Goedert, P. Horsfield, F. Rioux, and S. St. Pierre (1982) The regional distribution and chromatographic characterization of neurotensin-like immunoreactivity in the rat central nervous system. J. Neurochem. 38:992–999.

Fisione, G., C.F. Wu, S. Consolo, Ö. Nordström, N. Brynne, T. Bartfai, T. Melander, and T. Hökfelt (1987) Galanin inhibits acetylcholine release in the ventral hippocampus of the rat: histochemical, autoradiographic, in vivo and in vitro studies. Proc. Natl. Acad. Sci. USA 84:7339–7343.

Gall, C., and L. Selawski (1984) Supramammillary afferents to guinea pig hippocampus contain substance P-like immunoreactivity. Neurosci. Lett. 51:171–176.

Greenwood, R.S., S. Godar, and T.H. Reaves (1982) Cholecystokinin in hippocampal pathways. J. Comp. Neurol. 198:335–350.

Haas, H.L., A. Hermann, R.W. Greene, and V. Chan-Palay (1987) Action and location of neuropeptide tyrosine (Y) on rat hippocampal neurons in slice preparations. J. Comp. Neurol. 257:208–215.

Haglund, L., L.W. Swanson, and C. Köhler (1984) The projections of the supramammillary nucleus to the hippocampal formation: An immunohistochemical and anterograde transport study in the rat. J. Comp. Neurol. 229:171–185.

Handelman, G.E., D.U. Meyer, M.C. Beinfeld, and W.H. Oertel (1981) CCK-containing terminals in the hippocampal area. Brain Res. *224*:181–185.

Hara, Y., S. Shiosaka, E. Seraba, M. Sakanaka, S. Inagaki, H. Takagi, Y. Kawai, K. Takatsuki, and T. Matsuzaki (1982) Ontogeny of neurotensin containing neuron system of the rat: Immunohistochemical analysis. I. Forebrain and diencephalon. J. Comp. Neurol. *208*:177–195.

Hendry, S.H.C., and E.G. Jones (1985) Morphology of synapses formed by cholecystokinin-immunoreactive axon terminals in regio superior of rat hippocampus. Neuroscience *16*:57–68.

Hjorth-Simonsen, A. (1973) Some intrinsic connections of the hippocampus of the rat: An experimental analysis. J. Comp. Neurol. *147*:145–162.

Kataoka, K., N. Mizuno, and L.A. Frohman (1979) Regional distribution of immunoreactive neurotensin in monkey brain. Brain Res. Bull. *4*:57–60.

Köhler, C. (1986) Cytochemical architecture of the entorhinal area. In R. Schwarcz and Y. Ben-Ari (eds): Excitatory Amino Acids and Epilepsy. New York: Plenum, pp. 83–98.

Köhler, C., and V. Chan-Palay (1982) The distribution of cholecystokinin immunoreactive neurons and nerve terminals in the retrohippocampal region in the rat and guinea pig. J. Comp. Neurol. *210*:136–146.

Köhler, C., V. Chan-Palay, J.Y. Wu (1984a). Septal neurons containing glutamic acid decarboxylase immunoreactivity project to the hippocampal region in the rat brain. Anat. Embryol. *169*:41–44.

Köhler, C., H. Ericson, T. Watanabe, J. Polak, S. Palay, and V. Chan-Palay (1986a) Galanin immunoreactivity is present in hypothalamic histamine neurons: Further evidence for multiple messengers in the tuberomamillary nucleus. J. Comp. Neurol. *250*:58–65.

Köhler, C., L.G. Eriksson, S. Davies, and V. Chan-Palay (1986b) Neuropeptide Y innervation of the hippocampal region in the rat and monkey brain. J. Comp. Neurol. *244*:384–401.

Köhler, C., L. Haglund, and L.W. Swanson (1984b) A diffuse alpha melanocyte stimulating hormone-immunoreactive projection to the hippocampus and spinal cord from individual neurons in the lateral hypothalamic area and zona incerta. J. Comp. Neurol. *223*:501–514.

Köhler, C., H. Hallman, and A.C. Radesäter (1987a) Distribution of ^{3}H-cholecystokinin octapeptide binding sites in the hippocampal region of the rat brain as shown by in vitro receptor autoradiography. Neuroscience *21*:857:857–868.

Köhler, C., A.C. Radesäter, H. Hall, and B. Winblad (1985a) Autoradiographic localization of ^{3}H-neurotensin binding sites in the hippocampal region of the rat and primate brain. Neuroscience *16*:577–587.

Köhler, C., M. Schultzberg, A.C. Radesäter (1987b) Distribution of neuropeptide Y receptors in the rat hippocampal region. Neurosci. Lett. *75*:141–146.

Köhler, C., and H. Steinbusch (1982) Identification of serotonin and nonserotonin containing neurons of the midbrain raphe projecting to the entorhinal area and hippocampal formation: A combined fluorescence retrograde tracing study in the rat brain. Neuroscience *7*:951–957.

Köhler, C., L.W. Swanson, L. Haglund, and J.Y. Wu (1985b) The cytoarchitecture, histochemistry and projections of the tuberomammillary nucleus in the rat. Neuroscience *16*:85–110.

Kuhar, M.J., J.R. Unnerstall, and E.B. de Souza (1986) Neurotransmitter receptor mapping by autoradiography and other methods. Annu. Rev. Neurosci. *9*:27–59.

Lotstra, F., and J. Vanderhaegen (1987a) High concentration of cholecystokinin neurons in the newborn human entorhinal cortex. Neurosci. Lett. 80:191–196.

Lotstra, F., and J. Vanderhaegen (1987b) Distribution of immunoreactive cholecystokinin in the human hippocampus. Peptides 8:911–920.

Melander, T., T. Hökfelt, and Å. Rökaeus (1986a) Distribution of galanin-like immunoreactivity in the rat central nervous system. J. Comp. Neurol. 248:475–517.

Melander, T., C. Köhler, S. Nilsson, T. Hökfelt , E. Brodin, E. Theodorson, T. Bartfai (1988) Autoradiographic quantitation and anatomical mapping of ^{125}-galanin binding sites in the rat central nervous system. J. Chem. Neuroanat. 1:213–233.

Melander, T., and W.A. Staines (1986) A galanin-like peptide coexists in putative cholinergic somata of the septum basal forebrain complex and in acetylcholinesterase-containing fibers and varicosities within the hippocampus in the owl monkey. Neurosci. Lett. 68:17–22.

Melander, T., W.A. Staines, T. Hökfelt, Å. Rökaeus, F. Eckenstein, P.M. Salvaterra, and B.H. Wainer (1985) Galanin-like immunoreactivity in cholinergic neurons of the septum-basal forebrain complex projecting to the hippocampus of the rat. Brain Res. 360:130–138.

Melander, T., W.M. Staines, and Å. Rökaeus (1986b) Galanin-like immunoreactivity in hippocampal afferents in the rat with special reference to cholinergic and noradrenergic inputs. Neuroscience 19:223–240.

Michel, J.P., N. Sakamoto, N. Kopp, and J. Pearson (1986) Neurotensin immunoreactive structures in the human infant striatum, septum, amygdala and cerebral cortex. Brain Res. 397:93–102.

Mühlethaler M., S. Charpak, M.M. Manning, and Dreifuss (1984) Contrasting effects of neurohypophysial peptides on pyramidal and non-pyramidal neurons in the rat hippocampus. Brain Res. 308:97–101.

Nunzi, M.G., A. Gorio, F. Milan, J.F. Freund, P. Somogyi, and A.D. Smith (1985) Cholecystokinin immunoreactive cells form symmetrical synaptic contacts with pyramidal and non-pyramidal neurons in the hippocampus. J. Comp. Neurol. 237:485–505.

Roberts, G.W., P.L. Woodhams, J.M. Polak, and T.J. Crow (1984) Distribution of neuropeptides in the limbic system of the rat: the hippocampus. Neuroscience 11:35–77.

Scatton, B., H. Simon, M. Le Moal, and S. Bischoff (1980) Origin of dopamine innervation of the rat hippocampal formation. Neurosci. Lett. 18:125–131.

Shipley M.T., (1975) The topographical and laminar organization of the presubiculum projection to the ipsi- and contralateral entorhinal cortex in the guinea pig. J. Comp. Neurol. 160:127–146.

Skofitsch, G., and D. Jacobiwitz (1985) Immunohistochemical mapping of galanin like neurons in the rat central nervous system. Peptides 6:509–546.

Sloviter, R.S., and G. Nilaver (1987) Immunocytochemical localization of GABA-, cholecystokinin-, vasoactive intestinal polypeptide and somatostatin like immunoreactivity in the area dentata and hippocampus of the rat. J. Comp. Neurol. 256:42–61.

Steward, O., (1975) Topographic organization of the projections from the entorhinal area to the hippocampal formation of the rat. J. Comp. Neurol. 167:285–314.

Steward, O., S.A. Scoville (1976) Cells of origin of entorhinal cortical afferents to the hippocampus and fascia dentata of the rat. J. Comp. Neurol. 169:347–370.

Storm-Mathisen, J., and L.L. Iversen (1979) Uptake of ^{3}H-glutamic acid in excitatory nerve endings: Light and electron microscopic observations in the hippocampal formation of the rat. Neuroscience 4:1237–1253.

Swanson, L.W., and B. Hartman (1975) The central adrenergic system. An immunofluorescence study of the location of cell bodies and their efferent connections in the rat utilizing dopamine-B-hydroxylase as a marker. J. Comp. Neurol. *163*:467–506.
Swanson, L.W., C. Köhler, and A. Bjöklund (1988) The limbic region. I: The septohippocampal system. In L.W. Swanson, A. Björklund, and T. Hökfelt (eds): Handbook of Chemical Neuroanatomy, Vol. 5, pp. 125–255.

The Hippocampus—New Vistas, pages 189–205

13

Codistribution of Transmitter Receptors in the Human and Rat Hippocampus

KARL ZILLES

Anatomical Institute, University of Cologne, Cologne, Federal Republic of Germany

INTRODUCTION

Quantitative receptor autoradiography has developed into an important tool with which to study the chemical anatomy of the hippocampus. A rapidly increasing number of observations describes the regional distribution of various types of receptors in selected hippocampal subregions and layers in different animals and, less numerously, in the human brain as well. While each of these studies gives valuable information about single receptors or subregions, it is difficult to reach an integrative view.

This study, therefore, tries to achieve a more complex insight into receptor distributions by analyzing similarities and dissimilarities of the regional patterns of seven different receptor types on the basis of an identical parcellation of the anatomical structure of the human and rat hippocampus, respectively. Similarities between the regional distributions indicate codistribution on the laminar level. The hippocampus offers a clearly laminated structure, only comparable with the situation in the cerebellum, and the various presynaptic elements terminate in the different layers and sublayers almost without overlapping. For that reason the finding of eventual codistributions of different receptors can give information about possible interactions between neurochemically different systems on an anatomical level.

Codistribution should not be confused with colocalization in immunohistochemistry, because quantitative receptor autoradiography does not permit a local resolution down to the level of single neurons. It might be possible that two different codistributed receptors are colocalized in the same neuron and interact directly, but it is also possible that codistribution indicates similar regional preferences within the same lamina, but for different cells. Codistribution, as defined here, is not the random occurrence of high densities of two different receptors in one single layer, but the more complex aspect of statistically significant similar distribution patterns based on the receptor densities of *all* subregions and layers in a complex neuronal structure. Codistribution, therefore, reveals a structural principle indicative of putative integrated actions of different neurochemical systems.

MATERIALS AND METHODS

Pieces about $3 \times 3 \times 2$ cm large from the hippocampus of 14 human brains were excised between 6 and 40 h postmortem, frozen in isopentane at $-50°C$, and stored at $-70°C$. The ages of the patients were between 26 and 77 years, and all died because of diseases not primarily affecting the central nervous system. The cortical pieces were cut in a cryostat microtome at $-15°C$ (section thickness, 20 μm). The sections were mounted on gelatine-coated slides, dried at $-25°C$ overnight, and used for the different labeling procedures summarized in Table I. Adjacent sections were taken for staining of cell bodies with a modified silver stain (Merker, 1983). Complete rat brains from ten male and female Wistar rats were processed in the same way.

The measurement of the concentration of binding sites was performed by means of the IBAS 1 + 2 image analyzer (Kontron, Munich, FRG). Detailed descriptions of the equipment, quantitation procedure, and autoradiography have already been published (Zilles, 1988; Zilles et al., 1986, 1988). The absolute values of local receptor densities (fmol/mg protein) vary in dimension up to 10^3 between different receptor types. Additionally, the absolute values of human hippocampi are also extremely variable between different individuals, depending on biological differences and methodical problems in estimating absolute values (cf. Zilles et al., 1988). Since the aim of the present study was to compare the laminar distribution *patterns* of different receptors, the mean absolute receptor density in the entire hippocampus of each brain and receptor type was set at 100% and the actual layer specific values are expressed as relative values on this basis. Similarities between the distribution pattern of different receptors were tested with the Spearman rank correlation test. A significant similarity was found when the different receptors were codistributed on the level of hippocampal layers.

RESULTS

The regional distributions of five different binding sites were observed in the rat hippocampus (Fig. 1). The 5-HT$_1$ receptors show the highest densities in the radiatum and lacunosum-moleculare layers of subfield CA1, the molecular and granular layers of fascia dentata (FD), and the hilus region. The M1 receptors are found most densely packed in the oriens, pyramidal, and radiatum layers of CA1 and in the molecular layer of FD. Quite different is the regional distribution of M2 receptors, with values above the mean in all layers of CA1–CA4 with the exception of the lacunosum-moleculare layer of CA1 and the oriens layer of CA2. The [^{3}H]N-methyl-scopolamine (NMS) binding sites that comprise both M1 and M2 receptors show the highest densities in the pyramidal and radiatum layers of CA1. The glutamate binding sites are densest in the oriens, pyramidal and radiatum layers of CA1 and in the molecular layer of FD.

The distributional patterns were tested for similarities (Table II). The best codistribution is found for NMS and M1 binding sites. This is not surprising, because M1 receptors are the prevailing subset of binding sites labeled with [^{3}H]NMS. Even more interesting are the codistributions between the receptors of different neurotransmitters, i.e. 5-HT$_1$ with M1 receptors and M1 receptors with glutamate binding sites. The M2 receptors do not show a regional distribution significantly similar to any of the other binding sites analyzed in the rat hippocampus.

In the human hippocampus the distributional patterns of six different binding sites were evaluated (Fig. 2). The 5-HT$_1$ receptors show the highest relative densities in the pyramidal and radiatum layers of CA1 (Fig. 3). The GABA$_A$ receptors are most densely packed in the pyramidal and radiatum layers of CA1 and in the molecular layer of FD. The patterns of M1 receptors and NMS (M1 + M2) binding sites are very similar, with the highest values in the pyramidal layers of CA1 and, additionally in the case of the NMS binding sites, in the pyramidal layer of CA2. The glutamate binding sites show readings above the mean level in the pyramidal layer of CA1 and the molecular layer of FD. The D1 receptors are most densely packed in the pyramidal and radiatum layers of CA1 (as are the 5-HT$_1$ and GABA$_A$ receptors), but, in contrast to all other receptors, higher values than the mean density can also be observed in the CA3 (pyramidal and radiatum-lacunosum-moleculare layers) and CA4 subregions.

The comparison of distributions in the human hippocampus demonstrates, as found in the rat, a high degree of similarity between the patterns of M1 receptors and NMS binding sites (Table III). Also in agreement with the rat findings is the fact that 5-HT$_1$ and M1 receptors as well as M1 and glutamate binding sites are codistributed in man. The regional patterns of GABA$_A$ and 5-HT$_1$, respectively M1 and glutamate binding sites, show significant correspondence. The regional distribution of D1 receptors does not correlate with any of the other receptors analyzed here.

Finally, a comparison can be made between human and rat patterns. In this case 5-HT$_1$, NMS, M1, and glutamate binding sites can be tested for resemblance in regional distribution patterns. Only for the glutamate binding sites was a significant similarity in laminar distribution found (Spearman rank correlation: r = 0.72; $P < 0.01$).

DISCUSSION

The aim of this study was to search for codistributions between different neurotransmitter receptors within rat and human hippocampi. Codistribution means that two different receptor types show similar local preferences in all hippocampal subregions and layers.

An analysis of codistribution cannot be performed by comparing results of different studies on selected subregions and layers, because widely differing absolute values and scaling systems for receptor densities in the same region are published, and the generally incomplete mapping of the hippocampus in-

TABLE I. Short Summary of the Labeling Procedures for the Different Receptors Used in the Present Investigation

Ligand concentration	Incubation buffer	Preincubation	Incubation	Washing
[³H]5-HT 0.5 nM	0.17 M Tris-HCl (pH 7.7), 4 mM $CaCl_2$, 0.01% ascorbic acid, 1 μM fluoxetine, 10 μM pargyline	30 min at 25°C in 0.17 M Tris HCl (pH 7.7)	60 min at 25°C in incubation buffer	4 × 15 sec (4°C) in incubation buffer
[³H]N-methyl-scopolamine 0.2 nM	0.17 M Tris-HCl (pH 7.7), 10 mM $MgCl_2$	20 min at 25°C in incubation buffer	60 min at 25°C in incubation buffer	1 × 10 min (4°C) in incubation buffer
[³H]pirenzepine 2–3 nM	Modified Krebs' buffer (pH 7.4), 7 mM K^+, 37 mM Na^+	20 min at 25°C in incubation buffer	60 min at 25°C in incubation buffer	1 × 5 min (4°C) in incubation buffer
[³H]oxotremorine-M 1–2 nM	0.02 M HEPES-Tris (pH 7.5), 10 mM $MgCl_2$	20 min at 25°C in incubation buffer	30 min at 25°C in incubation buffer	2 × 2 min (4°C) in incubation buffer

Ligand	Buffer	Preincubation	Incubation	Washing
[³H]glutamate 100–150 nM	0.05 M Tris-HCl (pH 7.4), 2.5 mM $CaCl_2$	30 min at 4°C in incubation buffer	45 min at 4°C in incubation buffer (the ligand is diluted to 10 Ci/mmol)	4 × 2 sec with buffer (4°C) and 1 × 2 sec with acetone
[³H]glutamate 100–150 nM	0.05 M Tris-acetate (pH 7.4)	30 min at 4°C in incubation buffer	45 min at 4°C in incubation buffer (the ligand is diluted to 10 Ci/mmol)	4 × 2 sec with buffer (4°C) and 1 × 2 sec with acetone
[³H]muscimol 5–8 nM	0.05 M Tris-citrate (pH 7.0)	3 × 5 min at 4°C in incubation buffer	40 min at 4°C in incubation buffer	3 × 2 sec (4°C) in incubation buffer
[³H]SCH 23390 1 nM	0.05 M Tris-HCl, 0.12 M NaCl, 0.005 M KCl, 0.002 M $CaCl_2$, 0.001 M $MgCl_2$ (pH 7.7)	30 min at 25°C in incubation buffer	20 min at 25°C in incubation buffer	2 × 5 min (4°C) in incubation buffer

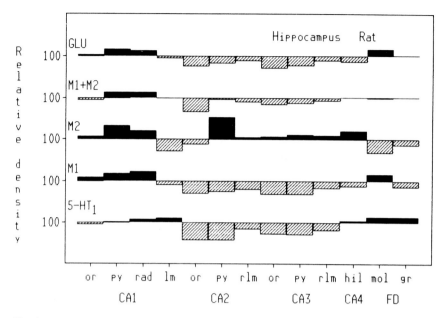

Fig. 1. Laminar distribution of receptor densities in the rat dorsal hippocampus (CA1–CA4 and fascia dentata). Binding sites for [³H]5-HT (5-HT₁), [³H]pirenzepine (M1), [³H]oxotremorine-M (M2), [³H]N-methyl-scopolamine (M1 + M2), and [³H]glutamate (GLU) are analyzed, and the mean receptor density in the entire hippocampus of each receptor is set at 100%. The relative receptor density is given for each subregion and layer and results in values higher (black columns) or lower (hatched columns) than the respective mean density. gr, granular layer; hil, hilus (=CA4); lm, lacunosum-moleculare layer; mol, molecular layer; or, oriens layer; py, pyramidal layer; rad, radiatum layer; rlm, radiatum-lacunosum-moleculare layer.

TABLE II. Spearman Rank Correlations of the Laminar Distributions of Transmitter Receptors in the Rat Hippocampus*

	5-HT₁	NMS	M1	M2	Glutamate binding sites
5-HT₁	—	0.78 0.01	0.74 0.01	NS	NS
NMS	—	—	0.87 0.005	NS	NS
M1	—	—	—	NS	0.65 0.025
M2	—	—	—	—	NS

*The regional and layer-specific patterns are compared. NS, not significant; first line, rank correlation coefficient; second line, error probability.

hibits transformation of absolute into relative densities on a common basis. The situation is even more complicated by the fact that the measurements of anatomical structures often lack a clear architectural definition. Therefore, the present study was founded on measurements of receptor densities in all layers of the hippocampus, the absolute values were transformed into relative values, and the delineation of layers was controlled by overlying immediately adjacent Nissl-stained sections (Zilles, 1988; Zilles et al., 1986, 1988). This permits an easy and reliable comparison of regional distribution patterns between receptor types of widely differing absolute scales.

The 5-HT$_1$ receptors were labeled with [^{3}H]5-HT in nM concentrations and in the presence of ascorbic acid, the monoamine oxydase (MAO) inhibitor pargyline, and the uptake inhibitor fluoxetine. This prevents degradation of the ligand and uptake into neurons and astrocytes (Kimelberg and Katz, 1985; Köhler, 1984). Since 5-HT$_{1B}$ and 5-HT$_{1C}$ receptors were found in very low concentrations or were missing in the hippocampus (Marcinkiewicz et al., 1984; Pazos and Palacios, 1985; Verge et al., 1986), the 5-HT binding sites represented almost exclusively the 5-HT$_{1A}$ subtype (Zilles, 1988). The present results for the regional distribution pattern of this receptor in the rat hippocampus corroborate and extend results of other observers (Biegon et al., 1982; Fischette et al., 1987; Glaser et al., 1985; Köhler, 1984; Marcinkiewicz et al., 1984; Pazos and Palacios, 1985). A comparison of the present results concerning the 5-HT$_1$ receptors in the human hippocampus shows a clear disagreement with the report of Biegon et al. (1986), who found the highest values in the dentate gyrus and about 45% lower densities in the pyramidal layers of CA1 and CA3. The receptor densities in CA1, CA3, and dentate gyrus described by our data (Fig. 3) are well comparable with the observations of Hoyer et al. (1986) and Pazos et al. (1987) on the level of subregions.

Experimental data argue against an autoreceptor role for the 5-HT$_1$ binding site in the hippocampus (Blackshear et al., 1981; Cross and Deakin, 1985; Fischette et al., 1987; Hall et al., 1985; Nelson et al., 1978; Quirion et al., 1985; Verge et al., 1985). Some of these receptors are found on cholinergic terminals (Cross and Deakin, 1985; Maura and Raiteri, 1986; Quirion et al., 1985; Quirion and Richard, 1987), where they inhibit acetylcholine release. The codistribution of 5-HT$_1$ and muscarinic M1 receptors in both rat and human described here may reflect this close relation between both binding sites, since the postsynaptic muscarinic receptors must be localized very near to the cholinergic terminal equipped with 5-HT$_1$ receptors because of the rapid degradation of acetylcholine by acetylcholinesterase. M2, glutamate, and D1 receptors are not codistributed with 5-HT$_1$ receptors. A lack of association between 5-HT$_1$ receptors and dopaminergic innervation was also found by Quirion and Richard (1987) in experimental studies. A similarity in the laminar pattern was found between GABA$_A$ and 5-HT$_1$ receptors in the human hippocampus. Interestingly, a very close relation between the serotonergic and gabaergic system was reported by Andrade et al. (1986) for the hippocampal pyramidal cells. 5-HT$_1$ and GABA$_B$ receptors are coupled by a G protein to the same K$^+$ channel in these cells. This example shows that interactions between different neurochemical systems can

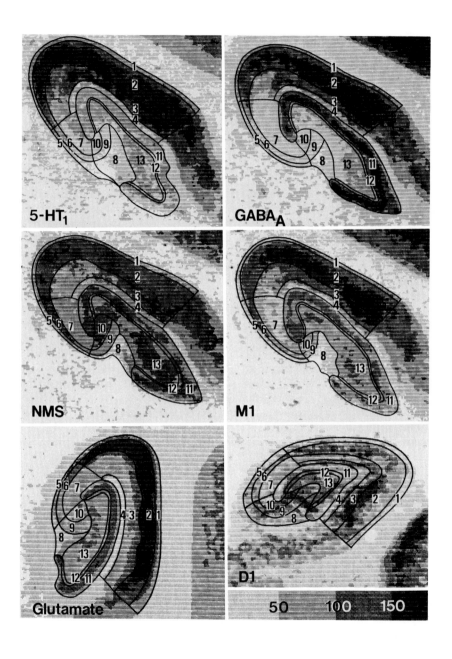

be structurally organized also by colocalization of different receptors in the same cell. Although direct evidence is lacking for a coupling of GABA$_A$ and 5-HT$_1$ receptors, the codistribution of both receptors as demonstrated here points to a close relationship of both systems.

Muscarinic receptors can be subdivided into M1 and M2 subtypes labeled with the antagonist [^{3}H]pirenzepine or the agonist [^{3}H]oxotremorine-M (Mash et al., 1985; Spencer et al., 1986; Wamsley et al., 1980, 1984). Both subtypes together can be labeled with the antagonist [^{3}H]NMS. M1 and M2 subtypes show completely different distributions in the rat hippocampus. The finding corroborates and extends earlier nonquantitative studies of Spencer et al. (1986). M1 receptors are most densely packed in regions where the proximal apical and basal dendrites of CA1 pyramidal cells (Zilles, 1988) and the dendrites of granule cells are found, whereas the M2 receptors reach their highest values in the pyramidal cell layers of CA1/2. The regional distribution of muscarinic and directly labeled M1 receptors in all subregions and layers of the human hippocampus is described here for the first time. So far as Cortés et al. (1987) and Lang and Henke (1983) have reported the laminar pattern of NMS and indirectly labeled M1 receptors, these and our observations are in agreement. The pyramidal layer of CA1 represents the highest density of muscarinic and especially M1 receptors. The M1 subtype is the quantitatively dominating muscarinic receptor in the hippocampus (Cortés et al., 1987; Messer and Hoss, 1987; Spencer et al., 1986; Watson et al., 1983). This explains the codistribution of [^{3}H]NMS binding sites with M1, but not with M2 receptors. The muscarinic receptors are found both pre- and postsynaptically and on astrocytes (Murphy et al., 1986). Presynaptic receptors, most probably M2 receptors, are located at cholinergic terminals (autoreceptors) in the striatum and the neocortex, where they inhibit cholinergic neurotransmission (Dodt and Misgeld, 1986; Mash et al., 1985). In the hippocampus M1 receptors mediate excitation on CA3 pyramidal cells and granule cells of the dentate gyrus (Müller and Misgeld, 1986). The affiliation of M2 receptors with cholinergic terminals and their decline in Alzheimer's disease and after experimental cholinergic denervation (Mash et al., 1985) argue for the position as autoreceptors, whereas the lack of changes in M1 receptors under these conditions supports the assumption that this subtype is not an autoreceptor. A presynaptic localization of muscarinic or M1 receptors on other than cholinergic terminals has been shown for 5-HT–con-

---

Fig. 2. Standardized receptor densities in the human hippocampus measured by image analysis. The laminar distribution of 5-HT$_1$, GABA$_A$, muscarinic (M1 + M2), M1, glutamate, and D1 receptors together with the delineations of subregions and layers are shown. The scale at the right lower corner gives the graphic symbols for the relative density ranges. The 50%, 100% (mean density of the entire hippocampus), and 150% limits are marked. 1–4, oriens, pyramidal, radiatum, and lacunosum-moleculare layers of CA1; 5–7, oriens, pyramidal, and radiatum-lacunosum-moleculare layers of CA2; 8–10, oriens, pyramidal, and radiatum-lacunosum-moleculare layers of CA3; 11,12, molecular and granular layers of the dentate gyrus; 13, hilus region (=CA4).

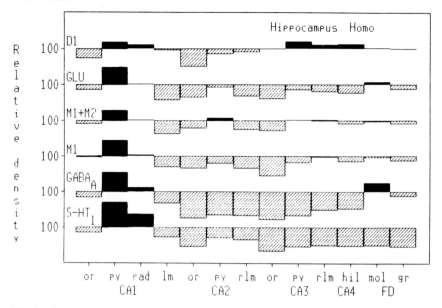

Fig. 3. Laminar distribution of receptor densities in the human hippocampus. Binding sites for [³H]5-HT (5-HT₁), [³H]muscimol (GABA_A), [³H]pirenzepine (M1), [³H]N-methyl-scopolamine (M1 + M2), [³H]glutamate (GLU), and [³H]SCH 23390 (D1) are analyzed. For further explanations and abbreviations, see Figure 1.

taining fibers (Marchi et al., 1986) and glutamatergic afferents from the entorhinal area to the hippocampus (Monaghan et al., 1982; Ulas et al., 1986; Valentino and Dingledine, 1981). The subtype of the muscarinic receptors has not been identified in all cases. The present results demonstrate a codistribution of M1 receptors with both 5-HT₁ and glutamate binding sites in the human and

TABLE III. Spearman Rank Corrlelations of the Laminar Distributions of Transmitter Receptors in the Human Hippocampus*

	5-HT₁	NMS	M1	GABA_A	Glutamate	D1
5-HT₁	—	NS	0.63 0.025	0.64 0.025	NS	NS
NMS	—	—	0.71 0.005	NS	0.82 0.001	NS
M1	—	—	—	0.82 0.001	0.75 0.005	NS
GABA_A	—	—	—	—	0.70 0.005	NS
Glutamate	—	—	—	—	—	NS

*The regional and layer-specific patterns are compared. NS, not significant; first line, rank correlation coefficient; second line, error probability.

rat hippocampus. Although these findings do not permit the identification of the precise cellular position, a near spatial relationship between serotoninergic, glutamatergic, and muscarinic systems can be stated.

[^{3}H] glutamate binding sites can present N-methyl-D-aspartate (NMDA), quisqualate, and kainate receptors (Greenamyre et al., 1983, 1984), glutamate uptake sites (Baudry and Lynch, 1984; Danbolt and Storm-Mathisen, 1986), and a chloride-dependent glutamate exchange system (Kessler et al., 1987). By using Tris-acetate buffer without Na$^+$, Cl$^-$, and Ca^{2+} and incubation at low temperatures, essentially all [^{3}H]glutamate binding sites are NMDA, quisqualate, and kainate receptors (Cotman et al., 1987). In a previous study (Zilles, 1988) it was shown that the regional pattern of [^{3}H]glutamate binding does not significantly differ between incubation procedures with or without Ca^{2+}/Cl$^-$ ions if the incubation is performed at low temperature (cf. Kessler et al., 1987). However, it has been shown that the absolute density of binding sites is clearly increased in the presence of Ca^{2+}/Cl$^-$ ions and the relative amount of binding sites in the lucidum layer of CA3 is decreased (Zilles, 1988). This is in agreement with reports about the inhibition of kainate binding in the presence of Ca^{2+} (Monaghan et al., 1983) and about an unmasking of glutamate receptors by stimulation of a membrane-bound, calcium-sensitive protease (Baudry et al., 1983; Greenamyre et al., 1985). The regional distribution pattern reported in the present investigation is compatible with the distribution of NMDA and quisqualate receptors (e.g. Monaghan et al., 1983; Cotman et al., 1987) in the rat and with NMDA displacable glutamate binding sites in the human hippocampus (Geddes et al., 1986). Since NMDA receptors (Monaghan and Cotman, 1985) show a much higher absolute density than quisqualate receptors (Monaghan et al., 1984), the distribution pattern in the rat and human hippocampus presented here emphasizes NMDA receptors. The regional distribution of these receptors matches that of the terminals of the glutamatergic perforant pathway and Schaffer collaterals (Nadler and Smith, 1981; Storm-Mathisen, 1977; White et al., 1977). Codistributions have been found (Tables 2, 3) between [^{3}H]glutamate binding sites and M1 receptors (for GABA$_A$ receptors, see below).

GABA$_A$ receptors can be labeled with the agonist [^{3}H]muscimol (Enna and Karbon, 1986), which is bound to the β subunit and activates the opening of the chloride channel. This increases membrane conductance to Cl$^-$ and stabilizes the cell's resting potential (for review, see Bormann, 1988). The binding sites for this ligand have been studied with both light and electron microscopic autoradiography (Chan-Palay, 1978a,b; Chan-Palay and Palay, 1978). They were found to be localized predominantly at synapses, but also at places without any visible synaptic structure (extrasynaptic sites). According to Alger and Nicoll (1982), the synaptic receptors mediating hyperpolarizing responses are located on the soma and proximal dendritic shafts of CA1 pyramidal cells, whereas the extrasynaptic portion of GABA$_A$ receptors is mainly found at the distal dendritic parts and leads to depolarization. The position of the synaptic fraction is matching the localization reported for GABAergic synapses (Anderson et al., 1986). [^{3}H]muscimol does not label uptake sites (Chan-Palay, 1978b) or glial cells (for review, see de Freudis, 1980).

A study on the distribution of [³H]muscimol binding sites with quantitative autoradiography (Palacios et al., 1981) shows the highest density in the molecular layer of FD, followed by the CA1 region of the rat hippocampus. The lowest values are found in the CA2/3 regions. An immunohistochemical study with antibodies against the GABA/benzodiazepine binding sites (Richards et al., 1987) reveals a very similar distribution pattern, with the highest values in the molecular and radiatum layers of FD and CA1 respectively, and the lowest densities of immunoreactive structures in the pyramidal and granular layers of the rat hippocampus.

The present results on the human hippocampus reveal a similar distribution if the subregions are compared with the rat pattern. A clear difference, however, is found between the pyramidal layers in both species. In man, the highest GABA$_A$ receptor densities occur in the pyramidal layer of CA1, where low densities are found in the rat. This difference can be explained by the structural differences between the pyramidal layers in humans and rats (Zilles, 1888). The rat pyramidal layer is very small and contains almost exclusively pyramidal cell somata in an extremely high packing density, whereas the human pyramidal layer is much wider and comprises not only the somata but also larger portions of apical and basal dendrites. These latter structures are restricted to the oriens and radiatum layers in the rat. Thus the human pyramidal layer integrates receptor distributions of the upper oriens, the pyramidal, and the deeper radiatum layers of the rat. Two of these layers show very high GABA$_A$ receptor densities (Palacios et al., 1981) in the rat; this means that the same cellular localization on basal and apical dendritic portions near to the soma, on initial parts of the axon, and on the soma will sum up to the very high density in the human pyramidal layer. The codistribution of GABA$_A$ receptors with glutamate binding sites is an indication for inhibitory influences on places where excitation is mediated by the glutamatergic perforant pathway and Schaffer collaterals. Although the cellular localization of both receptor types needs further elucidation, the present findings emphasize the integrative structure of two chemically and functionally different systems.

D1 receptors (for review, see Creese and Fraser, 1987; Clark and White, 1987) can be labeled with the antagonist [³H]SCH 23390 (Dawson et al., 1985), a tetrahydro-3-benzazepine derivative. These receptors lead to a hyperpolarization following a dopamine-mediated stimulation (Clark and White, 1987). Although there is some evidence that the D1 receptor in neocortical areas of the rat brain is situated postsynaptically (Dawson et al., 1986), preliminary evidence for a presynaptic localization is also reported by the same authors. The present data about the regional D1 receptor distribution in the human hippocampus seem to be the first description of this issue. The regional pattern shows the highest values in the pyramidal and radiatum layers of CA1 and CA3 and in the hilus region. This pattern is completely different from any other receptor distribution analyzed in this study. Verney et al. (1985) described the regional distribution of dopaminergic fibers and terminal fields in the rat hippocampus. Within a low overall density of these fibers the oriens and pyramidal layers of CA1 and CA3 together with the hilus region displayed the relatively highest concentrations of dopaminergic fibers. This regional pattern shows striking similarities with the D1 receptor distribution in the equivalent subregions of the human hippocampus, especially when the above-mentioned inclusion of parts of the oriens layer within the human pyramidal layer is taken into consideration.

The present data show a consistent codistribution of M1 with 5-HT_1 or glutamate binding sites in both the human and rat hippocampi. The GABA_A receptor (not studied in the rat) is codistributed with M1, 5-HT_1, and glutamate binding sites. M2 and D1 receptors do not show codistribution in the rat (M2; D1 not studied) or human (D1; M2 not studied) hippocampus. Since similar constellations of codistribution are found in the human striate and agranular frontal cortices (our unpublished observations), these correlations in laminar patterns may indicate a specific integration of different neurochemical systems on the level of receptors.

SUMMARY

Using receptor autoradiography and image analysis, the regional distribution of the following receptors in the human and rat hippocampus was evaluated: The 5-HT_1 type of the serotonin receptors, the muscarinic receptors and either of the subtypes M1 and M2, the glutamate binding sites, the GABA_A type of the GABA receptors, and the D1 type of the dopamine receptors. The hippocampal subregions and layers were delineated on the basis of adjacent histological sections, and the degree of similarity between the laminar patterns of different receptors was tested with the Spearman rank correlation test. Codistribution of two different receptors is indicated by a significantly positive correlation, i.e. they are both distributed with the same preferences for different hippocampal layers. 5-HT_1 receptors are codistributed with M1 receptors and M1 receptors with glutamate binding sites in both human and rat hippocampi. Only in the human brain (not investigated in the rat) were further codistributions found between GABA_A and 5-HT_1 or M1 or glutamate binding sites. M2 and D1 receptors were not codistributed with any of the other receptors. The analysis of receptor distribution reveals specific concurrence of different neurochemical systems, which give an integrative insight into possible local interactions.

ACKNOWLEDGMENTS

This work was supported by the Deutsche Forschungsgemeinschaft (Zi 192/8-1). The author thanks Dr. A. Schleicher, M. Rath, G. Selbach, and A. Bauer for technical support; A. van der Zander for help with the English version; and Dr. J. Traber, Troponwerke, Köln, for a gift of some of the labeled ligands.

REFERENCES

Alger, B.E., and R.A. Nicoll (1982) Pharmacological evidence for two kinds of GABA receptor on rat hippocampal pyramidal cells studied in vitro. J. Physiol. [Lond.] 328:123–141.

Anderson, K.J., B.E. Maley, and S.W. Scheff (1986) Immunocytochemical localization of γ-aminobutyric acid in the rat hippocampal formation. Neurosci. Lett 69:7–12.

Andrade, R., R.C. Malenka, and R.A. Nicoll (1986) A G protein couples serotonin and GABA_B receptors to the same channels in hippocampus. Science, 234:1261–1265.

Baudry, M., K. Kramer, and G. Lynch (1983) Irreversibility and time course of calcium stimulated (^{3}H) glutamate binding to rat hippocampal membranes. Brain Res. 270:142–145.

Baudry, M., and G. Lynch (1984) Glutamate receptor regulation and the substrates of memory. In G. Lynch, J.L. McGaugh, and N.M. Weinberger Neurobiology of Learning and Memory. New York: Guilford Press, pp. 431–446.

Biegon, A., S. Kargman, L. Snyder, and B.S. McEwen (1986) Characterization and localization of serotonin receptors in human brain postmortem. Brain Res. 363:91–98.

Biegon, A., T.C. Rainbow, and B.S. McEwen (1982) Quantitative autoradiography of serotonin receptors in the rat brain. Brain Res. 242:197–204.

Blackshear, M.A., L.R. Steranka, and E. Sanders-Bush (1981) Multiple serotonin receptors: Regional distribution and effect of raphe lesions. Eur. J. Pharmacol. 76:325–334.

Bormann, J. (1988) Electrophysiology of GABA_A receptor subtypes. TINS 11:112–116.

Chan-Palay, V. (1978a) Autoradiographic localization of γ-aminobutyric acid receptors in the central nervous system by using [^{3}H]muscimol. Proc. Natl. Acad. Sci. U.S.A. 75:1024–1028.

Chan-Palay, V. (1978b) Quantitative visualization of γ-aminobutyric acid receptors in hippocampus and area dentata demonstrated by [^{3}H]muscimol autoradiography. Proc. Natl. Acad. Sci. U.S.A. 75:2516–2520.

Chan-Palay, V., and S.L. Palay (1978) Ultrastructural localization of γ-aminobutyric acid receptors in the mammalian central nervous system by means of [^{3}H]muscimol binding. Proc. Natl. Acad. Sci. U.S.A. 75:2977–2980.

Clark, D., and F. White (1987) Review: D1 dopamine receptor—The search for a function: A critical evaluation of the D1/D2 dopamine receptor classification and its functional implications. Synapse 1:347–388.

Cortés, R., A. Probst, and J.M. Palacios (1987) Quantitative light microscopic autoradiographic localization of cholinergic muscarinic receptors in the human brain: Forebrain. Neuroscience 20:65–107.

Cotman, C.W., D.T. Monaghan, O.P. Otterson, and J. Storm-Mathisen (1987) Anatomical organization of excitatory amino acid receptors and their pathways. TINS 10:273–280.

Creese, I., and C.M. Fraser (eds) (1987) Dopamine Receptors. New York: Alan R. Liss.

Cross, A.J., and J.F.W. Deakin (1985) Cortical serotonin receptor subtypes after lesion of ascending cholinergic neurones in rat. Neurosci. Lett 60:261–265.

Danbolt, N.C., and J. Storm-Mathisen (1986) Na$^+$-dependent "binding" of D-aspartate in brain membranes is largely due to uptake into membrane-bounded saccules. J. Neurochem. 47:819–824.

Dawson, T.M., D.R. Gehlert, and J.K. Wamsley (1986) Quantitative autoradiographic localization of central dopamine D-1 and D-2 receptors. In G.R. Breese and J. Creese (eds): Neurobiology of Central D1- Dopamine Receptors. New York: Plenum Press, pp. 93–118.

de Freudis, F.V. (1980) Binding studies with muscimol: Relation to synaptic γ-aminobutyrate receptors. Neuroscience 5:675–688.

Dodt, H.U., and U. Misgeld (1986) Muscarinic slow excitation and muscarinic inhibition of synaptic transmission in the rat neostriatum. J. Physiol. 380:593–608.

Enna, S.J., and E.W. Karbon (1986) GABA receptors: An overview. In R.W. Olsen and J.C. Venter (eds): Benzodiazepine/GABA Receptors and Chloride Channels: Structural and Functional Properties. New York: Alan R. Liss, pp. 41–56.

Fischette, C.T., B. Nock, and K. Renner (1987) Effects of 5,7-dihydroxytryptamine on serotonin₁ and serotonin₂ receptors throughout the rat central nervous system using quantitative autoradiography. Brain Res. *421:*263–279.

Geddes, J.W., H. Chang-Chui, S.M. Cooper, I.T. Lott, and C.W. Cotmann (1986) Density and distribution of NMDA receptors in the human hippocampus in Alzheimer's disease. Brain Res. *399:*156–161.

Glaser, T., M. Rath, J. Traber, K. Zilles, and A. Schleicher (1985) Autoradiographic identification and topographical analyses of high affinity serotonin receptor subtypes as a target for the novel putative anxiolytic TVX Q 7821. Brain Res. *358:*129–136.

Greenamyre, J.T., J.M.M. Olson, J.B. Penney, and A.B. Young (1985) Autoradiographic characterization of N-methyl-D-aspartate-, quisqualate-, and kainate-sensitive glutamate binding sites. J. Pharmacol. Exp. Ther. *233:*254–263.

Greenamyre, J.T., A.B. Young, and J.B. Penney (1983) Quantitative autoradiography of L-(^{3}H)glutamate binding to rat brain. Neurosci. Lett *37:*155–160.

Greenamyre, J.T., A.B. Young, and J.B. Penney (1984) Quantitative autoradiographic distribution of L-(^{3}H)glutamate-binding sites in rat central nervous system. J. Neurosci. *4:*2133–2144.

Hall, M.D., S. El Mestikawy, M.B. Emerit, L. Pichat, M. Hamon, and H. Gozlan (1985) [^{3}H]8-hydroxy-2-(Di-n-propylamino)tetralin binding to pre- and postsynaptic 5-hydroxytryptamine sites in various regions of the rat brain. J. Neurochem. *44:*1685–1695.

Hoyer, D., A. Pazos, A. Probst, and J.M. Palacios (1986) Serotonin receptors in the human brain. I. Characterization and autoradiographic localization of 5-HT$_{1A}$ recognition sites. Apparent absence of 5-HT$_{1B}$ recognition sites. Brain Res. *376:*85–96.

Kessler, M., M. Baudry and G. Lynch (1987) Use of cystine to distinguish glutamate binding from glutamate sequestration. Neurosci. Lett. *81:*221–226.

Kimelberg, H.K., and D.M. Katz (1985) High-affinity uptake of serotonin into immunocytochemically identified astrocytes. Science *228:*889–891.

Köhler, C. (1984) The distribution of serotonin binding sites in the hippocampal region of the rat brain. An autoradiographic study. Neuroscience *13:*667–680.

Lang, W., and H. Henke (1983) Cholinergic receptor binding and autoradiography in brains of non-neurological and senile dementia of Alzheimer-type patients. Brain Res. *267:*271–280.

Marchi, M., P. Paudice, M. Bella, and M. Raiteri (1986) Dicyclomine- and pirenzepine-sensitive muscarinic receptors mediate inhibition of (^{3}H)serotonin release in different rat brain areas. Eur. J. Pharmacol. *129:*353–357.

Marcinkiewicz, M., D. Vergé, H. Gozlan, L. Pichat, and M. Hamon (1984) Autoradiographic evidence for the heterogeneity of 5-HT$_1$ sites in the brain. Brain Res. *291:*159–163.

Mash, D.C., D.D. Flynn, and L.T. Potter (1985) Loss of M2 muscarinic receptors in the cerebral cortex in Alzheimer's disease and experimental cholinergic denervation. Science *228:*1115–1117.

Maura, G., and M. Raiteri (1986) Cholinergic terminals in rat hippocampus posses 5-HT$_{1B}$ receptors mediating inhibition of acetylcholine release. Eur. J. Pharmacol. *129:*333–337.

Merker, B. (1983) Silver staining of cell bodies by means of physical development. J. Neurosci. Methods *9:*235–241.

Messer, W.S., and W. Hoss (1987) Selectivity of pirenzepine in the central nervous system. I. Direct autoradiographic comparison of the regional distribution of pirenzepine and carbamylcholine binding sites. Brain Res. *407*:27–36.

Monaghan, D.T., and C.W. Cotman (1982) The distribution of (^{3}H)kainic acid binding sites in rat CNS as determined by autoradiography. Brain Res. *252*:91–100.

Monaghan, D.T., and C.W. Cotman (1985) Distribution of N-methyl-D-aspartate-sensitive L-(^{3}H)glutamate binding sites in rat brain. J. Neurosci. *5*:2909–2919.

Monaghan, D.T., V.R. Holets, D.W. Toy, and C.W. Cotman (1983) Anatomical distribution of four pharmacologically distinct ^{3}H-L-glutamate binding sites. Nature *306*:176–178.

Monaghan, D.T., E.E. Mena, and C.W. Cotman (1982) The effect of entorhinal cortical ablation on the distribution of muscarinic cholinergic receptors in the rat hippocampus. Brain Res. *234*:480–485.

Monaghan, D.T., D. Yao, and C.W. Cotman (1984) Distribution of ^{3}H-AMPA binding sites in rat brain as determined by quantitative autoradiography. Brain Res. *324*:160–164.

Müller, W., and U. Misgeld (1986) Slow cholinergic excitation of guinea pig hippocampal neurons is mediated by two muscarinic receptor subtypes. Neurosci. Lett. *67*:107–112.

Murphy, S., B. Pearce, and C. Morrow (1986) Astrocytes have both M_1 and M_2 muscarinic receptor subtypes. Brain Res. *364*:177–180.

Nadler, J.V., and E.M. Smith (1981) Perforant path lesions deplete glutamate content of fascia dentata synaptosomes. Neurosci. Lett. *25*:275–280.

Nelson, D.L., A. Herbet S. Bourgoin, J. Glowinski, and M. Hamon (1978) Characteristics of central 5-HT receptors and their adaptive changes following intracerebral 5,7-dihydroxytryptamine administration in the rat. Mol. Pharmacol. *14*:983–995.

Palacios, J.M., J.K. Wamsley, and J. Kuhar (1981) High affinity GABA receptors—Autoradiographic localization. Brain Res. *222*:285–307.

Pazos, A., and J.M. Palacios (1985) Quantitative autoradiographic mapping of serotonin receptors in the rat brain. I. Serotonin-1 receptors. Brain Res. *34*:205–230.

Pazos, A., A. Probst, and J.M. Palacios (1987) Serotonin receptors in the human brain. III. Autoradiographic mapping of serotonin-1 receptors. Neuroscience *21*:97–122.

Quirion, R., and J. Richard (1987) Differential effects of selective lesions of cholinergic and dopaminergic neurons on serotonin-type 1 receptors in rat brain. Synapse *1*:124–130.

Quirion, R., J Richard and T.V. Dam (1985) Evidence for the existence of serotonin type-2 receptors on cholinergic terminals in rat cortex. Brain Res. *333*:345–349.

Richards, J.G., P. Schoch, B. Häring, B. Takacs, and H. Möhler (1987) Resolving $GABA_A$/benzodiazepine receptors: Cellular and subcellular localization in the CNS with monoclonal antibodies. J. Neurosci., *7*:1866–1886.

Spencer, D., E. Horvàth, and J. Traber (1986) Direct autoradiographic determination of M1 and M2 muscarinic acetylcholine receptor distribution in the rat brain: Relation to cholinergic nuclei and projections. Brain Res. *380*:59–68.

Storm-Mathisen, J. (1977) Localization of transmitter candidates in the brain: The hippocampal formation as a model. Prog. Neurobiol. *8*:119–181.

Ulas, J., M. Gradowska, M. Jezierska, M. Skup, and J. Skangiel-Kramska (1986) Bilateral changes in glutamate uptake, muscarinic receptor binding and acetylcholinesterase level in the rat hippocampus after unilateral entorhinal cortex lesions. J. Neurochem. Int. *9*:255–263.

Valentino, R.J., and R. Dingledine (1981) Presynaptic inhibitory effect of acetylcholine in the hippocampus. J. Neurosci. *1*:784–792.

Verge, D., G. Daval, M. Marcinkiewicz, A. Patey, S. El Mestikawy, H. Gozlan, and M. Hamon (1986) Quantitative autoradiography of multiple 5-HT1 receptor subtypes in the brain of control or 5,7-dihydroxytryptamine-treated rats. J. Neurosci. 6:3474–3482.

Verge, D., G. Daval, A. Patey, H. Gozlan, S. El Mestikawy, and M. Hamon (1985) Presynaptic 5-HT autoreceptors on serotonergic cell bodies and/or dendrites but not terminals are of the 5-HT$_{1A}$subtype. Eur. J. Pharmacol. 113:463–464.

Verney, C., M. Baulac, B. Berger, C. Alvarez, A. Vigny, and K.B. Helle (1985) Morphological evidence for a dopaminergic terminal field in the hippocampal formation of young and adult rat. Neuroscience 14:1039–1052.

Wamsley, J.K., D.R. Gehlert, W.R. Roeske, H.I. Yamamura (1984) Muscarinic agonist binding site heterogeneity as evidenced by autoradiography after direct labelling with (^{3}H)QNB and (^{3}H) pirenzepine. Life Sci. 34:1395–1402.

Wamsley, J.K., M.A. Zarbin, N.J.M. Birdsall, and M.J. Kuhar (1980) Muscarinic cholinergic receptors: Autoradiographic localization of high and low affinity agonist binding sites. Brain Res. 200:1–12.

Watson, M., H.I. Yamamura, and W.R. Roeske (1983) A unique regulatory profile and regional distribution of (^{3}H)pirenzepine binding in the rat provides evidence for distinct M1 and M2 muscarinic receptor subtypes. Life Sci. 32:3001–3011.

White, W.F., J.V. Nadler, A. Hamberger, C.W. Cotman, and J.T. Cummins (1977) Glutamate as a transmitter of hippocampal perforant path. Nature 270:356–357.

Zilles, K. (1988) Receptor autoradiography in the hippocampus of man and rat. Adv. Anat. Embryol. Cell Biol. 111:61–80.

Zilles, K., A. Schleicher, M. Rath, and A. Bauer (1988) Quantitative receptor autoradiography in the human brain. Methodical aspects. Histochemistry 90:129–137.

Zilles, K., A. Schleicher, M. Rath, T. Glaser, and J. Traber (1986) Quantitative autoradiography of transmitter binding sites with an image analyzer. J. Neurosci. Methods 18:207–220.

The Hippocampus—New Vistas, pages 207–224
© 1989 Alan R. Liss, Inc.

14

Radiohistochemistry of Receptors in the Hippocampus: Focus on the Cholinergic Receptors

J.M. PALACIOS AND G. MENGOD
Preclinical Research, Sandoz Ltd., Basel, Switzerland

INTRODUCTION

Understanding the mechanisms involved in neurotransmission requires the molecular characterization of both pre- and postsynaptic components. The enormous anatomical, cellular, and molecular complexity of the brain makes it difficult to analyze these mechanisms without techniques to acheive the appropriate anatomical, cellular, and subcellular resolutions. Some brain areas lend themselves better to detailed molecular analysis than do others. One of these privileged areas is the hippocampus. The application of a wealth of techniques to the understanding of neurotransmission in the hippocampus has generated an enormous amount of information about the working of this brain area. Many of these aspects are reviewed in other chapters of this book. In this chapter we will review our progress in the understanding of the anatomical organization of the receptors for neurotransmitters in the hippocampal formation.

Biochemical investigations have shown that the hippocampus is a brain area particularly enriched in receptors for neurotransmitters (for review, see Wamsley and Palacios, 1983). Biochemical methodology is, however, limited by its low level of anatomical resolution. In the last 10 years several techniques have been developed whose application has resulted in an improved understanding of the cellular and anatomical localization of receptors in the brain (see van Leeuwen et al., 1988). We will discuss three of these techniques. All three are based on the use of radiolabeled compounds detected using autoradiography. Collectively we call them *radiohistochemical procedures.* Historically, the first technique used to visualize the distribution of receptors at the light microscopic level was receptor autoradiography or radioligand binding autoradiography (Kuhar, 1985; Palacios, 1984). With our progress in the knowledge of receptor structure and in the purification of some neurotransmitter receptors it has been possible to develop both poly- and monoclonal antibodies against some of these receptor proteins. These antibodies have been used in the immunohistochemical visualization of receptors. Immunohistochemistry has a higher cellular resolution than receptor autoradiography as illustrated by the work of Richards et al., 1987. Finally, some genes coding for several neurotransmitter receptors have recently been isolated and characterized (Kubo et al., 1986a,b; Peralta et al., 1987b; Bonner et al., 1987; Schofield et al., 1987; Dixon et al., 1986). The availability of the sequence of cDNA or DNAs coding for neurotransmitter receptors has made possible the development of molecular probes for the analysis of the expression of these receptors in different tissues, using particularly the in situ hybridization technique. All of these techniques have been extensively used now for the study of receptors in the hippocampal formation. For the purposes of the present review, we will focus on the studies carried out until now on the receptors for the transmitter acetylcholine.

RECEPTOR LIGAND AUTORADIOGRAPHY

The prominence and significance of cholinergic input to the hippocampus is well documented. It is known that most of the cholinergic input to the hippocampus originates from the septum (Lewis and Shute, 1967, 1978; Butcher and Woolf, 1984). Pharmacological and electrophysiological studies have clearly shown that the hippocampus contains both nicotinic and muscarinic acetylcholine receptors. These two types of receptors have been characterized by ligand binding studies in the hippocampal formation, and some of them have been found to be particularly enriched there. We know now that several subtypes of both receptors are present in the brain. For example, muscarinic receptors have been classified pharmacologically into M_1 and M_2 according to the sensitivity of this receptor to the atypical antimuscarinic pirenzepine (Hammer and Giachetti, 1982). The multiplicity of nicotinic receptors is supported by different profiles of drug binding in the rat brain (Clarke et al., 1985). The ligands used in the study of cholinergic receptors in the hippocampal formation are summarized in Table I. Figures 1 and 2 illustrate some examples of the distribution of the different cholinergic ligands in the rat hippocampal formation.

Muscarinic Cholinergic Receptors

In the rat hippocampus the density of muscarinic cholinergic receptors as labeled with nonselective ligands such as [^{3}H]NMS or [^{3}H]QNB is one of the highest in the brain, only second to that seen in some components of the basal ganglia (Kuhar and Yamamura, 1976; Cortés and Palacios, 1986; Frey et al., 1985). In the mammalian hippocampus (Fig. 1) muscarinic cholinergic receptors present a differential regional localization. They are concentrated in the molecular layer of the dentate gyrus and also in the oriens and molecular layers of the CA1 area of the hippocampus. The CA2 presents clearly a lower concentration of these sites, and CA3 presents an intermediate density of muscarinic cholinergic receptors organized into parallel bands similar to the terminals of the mossy fibers. These two bands penetrate into the CA4 or hilus. The density of muscarinic cholinergic receptors is more or less homogenous in the anteroposterior and dorsoventral segments. Regarding the distribution

TABLE I. Autoradiographic Studies on Brain Nicotinic and Muscarinic Cholinergic Receptors

Ligand	Selectivity	Species	Labeling	Method	Selected references
Nicotinics					
[^{125}I]BTX	Muscle type	Rat, chick	In vitro	LM	Polz-Tejera et al. (1975)
		Rat	In vitro	EM + LM	Hunt and Schmidt (1978a)
		Mouse	In vitro	EM + LM	Arimatsu et al. (1978)
		Rat	In vitro	LM	Segal et al. (1978)
		Rat	In vitro	LM	
			In vivo	LM	Hunt and Schmidt (1978b)
		Human	In vitro	LM	Lang and Henke (1983)
[^{3}H]BTX	Muscle type	Rat	In vivo	LM	Silver and Billiar (1976)
[^{3}H]nicotine	Neural type	Rat	In vitro	LM	Clarke et al. (1984, 1985)
			In vitro	LM	London et al. (1985)
[^{3}H]ACh	Neural type	Rat	In vitro	LM	Rainbow et al. (1984)
			In vitro	LM	Clarke et al. (1985)
			In vitro	LM	Schwartz (1986)
[^{3}H]mChc	Neural type	Rat	In vitro	LM	Boksa and Quirion (1987)
Muscarinics					
[^{3}H]QNB	$M_1 + M_2$	Rat	In vivo	LM	Kuhar and Yamamura (1976)
		Rat	In vitro	LM	Wamsley et al. (1981)
		Human	In vitro	LM	Biegon et al. (1982)
[^{3}H]NMS	$M_1 + M_2$	Rat	In vitro	LM	Wamsley et al. (1980)
		Human	In vitro	LM	Palacios (1982)
[^{3}H]scopolamine	$M_1 + M_2$	Rat	In vivo	LM	Frey et al. (1985)
[^{3}H]PrBCh	$M_1 + M_2$	Rat	In vitro	LM	Rotter et al. (1979a,b)
		Rat	In vitro	EM	Kuhar et al. (1981)
[^{3}H]pirenzepine	M_1	Rat	In vitro	LM	Wamsley et al. (1984)
		Human	In vitro	LM	Cortés et al. (1986)
[^{3}H]ACh	M_2	Rat	In vitro	LM	Schwartz (1986)
		Rat	In vitro	LM	Quirion and Boksa (1986)
[^{3}H]Oxo-M	M_2	Rat	In vitro	LM	Potter et al. (1984)
[^{3}H]CD	M_2	Rat	In vitro	LM	Yamamura et al. (1985)

ACh, acetylcholine; BTX, α-bungarotoxin; CD, *cis*-methyldioxolane; EM, electron microscope; LM, light microscope; NMS, N-methyl-scopolamine; Oxo-M, oxotremorine-M; PrBCh, propylbenzilyl-choline mustard; QNB, quinuclidinylbenzilate; mChc, methyl-carbachol.

of the different pharmacological subtypes, the hippocampal formation is enriched in muscarinic cholinergic receptors of the M_1 subtype. Thus the distribution of [^{3}H]pirenzepine (Fig. 1) is similar to that seen with the nonselective ligands [^{3}H]NMS and [^{3}H]QNB. About 80% of the binding of these two nonselective ligands does in fact correspond to binding to the M_1 subtype. As will be seen later, this M_1 population is actually a very heterogeneous one, probably made up of at least three different subtypes. The agonist ligand [^{3}H]oxotremorine-M has been proposed to be a high-affinity ligand for the M_2 class of receptor. Potter and colleagues (1984) have shown that in the rat

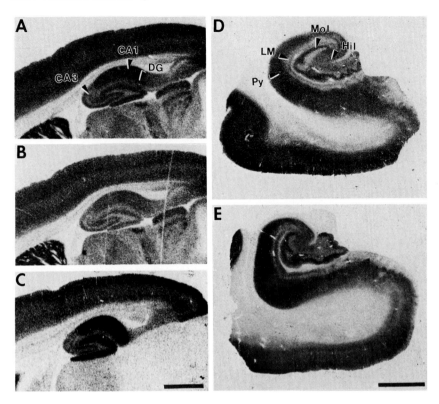

Fig. 1. The distribution of muscarinic cholinergic receptors in the rat and human hippocampus. Autoradiograms were obtained using [³H]NMS or [³H]pirenzepine as ligands and in vitro autoradiographic techniques. Dark areas represent those enriched in receptor binding. **A:** Distribution of [³H]NMS binding sites in the rat hippocampus. Note the high density of binding in the CA1 field and in the molecular layer of the dentate gyrus (DG) and the lower density in the CA3. [³H]NMS is not selective for the different subtypes of the mAChR. **B:** Pirenzepine was added to the incubation mixture to block the binding of [³H]NMS to the majority of the M_1 receptors, allowing the visualization of the M_2 sites. M_1 receptors are directly labeled with [³H]pirenzepine in **C. D,E:** Binding of [³H]NMS (D) and [³H]pirenzepine (E) to the human hippocampus. See text for details. Py, stratum pyramidalis; LM, stratum lacunosum-moleculare; Hil, hilus; Mol, molecular layer. A–C, bar = 2 mm; D,E, bar = 5 mm.

hippocampal formation [³H]oxotremorine labels a much lower density of receptor sites than does [³H]pirenzepine or [³H]NMS and that these receptors are mainly localized to the stratum oriens of the CA1 and CA2 regions. A lower density was also seen in the CA3 and hilar regions, while low to undetectable concentrations were seen in the molecular layer of the dentate gyrus. These results emphasize the differential distribution of the two groups (M_1 and M_2) of muscarinic receptors.

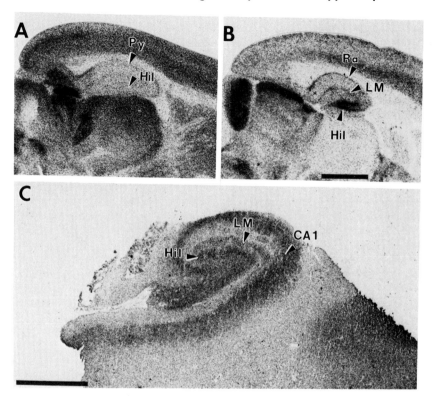

Fig. 2. The distribution of [³H]nicotine and [¹²⁵I]α-bungarotoxin binding sites in the rat and human hippocampus. **A,B:** Distribution of [³H]nicotine (A) and [¹²⁵I]α-bungarotoxin (B) binding sites in the rat hippocampus. Note the low density of [³H]nicotine sites, whereas [¹²⁵I]α-bungarotoxin sites were more abundant in the strata radiatum (Ra) and lacunosum-moleculare (LM) and in the hilus (Hil) Py, stratum pyramidalis. **C:** Distribution of [¹²⁵I]α-bungarotoxin binding sites in the human hippocampus. A,B, bar = 2 mm; C, bar = 5 mm.

The distribution of muscarinic cholinergic receptors appears to be very well preserved throughout the mammalian species. Studies in human postmortem tissue have shown that the distribution of muscarinic cholinergic receptors in the human hippocampal formation is comparable to that seen in the rat brain (Fig. 2) (Palacios, 1982; Lang and Henke, 1983; Cortés et al., 1986, 1987). Some small but significant differences were seen. In the human hippocampal formation the highest densities of muscarinic cholinergic receptors were associated with the strata oriens and pyramidalis of the CA1 subfield of the hippocampus proper and the molecular layer of the dentate gyrus. We also found low binding in the stratum lacunosum-moleculare in contrast with results of other investigators (Lang and Henke, 1983).

In the rat the topography of muscarinic cholinergic receptors is somewhat different in the sense that the highest densities are found in the strata oriens and radiatum of Ammon's horn and the molecular layer of the dentate gyrus, while almost no labeling occurs in the stratum pyramidalis. Nevertheless, in both species the layers containing high muscarinic cholinergic receptor densities correspond to the dendritic area of the pyramidal and granule cells, which are differently organized in rat and man. These layers have been shown to be the target of septal cholinergic fibers (Mosko et al., 1973). However, these projections terminate predominantly in CA2 and CA3 areas, which contain markedly lower densities of muscarinic cholinergic receptors when compared with the CA1. It is interesting to compare the distribution of muscarinic cholinergic receptors in the hippocampal formation with that observed using staining for the enzyme acetylcholinesterase. Important differences between species have been found in the staining of this enzyme. While in the rat intense staining is seen throughout the hippocampus, with sparing of the cell body layers, i.e. the pyramidal and granule cell layers and also the area of pyramidal cells in the CA3 area, in the human the hippocampus acetylcholinesterase staining is very weak, although concentrated in the strata oriens and radiatum of the CA2 and CA3. Therefore, it appears that there is not good parallelism between the patterns of distribution of acetylcholinesterase and muscarinic cholinergic receptors in the hippocampus.

Nicotinic Cholinergic Receptors in the Hippocampal Formation

Several ligands have been proposed for the labeling of central nicotinic receptors. The first one to be used was the toxin α-bungarotoxin (BTX) (Hunt and Schmidt, 1978a). The binding of $[^{125}I]$BTX is displaced differentially by nicotinic agents and hence the BTX binding sites have been named *nicotinic*. The displacement potency of nicotine in vitro suggests that it could act at the BTX site in vivo. However, other high-affinity ligands have been developed more recently, particularly $[^{3}H]$nicotine and $[^{3}H]$acetylcholine (Rainbow et al., 1984; Clarke et al., 1985; London et al., 1985). The binding of these two ligands has been shown to be potently displaced by nicotinic agents. In the case of $[^{3}H]$acetylcholine, binding is also observed to muscarinic receptors, so that this ligand has to be used in the presence of high concentrations of atropine to block the binding to these receptors. The three ligands have been used to label nicotinic sites in tissue sections from the rat brain and to localize autoradiographically the distribution of these binding sites. Clarke and colleagues (1985) have reported the differential localization of these three ligands throughout the rat brain. The hippocampal formation was characterized by extremely low binding densities of both $[^{3}H]$acetylcholine and $[^{3}H]$nicotine. Most of the binding was visualized in the molecular layer of the dentate gyrus, with a lower density being seen in the stratum lacunosum-moleculare of the hippocampus proper. In contrast, a somewhat higher binding was seen with $[^{125}I]$BTX in the rat hippocampal formation. $[^{125}I]$BTX binding was localized to the stratum albeus and the stratum lacunosum-moleculare and was particularly high in the hilus of the dentate gyrus. These results have been interpreted to be an indication of the presence of distinct populations of nicotinic receptors in the rat brain. As it will be discussed later, this hypothesis has been confirmed recently through the cloning of different types of mammalian nicotinic receptor genes.

Cellular Localization of Cholinergic Receptors in the Hippocampal Formation: Limitations of Receptor Autoradiography

An important limitation of receptor autoradiography is the low level of cellular resolution obtained. This is related to the use of emulsions and to radioactivity. Studies by Salpeter and colleagues (1969) have shown that the resolution of electron microscopic autoradiography is still too low to allow the assignment of autoradiographic grains to defined subcellular membranes. Kuhar and colleagues (1981) have demonstrated this for muscarinic cholinergic receptors in the rat hippocampus and concluded that other techniques are necessary to localize receptors to subcellular structures using electron microscopy.

An alternative to EM autoradiography is the combination of light microscopic receptor autoradiography with selective cellular lesions. The hippocampal formation is particularly well suited for this type of study. It is possible to abolish both intrinsic and extrinsic connections to the hippocampus by producing different types of cellular lesions, i.e. one can electrolytically lesion the septal nucleus and eliminate in this way the well-known septohippocampal cholinergic pathway (Fig. 3A,B). By studying the distribution of density of cholinergic receptors in the tissues of animals bearing such lesions it is possible to assign these receptor sites to different components of the hippocampus. Using neurotoxins such as ibotenic or kainic acid, one can selectively lesion the cell bodies in both the hippocampus proper and the dentate gyrus. On the other hand, local colchicine injections into the hippocampal formation have been shown to destroy selectively the granule cells. Other inputs to the hippocampus such as the one coming from the entorhinal cortex or the noradrenergic or serotonergic inputs can be abolished with other types of lesions both mechanical and chemical. We and others have examined the effects of such lesions in the distribution of cholinergic receptors. When the intrinsic neuronal cell bodies of the hippocampal formation are destroyed using local injections of ibotenic acid or colchicine, a marked decrease of muscarinic binding is observed in the hippocampus proper and/or the molecular layer of the dentate gyrus. These results can be interpreted as an indication that the majority of receptors in the hippocampal formation are localized to processes of intrinsic neurons, particularly pyramidal and granule cell layers. However, pharmacological and biochemical evidence supports the presence of a population of homo- or heteropresynaptic receptors. When septal lesions were placed in rats and the effects of these lesions were examined in the hippocampal formation, contradictory results were found. In some animals a decrease of [^{3}H]NMS binding to muscarinic receptors in the CA1 zone was seen (Fig. 3C–F). However, this was not a reproducible result. Furthermore the results are in contradiction

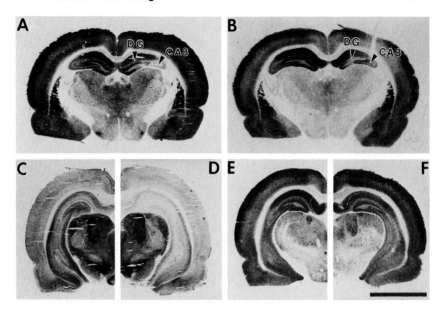

Fig. 3. Effects of different lesions on the distribution of muscarinic acetylcholine receptors in the rat hippocampus. **A:** Effects of the stereotaxic injection of 0.75 μg of kainic acid. Note the decrease of [³H]NMS binding in the CA3 area without effects in the dentate gyrus (DG). **B:** In contrast, colchicine injection (3.5 μg) results in decreased binding in the dentate gyrus but not in the CA3. **C,D:** Acetylcholinesterase (AChE) staining of a control (C) and a rat with an electrolytic lesion in the septum (D). Note the marked decrease of AChE in the lesioned animal. In contrast, receptor binding was unaltered (**E** vs. **F**) in these animals. Bar = 2 mm.

with the results obtained with ibotenic or colchicine lesions. The variability of the effects of septal lesions in the density of hippocampal muscarinic receptors is an illustration of the limitation of the lesion approach. Similar contradictory results have been seen with other receptors in the hippocampus, i.e. serotonin receptors.

The effects of the removal of entorhinal cortical projections to the hippocampus on hippocampal muscarinic receptors have been examined by Monaghan et al. (1982), who reported a biphasic effect. In adult rats a decreased density of receptors was observed 2 days after lesion in the denervated outer molecular layer of the dentate gyrus, suggesting the presence of presynaptic receptors in the entorhinal cortical fibers. Thirty days after lesion, a small increase in receptor density was observed in this layer. Furthermore, a larger increase was seen in the stratum lacunosum-moleculare. The investigators interpreted these results to be an indication that entorhinal cortical fibers are normally responsible for determining the lamination pattern of muscarinic acetylcholine receptors (mAChR) in the hippocampus, in agreement with the

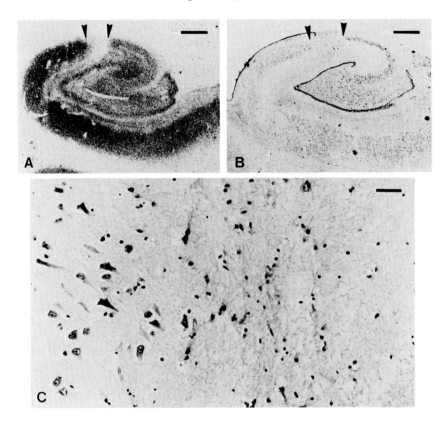

Fig. 4. Effects of a vascular lesion on muscarinic receptor binding in the human hippocampus. **A:** Loss of [³H]NMS binding in a small vascular lesion (arrowheads) in the CA1 field. **B:** A loss of pyramidal neurons in the infarct area (arrowheads) is observed with Cresyl violet staining. **C:** A higher magnification microphotograph of the border of the infarct zone illustrates the disappearance of neurons and the increase in glial cells in the lesion. A,B, bar = 2 mm; C, bar = 0.2 mmm.

suggestions of Rotter et al. (1979a,b). These results imply a noncholinergic afferent-mediated control of cholinergic receptor density.

In the human hippocampus a localization of the mAChRs to processes of the pyramidal cells is suggested by the observation of a marked decrease of these receptors in small vascular infarct zones where neurons degenerate and glial cells proliferate (Fig. 4). Furthermore, studies on the hippocampus of Alzheimer's disease patients have shown that while the presence of neuritic plaques did not alter the distribution of mAChRs, there was a significant positive correlation between the total concentration of mAChRs and the density of pyramidal cells (Palacios, 1982; Probst et al., 1988). To our knowledge, until now no lesion studies have been carried out to examine the localization of nicotinic receptors.

NICOTINIC RECEPTORS: IMMUNOHISTOCHEMISTRY AND IN SITU HYBRIDIZATION

Radioligand binding techniques are limited not only because of their low anatomical resolution but also because of the limited and in some cases unsuspected selectivity of the available ligands. Advances in receptor biochemistry and molecular biology, however, have provided new tools that can overcome these problems. The main new tools are antibodies against purified receptor proteins and nucleic acid probes derived from the cloning of the receptor genes.

Nature has favored the research of the nicotinic receptors with two exceptional gifts: an organ in which nicotinic acetylcholine receptors (nAChR) are enormously enriched (the electric organ of the electric fishes) and high-affinity ligands (the peptide toxins such as α-bungarotoxin). Because of these gifts, several laboratories have purified the nicotinic receptors to homogeneity and found them to consist of four different subunits. Purified receptors have been used to generate two important tools for receptor visualization: antibodies and cDNA probes.

IMMUNOHISTOCHEMICAL LOCALIZATION OF CHOLINERGIC RECEPTORS

Immunohistochemical localization of receptors, because of their greater anatomical resolution, is a necessary complement to both receptor ligand autoradiography and in situ hybridization. Antibodies raised against purified nAChRs have been important probes in the study of these receptors. Monoclonal antibodies (Lindstrom, 1987) to both muscle and fish electric organs, which bind to neuronal receptors and do not recognize BTX sites (Whiting and Lindstrom, 1987), have proved particularly useful in the study of nAChRs in the mammalian CNS. Classical immunoperoxidase (Deutch et al., 1987) and radioimmunohistochemistry (Swanson et al., 1987) have been used to visualize receptors in the rodent brain. Two monoclonal antibodies to chicken and rat brain nAChRs radiolabeled with[1];[25]I were shown to label sites with a distribution similar to that found with [^{3}H]nicotine as a ligand but different from that of [^{125}I]BTX binding sites. As with the radioligands, relatively low densities of nAChRs were seen in the hippocampal formation. The densest labeling was seen in the molecular layer of Ammon's horn centered over the stratum lacunosum-moleculare and in the middle one-third of the dentate molecular layer and in the terminal region of the medial perforant pathway from the entorhinal area. The subiculum, presubiculum, and parasubiculum were also labeled (Swanson et al., 1987). To our knowledge no immunohistochemical study has been published with antibodies against mAChRs.

CLONING OF THE NICOTINIC RECEPTORS: VISUALIZATION OF EXPRESSION BY IN SITU HYBRIDIZATION

The sequence of peptides from the different subunits was established chemically and used to synthesize oligonucleotides that were used for the cloning of the nicotinic receptor of the electric organ of the *Torpedo californica*.

The cDNA sequences of the genes coding for the α, β, γ, and σ polypeptide chains of the nicotinic AChR from *T. californica* were the first determined (for reviews, see McCarthy et al., 1986; Hucho, 1986). The amino acid sequence of the α subunits from *Torpedo*, mouse, bovine, and human sources showed the receptors to be close evolutionary homologs of one another (Boulter et al., 1985). The α, β, γ, and σ chains within any one species are more distantly related to each other than is the α subunit between human and *Torpedo* (McCarthy et al., 1986).

Mammalian nicotinic AChR were cloned based on the homologies between sequences of the nicotinic receptor from the skeletal muscle and those of neuronal receptors. The results obtained until now have confirmed the ligand binding studies and suggest the existence of a family of related nicotinic receptor subtypes in the mammalian brain. Several cDNA clones were isolated that appeared to code for α subunits of different acetylcholine receptors. One of them (the α-1 clone) was isolated from a mouse muscle cell line and coded for the α subunit of skeletal muscle nicotinic AChR (Boulter et al., 1985). The α-2 clone has been identified as a neuronal nAChR gene in rat (Wada et al., 1988). The α-3 clone was obtained from a rat pheochromocytoma cell line, PC12, and coded for another neural nicotinic receptor α subunit (Boulter et al., 1986; Goldman et al., 1986). A fourth neural nicotinic AChR (α-4) was isolated from a cDNA library from rat hypothalamus and hippocampus (Goldman et al., 1987).

In situ hybridization studies using probes derived from these four genes have shown that these receptors are expressed differentially throughout the rat brain (Wada et al., 1988; Boulter et al., 1986; Goldman et al., 1986, 1987). In the rat brain only weak signals for α-2 are visualized in the diencephalon, where α-3 and α-4 transcripts are highly expressed, particularly in several thalamic nuclei and especially in the medial habenula. The most intense signal for α-2 has been detected in the interpeduncular nucleus. With probes for the α-3 clone, strong signals were observed in the dentate gyrus and hippocampus. However, high levels of nonspecific hybridization were also seen in these regions. Although not discussed in the published data, hybridization of both α-3 and α-4 subunits was evident in the dorsal subiculum in the published autoradiograms. The demonstration of specific hybridization signals in the rat hippocampal formation with probes for the different nicotinic receptors has proven difficult, in part because of the high levels of nonspecific hybridization and the apparent low levels of expression in these regions. The expression of the nAChR in the hippocampus is supported by Northern hybridization, which has shown the presence of specific transcripts homologous to both the muscle α-1 and the neuronal α-3 subunits (Goldman et al., 1986). On the other hand, the α-4 subtype was cloned from a hippocampal cDNA library, suggesting that even at low levels this subtype is also expressed in the rat hippocampus. Thus, although all the available evidence indicates that the mammalian hippocampus contains several subtypes of the nAChR, a definitive demonstration of the cells expressing these receptors is still missing.

MUSCARINIC RECEPTORS: IN SITU HYBRIDIZATION

Both the M_1 subtype of the mAChR of the porcine brain and the M_2 of the porcine atria have been purified to homogeneity, partially sequenced, and these sequences used to clone cDNAs encoding these receptors (Kubo et al., 1986a,b; Peralta et al., 1987b). Bonner et al. (1987) were able to clone three different mAChR subtypes (m_1, m_3, and m_4) from a rat cerebral cortex library by cross hybridization with probes derived from highly conserved regions among the receptors coupled to G proteins. Independently, Peralta et al. (1987a) cloned the human counterpart of the rat and porcine receptors. All four receptors are highly homologous proteins similar to the adrenergic receptor family (Dixon et al., 1986; Kobilka et al., 1987). Their amino acid sequences suggest a structure of seven transmembrane segments and a large intracellular loop, unique to each subtype. The four different subtypes, when expressed by transfection of mammalian cells, presented clear pharmacological differences. However, pirenzepine was unable to differentiate among M_1, M_3, and M_4 subtypes. These results indicate that the autoradiographic experiments performed until now have failed to differentiate these three receptor subtypes. No selective ligand is yet available.

Probes derived from the porcine M_1 and rat M_1, M_3, and M_4 mAChR genes have been used to visualize by in situ hybridization the cells in the hippocampus expressing these receptors. We have used oligonucleotide probes from the porcine M_1 receptor and found high levels of expression in the pyramidal, granular, and hilar cell bodies in the porcine hippocampus (Fig. 5). Similar results were obtained in the rat hippocampus using rat probes. A comparison of the expression of the four subtypes has been done by in situ hybridization using oligonucleotides from the sequences of the four genes (Bonner et al., 1987; Brann et al., 1988; our unpublished results). These experiments have clearly shown that three subtypes of the mAChR are expressed by intrinsic neurons of the hippocampus. High levels of expression of the M_1 receptor are found in the pyramidal cell layer of CA1, CA2, and CA3, in the hilus, and in the granule cells of the dentate gyrus. The M_3 receptor as defined by Bonner et al. (1987) is expressed in the pyramidal cells of the hippocampus proper and in the hilus, but only at very low levels in the granule cells of the dentate gyrus. The M_4 subtype also presents very low levels of expression in the hippocampus. No signal was found with either the porcine or human M_2 probes in the hippocampal formation of the rat, pig, or human brains. A low expression of the M_2 receptor mRNA was seen, however, in the septum and diagonal band of Broca. In addition to these areas, M_1 receptor expression has been visualized in the entorhinal cortex in the human, rat, and pig brains (Vilaró, Cortés, Palacios, and Mengod, unpublished observations).

The results of the in situ hybridization experiments show, first, a good agreement with the results obtained by receptor autoradiography with nonselective ligands and confirm the lesion experiments previously discussed that suggested that the majority of mAChR in the hippocampal formation are synthesized by neurons intrinsic to the hippocampal formation. Furthermore, these results clearly indicate that mAChR are synthesized by cells such as those in

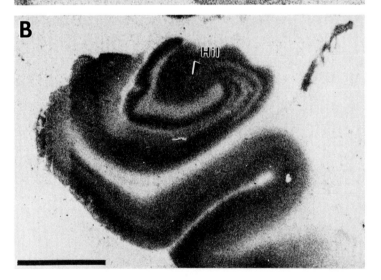

Fig. 5. Visualization of the expression of the M_1 muscarinic receptor mRNA and receptor binding sites in the porcine hippocampus. A: Photomicrograph from a porcine hippocampal section hybridized with a synthetic oligonucleotide complementary to the sequence of the porcine M_1 mRNA. High levels of expression can be seen in the pyramidal cell layer (Py), the granule cell layer of the dentate gyrus (Gy), and in scattered cells in the hilus (Hil). B: The distribution of muscarinic receptor binding is visualized with [^{3}H]NMS as a ligand. Hil, hilus. Bar = 5 mm.

the septum, diagonal band, and entorhinal cortex, which are known to project to the hippocampus. Thus the existence of a small population of presynaptic M_2 receptors in the hippocampus, which has been postulated on the basis of pharmacological experiments, is supported by these findings. It is interesting that a population of presynaptic M_1 receptors, not yet pharmacologically characterized, probably exists in the terminals of the perforant pathway from the entorhinal cortex to the dentate gyrus, which is known to use glutamate as neurotransmitter. Second, the hybridization histochemistry results demonstrate that the hippocampal neurons, particularly the pyramidal cells, express more than one mAChR at the same time and that in the absence of selective ligands for these receptors a clear visualization and characterization of the different subtypes cannot be achieved at the present time.

CONCLUSIONS AND FUTURE TRENDS

The studies reviewed in this chapter illustrate the power of radiohistochemical techniques in studying chemically characterized neuronal pathways in the brain and particularly in the hippocampus. The progress in our knowledge at the molecular level of the neurotransmitter receptors can be rapidly translated, because of these techniques, into an increased understanding of the chemical neuroanatomy of the brain. Each of the techniques reviewed has limitations and also promises for the future. To list a few: Neurotransmitter receptors can now be visualized in the living human being using positron emission tomography. Although the resolution of the currently available systems is still low, recent technical development in this field will soon provide a much-improved high-resolution system. The cloning of the genes for neurotransmitter receptors has allowed us to predict the primary structure of these proteins. Antibodies can be raised against synthetic peptides made from selected regions of these receptors. These antibodies could be used to examine further at the subcellular level the localization and processing of these receptors. This, combined with in situ hybridization, could provide insights into the regulatory mechanisms controlling receptor synthesis and degradation. The application of these new approaches to the study of normal and pathological human brain will hopefully result in the development of new therapeutic approaches for the treatment of psychiatric and neurodegenerative diseases.

ACKNOWLEDGMENTS

We gratefully acknowledge Dr. R. Cortés, Dr. A. Probst, and Ms. T. Vilaró for their collaboration in some of the studies described in this chapter and for allowing the use of unpublished material. We also thank K.H. Wiederhold for his unvaluable help with the photography.

REFERENCES

Arimatsu, Y., A. Seto, and T. Amano (1978) Localization of α-bungarotoxin binding sites in the mouse brain by light and electron microscopic autoradiography. Brain Res. *147*:165–169.

Biegon, A., T.C. Rainbow, J.J. Mann, and B.S. McEwen (1982) Neurotransmitter receptor sites in human hippocampus: A quantitative autoradiographic study. Brain Res. *247*:379–382.

Boksa, P., and R. Quirion (1987) ³H-methyl-carbamylcholine: A new radioligand specific for nicotinic acetylcholine receptors in brain. Eur. J. Pharmacol. *139*:323–333.

Bonner, T.I., N.J. Buckley, A.C. Young, and M.R. Brann (1987) Identification of a family of muscarinic acetylcholine receptor genes. Science *237*:527–532.

Boulter, J., K. Evans, D. Goldman, G. Martin, D. Treco, S. Heinemann, and J. Patrick (1986) Isolation of a cDNA clone coding for a possible neural nicotinic acetylcholine receptor α-subunit. Nature *319*:368–374.

Boulter, J., W. Luyten, K. Evans, P. Mason, M. Ballivet, D. Goldman, S. Stengelin, G. Martin, S. Heinemann, and J. Patrick (1985) Isolation of a clone coding for the α-subunit of a mouse acetylcholine receptor. J. Neurosci. *5*:2545–2552.

Brann, M.R., N.J. Buckley, and T.I. Bonner (1988) The striatum and cerebral cortex express different muscarinic receptor mRNAs. FEBS Lett. *230*:90–94.

Butcher, L.L., and N.J. Woolf (1984) Histochemical distribution of acetylcholinesterase in the central nervous system: Clues to the localization of cholinergic neurons. In A. Björklund, T. Hökfelt, and M.J. Kuhar (eds): Handbook of Chemical Neuroanatomy, Vol. 3, Classical Transmitters and Transmitter Receptors in the CNS, Part II. Amsterdam: Elsevier, pp. 1–50.

Clarke, P.B.S., C.B. Pert, and A. Pert (1984) Autoradiographic distribution of nicotine receptors in rat brain. Brain Res. *323*:390–395.

Clarke, P.B.S., R.D. Schwartz, S.M. Paul, C.B. Pert, and A. Pert (1985) Nicotinic binding in rat brain: Autoradiographic comparison of [³H]acetylcholine, [³H]nicotine, and [¹²⁵I]-α-bungarotoxin. J. Neurosci. *5*:1307–1315.

Cortés, R., and J.M. Palacios (1986) Muscarinic cholinergic receptor subtypes in the rat brain. I. Quantitative autoradiographic studies. Brain Res. *362*:227–238.

Cortés, R., A. Probst, and J.M. Palacios (1987) Quantitative light microscopic autoradiographic localization of cholinergic muscarinic receptors in the human brain: Forebrain. Neuroscience *20*:65–107.

Cortés, R., A. Probst, H.-J. Tobler, and J.M. Palacios (1986) Muscarinic cholinergic receptor subtypes in the human brain. II. Quantitative autoradiographic studies. Brain Res. *362*:239–253.

Deutch, A.Y., J. Holliday, R.H. Roth, L.L.Y. Chun, and E. Hawrot (1987) Immunohistochemical localization of a neuronal nicotinic acetylcholine receptor in mammalian brain. Proc. Natl. Acad. Sci. U.S.A. *84*:8697–8701.

Dixon, R.A.F., B.K. Kobilka, D.J. Strader, J.L. Benovic, H.G. Dohlman, T. Frielle, M.A. Bolanowski, C.D. Bennet, E. Rands, R.E. Diehl, R.A. Munford, E.E. Slater, I.S. Sigal, M.G. Caron, R.J. Lefkowitz, and C.D. Strader (1986) Cloning of the gene and cDNA for mammalian β-adrenergic receptor and homology with rhodopsin. Nature *321*:75–79.

Frey, K.A., R.L.E. Ehrenkaufer, and B.W. Agranoff (1985) Quantitative in vivo receptor binding. II. Autoradiographic imaging of muscarinic cholinergic receptors. J. Neurosci. *5*:2407–2414.

Goldman, D., D., Simmon, L.W. Swanson, J. Patrick, and S. Heinemann (1986) Mapping of brain areas expressing RNA homologous to two different acetylcholine receptor α-subunit cDNAs. Proc. Natl. Acad. Sci. U.S.A. *83*:4076–4080.

Goldman, D., E. Deneris, W. Luyten, A. Kochhar, J. Patrick, and S. Heinemann (1987) Members of a nicotinic acetylcholine receptor gene family are expressed in different regions of the mammalian central nervous system. Cell *48*:965–973.

Hammer, R., and A. Giachetti (1982) Muscarinic receptor subtypes: M_1 and M_2 biochemical and functional characterization. Life Sci. *31:*2991–2998.

Hucho, F. (1986) The nicotinic acetylcholine receptor and its ion channel. Eur. J. Biochem. *158:*211–226.

Hunt, S., and J. Schmidt (1978a) Some observations on the binding patterns of α-bungarotoxin in the central nervous system of the rat. Brain Res. *157:*213–232.

Hunt, S., and J. Schmidt (1978b) The electron microscopic autoradiographic localization of α-bungarotoxin binding sites within the central nervous system of the rat. Brain Res. *142:*152–159.

Kobilka, B.K., R.A.F. Dixon, T. Frielle, H.G. Dohlman, M.A. Bolanowski, I.S. Sigal, T.L. Yang-Fen, U. Francke, M.G. Caron, and R.J. Lefkowitz (1987) cDNA for the human β₂-adrenergic receptor: A protein with multiple membrane spanning domains and encoded by a gene whose chromosomal location is shared with that of the receptor for platelet derived growth factor. Proc. Natl. Acad. Sci. U.S.A. *84:*46–50.

Kubo, T., K. Fukuda, A. Mikami, A. Maeda, H. Takahashi, M. Mishina, T. Haga, K. Haga, A. Ichiyama, K. Kangawa, M. Kojima, H. Matsuo, T. Hirose, and S. Numa (1986a) Cloning, sequencing and expression of complementary DNA encoding the muscarinic acetylcholine receptor. Nature *323:*411–416.

Kubo, T., A. Maeda, K. Sugimoto, I. Akiba, A. Mikami, H. Takahashi, T. Haga, K. Haga, A. Ichiyama, K. Kangawa, H. Matsuo, T. Hirose, and S. Numa (1986b) Primary structure of porcine cardiac muscarinic acetylcholine receptor deduced from the cDNA sequence. FEBS Lett. *209:*367–372.

Kuhar, M.J. (1985) Receptor localization with the microscope. In H. Yamamura, S. Enna, and M.J. Kuhar (eds): Neurotransmitter Receptor Binding, ed 2. New York: Raven Press.

Kuhar, M.J., and H.I. Yamamura (1976) Localization of cholinergic muscarinic receptors in rat brain by light microscopic radioautography. Brain Res. *110:*229–243.

Kuhar, M.J., N. Taylor, J.K. Wamsley, E.C. Hulme, and N.K.M. Birtsall (1981) Muscarinic cholinergic receptor localization in brain by electron microscopic autoradiography. Brain Res. *216:*1–9.

Lang, W., and H. Henke (1983) Cholinergic receptor binding and autoradiography in brains of non-neurological and senile dementia of Alzheimer type patients. Brain Res. *267:*271–280.

Lewis, P.R., and C.C.D. Shute (1967) The cholinergic limbic system: Projections to hippocampal formation, medial cortex, nuclei of the ascending cholinergic reticular system, and the subfornical organ and supra-optic crest. Brain *90:*521–542.

Lewis, P.R., and C.C.D. Shute (1978) Cholinergic pathways in CNS. In L.L. Iversen, S.D. Iversen, and S.H. Snyder (eds): Handbook of Psychopharmacology, Vol. 9, Chemical Pathways in the Brain. New York: Plenum Press, pp. 315–355.

Lindstrom, J.M. (1986) Probing nicotinic acetylcholine receptors with monoclonal antibodies. Trends Neurosci. *9:*401–407.

London, E.D., S.B. Waller, and J.K. Wamsley (1985) Autoradiographic localization of ³H-nicotine binding sites in the rat brain. Neurosci. Lett. *53:*179–184.

McCarthy, M.P., J.P. Earnest, E.F. Young, S. Choe, and R.M. Stroud (1986) The molecular neurobiology of the acetylcholine receptor. Annu. Rev. Neurosci. *9:*383–413.

Monaghan, D.T., E.E. Mena, and C.W. Cotman (1982) The effect of entorhinal cortical ablation on the distribution of muscarinic cholinergic receptors in the rat hippocampus. Brain Res. *234:*480–485.

Mosko, S., G. Lynch, and C.W. Cotman (1973) The distribution of septal projections to the hippocampus of the rat. J. Comp. Neurol. *152:* 163–174.

Palacios, J.M. (1982) Autoradiographic localization of muscarinic cholinergic receptors in the hippocampus of patients with senile dementia. Brain Res. *243*:173–175.

Palacios, J.M. (1984) Receptor autoradiography: The last ten years. J. Receptor Res. *4*:633–644.

Peralta, E.G., A. Ashkenazi, J.W. Winslow, D.H. Smith, J. Ramachandran, and D.J. Capon (1987a) Distinct primary structures, ligand-binding properties and tissue-specific expression of four human muscarinic acetylcholine receptors. EMBO J. *6*:3923–3929.

Peralta, E.G., J.W. Winslow, G.L. Peterson, D.H. Smith, A. Ashkenazi, J. Ramachandran, M.I. Schimerlik, and D.J. Capon (1987b) Primary structure and biochemical properties of an M_2 muscarinic receptor. Science *236*:600–605.

Polz-Tejera, G., J. Schmidt, and H.J. Karten (1975) Autoradiographic localization of α-bungarotoxin binding sites in the central nervous system. Nature *258*:349–351.

Potter, L.T., D.D. Flynn, H.E. Hanchet, D.L. Kalinoski, J. Luber-Narod, and D.C. Mash (1984) Independent M_1 and M_2 receptors: Ligands, autoradiography and function. Trends Pharmacol. Sci. [Suppl.] pp. 22–31.

Probst, A., R. Cortés, J. Ulrich, and J.M. Palacios (1988) Differential modification of muscarinic cholinergic receptors in the hippocampus of patients with Alzheimer's disease: An autoradiographic study. Brain Res. *450*:190–201.

Quirion, R., and P. Boksa (1986) Autoradiographic distribution of muscarinic ^{3}H-acetylcholine receptors in the rat brain: Comparison with antagonists. Eur. J. Pharmacol. *123*:170–172.

Rainbow, T.C., R.D. Schwartz, B. Parsons, and K.J. Kellar (1984) Quantitative autoradiography of nicotinic [^{3}H]acetylcholine binding sites in rat brain. Neurosci. Lett. *50*:193–196.

Richards, J.G., P. Schoch, P. Häring, B. Takacs, and H. Möhler (1987) Resolving $GABA_A$/benzodiazepine receptors: Cellular and subcellular localization in the CNS with monoclonal antibodies. J. Neurosci. *7*:1866–1886.

Rotter, A., N.J.M. Birdsall, A.S.V. Burgen, P.M. Field, E.C. Hulme, and G. Raisman (1979a) Muscarinic receptors in the central nervous system of the rat. I. Technique for autoradiographic localization of the binding of [^{3}H]propylbenzilylcholine mustard and its distribution in the forebrain. Brain Res. Rev. *1*:141–165.

Rotter, A., N.J.M. Birdsall P.M. Field, and G. Raisman (1979b) Muscarinic receptors in the central nervous system of the rat. II. Distribution of binding of ^{3}H-propylbenzilylcholine mustard in the midbrain and hindbrain. Brain Res. Rev. *1*:167–183.

Salpeter, M.M., L. Bachmann, and E.E. Salpeter (1969) Resolution in electron microscope autoradiography. J. Histochem. Cytochemn. *24*:1204.

Schofield, P.R., M.G. Darlison, N. Fujita, D.R. Burt, F.A. Stephenson, H. Rodriguez, L.M. Rhee, J. Ramachandran, V. Reale, T.A. Glencores, P.H. Seeburg, and E.A. Barnard (1987) Sequence and functional expression of the $GABA_A$ receptor shows a ligand-gated receptor super-family. Nature *328*:221–227.

Schwartz, R.D. (1986) Autoradiographic distribution of high affinity muscarinic and nicotinic cholinergic receptors labeled with ^{3}H-acetylcholine in rat brain. Life Sci. *38*:2111–2119.

Segal, M., Y. Dudai, and A. Amsterdam (1978) Distribution of an α-bungarotoxin binding cholinergic nicotinic receptor in rat brain. Brain Res. *148*:105–119.

Silver, J., and R.B. Billiar (1976) An autoradiographic analysis of ^{3}H-α-bungarotoxin distribution in the rat brain after intraventricular injection. J. Cell Biol. *71*:956–963.

Swanson, L.W., D.M. Simmons, P.J. Whiting, and J. Lindstrom (1987) Immunohistochemical localization of neuronal nicotinic receptors in the rodent central nervous system. J. Neurosci. *7*:3334–3342.

van Leeuwen, F.W., R.M. Buijs, C.W. Pool, and O. Pach (eds) (1988) Molecular Neuroanatomy. Amsterdam: Elsevier.

Wada, K., M. Ballivet, J. Boulter, J. Connolly, E. Wada, E.S. Deneris, L.W. Swanson, S. Heinemann, and J. Patrick (1988) Functional expression of a new pharmacological subtype of brain nicotinic acetyl-choline receptor. Science 240:330–334.

Wamsley, J.K., D.R. Gehlert, W.R. Roeske, and H.I. Yamamura (1984) Muscarinic antagonist binding site heterogeneity as evidenced by autoradiography after direct labeling with [^{3}H]QNB and [^{3}H]pirenzepine. Life Sci. 34:1395–1402.

Wamsley, J.K., M.S. Lewis, W.S. Young III, and M.J. Kuhar (1981) Autoradiographic localization of muscarinic cholinergic receptors in rat brainstem. J. Neurosci. 1:176–191.

Wamsley, J.K., and J.M. Palacios (1983) Receptor mapping by histochemistry. In A. Lajtha (ed): Handbook of Neurochemistry, Vol. 2, ed 2. London: Plenum Press Co., pp. 27–51.

Wamsley, J.K., M.A. Zarbin, N.J.M. Birdsall, and M.J. Kuhar (1980) Muscarinic cholinergic receptors: Autoradiographic localization of high and low affinity agonist binding sites. Brain Res. 200:1–12.

Whiting, P., and J. Lindstrom (1987) Purification and characterization of a nicotinic acetylcholine receptor from rat brain. Proc. Natl. Acad. Sci. U.S.A. 84:595–599.

Yamamura, H.I., T.W. Vickroy, D.R. Gehlert, J.K. Wamsley, and W.R Roeske (1985) Autoradiographic localization of muscarinic agonist binding sites in the rat central nervous system with (+)-cis-^{3}H-methyldioxolane. Brain Res. 179:255–270.

The Hippocampus—New Vistas, pages 225–236
© 1989 Alan R. Liss, Inc.

15
Mechanisms Underlying the Lability of GABAergic Inhibition in the Hippocampus

SCOTT M. THOMPSON

Brain Research Institute, University of Zürich, Zürich, Switzerland

INTRODUCTION

Epilepsy is a disease characterized by the excessive, synchronous discharge of a large population of nerve cells. Much of our understanding of the cellular events underlying epileptiform discharge has come from the study of acute, experimental epileptic foci made with the topical application of convulsant drugs, such as penicillin (for reviews, see Dichter and Ayala, 1987; Prince, 1978). Many of these drugs have been shown to act as antagonists of inhibitory synaptic transmission mediated by γ-aminobutyric acid (GABA) (Krnjević, 1983), leading to the suggestion that epilepsy results from a pathological decrease in the effectiveness of GABAergic inhibitory synaptic transmission. This suggestion is complemented by recent findings that a long-term loss of GABAergic inhibition occurs in some models of chronic epilepsy, as well (Stelzer et al., 1987; Sloviter, 1987). A fundamental question remaining to be answered is: How do cell populations become disinhibited in situ?

In some of the earliest experiments with application of exogenous GABA, it was noted that there was a fading of its inhibitory effects during repeated or prolonged application (Curtis et al., 1959). Lability of the intracellularly recorded inhibitory postsynaptic potential (IPSP) was later shown by Andersen and Lømo (1968), who found that the IPSP was reduced in amplitude following trains of synaptic stimuli in situ. For example, repetitive stimulation in organotypic hippocampal slice cultures at frequencies of 2–5 Hz for 30–60 s produces decreases in IPSP amplitude of 50–90% (Fig. 1B), similar to previous findings in situ (Andersen and Lømo, 1968; Ben-Ari et al., 1979) and in acute slices (McCarren and Alger, 1985; Wong and Watkins, 1982). Furthermore, at higher intensities of stimulation, repetitive stimulation results in pronounced epileptiform afterdischarges, synchronized throughout the cell population. These afterdischarges can occur both spontaneously and in response to synaptic stimuli that previously elicited pronounced IPSPs (Fig. 1A). Afterdischarges become progressively shorter following the end of the stimulus train and cease

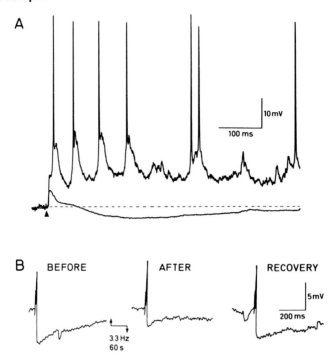

Fig. 1. Effects of repetitive stimulation on IPSPs under current-clamp. **A:** At high stimulus intensities, a compound synaptic potential is evoked (lower trace) consisting of a short latency excitatory postsynaptic potential, the IPSP, and a late postsynaptic potential. Membrane potential (V_M) = -72 mV, slightly hyperpolarized to the reversal potential of synaptic current underlying IPSPs (E_{IPSC}). Repetitive stimulation (5 Hz for 30 s) results in loss of the IPSP and the development of evoked epileptiform afterdischarge. **B:** Excitatory postsynaptic potentials and IPSPs in another cell at V_M = -55 mV before, immediately after a train of stimuli at low intensity (3.3 Hz for 60 s), and after 2–3 min recovery. The amplitude of the IPSP is decreased 70% by such repetitive stimulation.

after 1–3 min, coincident with recovery of the IPSP. Such hyperexcitability resulting from repetitive stimulation suggests that this *activity-dependent disinhibition* could be an important mechanism in the genesis of epileptiform discharge.

To understand how GABA responses and IPSPs become decreased in effectiveness with repetitive use, it is important to understand their underlying mechanisms. Considerable evidence suggests that release of GABA from inhibitory interneurons activates ion channels in pyramidal cells that are selectively permeable to Cl⁻ ions. First, both IPSPs and GABA responses are blocked by bath-applied bicuculline. Second, the reversal potentials of the IPSP and of responses to exogenously applied GABA (E_{GABA}) are shifted in the depolarizing direction if the intracellular Cl⁻ concentration is increased by iontophoresis of Cl⁻ from KCl-filled recording electrodes. Likewise, in hippocampal slice cultures, the dependence of E_{GABA} on the extracellular Cl^- concentration is close to that predicted by the Nernst equation for Cl^- (Thompson and Gähwiler, 1989a). These data allow us to assume that the IPSP is GABA mediated and that the equilibrium potentials of both are approximately equal to the Cl^- equilibrium potential (E_{Cl^-}). The efficacy of GABA-mediated inhibitory transmission therefore depends on two key factors: 1) the size of the conductance activated by GABA, a function of the amount of GABA released by presynaptic elements and the postsynaptic sensitivity to GABA; and 2) the driving force for Cl^- ion flow across this conductance, i.e. the difference between the membrane potential and E_{Cl^-}.

Disinhibition has been described in hippocampus as a consequence of interference at each of these steps. For example, opiate peptides are potent convulsants because they decrease GABA release from presynaptic interneurons (e.g. Nicoll et al., 1979). Likewise, decreasing IPSP driving force by lowering the extracellular Cl^- concentration results in synchronous, epileptiform discharge (Yamamoto and Kawai, 1967). Indeed, there is evidence to support alterations of each of these aspects of synaptic inhibition as a consequence of repetitive stimulation. Ben-Ari et al. (1979) measured a decrease in the conductance underlying IPSPs following repetitive stimulation of hippocampal pyramidal cells in situ. More recently, under more stable conditions in acute slices, McCarren and Alger (1985) suggested that IPSPs are reduced in amplitude because of both a decrease in IPSP conductance and a decrease in IPSP driving force. Unfortunately, these observations were made with current-clamp recording techniques, thus precluding a quantitative analysis of the relative importance of each of these factors.

The effects of repetitive stimulation were recently re-examined (Thompson and Gähwiler, 1989a) using single-electrode voltage-clamp recording from pyramidal cells in organotypic hippocampal slice cultures (for a complete description of this preparation, see Gähwiler, 1984). These cultures are particularly advantageous for single-electrode voltage-clamp experiments because of the excellent visibility of live neurons under phase contrast microscopy, facilitating impalement, and the relative lack of diffusional barriers between the cells and the bathing saline, facilitating rapid application of drugs and alteration of the ionic millieu. CA3 cells were chosen for these studies because of the importance of this cell population as a pacemaker in the genesis of epileptiform discharge (Wong and Traub, 1983). IPSPs were indirectly evoked by stimulation of the mossy fiber afferent pathway. Under voltage-clamp, both the reversal potential of the IPSP (E_{IPSC}) and the conductance of the IPSP (g_{IPSC}) may be directly assessed by measuring the current underlying the IPSP at several different membrane potentials and plotting the amplitude of these synaptic currents as a function of the membrane potential (V_M) at which they were evoked (e.g. Fig. 2B). With this method, E_{IPSC} is given as the zero current intercept, and g_{IPSC} is the slope of the "best fit" line.

Repetitive stimulation in hippocampal slice cultures at frequencies of 2–5 Hz for 30–60 s, while the membrane potential is voltage-clamped 5–15 mV depolarized with respect to E_{IPSC}, consistently produces two effects. First, there

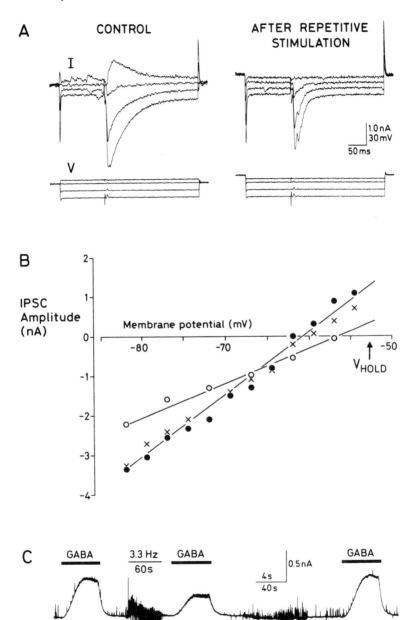

A

CONTROL

AFTER REPETITIVE
STIMULATION

I

V

1.0 nA
30 mV

50 ms

B

IPSC
Amplitude
(nA)

Membrane potential (mV)

V_{HOLD}

C

GABA

3.3 Hz
60s

GABA

GABA

0.5 nA

4 s
40 s

is a depolarizing shift in E_{IPSC} of 2–8 mV toward the membrane potential maintained by the voltage-clamp. The result of this shift is a decrease in IPSP driving force of 20–90% (mean decrease in driving force = 49%, N = 15). Second, there is a decrease in g_{IPSC} averaging 22%. Together these two effects would be expected to produce decreases in the amplitude of IPSPs of as much as 90% and can thus account for previous observations made with current-clamp recording techniques. Further experiments were performed to describe the mechanisms underlying these changes in IPSPs.

MECHANISMS OF ACTIVITY-DEPENDENT DECREASES IN IPSP DRIVING FORCE

Decreases in IPSP driving force as a result of depolarizing shifts of E_{IPSC} could reflect either a true depolarizing shift of E_{Cl}^- or an enhancement of some other partially overlapping component of the compound synaptic response that has a reversal potential less negative than E_{IPSC}. For example, Andersen and Lømo (1968) suggested that potentiation of the EPSP could result in an apparent depolarizing shift in E_{IPSC}. This possibility can be tested with iontophoretic application of GABA. Consistent with a true decrease in the driving force for Cl^-, GABA-activated outward currents are always reduced in amplitude following a train of stimuli given while maintaining V_M depolarized with respect to E_{IPSC} (Fig. 2C).

A depolarizing shift in E_{Cl}^-, as defined by the Nernst equation, may reflect either a decrease in the extracellular Cl^- concentration or an increase in the intracellular Cl^- concentration ($[Cl^-]_i$). Measurements made with ion-selective microelectrodes have shown that the extracellular Cl^- concentration is effec-

---

Fig. 2. Effects of repetitive stimulation under voltage-clamp on E_{IPSC} and g_{IPSC}. **A:** Membrane currents (I, upper traces) and sampled membrane potential (V, lower traces) in response to step voltage commands (to -58, -63, -73, and -83 mV in both). Synaptic currents, evoked 120 ms after the start of the step commands, are outward (plotted upward in this and subsequent figures) at depolarized V_M and inward (plotted downward in this and subsequent figures) at hyperpolarized V_Ms. Comparison of control synaptic currents with those after repetitive stimulation (3.3 Hz for 60 s at a holding potential of -53 mV) shows that synaptic currents were depressed by the stimulus train. **B:** Calculation of E_{IPSC} and g_{IPSC}, by plotting the amplitude of the inhibitory postsynaptic current (IPSC, measured at a latency of 35 ms after stimulation) as a function of the V_M at which it was evoked, before (filled circles), after repetitive stimulation (open circles), and after recovery (crosses). Driving force was reversibly decreased 50% because of a 4 mV depolarizing shift in E_{IPSC} toward the holding potential (V_{HOLD}), and g_{IPSC} was decreased 44% following repetitive stimulation. Same cell as in A. **C:** Effects of repetitive stimulation at depolarized V_M on outward currents activated by GABA are shown in this continuous chart recording from another cell. Responses to iontophoretic application of GABA were obtained before and at varying times after a train of repetitive synaptic stimuli (3.3 Hz for 60 s) at $V_M = -50$ mV. Repetitive stimulation clearly resulted in a transient depression of the GABA-activated current. The chart speed was reduced between GABA responses as indicated. Vertical deflections result from spontaneous synaptic potentials.

tively constant even in the face of intense neuronal discharge (Dietzel et al., 1982). In contrast, Huguenard and Alger (1986) have suggested that Cl^- influx, as the charge-carrying ion of the outward current underlying the IPSP itself, may be sufficient to alter $[Cl^-]_i$ significantly. Such a source of Cl^- influx would be especially relevant during the maintained increase in Cl^- conductance, resulting from the partial summation of IPSPs, during a train of repetitive stimuli. This was indeed shown to be the source of Cl^- influx by delivering the train of stimuli while holding V_M hyperpolarized with respect to E_{IPSC}. Under this condition, with the direction of Cl^- flux reversed from inward to outward, no activity-dependent depolarizing shift in E_{IPSC} was observed (Thompson and Gähwiler, 1989a). We may therefore conclude that Cl^- passively enters the cell during the IPSP when V_M is less negative than E_{IPSC}, i.e. as is normally observed in situ, and accumulates during the train of stimuli. This produces an increase in the intracellular Cl^- concentration that accounts for the activity-dependent depolarizing shift in E_{Cl^-}.

One well-characterized consequence of repetitive stimulation in the hippocampus is for neurons to release K^+ into the extracellular space, leading to an increase in its concentration from 3 to 12 mM (Heinemann and Lux, 1977). McCarren and Alger (1985) have noted a close correlation between the amount of K^+ that accumulates in the extracellular space following repetitive stimulation in acute slices and the decrease in IPSP driving force. Similarly, in hippocampal slice cultures, when the resting extracellular K^+ concentration was reduced from control (5.8 mM) to 1 mM, the activity-dependent decrease in IPSP driving force was significantly reduced from 78% to only 19% of control ($N = 5$) (Thompson and Gähwiler, 1989a). Presumably, the maximum concentration of K^+ reached during the stimulus train was reduced by lowering the initial K^+ concentration (Heinemann and Lux, 1977).

Elevated extracellular K^+ has recently been shown to inhibit outward Cl^- transport from several cell types by inhibiting a furosemide-sensitive, potassium/chloride cotransport system (Aickin et al., 1982; Deisz and Lux, 1982; Misgeld et al., 1986; Thompson et al., 1988). This outward Cl^- transport process is responsible for maintaining E_{Cl^-} more negative than the resting V_M, as shown by the depolarizing shift in E_{IPSC} in the presence of either furosemide or elevated extracellular K^+ in hippocampal slice cultures (Thompson and Gähwiler, 1989b). Inhibition of outward chloride transport by the increased extracellular K^+ following the stimulus train will act to "trap" the Cl^- that passively entered the cell during the partially summated IPSPs and thus significantly enhance the activity-dependent increase in $[Cl^-]_i$.

MECHANISMS OF ACTIVITY-DEPENDENT DECREASES IN IPSP CONDUCTANCE

Decreases in g_{IPSC} could result from either a decreased sensitivity of postsynaptic receptors to a constant release of GABA, i.e. desensitization, or a decreased release of GABA from presynaptic elements. Desensitization of GABA receptors following a stimulus train will also decrease the sensitivity of a cell to exogenously applied GABA, an effect reported by Ben-Ari et al. (1979) in situ. As described above, GABA-activated outward currents were decreased in amplitude following repetitive stimulation at depolarized holding potentials (Fig. 2C); however, the decrease in the Cl^- driving force under these conditions will also reduce GABA responses. GABA was therefore applied after a train of stimuli delivered with the membrane potential voltage-clamped hyperpolarized to E_{IPSC}. Under these conditions, in which there is no change in E_{IPSC}, repetitive stimulation has no effect on GABA responses (Thompson and Gähwiler, 1989a), demonstrating that the postsynaptic sensitivity to GABA has not changed. We may therefore rule out significant activity-dependent desensitization as the cause of the decrease in g_{IPSC}. In other experiments in which the "fading" of the GABA-activated conductance was measured during prolonged iontophoretic applications, the rate of desensitization was observed to be quite slow (mean time constant = 51 s) (Thompson and Gähwiler, 1989c; Wong and Watkins, 1982), perhaps explaining why significant desensitization does not occur during a stimulus train.

If the postsynaptic GABA sensitivity has not changed, then the activity-dependent decrease in g_{IPSC} must result from a decrease in GABA release. Iontophoretically applied GABA itself has a potent depressant action on IPSPs. This effect is strongly dose dependent: With small iontophoretic currents, IPSPs are depressed by 30%; with large iontophoretic currents, IPSPs may be almost entirely blocked. Complete recovery requires some 60–90 s (Thompson and Gähwiler, 1989c). Several different mechanisms can be postulated to account for these effects of GABA: Postsynaptic GABA receptors could be desensitized, E_{Cl^-} could have been shifted in the depolarizing direction as a result of Cl^- influx, or presynaptic GABA release could have been decreased. These possibilities were examined by testing the effect of such an application of GABA on a second, paired pulse of GABA (Thompson and Gähwiler, 1989c). For small iontophoretic currents, which caused a decrease in IPSP amplitude <40% when applied singly, there was no change in the amplitude of the second pulse (Fig. 3). For larger iontophoretic currents, which caused a decrease in IPSP amplitude >60% when applied singly, the amplitude of a second, identical iontophoretic pulse was always decreased in amplitude (Fig. 3). This decrease in amplitude could be shown to result from a decrease in Cl^- driving force and never from a decrease in evoked conductance. The smaller iontophoretic pulses were thus capable of decreasing the amplitude of IPSPs without altering either E_{IPSC} or the postsynaptic sensitivity to GABA. GABA must therefore be capable of decreasing its own release.

Deisz and Prince (1986) have presented evidence that activity-dependent decreases in g_{IPSC} in the neocortex result from a negative feedback of GABA onto presynaptic $GABA_B$ receptors that inhibit subsequent release. In the neocortex, inhibition of GABA uptake with nipecotic acid enhanced the activity-dependent decrease in g_{IPSC} by prolonging the time course of GABA in the synaptic cleft (Desiz and Prince, 1986). In the neocortex and hippocampus, both iontophoretic and bath applications of the selective $GABA_B$-receptor agonist baclofen have been shown to result in a depression of IPSPs (Fig. 4A) (Bowery et al., 1980; Howe et al., 1987; Misgeld et al., 1984). Under voltage-

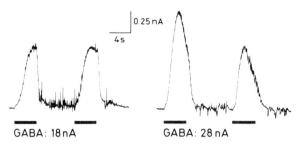

Fig. 3. Chart recordings of outward currents at $V_M = -55$ mV activated by identical, paired 6 s applications of GABA at two iontophoretic current intensities. The amplitude of the current evoked by GABA is greater for the higher iontophoretic current intensity. However, note that only for the larger iontophoretic dose is there a decrement in the amplitude of the second response relative to the first. When ramp voltage commands were used to measure the GABA-activated conductance and E_{GABA} simultaneously, there was no difference in either E_{GABA} or conductance for the two 18 nA pulses, as expected from their identical amplitudes. However, for the 28 nA iontophoretic pulses, there was a significant depolarizing shift in the E_{GABA} of the second pulse toward the holding V_M, although the evoked conductance was not different for the two pulses (see Thompson and Gahwiler, 1989c). Therefore, a decrease in driving force, and not receptor desensitization, is responsible for the decrease in amplitude of the second pulse relative to the first.

clamp it can be seen that this results purely from a decrease in g_{IPSC} (Fig. 4B) (Thompson and Gähwiler, 1989c). This effect is rapid in onset, can produce a complete block of synaptic transmission, and is seen with concentrations of $(-)$-baclofen as low as 10^{-7} M. Since postsynaptic GABA responsiveness is unaffected (Howe et al., 1987; Thompson and Gähwiler, 1989c), baclofen must decrease g_{IPSC} by decreasing presynaptic GABA release. It is likely that the activity-dependent decrease in g_{IPSC} results from a negative feedback of GABA, which accumulates in the synaptic cleft during the stimulus train, onto these presynaptic $GABA_B$ receptors.

The ionic mechanism of this presynaptic baclofen action is uncler. Baclofen has been shown to inhibit Ca^{2+} current directly in some peripheral cells (e.g. Deisz and Lux, 1985). In hippocampus, however, baclofen increases pyramidal cell K^+ conductance but does not effect pyramidal cell Ca^{2+} current (Gähwiler and Brown, 1985; Newberry and Nicoll, 1985). Either mechanism could reduce GABA release if present at presynaptic elements. However, pertussis toxin has recently been shown to block the ability of baclofen to increase K^+ conductance but not to block the ability of baclofen to decrease synaptic transmission. Likewise, the $GABA_B$ receptor antagonist phaclofen prevents activation of the postsynaptic K^+ conductance but not the presynaptic action (Dutar and Nicoll, 1988).

In summary, repetitive stimulation leads to a short-term reduction in the efficacy of GABA-mediated inhibitory synaptic transmission. Miles and Wong (1987) have shown that such partial disinhibition may be enough to unleash powerful, latent excitatory interactions between pyramidal cells that serve to

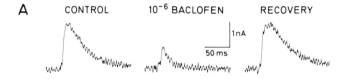

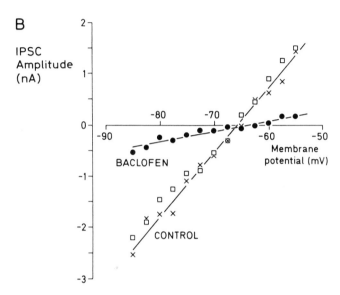

Fig. 4. Effects of the GABA$_B$-receptor agonist baclofen on IPSPs. **A:** Outward synaptic currents evoked at $V_M = -55$ mV before, 3 min after bath application of 10^{-6} M $(-)$-baclofen, and 3 min after washout of baclofen. **B:** Calculation of E_{IPSC} and g_{IPSC}, as in Figure 2, before (open squares), in the presence of baclofen (filled circles), and after washout of baclofen (crosses) for same experiment as A. At 10^{-6} M, baclofen reduced g_{IPSC} from 127 to 20 nS, without changing E_{IPSC}. g_{IPSC} fully recovered upon washout.

synchronize discharge throughout the population. Repeated applications of such stimulus trains might both strengthen excitation, perhaps through the mechanisms of long-term potentiation, and lead to a chronic decrease in GABA-mediated inhibition (e.g. Stelzer et al., 1987). Activity-dependent disinhibition thus results from several potent endogenous mechanisms that can transiently or chronically increase excitability. This lability of GABAergic inhibitory transmission may therefore be an important factor in the pathology of epilepsy.

SUMMARY

Repetitive stimulation of afferent synaptic pathways in the hippocampus at low frequencies leads to a depression of inhibitory postsynaptic potentials and to hyperexcitability. In single-electrode voltage-clamp recordings from CA3 pyramidal cells, it was shown that this depression results from decreases in both the driving force of the IPSP and the evoked conductance underlying the IPSP. The *decrease in IPSP driving force* is produced by accumulation of Cl$^-$ inside the cell that consequently shifts E_{Cl}^- in the depolarizing direction towards the resting membrane potential. This Cl$^-$ is then trapped in the cell, because active outward potassium/chloride cotransport is partially inhibited by activity-dependent increases in the extracellular K$^+$ concentration. The *decrease in IPSP conductance* results from a decrease in the presynaptic release of GABA, not from desensitization of postsynaptic receptors. Both exogenous GABA and baclofen can block IPSPs by decreasing GABA release from presynaptic elements. A negative feedback of GABA onto these GABA$_B$ receptors during the stimulus train could therefore account for the decrease in IPSP conductance. Activity-dependent disinhibition thus results from several endogenous mechanisms that might be important in the genesis or spread of epilepsy.

ACKNOWLEDGMENTS

It is a pleasure to thank Dr. B.H. Gähwiler for his active collaboration and support of the experiments described here, as well as for critically reading this manuscript; Dr. R.A. Deisz for many stimulating discussions; and Ms. L. Rietschin for help with the cultures. This work was supported by a NATO Postdoctoral Fellowship (1986), the Swiss National Funds, the Dr. Eric Slack-Gyr Foundation, and M.E. Leasca.

REFERENCES

Aickin, C.C., R.A. Deisz, and H.D. Lux (1982) Ammonium action on post-synaptic inhibition in crayfish neurones: Implications for the mechanism of chloride extrusion. J. Physiol. [Lond.] *329*:319–339.

Andersen, P., and T. Lømo (1968) Counteraction of powerful recurrent inhibition in hippocampal pyramidal cells by frequency potentiation of excitatory synapses. In C. von Euler, S. Skoglund, and U. Soderberg (eds): Structure and Function of Inhibitory Neuronal Mechanisms. Oxford: Pergamon Press, pp. 335–342.

Ben-Ari, Y., K. Krnjević, and W. Reinhardt (1979) Hippocampal seizures and failure of inhibition. Can J. Physiol. Pharmacol. *57*:1462–1466.

Bowery, N.G., D.R. Hill, A.L. Hudson, A. Doble, D.N. Middlemiss, J. Shaw, and M. Turnbull (1980) (-) Baclofen decreases neurotransmitter release in the mammalian CNS by an action at a novel GABA receptor. Nature *283*:92–94.

Curtis, D.R., J.W. Phillis, and J.C. Watkins (1959) The depression of spinal neurones by gamma-amino-n-butyric acid and β-alanine. J. Physiol. [Lond.] *146*:185–203.

Deisz, R.A., and H.D. Lux (1982) The role of intracellular chloride in hyperpolarizing post-synaptic inhibition of crayfish stretch receptor neurones. J. Physiol. [Lond.] *326*:123–138.

Deisz, R.A., and H.D. Lux, (1985) Gamma-aminobutyric acid-induced depression of calcium currents of chick sensory neurons. Neurosci. Lett. *56*:205–210.

Deisz, R.A., and D.A. Prince (1989) Frequency dependent depression of inhibition in the guinea pig neocortex in vitro by GABA$_B$ receptor feedback on GABA release. J. Physiol. [Lond.] (in press).

Dichter, M.A., and G.F. Ayala (1987) Cellular mechanisms of epilepsy: A status report. Science *237*:157–164.

Dietzel, I., U. Heinemann, G. Hofmeier, and H.D. Lux (1982) Stimulus-induced changes in extracellular Na$^+$ and Cl$^-$ concentration in relation to changes in the size of the extracellular space. Exp. Brain Res. 46:73–84.

Dutar, P., and R.A. Nicoll (1988) Pre- and postsynaptic GABA$_B$ receptors in the hippocampus have different pharmacological properties. Neuron 1:585–591.

Gähwiler, B.H. (1984) Development of the hippocampus in vitro: Cell types, synapses, and receptors. Neuroscience 11:751–760.

Gähwiler, B.H., and D.A. Brown (1985) GABA$_B$-receptor-activated K$^+$ current in voltage-clamped CA$_3$ pyramidal cells in hippocampal cultures. Proc. Natl. Acad. Sci. U.S.A. 82:1558–1562.

Heinemann, U., and H.D. Lux (1977) Ceiling of stimulus induced rises in extracellular potassium concentration in the cerebral cortex of the cat. Brain Res. 120:231–249.

Howe, J.R., B. Sutor, and W. Zieglgänsberger (1987) Baclofen reduces post synaptic potentials of rat cortical neurones by an action other than its hyperpolarizing action. J. Physiol. [Lond.] 384:539–569.

Huguenard, J.R., and B.E. Alger (1986) Whole-cell voltage-clamp study of the fading of GABA-activated currents in acutely dissociated hippocampal neurons. J. Neurophysiol. 56:1–18.

Krnjević, K. (1983) GABA-mediated inhibitory mechanisms in relation to epileptic discharges. In H.H. Jasper, and N.M. van Gelder (eds): Basic Mechanisms of Neuronal Hyperexcitability. New York: Alan R. Liss, pp. 249–280.

McCarren, M., and B.E. Alger (1985) Use-dependent depression of IPSPs in rat hippocampal pyramidal cells in vitro. J. Neurophysiol. 53:557–571.

Miles, R., and R.K.S. Wong (1987) Latent synaptic pathways revealed after tetanic stimulation in the hippocampus. Nature 329:724–726.

Misgeld, U., R.A. Deisz, H.U. Dodt, and H.D. Lux (1986) The role of chloride transport in postsynaptic inhibition of hippocampal neurons. Science 232:1413–1415.

Misgeld, U., M.R. Klee and M.L. Zeise (1984) Differences in baclofen-sensitivity between CA3 neurons and granule cells of the guinea pig hippocampus in vitro. Neurosci. Lett. 47:307–311.

Newberry, N.R., and R.A. Nicoll (1985) Comparison of the action of baclofen with gamma-aminobutyric acid on rat hippocampal pyramidal cells in vitro. J. Physiol. [Lond.] 360:161–185.

Nicoll, R.A., B.E. Alger, and C.E. Jahr (1979) Enkephalin blocks inhibitory pathways in the vertebrate central nervous system. Nature 281:315–317.

Prince, D.A. (1978) Neurophysiology of epilepsy. Annu. Rev. Neurosci. 1:395–415.

Sloviter, R.S. (1987) Decreased hippocampal inhibition and a selective loss of interneurons in experimental epilepsy. Science 235:73–76.

Stelzer, A., N.T. Slater, and G. ten Bruggencate (1987) Activation of NMDA receptors blocks GABAergic inhibition in an in vitro model of epilepsy. Nature 326:698–701.

Thompson, S.M., R.A. Deisz, and D.A. Prince (1988) Outward chloride/cation co-transport in mammalian cortical neurons. Neurosci. Lett. 89:49–54.

Thompson, S.M., and B.H. Gähwiler (1989a) Activity-dependent disinhibition. I. Repetitive stimulation reduces IPSP driving force and conductance in the hippocampus in vitro. J. Neurophysiol. (in press).

Thompson, S.M., and B.H. Gähwiler (1989b) Activity-dependent disinhibition. II. Effects of extracellular potassium, furosemide, and membrane potential on E$_{Cl}$$^-$ in hippocampal CA3 neurons. J. Neurophysiol. (in press).

Thompson, S.M., and B.H. Gähwiler (1989c) Activity-dependent disinhibition. III. Desensitization and GABA$_B$ receptor-mediated presynaptic inhibition in the hippocampus in vitro. J. Neurophysiol. (in press).

Wong, R.K.S., and R.D. Traub (1983) Synchronized burst discharge in disinhibited hippocampal slice. I. Initiation in CA2-CA3 region. J. Neurophysiol. 49:442–458.

Wong, R.K.S., and D.J. Watkins (1982) Cellular factors influencing GABA response in hippocampal pyramidal cells J. Neurophysiol. 48:938–951.

Yamamoto, C., and N. Kawai (1967) Seizure discharge evoked in vitro in thin sections from guinea-pig hippocampus. Science 155:341–342.

16
Neuronal Grafting to the Damaged Adult Hippocampal Formation

FRED H. GAGE AND GYÖRGY BUZSÁKI

Department of Neurosciences, University of California at San Diego, La Jolla, California

INTRODUCTION

The hippocampal formation (HF), as exemplified in this volume, has been extensively used as a model brain system in which to investigate neuronal and behavioral plasticity following damage. The success of this work is predicted on the basis of the wide body of anatomical, biochemical, electrophysiological, and behavioral knowledge about the HF that has been accumulated. Thus, with this background, the deafferented HF has been emploved to investigate the viability of brain tissue grafting, using the anatomical, electrophysiological, biochemical, and behavioral parameters already available as indices of morphological integration, specificity of axonal ingrowth, biochemical restoration, electrophysiological function, and behavioral recovery. Other investigators have used the neonatal HF as host tissue for neural grafting with excellent results (see Zimmer et al., Chapter 17, this volume). In this review, we will focus on the grafting of central nervous system tissue to the adult denervated HF as a model system for studies of graft integration and function.

GRAFTING PROCEDURE

Two principal techniques have been used to graft fetal CNS tissue to the denervated adult hippocampus (HPC). The first one involves the transplantation of solid pieces of tissue to a surgically prepared transplantation cavity. In this procedure good graft survival is ensured by preparing the cavity in such a way that the graft can be placed on a richly vascularized surface (e.g. the pia in the choroidal fissure) that can serve as a "culturing bed" for the graft (Stenevi et al., 1976). Both the fimbria-fornix lesion and the perforant pathway aspirative lesion (Stenevi et al., 1976) provide such "culturing beds." These cavities are in direct communication with the lateral ventricle, which may allow for the CSF to circulate through the graft cavity and thus possibly help the graft to survive, particularly during the early postoperative period.

The second technique used in drafting CNS fetal tissue to the denervated HF involves the implantation of a dissociated cell suspension (Schmidt et al., 1981; Björklund et al., 1983c). In this technique pieces of fetal CNS tissue are trypsinized and mechanically dissociated into a milky cell suspension. Small volumes of the suspension can then be stereotaxically injected into the desired site of the HPC, using a microsyringe. The main advantage of this technique is that it allows precise and multiple placements of the cells. The technique also makes possible accurate monitoring of the number of cells injected by counting the density of cells in the suspension. For the remainder of this chapter the first technique will be referred to as the "solid graft" technique and the second technique will be referred to as the "cell suspension" technique.

GRAFT STRATEGIES

Three separate grafting strategies have used the denervated HF as a target tissue. The first strategy, that of "reafferentation," uses fetal cells from brain regions that normally send axons to the hippocampus, but that have been transected by the lesion. This strategy permits the evaluation of the extent to which donor tissue can grow axons into the host brain and accurately reestablish a new terminal network in the host hippocampus. The second strategy, that of "bridging," uses pieces of tissue placed in the cavity made by the fimbria-fornix lesion to promote regeneration of the septohippocampal pathway by serving as a bridge between the denervated axons passing through the septal area to the HPC. The third strategy is to use the transplantation cavities as culture beds or "in vivo explants" to investigate graft growth and development without special reference to its connectivity to the HPC. The results from each of these strategies will be briefly reviewed, summarizing data from solid grafts as well as cell suspensions.

Reafferentation

The aims of this approach are to test to what extent, and with what degree of precision, neuron transplants are able to re-establish normal terminal innervation patterns in the previously denervated HPC. In the studies reviewed below, solid grafts were obtained from 16- to 17-day-old rat fetuses, while cell suspensions were taken from 13- to 15-day-old rat fetuses. The fetal donor brain regions used were 1) the septal-diagonal band area, containing developing cholinergic neurons that normally innervate the HF and neocortex; 2) the locus coeruleus region of the pons, containing the cells of origin for the noradrenergic innervation of the HF; and 3) the pontine and mesencephalic raphe region, containing serotonergic cells that also innervate the HF.

The fetal septal-diagonal band area has been transplanted both as solid grafts (Björklund and Stenevi, 1977; Björklund et al., 1983b) and as cell suspensions (Schmidt et al., 1981; Dunnett et al., 1982; Björklund et al., 1983a,b) to the HPC in rats that had received prior fimbria-fornix lesions. They gave rise to a pattern of innervation in the HF that closely mimicked the normal cholinergic innervation (as assessed by acetylcholinesterase [AChE] staining) (see Fig. 1A,B). Several features of this reinnervation attest to its specificity. Specifically, suspension grafts approximately double their volume in the denervated hippocampus, and individual cholinergic neurons in the grafts grow to the approximate size of adult cholinergic neurons within several months after grafting. In addition, about 60% of the cholinergic neurons initially grafted will ultimately survive. All of these measures of growth are dependent on prior or simultaneous fimbria-fornix transection. Grafting into the intact hippocampus is much less supportive of graft growth and survival (Gage and Björklund, 1986). Several features of this reinnervation attest to its specificity. First, when ingrowing axons are given a choice between different denervated terminal fields, they show a clear preference for the zones denervated of the homologous fiber type. For example, septal solid grafts or cell suspensions implanted in the hippocampal formation after fimbria-fornix lesions extend cholinergic axons from the graft restrictively to the normal cholinergic terminal fields, even though the lesion denervates the extensive system of noncholinergic commissural afferents (see Fig. 1C). Zones receiving dense commissural (but sparse septal) innervation, such as the striatum layer, are largely devoid of fibers from the transplant. In addition, Clarke et al. (1986) have demonstrated that septal grafts make synaptic contacts on granular cells (the normal target cells) in the dentate gyrus of a denervated host hippocampus. The specificity of these contacts is not exact, for the normal cholinergic neurons synapse predominantly on the dendrites and spines of the granular cells, while the grafted cholinergic neurons synapse also on the somata of the granular cells. The reason for this inappropriate synaptic connectivity is not known. A third example of this specificity of growth of the cholinergic grafts is provided by taking advantage of the fact that, after perforant pathway lesion, the intrinsic septal afferents will sprout selectively into the outer molecular layer of the dentate gyrus. By lesioning both the perforant pathway and the fimbria-fornix, and then transplanting either solid septal grafts (Björklund et al., 1979a) or septal cell suspensions, one observes that the grafts innervate not only the normal terminal fields but also the outer molecular layer of the dentate gyrus. Thus, the fiber outgrowth from septal cholinergic grafts illustrates a remarkable selectivity, and yet the same plasticity as the intrinsic septal afferents.

The locus coeruleus solid grafts appear to re-establish a "coeruleohippocampal" noradrenergic pathway in animals initially denervated of their hippocampal noradrenaline input by a 6-hydroxydopamine lesion (Björklund et al., 1976, 1979b, 1986). Up to 330 surviving noradrenaline neurons were found at each implantation site (injected with 2–3 μl of cell suspension), which represents an estimated survival rate of about 40%. In the most successful cases the entire dorsal hippocampal formation was supplied with a new noradrenaline-containing network that reaches normal densities in regions closest to the grafts. The ingrowing axons re-established a laminar innervation pattern that resembled that of the normal locus coeruleus afferents. In the hippocampus, two 2-μl injections of locus coeruleus cell suspension restored the total hippocampal noradrenaline content to an average of 55%, and the noradrenaline

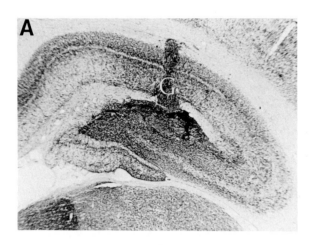

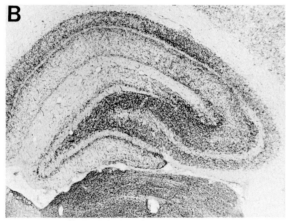

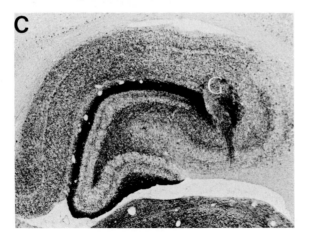

synthesis rate (as assessed by the rate of DOPA accumulation after synthesis inhibition) was found to be close to normal in the graft-reinnervated specimens (Björklund et al., 1986).

The selectivity of the patterning of the ingrowing noradrenergic fibers is emphasized by the dense innervation of the hilar zone of the dentate gyrus, the area most densely innervated by the intrinsic noradrenergic fibers. However, other regions of the HF that are also denervated by the fimbria-fornix lesion are not densely innervated by locus coeruleus (LC) grafts.

To evaluate serotoninergic graft survival and growth in the hippocampus, suspensions of cells were taken from the mesencephalic raphe regions, injected into the hippocampus of adult rats previously denervated of its serotoninergic input by 5,7-dihydroxytryptamine, and processed at periods of up to 14 months after implantation, for 5-hydroxytryptamine (5-HT) (Foster et al., 1986). Surviving grafts were found in all animals. The implants contained neurons immunoreactive to 5-HT, substance P (SP), and to both substances together. On average, 19% of the potential number of mesencephalic 5-HT neurons were found in the grafts. Outgrowth of 5-HT-immunoreactive fibers was extensive and displayed the typical pattern of 5-HT innervation in the normal hippocampus; the densest plexuses were found in the dentate gyrus, with sparser networks in the CA1 and CA2 regions. From a morphological perspective the reafferentation strategy has thus demonstrated the capacity of grafted monoaminergic and cholinergic brain stem or basal forebrain neurons to reestablish innervation patterns in the previously denervated HPC, leading to selective terminal patterns and synaptic contacts with the host target neurons.

Bridge

Grafted peripheral tissues have been used as bridges to promote axonal regeneration across damaged tissue or tissue defects in the nervous system (Tello, 1911; Svendgaard et al., 1975; Aguayo et al., 1982). The specific issue being addressed in the bridge strategy as it relates to the denervated HPC is to determine to what extent a fetal hippocampal implant can replace the normal hippocampus as a target for the formation of connections with the host septum and to what extent the same implant can promote a regeneration of the septohippocampal pathway and serve as a bridge for the regeneration of the axons from the damaged septal afferents to the HPC. Previous research showed that

---

Fig. 1. Photomicrographs of acetylcholinesterase (AChE)-positive sections through the dorsal hippocampus. **A:** Suspension graft of fetal basal forebrain injected into the hippocampus 6 weeks earlier. This animal received a fimbria-fornix lesion at the time of grafting; thus all the innervation observed is derived from the graft. **B:** Same animal as in A, but from a section rostral to the graft. Note the innervation distinct laminated pattern within the hippocampus. **C:** Suspension of fetal basal forebrain injected into the hippocampus 3 months earlier. This animal received a fimbria-fornix lesion and a perforant pathway lesion at the time of grafting. Note the intense AChE staining derived from the graft in the outer molecular layer of the dentate gyrus, characteristic of the sprouting of the intrinsic cholinergic septal fibers following perforant pathway transection. G, graft. × 120.

implants of denervated iris to the fimbria-fornix could stimulate the cholinergic septal neurons of the host to reinnervate large portions of the denervated iris in a homotypic manner (Svendgaard et al., 1976). With the same paradigm, but using fetal hippocampal tissue as a bridge between septum and hippocampus (Kromer et al., 1981a,b; Buzsáki et al., 1987a,b), AChE-positive fibers from the septal region were seen to innervate the entire implant with time. Parallel biochemical studies revealed a dramatic increase in choline acetyltransferase (ChAT) activity in the implant. In addition, by 4 to 6 weeks after transplantation, new AChE-positive fibers appeared in parts of the subiculum, hippocampus, and dentate gyrus, immediately bordering the implant, and at later time periods new fibers from the graft had expanded 2.5 to 3.5 mm into the dorsal HPC. Again these histochemical observations were confirmed by measuring a recovery of up to about 50% of control in ChAT levels in the dorsal HF.

Lesions of the septum-diagonal band area in the regenerated grafted animals and horseradish peroxidase (HRP) injections into the host HPC caudal to the hippocampal bridge graft showed that the origin of the regenerated cholinergic axons was predominantly the ipsilateral ventral medial septum and diagonal band area. These results suggest that a piece of fetal CNS tissue (Kromer et al., 1981a,b; Buzsáki et al., 1987a,b), in addition to mature peripheral tissue (Svendgaard et al., 1975, 1976), can promote regeneration of axotomized central neurons both into the implant tissue and through the implant tissue to innervate the denervated host tissue in a homotypic manner.

To better understand the mechanisms and molecules that are necessary and sufficient for regeneration, or bridging in the CNS, human amnion membrane matrix (HAMM) was used as a substratum for the cholinergic axonal growth in the fimbria-fornix (FF) cavity. Davis et al. (1987) had shown that HAMM contained a dense laminin layer on the basement surface of the membrane that could induce axonal growth in vitro. To test the in vivo properties of the HAMM, we transplanted this tissue-attached nitrocellulose paper to the FF cavity in the same way we transplanted fetal hippocampal tissue above (Gage et al., 1988).

AChE-positive fibers grew out from the septum onto the HAMM by 2 weeks, and by 8 weeks more extensive growth was observed on the HAMM (see Fig. 2 A,B,C). By 8 weeks AChE fibers could be clearly seen coming off the membrane and entering the host hippocampus (see Fig. 2D). By double labeling for the basement membrane side of the HAMM (using antihuman laminin antibodies) and for cholinergic fibers (using AChE histochemistry) in the same sections, it was possible to see fibers clearly growing on the laminin-positive side of the HAMM, but little or no growth on the opposing laminin-negative stromal side. The HAMM represents a useful, regeneration-promoting grafting material for central nervous system "bridging" studies. This type of bridge falls into the category of *passive* rather than *active* bridge exemplified by the fetal hippocampal tissue, since the HAMM contributes no cell connectivity itself.

In Vivo Explant

The objective of this strategy is to utilize the richly vascularized pial surface provided by the hipppocampal transplantation cavities to address develop-

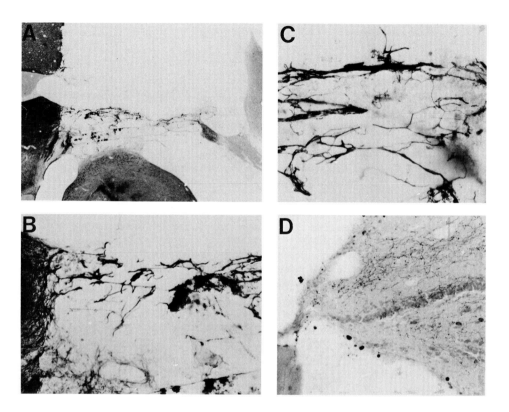

Fig. 2. Photomicrographs of acetylcholinesterase (AChE)-positive staining in sagittal sections through a rat forebrain 12 weeks following implantation of human amnionic membrane (HAMM) attached to nitrocellulose paper in a fimbria-fornix cavity between the septum on the left and the hippocampus on the right. **A:** Low-power magnification showing AChE fibers coursing from the denervated septum to the hippocampus. ×44. **B:** Higher power magnification showing the AChE fiber emerging from the septum onto the HAMM. ×220. **C:** Same magnification as in B showing AChE fibers on the HAMM. ×220. **D:** AChE fiber entering the denervated hippocampus.

mental questions, similar to what has previously been done in in vitro explant or reaggregation cultures and with the intraocular grafting technique. The intracerebral grafting technique should therefore provide a useful tool for obtaining additional information concerning the cellular events that determine the organization of the developing CNS. This approach is also reviewed in this volume by Zimmer et al. (Chapter 17).

An additional application of the in vivo explant strategy is one that uses the denervated HF as a system that may release neurotrophic factors upon damage. Thus, by transplanting different cell types that may or may not have a dependency on neurotrophic factors, survival of grafted cells can be assessed as a quantitative in vivo bioassay of the alleged factors. Experiments with grafts of adult and neonatal sympathetic ganglia have already provided some evidence for such denervation-dependent neurotrophic effects (Björklund and Stenevi, 1979a; Gage et al., 1984a,b).

Additionally, the trophic effects of denervation on the survival of fetal cholinergic neuronal cell suspensions grafted to the hippocampal formation of the rat have been assessed (Gage and Björklund, 1986). Young adult female rats were injected with cell suspensions of neurons obtained from the fetal basal forebrain region into the hippocampal formation simultaneously with (or without) a fimbria-fornix transection. Four to 6 months later, one group of grafted animals was evaluated histochemically for 1) transplant volume, 2) number of AChE-positive cells, and 3) size of AChE-positive cells in the graft. A parallel study was conducted to determine the total number and size of the AChE-positive cells in the septal-diagonal band–substantia innominata complex of the adult rat, to match with the cell survival and growth in the grafts. A second group of grafted rats was taken in parallel for biochemical analysis of ChAT activity in the grafted hippocampus. The transplant volume in the rats with fimbria-fornix transection was greater than twice the volume seen in animals without fimbria-fornix lesion (see Fig. 3). In addition, the number of AChE-positive cells in the transplant was twice as great in the denervated animals as in the nondenervated ones. However, the number of AChE-positive cells per mm^3 of graft volume did not differ between the two groups, suggesting that the trophic effect of the denervation was not specific for the cholinergic neurons, but affected the entire grafted tissue. The hippocampal ChAT activity of the animals that received the fimbria-fornix lesion simultaneously with transplantation was about three times higher than that of the rats that received grafts but no simultaneous fimbria-fornix transection. A control experiment with animals that received an aspirative lesion of the retrosplenial cortex, transecting the perforant pathway input, revealed no enhancing effect of hippocampal ChAT activity over nonlesioned grafted animals. Thus, the denervation-enhancing effects of the fimbria-fornix lesion appear to be selective and not the result of a general wound-induced mechanism.

These results strongly support the contention that neurotrophic factors are released as a result of denervation in the adult hippocampal formation and that these neurotrophic factors can support survival and growth of central cholinergic neurons. However, the factors involved do not appear to be specific for the cholinergic neurons, but rather have their trophic effects on many types of cells.

GRAFT FUNCTION

The survival and growth of solid grafts and cell suspensions in the denervated HPC have thus been well characterized for several different neuronal cell types, and intrahippocampal grafting has received interesting applications to the understanding of neural plasticity and development in the HPC. However, methods different from those required to assess survival and growth are needed to determine whether the grafted cells can function in their new environment. In

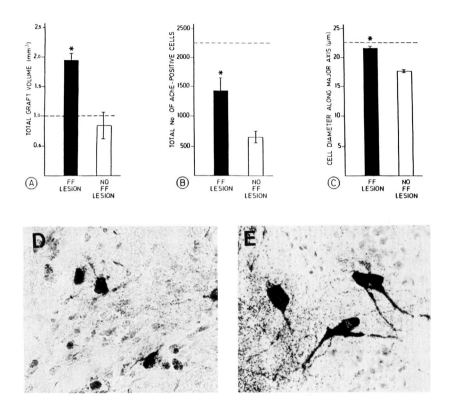

Fig. 3. **A:** Total graft volume from animals with or without fimbria-fornix (FF) lesion, expressed in mm³, relative to the estimated volume of tissue injected. **B:** Total number of AChE-positive cells in transplants of diisopropylfluorophosphate (DFP)-treated rats with or without FF lesion, expressed relative to the estimated total number of potential AChE-positive cells grafted. **C:** Cell diameter of AChE-positive cells along their major axis in suspension grafts from DFP-treated animals with or without FF lesions, expressed in μm relative to the mean size of AChE-positive neurons in the normal septal-diagonal band complex in situ. Means ± S.E.M. of values from six to eight rats in each group. Two independent observers measured the cell sizes of a total of 60 cells from randomly selected sections from four rats in each group. Asterisks indicate significant differences between FF lesioned and non-FF lesioned animals. Dotted lines indicate estimated baseline values. The top two panels are photomicrographs of AChE-positive cells from a fetal basal forebrain graft implanted 4 months earlier in a rat treated with DFP at the time of sacrifice. **D:** Intact hippocampus. **E:** Denervated hippocampus. The magnification is the same for both photographs.

addition, "function" itself can be assessed at several different levels, each of which provides important information about the quality and quantity of information that is communicated between the graft and the host tissue. At present three general types of functional procedures have been applied to this issue: 1) biochemical, 2) behavioral, and 3) electrophysiological. Each of these will be discussed separately.

Biochemical Measures

The biochemical activity of the cholinergic innervation of the denervated HF, derived from solid or suspension grafts of the septal-diagonal band area, has been studied fairly extensively. Graft-derived ChAT activity was barely detectable 10 days after cell suspension grafts, but sharply increased between 10 days and 1 month in the HF regions close to the graft. By 6 months, ChAT activity was restored to near normal levels in all segments of the previously denervated HF. When comparing the total amount of ChAT activity derived from the solid grafts and the cell suspension grafts, the cell suspension grafts appeared to be about twice as effective as the solid grafts, although the amount of tissue grafted was about the same in each case.

The functional activity of the cell suspension grafts was further assessed by measurements of $[^{14}C]$acetylcholine synthesis from $[^{14}C]$glucose in vitro. The overall hippocampal $[^{14}C]$acetylcholine synthesis was restored to normal levels in the grafted animals, and estimates of the acetylcholine turnover rate suggested that the transmitter machinery of the newly established septohippocampal connections operated at a rate similar to that of the intrinsic septohippocampal pathway. Thus, these septal cell suspensions seem capable of maintaining function at a relatively "physiological" level despite their abnormal position.

Kelly et al. (1985) investigated the magnitude of lesion-induced alterations in the HF as reflected in the local rates of $[^{14}C]$2-deoxy-glucose (2-DG) utilization, and the degree to which the index of functional activity could be normalized following reinnervation by solid septal grafts. Six months after unilateral fimbria-fornix lesion the 2-DG utilization was markedly reduced in the HF of the nongrafted aminals. Rats that received the solid grafts displayed a significant increase in 2-DG use as compared with the rats with lesion alone. In addition, the changes in 2-DG utilization were significantly correlated with the density of AChE staining in adjacent sections from the same brains, thus suggesting a relationship between the cholinergic innervation from the septal grafts and the restoration of functional glucose utilization. Though it is difficult to generalize beyond the septal grafts in the denervated hippocampus to other transmitter systems, these results at least strongly suggest that the cholinergic component of the grafts is functioning at the biochemical level and influencing, or normalizing, the function of the deafferented HPC.

Behavioral Studies

Bilateral fimbria-fornix lesions in rats are known to result in severe impairments in working memory (Olton et al., 1978) or spatial memory (O'Keefe and Nadel, 1978). In addition, the same types of impairments can be obtained by pharmacological blockade of cholinergic transmission in a variety of tests (Sutherland et al., 1982; Eckerman et al., 1980). Using several standard behavioral tests of learning and memory, researchers have demonstrated the ability of the fetal septal grafts to reverse these impairments. In the eight-arm radial maze (Low et al., 1982) rats with septal grafts showed a positive linear trend in maze performance over days of testing, but did not differ significantly from nongrafted rats with lesions overall. However, potentiation of the cholinergic transmission by pretreatment with physostigmine produced a significant enhancement of maze performance in the grafted group, but not in the lesioned control group, and in some cases the grafted rats performed as well as the nonlesioned control animals. In another study (Dunnett et al., 1982) using a T-maze forced-choice alternation test, seven of nine rats with solid septal grafts and four of five rats with septal cell suspensions learned the task, some of them up to the level of the control rats. The remaining rats with septal grafts, and a separate group of rats with locus coeruleus grafts, performed at chance level, similar to the rats that only received the fimbria-fornix lesion. In this study there was a positive and significant correlation between performance of the grafted rats and the amount of graft-derived AChE-positive staining in the previously denervated HF. In a more recent study (Nilsson et al., 1987) septal cell suspension grafts, implanted into the hippocampal formation in rats with bilateral fimbria-fornix lesions, were found to improve spatial learning also in the Morris (1984) water maze task. This was seen both in rats that had been pretrained in the task prior to lesion and grafting and in rats that had not been exposed to the water maze prior to lesion and transplantation. In the pretrained rats, the bilateral fimbria-fornix lesion completely abolished the acquired performance, and while the lesioned rats could partially solve the task using nonspatial strategies, most of the septal grafted rats were able to show evidence of learning the location of the platform. Interestingly, atropine (50 mg/kg) completely abolished the reacquired spatial learning in the grafted animals. This atropine effect was seen also in the normal control rats, but to a lesser extent. Together these studies strongly suggest not only that the grafts can partially ameliorate deficits in spatial learning that result from fimbria-fornix lesions but also that the amelioration shows some specificity for the septal grafts that provide a cholinergic reinnervation of the deafferented hippocampal formation.

Electrophysiological Studies

In an attempt to reveal the physiological mechanisms for the behavioral improvements observed in bilaterally lesioned and grafted animals, we investigated the electrophysiological activity of the deafferented host hippocampus of freely moving animals after transplanting fetal tissue into the lesion cavity or directly into the host hippocampus. The most striking reparative change we observed was the reappearance of hippocampal rhythm in slow wave activity, or theta (RSA) with septal and hippocampal bridges (Buzsáki et al., 1987a,b) (see Fig. 4). Concurrent with RSA, granule cells and interneurons fired rhythmically, phase-locked to RSA. Cross-correlation of EEG from the transplanted and intact sides revealed that RSA in both hippocampi was in-

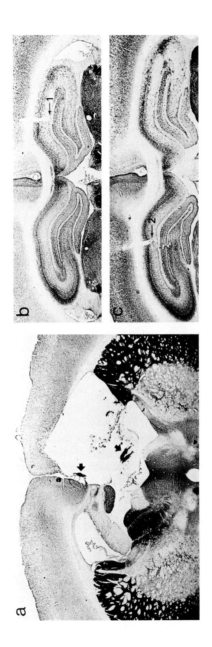

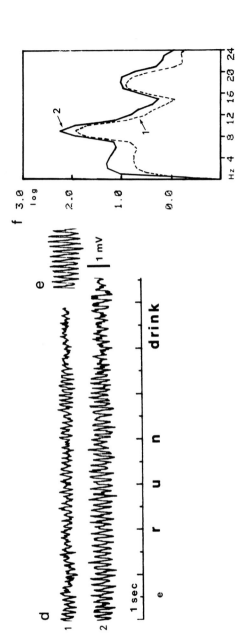

Fig. 4. Restoration of hippocampal theta activity by solid septal grafts. **a–c:** AChE-staining. **a:** Transection of the right fimbria-fornix. Arrows indicate darkly stained AChE-positive fetal septal bridge 8 months after transplantation. b,c: AChE-stained sections of the host hippocampus at the level of the recording electrodes (1,2). **d:** EEG activity recorded during running and drinking. Note the similar waveforms on the reafferented (1) and intact (2) sides. **e:** Sample of EEG during running recorded from an identical location as 1 in an intact rat. **f:** Power spectra of EEG recorded from the reafferented (1) and intact (2) hemispheres.

phase, suggesting that both hippocampi were modulated by the same "pacemaker" group of neurons. Similiar to normal rats, RSA was present only during running and walking and was absent during behavioral immobility and drinking. The depth profile and the septotemporal distribution of the power of RSA correlated with the density and distribution of the graft-mediated AChE-positive reinnervation of the host hippocampus. Considerably better restoration was found with solid septal than with solid hippocampal graft bridges. Suspension grafts of fetal septal or locus coeruleus cells did not restore behavior-dependent RSA in the host hippocampus.

The findings that RSA recorded from the intact and reinnervated hippocampi was highly coherent, and temporally related, and that septal cells injected directly into the host hippocampus did not produce behavior-dependent RSA led us to hypothesize that axons of the host septal neurons grew back across the fetal tissue bridge and contacted their normal target cells. According to this passive bridge model the graft tissue merely served as a scaffold to induce and guide regeneration of the severed septohippocampal connections.

Following fimbria-fornix transection, 60 to 80% of the cells in the medial septum and diagonal band of Broca undergo degeneration (Gage et al., 1986). Consequently, we assumed that the few remaining septal cholinergic cells were sufficient for maintaining a pacemaker rhythmicity, and through their regrown axon terminals they were able to modulate the synaptic membranes of a sufficient number of hippocampal neurons to result in rhythmic extracellular current flow.

In all of the "bridging" experiments above, restoration of normal or near-normal electrophysiological patterns was observed only in the anterior part of the hippocampal formation. The remaining part displayed electrical patterns similar to those observed in rats with lesion only. Also, peripheral administration of the cholinergic blocker scopolamine completely abolished the graft-mediated RSA (Buzsáki et al., 1987a). In the behaving rat, scopolamine cannot eliminate all theta activity from the intact hippocampus (Vanderwolf and Baker, 1986).

In a separate series of experiments we investigated the ability of grafted cells to modulate the excitability of the deafferented hippocampus (Buzsáki et al., 1988, 1989). In rats with bilateral fimbria-fornix lesion and suspension grafts of locus coeruleus neurons, the incidence of epileptic spikes was much lower than in the lesion-only group. In addition, locus coeruleus grafts virtually eliminated the picrotoxin (1 mg/kg)-induced behavioral seizures. In contrast, in animals with suspension grafts of hippocampal cells, the frequency of epileptic interictal transients was several times higher than in the control group. In 50% of the animals with hippocampal grafts, spontaneous EEG and/or behavioral grand mal seizures were observed (Buzsáki et al., 1988). These findings are in agreement with independent observations that locus coeruleus grafts may delay the onset of behavioral seizures in a kindling model of epilepsy (Barry et al., 1987).

POSSIBLE MECHANISM OF GRAFT ACTION

Neuronal replacement by intracerebral implants in brain-damaged young rats is a striking example of how the brain can allow new elements to be inserted and linked into its own functional subsystems. Obviously there must be definite limitations as to which types of neurons or functional subsystems can successfully be manipulated in this way. Neuronal implants would seem most likely to have behaviorally meaningful functional effects with types of neurons that normally do not convey, or link, specific pattern messages, e.g. in sensory or motor input and output systems. Indeed functional recovery using the reafferentation strategy has so far been demonstrated primarily for neurons of the types that normally appear to act as tonic regulatory or level-setting systems. The basal forebrain cholinergic neurons and the ascending aminergic neurons are commonly conceived of as modulatory or level-setting systems that tonically regulate the activity of the hippocampal neuronal machinery. Functional recovery observed after reinstatement of impaired cholinergic transmission by implants can thus be interpreted as a reactivation or inhibition of otherwise intact neuronal circuits. This view is complicated, however, by recent observations and conclusions summarized below.

The major input to the hippocampus arrives from the entorhinal cortex. In the absence of the subcortical direct or feed-forward inhibition, the afferent neuronal template from the entorhinal input is amplified within the trisynaptic circuitry, and the unprocessed signal pattern is fed back to the entorhinal cortex via the subiculum (Buzsáki, 1986; Buzsáki et al., 1983). The returned and magnified afferent template may interfere with the activity of the entorhinal cortex as well. This mechanism may explain why sectioning of the fimbria-fornix is more devastating to behavior than selective removal of 90% of the neurons from the hippocampus by ibotenic acid lesion (Jarrard, 1986).

Viewed from this perspective, grafts restoring the subcortical control of the hippocampus appear ideal for behavioral recovery. Thus, the nearly perfect reappearance of the electrical activity of the host hippocampus in some animals with solid grafts could be taken to indicate that the "bridging" technique may be more efficient than suspension grafts in attempts to restore behavioral deficits. Indeed, behavioral deficits in different types of spatial tasks in fimbria-fornix-damaged rats were significantly improved by solid septal grafts placed into the lesion cavity, although subcortical afferents were not restored in these animals, and the electrophysiological consequences of septal graft bridges and suspension injections, as shown above, are very different.

It should be emphasized, however, that reinnervation and restoration of RSA from graft bridges were restricted to the septal pole of the host hippocampus. Thus, even if normal function reappeared completely in the anterior part of the host hippocampus, the physiological activity of the major portion of the structure remained similar to fimbria-fornix-lesioned animals.

On the other hand, in rats with suspension grafts of septal tissue at two or three levels along the septotemporal axis of the hippocampus, subcortical control is not re-established, but reinnervation of the host hippocampus by AChE-positive fibers is nearly complete (Dunnett et al., 1982; Nilsson et al., 1987; Björklund et al., 1983a,c; Gage et al., 1984b; Gage and Björklund, 1986). It is possible that the nonregulated cholinergic and/or GABAergic cells of the graft suppressed the deleterious amplifying action of the host hippocampus.

An additional cause of the behavioral deficit seen in fimbria-fornix animals may be the lack of synaptic plasticity in the deafferented hippocampus. Indeed, in a recent series of experiments we consistently failed to produce long-term potentiation in the dentate gyrus by high-frequency activation of the perforant pathway input (Buzsáki and Gage, 1989). Long-term potentiation is thought to represent a laboratory model for memory trace formation (McNaughton and Morris, 1987; Goddard, 1980). Based on these findings, we hypothesize that suspension grafts placed directly into the hippocampus may restore the impaired synaptic plasticity and thereby may facilitate behavioral recovery.

Our electrophysiological analyses, as summarized above, suggest that behavioral improvement may be obtained by merely suppressing the pathological electrical patterns of the denervated hippocampus that may interfere with the normal activity of its target structures. This mechanism of behavioral improvement would thus not necessarily reflect real restoration, but rather suppression of abnormal activity. The graft may work as a regulated short circuit that may reduce damage-induced "noise-producing" neuronal circuits. It remains an exciting challenge for future transplantation experiments to produce more extensive behavioral recovery by more complete and normal brain reconstruction.

ACKNOWLEDGMENTS

We thank Sheryl Christenson for her assistance in typing and editing the manuscript. The research presented in this chapter was supported by NIH AGO6088, NIH AGO5344, the J.D. French Foundation, The Sandoz Foundation, The Herbert Hoover Foundation, and the Office of Naval Research.

REFERENCES

Aguayo, A., P.M. Richardson, S. David, and M. Benfrey (1982) Transplantation of neurons and sheath cells—A tool for the study of regeneration. In: J.G. Nicholls (ed): Repair and Regeneration of the Nervous System. New York: Springer-Verlag, pp. 91–105.

Barry, D.I., I. Kikvadze, P. Brundin, T.G. Bolwig, A. Björklund, and O. Lindvall (1987) Grafted noradrenergic neurons suppress seizure development in kindling-induced epilepsy. Proc. Natl. Acad. Sci. U.S.A. *84*:8712–8715.

Björklund, A., F.H. Gage, R.H. Schmidt, Y. Stenevi, and S.B. Dunnett (1983a) Intracerebral grafting of neuronal cell suspensions. VII. Recovery of choline acetyltransferase activity and acetylcholine synthesis in the denervated hippocampus reinnervated by septal suspension implants. Acta Scand. Physiol. [Suppl.] *522*:59–66.

Björklund, A., F.H. Gage, U. Stenevi, and S.B. Dunnett (1983b) Intracerebral grafting of neuronal cell suspensions. VI. Survival and growth of intrahippocampal implants of septal cell suspensions. Acta Physiol. Scand. [Suppl.] *522*:49–58.

Björklund, A., L.F. Kromer, and U. Stenevi (1979a) Cholinergic reinnervation of the rat hippocampus by septal implants is stimulated by perforant path lesion. Brain Res. *173*:57–64.

Björklund, A., H. Nornes, and F.H. Gage (1986) Cell suspension grafts of noradrenergic locus coeruleus neurons in rat hippocampus and spinal cord: Reinnervation and transmitter turnover. Neuroscience *18:(3)*685–698.

Björklund, A., M. Segal, and U. Stenevi (1979b) Functional reinnervation of rat hippocampus by locus coeruleus implants. Brain Res. *170:*409–426.

Björklund, A., and U. Stenevi (1977) Reformation of the severed septohippocampal cholinergic pathway in the adult rat by transplanted septal neurons. Cell Tissue Res. *185*:289–302.

Björklund, A., U. Stenevi, R.H. Schmidt, S.B. Dunnett, and F.H. Gage (1983c) Intracerebral grafting of neuronal cell suspensions. I. Introduction and general methods of preparation. Acta Physiol. Scand. [Suppl.] *522:*1–10.

Björklund, A., Y. Stenevi, and N.-A. Svendgaard (1976) Growth of transplanted monoaminergic neurones into the adult hippocampus along the perforant path. Nature *262:*787–790.

Buzsáki, G. (1986) Hippocampal sharp-waves: Their origin and significance. Brain Res. *398*:242–252.

Buzsáki, G., R.G. Bickford, S. Varon, D.M. Armstrong, and F.H. Gage (1987a) Reconstruction of the damaged septohippocampal circuitry by combination of fetal grafts and transient NGF infusion. Soc. Neurosci. Abstr. (13:681).

Buzsáki, G., and F.H. Gage (1989) Absence of long-term potentiation in the subcortically deafferented dentate gyrus. Brain Res. (in press).

Buzsáki, G., F.H. Gage, J. Czopf, et al. (1987b) Restoration of rhythmic slow activity in the subcortically denervated hippocampus by fetal CNS transplants. Brain Res. *400:*334–347.

Buzsáki, G., F.H. Gage, L. Kellenyi, and A. Björklund (1987c) Behavioral dependence of the electrical activity of intracerebrally transplanted fetal hippocampus. Brain Res *400:*321–333.

Buzsáki, G., L.S. Leung, and C.H. Vanderwolf (1983) Cellular basis of hippocampal EEG in the behaving rat. Brain Res. Rev. *6:*139–171.

Buzsáki, G., G.L. Ponomareff, F. Bayardo, et al. (1989) Neuronal activity in the subcortically denervated hippocampus: A chronic model for epilepsy. Neuroscience (in press).

Buzsáki, G., G. Ponamareff, F. Bayardo, T. Shaw, and F.H. Gage (1988) Suppression and induction of epileptic activity by neuronal grafts. Proc. Natl. Acad. Sci. USA *85:*9327–9330.

Clarke, D.J., F.H. Gage, O.G. Nilsson, and A. Björklund (1986) Grafted septal neurons from cholinergic synaptic connections in the dentate gyrus of behaviorally impaired aged rats. J. Comp. Neurol. *252:*483–492.

Davis, G.E., S.N. Blaker, E. Engvall, S. Varon, M. Manthorpe and F.H. Gage (1987) Human amnion membrane serves as a substratum for growing axons in vitro and in vivo. Science *236:*1106–1109.

Dunnett, S.B., W.C. Low, S.D. Iversen, Y. Stenevi, and A. Björklund (1982) Septal transplants restore maze learning in rats with fimbria-fornix lesions. Brain Res. *251:*335–348.

Eckerman, D.A., W.A. Gordon, J.D. Edwards R.C. MacPhail, and M.I. Gage (1980) Effects of scopolamine, pentobarbital and amphetamine on radial arm maze performance in the rat. Pharmacol. Biochem. Behav. *12:*595–602.

Foster, G.A., M. Schultzberg, F.H. Gage, A. Björklund, T. Hökfelt, A.C. Cuello, A.A.J. Verhofstad, and T.J. Visser (1986) Transmitter expression and morphological development of embryonic medullary and mesencephalic raphe neurones after transplantation to the adult rat central nervous system. II. Grafts to the hippocampus. Exp. Brain Res. 24:77–84.

Gage, F.H., and A. Björklund (1986) Enhanced graft survival in the hippocampus following selective denervation. Neuroscience 17(1):89–98.

Gage, F.H., A. Björklund, U. Stenevi, et al. (1984a) Intrahippocampal septal grafts ameliorate learning impairments in aged rats. Science 225:533–536.

Gage, F.H., A. Björklund, and U. Stenevi (1984b) A neuronal survival factor in the adult hippocampal formation is released by denervation. Nature 308:637–639.

Gage, F.H., S.N. Blaker, G.E. Davis, E. Engvall, S. Varon, and M. Manthorpe (1988) Human amnion membrane matrix as a substratum for axonal regeneration in the central nervous system. Exp. Brain Res. 72:321–380.

Gage, F.H., K. Wictorin, W. Fisher, L.R. Williams, S. Varon, and A. Björklund (1986) Retrograde cell changes in medial septum and diagonal band following fimbria-fornix transection: Quantitative temporal analysis. Neuroscience 19:241–255.

Goddard, G.V. (1980) Component properties of memory machines: Hebb revisited. In P.W. Jusczyk and R.M. Klein (eds): The Nature of Thought: Essays in Honour of D.O. Hebb. Hillsdale, N.J.: Lawrence Erlbaum.

Jarrard, L. (1986) Selective hippocampal lesions and behavior: Implications for current research and theorizing. In: R.S. Isaacson and K.M. Pribram (eds): The Hippocampus. New York: Plenum.

Kelly, P.A.T., F.H. Gage, M. Ingvar, O. Lindvall, U. Stenevi, and A. Björklund (1985) Functional reactivation of the deafferented hippocampus by embryonic septal grafts as assessed by measurements of local glucose utilization. Exp. Brain Res. 58:570–579.

Kromer, L.F., A. Björklund, and U. Stenevi, (1981a) Innervation of embryonic hippocampal implants by regenerating axons of cholinergic septal neurons in the adult rat. Brain Res. 210:153–171.

Kromer, L.F., A. Björklund, and U. Stenevi, (1981b) Regeneration of the septohippocampal pathway in adult rats is promoted by utilizing embryonic hippocampal implants as bridges. Brain Res 210:173–200.

Low, W.C., P.R. Lewis, S.T. Brunch, S.B. Dunnett, S.R. Thomas, S.D. Iversen, A. Björklund, and U. Stenevi (1982) Functional recovery following neural transplantation of embryonic septal nuclei in adult rats with septohippocampal lesions. Nature 300:260–262.

McNaughton, B.L., and R.G.M. Morris (1987) Hippocampal synaptic enhancement and information storage within a distributed memory system. Trends Neurosci. 10:408–415.

Morris, R. (1984) Development of a water-maze procedure for studying learning in the rat. J. Neurosci. Methods 11:47–60.

Nilsson, O.B., M.L. Shapiro, F.H. Gage, D.S. Olton, and A. Björklund (1987) Spatial learning and memory following fimbria-fornix transection and grafting of fetal septal neurons to the hippocampus. Exp. Brain Res. 67:195–215.

O'Keefe, J., and L. Nadel (1978) The Hippocampus as a Cognitive Map. Oxford: Clarenden Press.

Olton, D.S., J.A. Walker, and F.H. Gage (1978) Hippocampal connections and spatial discriminations. Brain Res. 139:295–308.

Schmidt, R.H., A. Björklund, and U. Stenevi (1981) Intracerebral grafting of dissociated CNS tissue suspensions: A new approach for neuronal transplantation to deep brain sites. Brain Res. 218:347–356.

Stenevi, U., A. Björklund, and N.-A. Svendgaard (1976) Transplantation of central and peripheral monoamine neurons to the adult rat brain: Techniques and conditions for survival. Brain Res. *114:*1–20.

Sutherland, R.J., I.Q. Whishaw, and J.C. Regeher (1982) Cholinergic receptor blockade impairs spatial localization using distal cues in the rat. J. Comp. Physiol. Psychol. *96:*563–573.

Svendgaard, N.A., A. Björklund, and U. Stenevi (1975) Regenerative properties of central monoamine neurons as revealed in studies using iris transplants as targets. Adv. Anat. Embryol. Cell Biol. *51:*1–77.

Svendgaard, N.A., A. Björklund, and U. Stenevi (1976) Regeneration of central cholinergic neurons in the adult rat brain. Brain Res. *102:*1–22.

Tello, F. (1911) La influencia del neurotropismo en la regeneracion de los centros nerviosos. Trab Lab Invest. Biol *9:*123–159.

Vanderwolf, C.H., and G.B. Baker (1986) Evidence that serotonin mediates noncholinergic neocortical low voltage fast activity, noncholinergic hippocampal rhythmical slow activity and contributes to intelligent behavior. Brain Res. *374:*342–356.

The Hippocampus—New Vistas, pages 257–285
© 1989 Alan R. Liss, Inc.

17
Hippocampus and Fascia Dentata Transplants: Anatomical Organization and Connections

JENS ZIMMER, NIELS TØNDER, AND TORBEN SØRENSEN

Institute of Neurobiology, University of Aarhus, Aarhus, Denmark

INTRODUCTION

The laminar organization of the hippocampus and fascia dentata (Fig. 1) and their functional role in memory and learning have attracted students from almost all neurobiological disciplines. In restorative neurobiology previous and current studies of lesion-induced neuronal plasticity (collateral sprouting, aberrant axonal growth) have benefitted from the unique hippocampal structure (see Cotman, 1978, 1985; Zimmer, 1978; Zimmer et al., 1986). More recently the distinct laminar distribution of terminal fields have been used in reinnervation experiments, where the hippocampus has served as a target for transplantation of fetal nonhippocampal neurons of mainly cholinergic and catecholaminergic origin (see Gage and Buzsáki, Chapter 16, this volume). In parallel with these grafting experiments hippocampal and dentate tissue has itself been used for transplantation. These hippocampal and dentate transplants are the topic of this chapter, which again will illustrate how the unique hippocampal and dentate structure has facilitated the analysis of the intrinsic graft structure and the exchange of connections with the host brain.

DONOR AGE

Hippocampal and dentate neurons can only survive grafting when they are immature and have not fully developed their efferent and afferent connections. In the rat the hippocampal pyramidal cells (CA3 and CA1) and the dentate hilar neurons (CA4) form prenatally, mainly between embryonic days 16 and 19 (Bayer, 1980), and these cells show optimal survival and transplant growth when grafted during this period or within the next few days (Olson et al., 1983; Das, 1983). When grafted as tissue blocks they also survive grafting after birth (Sunde and Zimmer, 1983) and even after they have grown commissural axons (Tønder et al., 1986). The dentate granule cells have a normal long and in rodents mainly postnatal proliferative period (Bayer, 1980). In the rat most granule cells thus form during the first postnatal week. Granule cells therefore

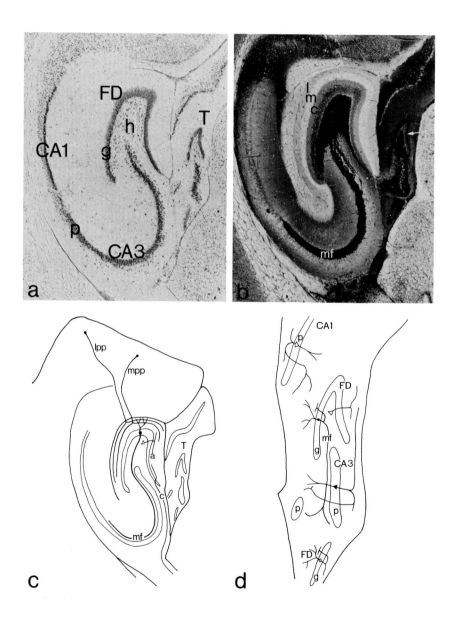

Fig. 1. Structure and main connections of normal and transplanted hippocampus and fascia dentata. **a:** Cell staining of normal adult rat hippocampus (CA3, CA1) and fascia dentata (FD) and adjacent organotypic, but isolated graft (T). Donor, 5-day-old rat; recipient, 8-day-old rat; survival, 8 weeks. ×22. **b:** Timm staining of adjacent section,

survive well in grafts from fetal rats and newborn rats up to at least postnatal day 9 (Sunde and Zimmer, 1983). The most commonly used donor age is between embryonic day 16 and birth. Mouse hippocampal tissue has been grafted at slightly earlier ages, but this has partially been due to the better survival of more immature tissue in xenograft experiments (see below) (Zimmer et al., 1988a–c). In a study including human hippocampal tissue grafted to the rat brain, 22- to 24-week-old human fetuses served as donors (Buzsáki and Gage, 1988).

RECIPIENT AGE

While the donor age for graft survival lies within a relatively narrow time period during development, such restrictions do not apply to recipient age. Hippocampal grafts survive well in both the developing and the mature brain

---

showing normal laminar terminal fields of the lateral (l) and medial (m) perforant pathways and the commissural-associational projections (c) in the host dentate molecular layer and the dentate mossy fiber projection to CA3 (mf). Note the absence of perforant path zones in the graft dentate molecular layer. The resulting reorganization includes ingrowth of CA3-associated afferents and aberrant supragranular mossy fibers (arrow) (for explanation, see d). ×22. **c:** Schematic illustration of normal, major dentate afferent and efferent connections. **d:** Schematic illustration of reorganized intrinsic connections of the isolated graft.

Abbreviations in figures

a	associational zone or fibers
c	commissural zone or fibers
CA1	hippocampal subfield CA1, regio superior
CA3	hippocampal subfield CA3, regio inferior
dc	host dentate commissural fibers
FD	fascia dentata
g	dentate granule cell layer
h	dentate hilus (CA4)
hc	hippocampal commissural fibers
HFD	host fascia dentata
l	lateral perforant path zone
lpp	lateral perforant path
m	medial perforant path zone
mf	mossy fiber layer
mpp	medial perforant path
p	hippocampal pyramidal cell layer
s	dendritic spine
sh	dendritic shaft
T	transplant
tg	transplant granule cell layer
XCA3	xenograft CA3
XFD	xenograft fascia dentata

(see below) and spinal cord (Bregman and Reier, 1986; our unpublished data). Like other neural grafts the hippocampal grafts seem to grow larger in developing brains. This may be due to the presence of more growth-stimulating substances in immature recipient brains, but there is also less mechanical restrains in the soft developing brains.

GRAFTING PROCEDURES

Three main grafting procedures are commonly used for intracerebral grafting: 1) placement of a donor tissue block in a cavity made by suction either immediately before or about 1 week earlier (cavity technique) (Stenevi et al., 1976); 2) injection of a donor tissue block by a glass capillary, usually mounted on a syringe (block injection technique) (Das, 1974; Sunde and Zimmer, 1981a, 1983); and 3) injection of a donor cell suspension by the fine cannula of a Hamilton syringe (Björklund et al., 1983). Each technique has its advantages and disadvantages regarding placement into superficial versus deep recipient brain areas, structural integration with the host brain, and access for later graft manipulation (lesioning, tracer injection, electrophysiological analysis). While a preceding lesion seems to improve graft survival in cavities of adult recipients through formation of a vascular bed (Stenevi et al., 1976; Kromer et al., 1981a) or production of growth factors (Nieto-Sampedro et al., 1983, 1987), such lesions are not necessary for graft survival with the injection techniques, although they may improve growth and formation of connections (see Gibbs et al., 1985; Tønder et al., 1989).

PRETREATMENT AND STORAGE OF DONOR TISSUE

For the labeling, manipulation, and storage of hippocampal donor tissue before transplantation, several methods have been used. In one study hippocampal neurons were prelabeled by retrograde axonal transport of the fluorescent dye Granular Blue. The dye was injected unilaterally into the hippocampus of neonatal rats 2 days before the contralateral hippocampus was grafted into uninjected littermates (Tønder et al., 1986). The subsequent detection of fluorescent neurons in the grafts served to identify these neurons as CA3 pyramidal cells and dentate hilar cells and at the same time demonstrated that developing hippocampal neurons can survive grafting even after axotomy.

Late embryonic and neonatal hippocampal tissue has also been grown in intermediate explant culture for 1 to 5 days before grafting into the hippocampus and fascia dentata of adult rats (Lindsay and Raisman, 1984). The culture step was used to eliminate granule cells by X-irradiation and/or to label the graft neurons and glial cells by tritiated thymidine for later identification in the host brain by autoradiography. Extensive migration of graft-derived glial cells into the adjacent host hippocampus was demonstrated in this way (Lindsay and Raisman, 1984; Lindsay et al., 1987).

Finally, blocks of fetal hippocampal tissue have been stored by cryopreservation in liquid nitrogen for from 1 day to 7 months before grafting to the anterior eye chamber (Jensen et al., 1984) and the hippocampal region of adult rats (Sørensen et al., 1986). The results showed that cryopreservation is a feasable method for storage of viable immature central nervous tissue, although the freezing and thawing narrow the span of donor ages with optimal graft survival (see also Das et al., 1983; Jensen et al., 1987).

CELLULAR ORGANIZATION OF TRANSPLANTS

In rat and mouse allografts of the fascia dentata with hilus (CA4), the hippocampus proper (CA3 and CA1), and sometimes adjacent parts of the subiculum, the individual areas and subfields retain their basic organotypic organization (Fig. 1). Both neurons and glial cells express cell- and area-specific morphological characteristics. The main cell and neuropil layers are usually preserved irrespective of the age of the recipient and the location in the recipient CNS (Sunde and Zimmer, 1981a, 1983; Kromer et al., 1981a). The same holds for grafts placed in the anterior eye chamber of adult rats (Olson et al., 1977; Goldowitz et al., 1982, 1984a,b; Jensen et al., 1984). Also the presence and distribution of neurons other than pyramidal cells and granule cells appear undisturbed. These neurons, which normally are located both within and outside the main cell layers, have been visualized in the intracerebral transplants by immunocytochemical staining for somatostatin, enkephalin/dynorphin and cholecystokinin (CCK) (Zimmer and Sunde, 1984), glutamate decarboxylase (GAD) (Frotscher and Zimmer, 1987), and γ-aminobutyric acid (GABA) (Robain et al., 1987) or staining with the diisopropylfluorophosphate-acetylcholinesterase (DFP-AChE) method for AChE-producing neurons, which at least partially overlap with the neuropeptidergic neurons (Zimmer et al., 1983; Zimmer and Sunde, 1984).

Light microscopic Golgi studies (Woodward et al., 1977; Frotscher and Zimmer, 1986; Robain et al., 1987), electron microscopic (EM) analysis (Robain et al., 1987; Sørensen and Zimmer, 1988a,b), and EM combined with Golgi impregnation (Frotscher and Zimmer, 1986) or immunocytochemical staining for GAD (Frotscher and Zimmer, 1987) have shown that hippocampal pyramidal cells, dentate granule cells, and GAD-positive, GABAergic interneurons retain their basic structural characteristics in the grafts. This includes dendrite organization, presence or absence of spines and spine types, appearance of axon terminals, and presence of nuclear rods in interneurons. There are also abnormal traits like narrowing of the cell and neuropil layers, quantitative changes in synaptic densities, appearance of greater numbers of somatic spines on dentate granule cells, and formation of aberrant supragranular mossy fibers, but these changes can be related to the presence or absence of afferent connections and the resulting connective reorganization (see below) (Frotscher and Zimmer, 1986; Sørensen and Zimmer, 1988a,b).

INTRINSIC GRAFT CONNECTIONS

The distribution of intrinsic graft nerve connections does of course depend on the cellular content and size of the individual grafts, but it also depends on the type and degree of host innervation (see below). From studies of the intrinsic connections of isolated intracerebral grafts using Timm's sulfide silver staining of terminal fields, silver staining of nerve fibers, and immunocytochemical staining of neuropeptides (somatostatin, CCK, and enkephalin/dynorphin) and GAD-positive fibers and terminals, it can be concluded that the reorganization and distribution of intrinsic graft connections are determined by the same factors that regulate the connective reorganization after lesions and denervation in situ (Fig. 1b,d) (Sunde and Zimmer, 1981a, 1983; Frotscher and Zimmer, 1986; Zimmer et al., 1985a,b). Both in the grafts and in the deafferented and de-efferented tissue in situ the cellular and connective differentiation is accordingly to a large extent regulated by factors intrinsic to the neurons and their local environment. The latter consists of glial cells and subsets of neurons that often connect normally, but also engage in synaptic reorganization by collateral sprouting and aberrant axonal growth in the absence of extrinsic afferents and target areas.

In nonisolated grafts, for example dentate grafts innervated by the host perforant path, the distribution of intrinsic graft connections becomes normalized. Under these conditions they must compete for synaptic sites with the ingrowing host afferents (see below).

Electron microscopic studies of fascia dentata transplants have confirmed the light microscopic observations on the cellular and the connective organizations of the isolated grafts (Frotscher and Zimmer, 1986; Sørensen and Zimmer, 1988a,b). In addition to the demonstration of normal cellular characteristics and to the presence of an aberrant supragranular mossy fiber projection, quantitation of the synapses in the graft dentate molecular layer has shown that all the normal morphological types of synaptic contacts are present, also in the absence of normal extrinsic afferent connections. The average synaptic density, expressed as number per unit area of neuropil, was, however, reduced by 16.4% from 23.89 to 19.97 per 100 μm^2. This was primarily due to a 17.6% reduction from 19.42 to 16.01 per 100 μm^2 of spine synapses of the simple, straight type, which is the most common synapse both normally and in the grafts. The most significant change regarding one type of synapse was a 43.4% reduction of symmetric synapses on dendritic shafts, a type that usually is associated with flattened synaptic vesicles and inhibitory function.

In relation to the last observation, three other morphological observations are of interest: 1) the positive immunocytochemical identification of GAD-positive GABAergic neurons and terminals in dentate and hippocampal grafts (Frotscher and Zimmer, 1987); 2) a reduction of GABAergic synapses on the initial axon segments of hippocampal graft pyramidal cells (Buzsáki et al., 1988); and 3) an increased incidence of asymmetrical, presumably excitatory, synapses on the graft dentate granule cell (Sørensen and Zimmer, 1988a,b) and pyramidal cell bodies (Freund and Buzsáki, cited by Buzsáki et al., 1988). Together these morphological observations suggest that inhibition of graft granule cells and pyramidal cells might be decreased, just as inhibition could be further outbalanced by the formation of reverberatory excitatory neural circuits by collateral sprouting and aberrant axonal growth (see Electrophysiological Studies of Hippocampal Grafts, below).

GRAFT–HOST NERVE CONNECTIONS

The formation of nerve connections between grafts of hippocampal and dentate tissue and the host CNS or PNS depends on the neuronal composition of the grafts, the graft location (hippocampal region, other brain areas, spinal cord, anterior eye chamber), determining which host fibers and targets are available, the nerve type (host cholinergic or catecholaminergic "global systems" versus fibers of the "point-to-point type," using amino acids as transmitters), the age and developmental stage of the recipient, and, finally, the conditions in the recipient area (intact or damaged with loss of neurons or afferents), which may prime the growth of host fibers or provide synaptic sites for graft fibers.

The results available on anatomical connections of hippocampal and dentate grafts will be presented below in the following order: homotopic grafts in intact recipients; restoring connections of the X-irradiated fascia dentata; improved host fiber ingrowth after grafting to axon-sparing ibotenic acid lesions; restoration of connections after grafting to ischemic CA1 lesions; host rat–mouse xenograft interconnections; and heterotopic grafts outside the hippocampal region. Most of the results in these experiments, performed in this and other laboratories, have been obtained using (alone or in combination) the histochemical Timm sulfide silver method, which differentially stains the terminals of the intrinsic and extrinsic fiber systems of the hippocampus and fascia dentata; histochemical staining of AChE for cholinergic afferents; immunocytochemical staining of neuropeptides (somatostatin, cholesystokinin [CCK], and enkephalin/dynorphin); Fink-Heimer silver staining or electron microscopy of anterograde axonal and terminal degeneration; and retrograde axonal tracing by fluorescent dyes or horseradish peroxidase (HRP).

Homotopic Grafts in Intact Recipients

Developing recipients

Host fibers. Hippocampal and dentate grafts placed in or encroaching on the hippocampus and fascia dentata or their white matter (fimbria, angular bundle) were all stained for AChE, suggesting an innervation by host cholinergic fibers of septal origin. The AChE staining was dense around the cell layers, as normally. In the neuropil the staining adapted to the distribution of the major noncholinergic intrinsic graft and extrinsic host pathways, showing affinities for some and disaffinities for others (Zimmer et al., 1986).

Regarding host noncholinergic afferents, in particular the dentate grafts have been analyzed. Depending on their location, these grafts received dense and extensive host brain projections (Fig. 2, cells 3–5). They included properly located, laminar host lateral and medial perforant path projections from the host lateral and medial entorhinal cortices, respectively, to the outer parts of the graft dentate molecular layer (Fig. 2, cell 3) and a correspondingly normal projection of host commissural fibers to the inner parts of the molecular layer (Sunde and Zimmer, 1983; Zimmer et al., 1985a,b). By immunocytochemical

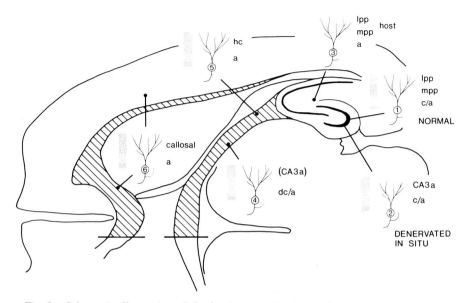

Fig. 2. Schematic illustration of the laminar innervation of dentate granule cells in normal rats (1), after in situ removal of the perforant pathways (2), and after transplantation to different sites in immature recipient brains, namely the hippocampus or fascia dentata, encroaching on host perforant path zones (3); the medial part of the fimbria, encroaching on the host commissural projection to the host dentate (4); the lateral part of the fimbria, encroaching on the commissural projection to the host hippocampus (5); and the neocortex or the corpus callosum (6). In the various situations the dentate granule cell afferents include normal (c) and host dentate commissural fibers (dc), associational fibers from the dentate hilus (a), aberrant associational fibers from the adjacent CA3 (CA3a), normal and host entorhinal lateral (lpp) and medial perforant path (mpp) fibers, host hippocampal commissural fibers (hc), and fibers from the host corpus callosum (callosal). The dotted panels to the left of the cells indicate the AChE patterns attained at the different locations. (Reproduced from Zimmer et al., 1985b, with permission of the publisher.)

staining for enkephalin/dynorphin and CCK, the host lateral and medial perforant pathways were seen to retain these respective neuropeptide characteristics as they innervated the grafts (Zimmer and Sunde, 1984). In cases in which the host perforant path was either weak or absent, the host commissural projection and intrinsic transplant associational afferents expanded into the graft dentate molecular layer (Fig. 2, cell 4). In dentate grafts located exclusively in the hippocampal CA3 and CA1 subfields or encroaching on white matter in the lateral fimbria or alveus, which convey commissural fibers to these areas, an aberrant host commissural projection from the contralateral hippocampus occupied the outer parts of the graft molecular layer (Fig. 2, cell 5) (Sunde and Zimmer, 1983).

Graft fibers. Outgrowth of graft mossy fibers into the developing host hippocampus has been shown for Timm-stained mossy fiber terminals into the host CA3 (Sunde and Zimmer, unpublished data) and CA1 (Sunde and Zimmer, 1981b). Since host and graft mossy fiber terminals are similar in Timm staining, graft mossy fiber terminals were only identified with certainty at an aberrant infrapyramidal location in CA3 next to fascia dentata transplants and along the pyramidal cell layer in CA1, where mossy fibers normally are absent. The terminals occupied positions near the pyramidal cell bodies, as they normally do in CA3.

The growth of graft commissural fibers from one side of the brain to the contralateral hippocampus in newborn rats was demonstrated by retrograde axonal tracing using the fluorescent dye Fluorogold (Tønder et al., 1988). Only graft CA3 pyramidal cells and CA4 hilar cells, which normally project to the contralateral hippocampus proper (CA3–CA1) and fascia dentata, respectively, have thus far been found to grow commissural axons (Fig. 3). The pro-

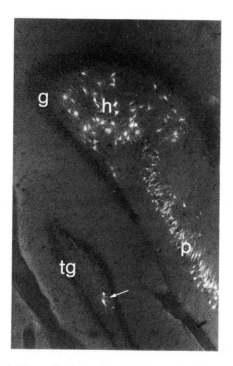

Fig. 3. Dentate graft hilar cells (arrow) with commissural projections shown by retrograde axonal transport of the fluorescent dye Fluorogold. Note normal commissural labeling of dentate hilar cells (h) and CA3 pyramidal cells (p) in adjacent host hippocampus. g, dentate granule cell layer; tg; transplant granule cell layer. Donor, newborn rat; recipient, newborn rat; survival, 6 weeks. ×42.

jecting cells were located in grafts that had been well incorporated into the recipient hippocampus or fimbria, and they usually laid opposite to host neurons and fibers with normal commissural projections. A possible regional specificity of the commissural termination of the graft neurons has not yet been established, although it appeared that the axonal outgrowth followed in the trail of fibers from adjacent host neurons.

In conclusion, hippocampal and dentate rat allografts can receive precise and normal cholinergic, perforant path, and commissural afferent connections from the developing recipient brains and send efferent projections as mossy fibers to the ipsilateral CA3 (and CA1) and commissural fibers to the contralateral hippocampus. Except for the cholinergic afferents, the formation of a normal type of connection does, however, depend on graft location. Aberrant, extrinsic, and intrinsic afferent connections will easily form in locations outside the reach of the normal types of input, as demonstrated in particular for the dentate grafts (Fig. 2, cells 4 and 5).

Adult recipients

Host fiber ingrowth. Hippocampal and dentate grafts placed into or encroaching on the hippocampus and fascia dentata of adult rat recipients have been found to receive AChE-positive, cholinergic afferents from the host septum (Kromer et al., 1981a; Sunde and Zimmer, 1981a, 1983; Wendt et al., 1983; Zimmer et al., 1985b; Sørensen et al., 1986) and even to provide a bridge for regenerating adult host cholinergic fibers across a fimbria lesion (Kromer et al., 1981b; Buzsáki et al., 1988). The origin of the fibers in the host septum and diagonal band was confirmed by retrograde axonal tracing with HRP (Kromer et al., 1981a,b). Similar results with host septal innervation of homotopic rat entorhinal cortex grafts were obtained by Gibbs et al. (1985). Adult host serotoninergic fibers of brain stem raphe origin have also been found by immunocytochemical staining to invade fetal hippocampal mouse isografts placed in the septal hippocampus and fimbria (Azmitia et al., 1981).

Following HRP and fluorochrome injections into hippocampal grafts placed in lesion cavities in the septal hippocampus, retrogradely labeled neurons were also found in the adjacent host hippocampus (Kromer and Björklund, 1980; Woodruff et al., 1987). The type and distribution of these neurons do, however, still need to be systematically analyzed.

A limited ingrowth of rat host dentate mossy fibers into small allografts of CA3 tissue encroaching on the host CA3 or fascia dentata has been demonstrated by Timm staining (Raisman and Ebner, 1983; Lindsay et al., 1987). Similarly, host perforant path projections to dentate grafts placed in or encroaching on the host rat fascia dentata have been demonstrated. From these results, obtained by the Timm method (Zimmer et al., 1985b; Sørensen et al., 1986) and by light and electron microscopic tracing of anterograde axonal degeneration (Sørensen et al., 1986; Tønder et al., 1989), it is evident that the host perforant pathway (and commissural) innervation of the dentate grafts is much less extensive than after grafting to developing recipients. In accordance with this, Gibbs et al. (1985) were unable to detect ingrowth of noncholinergic projections from the ipsilateral amygdala and contralateral entorhinal cortex into retrohippocampal entorhinal cortex grafts in adult recipients.

Graft fiber outgrowth. Efferent projections from hippocampal tissue grafted to the mature hippocampal region have been demonstrated by various methods in various studies. Gibbs et al. (1985) grafted embryonic entorhinal cortex to 8–10-day-old knife-cut lesions in the adult rat retrohippocampal area and traced graft efferent projections to the host hippocampus, fascia dentata, and amygdala by anterograde axonal transport of HRP injected into the grafts and retrograde transport of HRP and Fast Blue from injections into the host brain. By projecting to the hippocampus, fascia dentata, and amygdala, the grafts appeared able to locate areas normally receiving an entorhinal input, although the density of the graft projections was subnormal. With the homotopic location of the grafts it is likely that the outgrowth was guided or stimulated by the degeneration of the original host entorhinal projections (see also Nieto-Sampedro et al., 1987).

In another study by Zhou et al. (1985), immunocytochemical staining for a graft-specific Thy-1 membrane glycoprotein was used to visualize projections from mouse hippocampal and dentate allografts placed in the hippocampus of adult mice. These grafts also displayed what appeared to be cell type- and location-specific patterns of fiber outgrowth. Only grafts containing granule cells projected to the host mossy fiber layer. Grafts of hippocampal pyramidal cells avoided this layer and projected instead to the commissural and associational zones of fascia dentata, CA3, and CA1, depending on their exact location in the host hippocampus. The graft fiber outgrowth seemed to require or at least to be stimulated by some denervation of the respective host neuropil layers. Such denervation is almost inevitably caused by the insertion of the grafts.

Related results have been obtained using Timm staining to monitor graft efferents in the rat. They include the outgrowth of dentate mossy fibers to the host CA3 (Sørensen et al., 1986) and CA1 (Raisman and Ebner, 1983) pyramidal cell layers and the projection of CA1-subiculum and CA3-associated graft efferents into denervated parts of the perforant pathway zones of the adjacent host fascia dentata (Sunde and Zimmer, 1981a; Zimmer et al., 1985b; Sørensen et al., 1986).

Restoring Connections of the X-Irradiated Fascia Dentata

Most rat dentata granule cells form after birth, mainly during the first postnatal days (Bayer, 1980). X-irradiation of the hippocampal region of newborn rats, damaging the dividing cells, therefore induces a maldevelopment of the fascia dentata in which 50–90% of the granule cells are lost (Bayer and Altman, 1975; Laurberg and Hjorth-Simonsen, 1977). In such X-irradiated rats with the absence of particularly the free, medial blade of the fascia dentata, the perforant pathways project aberrantly to extend basal dendrites of the CA3c pyramidal cells, just as the dentate mossy fiber projection to CA3 is reduced (Fig. 4b) (Laurberg and Hjorth-Simonsen, 1977).

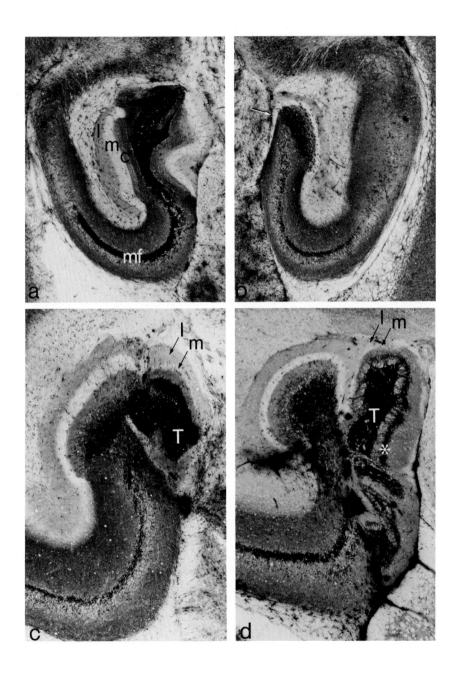

When neonatal dentate tissue was grafted to newborn rats immediately after irradiation, normal and precisely laminated serial nerve connections were established by host perforant path and host commissural hippocampodentate fibers projecting to the graft dentate granule cells, which in turn sent mossy fibers to the host hippocampal CA3 (Fig. 4a,b) (Sunde et al., 1984, 1985; Zimmer et al., 1985a, 1987). The formation of such serial connections did, however, require that the grafts be located in and just next to the residual host fascia dentata. Deviations from this position resulted in only partial restoration of the serial chain of connections through the grafts, as, for instance, the formation of a correct host perforant path input, but no graft to host mossy fiber projection, or vice versa. In the best cases the grafts normalized the host graft–host connections along about one-third of the longitudinal septotemporal axis of the hippocampus.

When the grafting was delayed by 3 weeks, and hence performed into 3-week-old, not fully matured recipient brains, properly located dentate grafts still became heavily innervated by host perforant path afferents and sent mossy fibers into the host CA3. When the grafting was delayed for 5 weeks or more, in some cases for up to 10 months, there was a marked decrease in both the host perforant path ingrowth and the growth of graft mossy fibers into the host CA3 (Fig. 4c,d) (Sunde et al., 1985; Zimmer et al., 1987, 1988c). Ingrowth of host commissural afferents were not detected in these cases. Corresponding to this recipient age-dependent decrease in exchange of connections, the location of the grafts became more crucial. For the host perforant path ingrowth, which has been confirmed at the ultrastructural level, it was characteristic that the terminal zones attained a more superficial position in the graft dentate molecular layer and finally vanished as one moved away from the host–graft interface (Fig. 4d). Corresponding to this, the Timm staining of the intrinsic graft associational systems expanded. Aberrant supragranular mossy fibers

---

Fig. 4. Grafts in X-irradiated rats. **a,b:** Grafted (a) and nongrafted (b) sides of adult 5-month-old rat subjected to bilateral hippocampal X-irradiation at birth, immediately followed by unilateral grafting of block of intact, neonatal fascia dentata. The well-integrated graft receives a normal laminar input of host lateral (l) and medial (m) perforant path and dentate commissural fibers (c) and sends mossy fibers with normal Timm-positive terminals to the host CA3 mossy fiber layer (mf). For control of radiation effects, see part b with aberrant perforant path projections (arrow) to CA3 in the absence of the late forming, medial blade of fascia dentata and a sparse mossy fiber projection. ×27. **c,d:** Delayed grafting to adult rats, irradiated at birth, results in less host lateral (l) and medial (m) perforant path ingrowth into even well-placed dentate transplants (T). Donor, newborn rat; recipients, 4-month-old (c) and 2-month-old (d) rats with bilateral hippocampal X-irradiation at birth. Survival 10 (c) and 2 (d) months. Notice in d the vanishing of the perforant path zones away from the host–graft interface, the corresponding spread of the Timm-stained inner zone, and the increase in aberrant supragranular mossy fiber terminals (asterisk). Also in d there is indication of some graft mossy fiber outgrowth with increased staining and width of the host CA3 mossy fiber layer. c, ×37; d, ×46.

were also consistently present in these grafts, with little host perforant path input, as in the isolated or weakly innervated grafts in immature recipients.

In contrast to the decrease in perforant path and commissural innervation, there was no obvious decrease in the AChE staining for cholinergic afferents after delayed grafting into adult rats (Fig. 5). The pattern of AChE staining, moreover, seemed to adapt to the distributions of the major, noncholinergic pathways (see above) (Zimmer et al., 1986).

Improved Host Fiber Ingrowth After Grafting to Axon-Sparing Ibotenic Acid Lesions

X-irradiation only affects dividing cells. Models for lesions and repair of the adult fascia dentata therefore call for other lesion methods. One useful lesion method is focal injection of the excitotoxic glutamate analog ibotenic acid, which by a so-called axon-sparing lesion kills the neurons in the injected area

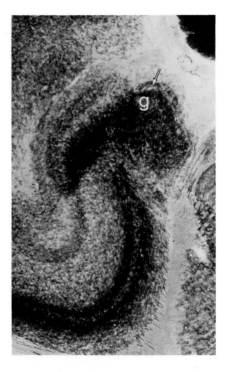

Fig. 5. AChE-stained section adjacent to the one shown in Figure 4c demonstrating apparently unrestrained ingrowth of AChE-positive, cholinergic host fibers into the dentate graft. Note the normal laminar staining pattern in the graft and host dentate molecular layers. Arrow, points to normal denser staining in the medial perforant path terminal zone; g, graft granule cell layer. × 37.

but saves the extrinsic afferents, which remain for extended periods of time (Coyle and Schwarcz, 1983; Tønder et al., 1989).

In a recent study we used such lesions followed by grafting of dentate tissue (Tønder et al., 1989). In brief, 0.5 μl of a 1% w/v solution of ibotenic acid in isotonic phosphate buffer was injected into the dorsal fascia dentata of young adult rats, followed after 1 week by injection of a block of neonatal fascia dentata. When the grafts were analyzed from 6 weeks to 9 months later they were found to have survived well, and they had often grown to large dimensions. They were organotypically organized with a distinct dentate hilus (CA4) and molecular and granule cell layers (Fig. 6a). They contained the normal cell types, including peptidergic somatostatin- and CCK-reactive cells in the hilus and enkephalin/dynorphin-reactive granule cells with mossy fiber terminals. The grafts were innervated not only by AChE-positive cholinergic fibers from the host systems (Fig. 6b) but also by perforant path fibers from the ipsilateral host entorhinal area. The latter, surprisingly extensive innervation was observed with Timm staining and confirmed by light and electron microscopy of anterograde axonal degeneration following acute entorhinal lesions (Fig. 6c). From the Timm staining and the mapping of host perforant path degeneration by electron microscopy, it was obvious that the dentate grafts placed in the ibotenic acid lesions received a more extensive and denser host perforant path innervation than similar grafts placed in the intact adult brain (Fig. 6d).

We conclude that under special conditions after axon-sparing lesions, mature host perforant path fibers can attain a growth ability approaching that observed for host fibers in developing brains. Primed by the removal of their normal target cells and without significant axonal damage, mature central nerve fibers of the point-to-point type can in this situation successfully compete with developing, intrinsic transplant fiber systems and establish extensive connections with the transplants.

Restoration of Connections After Grafting to Ischemic CA1 Lesions

In the hippocampal region of adult rats transient cerebral ischemia induced by the four-vessel occlusion technique (Pulsinelli and Brierly, 1979) damages the somatostatinergic neurons in the dentate hilus (Johansen et al., 1987) and the CA1 pyramidal cells in the dorsal CA1 (Johansen et al., 1984). The lesions are assumed to be of the excitotoxic type, with terminal efflux of glutamate as a major factor (Benveniste et al., 1984). In that sense, the ischemic lesions resemble the above-mentioned ibotenic acid lesions, with the exception that the ischemic lesions, besides sparing the extrinsic axons, also spare for instance the nonpyramidal cells in the dorsal CA1 (Johansen et al., 1983).

In an ongoing series of experiments we have examined whether grafts of embryonic CA1 cells can restore the anatomical connections of the ischemically lesioned CA1 region. For this purpose we grafted suspensions of CA1 cells from late fetal (E18–20) rats into 1-week-old ischemic lesions of the dorsal CA1 of adult rats (Tønder et al., 1987). When analyzed 6–9 weeks later, 80% of the grafts had survived and often grown to large sizes (Fig. 7a). The grafts

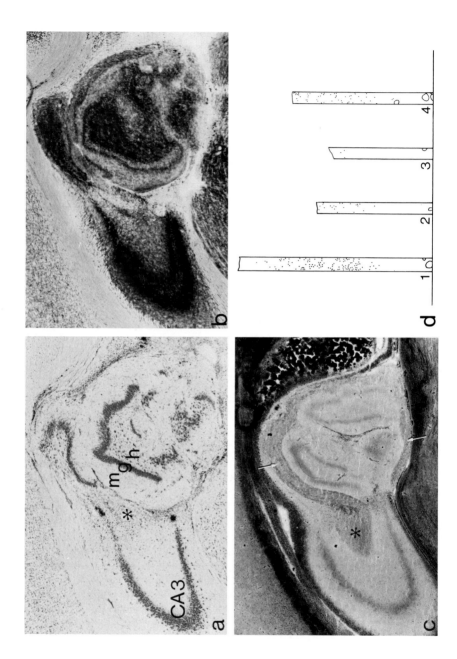

contained both pyramidal cells, arranged in small layers or clusters, and CCK- and somatostatin-reactive neurons of the nonpyramidal type and displayed a near-normal astrocyte staining for glial fibrillary acidic protein (GFAP), hence contrasting with the gliosis in the host ischemic lesion (Fig. 8a). Intimate structural and connective integration with the host brain was observed in semithin plastic sections and in silver-stained sections, showing dendrites and nerve fibers passing across the host–graft interface. AChE-positive host cholinergic fibers innervated the grafts with normal high density of AChE staining mainly around the cell bodies (Fig. 7b). Ingrowth of host hippocampal commissural fibers was demonstrated by Fink-Heimer staining and by electron microscopy following transection of the hippocampal commissures. At the ultrastructural level host commissural nerve terminals were also found deep inside the graft neuropil (Fig. 8b). Homotypic projections from graft to host were demonstrated by labeling of pyramidal-like graft neurons after injections of the retrograde fluorochrome tracer Fluorogold into the ipsilateral host CA1 and subiculum at posterotemporal levels (Fig. 7c,d). Minor abnormal graft projections to the host dentate molecular layer were evident in Timm staining where the CA1 grafts extended into the host fascia dentata.

From our results and the results obtained by Mudrick et al. (1987), we conclude that CA1 neurons from late fetal rat hippocampi can survive in the ischemically lesioned CA1 of adult rats. The grafts express the cellular morphology and neuron-specific markers of the cells they replace. They integrate well and can receive and send out homotypic nerve connections to the ipsilateral CA1 and subiculum.

Host Rat–Mouse Xenograft Interconnections

Neural and non-neural tissue grafted to the brain is less prone to be rejected than after grafting to most other areas of the body (Medawar, 1948). This so-called *immunological privilege* of the brain has been related to the sparse

---

Fig. 6. Dentate grafts in ibotenic acid lesion of adult fascia dentata. **a,b:** Large dentate graft with distinct granule cell layer (g), molecular layer (m), and hilus (h) and dense and basically normal AChE-staining (b), suggestive of innervation by cholinergic fibers from host septum. Asterisk in a indicates adjacent gliotic area in host hippocampus. Donor, newborn rat; recipient, adult rat with 1-week-old ibotenic acid lesion; survival, 6 weeks. ×25. **c:** Large dentate graft with dense host perforant path innervation of normal, outer parts of graft dentate molecular layer (arrows), shown by Fink-Heimer staining 3 days after lesion of ipsilateral host entorhinal cortex. Asterisk in c indicates normal perforant path degeneration in host CA3 molecular layer. Donor, newborn rat; recipient, adult rat with 1-week-old ibotenic lesion; survival, 6 weeks. ×25. **d:** Density and distribution of perforant path terminals represented by dots in columns made from electron micrographs taken of the dentate molecular layer of normal (1) and grafted (2–4) fascia dentata 3 days after entorhinal lesions. 1–3: Normal adult rat with predominantly medial perforant path degeneration. Dentate graft placed in intact adult fascia dentata, showing host perforant path innervation next to host graft interface (2) and decrease 200 μm away (3). 4: Dentate graft placed in axon-sparing, ibotenic acid lesion of adult fascia dentata (Tønder et al., 1988a).

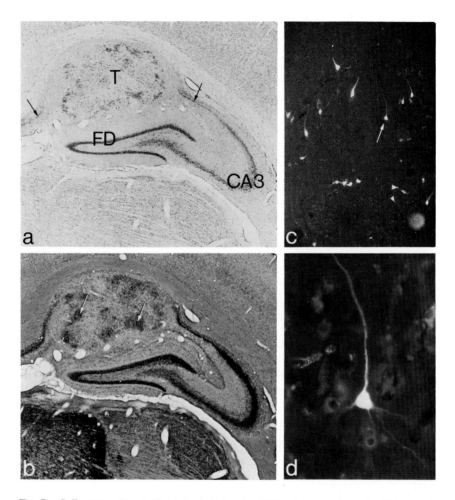

Fig. 7. Cell suspension graft of fetal CA1 cells (E21) placed in 1-week-old ischemic lesion of dorsal CA1 of adult rat. Survival, 5 months. **a:** Cell staining of large transplant (T) with cell clusters. Arrows point to lesioned host CA1 pyramidal cell layer. **b:** AChE staining predominantly around cell clusters (arrows) in the same graft as shown in a. The subnormal density of AChE staining in the section is due to formaldehyde fixation of the animal to preserve the fluorescent labeled cells (c,d). **c:** Fluorescent neurons, predominantly of the pyramidal shape in the graft shown in a and b. The cells were labeled by retrograde axonal transport of Fluorogold injected into the ipsilateral CA1 and subiculum at more posterotemporal levels 6 days before sacrifice. A cell (at arrow) in c is shown at higher magnification in **d.** a,b, × 19; c, × 56; d, × 290.

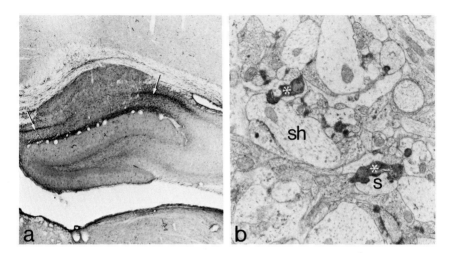

Fig. 8. **a:** GFAP staining for astroglia in graft of fetal (E21) CA1 cells placed in 1-week-old ischemic CA1 lesion of adult rat; survival, 8 weeks. Note dense gliosis in lesioned CA1 (arrows) with shrinkage of cell and neuropil layers, but near-normal astroglia staining in transplants (between arrows). ×19. **b:** Electron micrograph of degenerating, electron-dense nerve terminals of host commissural origin (asterisks) in synaptic contact with dendritic shaft (sh) and spine (s) in fetal (E21) CA1 graft placed in 1-week-old ischemic lesion of adult rat CA1; survival, 8 weeks. ×8,400.

lymphatic drainage of the brain, the blood–brain barrier, the absence in normal brain tissue of antigen-presenting cells (dendritic cells), and, in cases with neural grafts, the low antigenicity of nerve tissue (Mason et al., 1985). The contribution of these and other factors to what now appears to be a delayed and reduced immune response rather than a "privilege" is being studied intensely in several laboratories. The studies involve neural grafting between different inbred strains of rats (allografting) as well as grafting between rats and mice (xenografting) and include immunosuppression by Cyclosporin A (Brundin et al., 1985; Finsen et al., 1988a), characterization of the cellular infiltration in and around the grafts (Finsen et al., 1987, 1988a,b), and analysis of the cellular and humoral immune responses in the recipient animals in general.

Other xenograft studies, although aware of the brain-specific immune conditions, have focused on the formation of host brain–xenograft nerve connections. In the hippocampus such studies have included grafting of fetal mouse and human septal tissue with cholinergic neurons into the adult rat hippocampus (Daniloff et al., 1984, 1985; Nilsson et al., 1988a) and grafting of mouse hippocampal and in particular dentate tissue to adult (Finsen et al., 1988a,b) and newborn rats (Finsen and Zimmer, 1986; Sørensen et al., 1987; Zimmer et al., 1987, 1988a–c). In this relation, cross-species (or sometimes cross-strain) transplantations have benefitted from the use of species-specific (or strain-specific) membrane or cell markers for identification and distinction of donor and recipient cells and tissue (Fig. 9) (Lund et al., 1985; Zhou et al., 1985; Finsen and Zimmer, 1986; Lindsay et al., 1987; Sørensen et al., 1987; Zimmer et al., 1987, 1988a,b). Recently we used the difference in the expression of CCK immunoreactivity between mouse and rat mossy fiber terminals to demonstrate the formation of CCK-reactive mouse mossy fibers to the otherwise CCK-poor mossy fiber layer of the host rat CA3 (Zimmer et al., 1988a–c).

From our xenograft experiments with grafting of blocks of fetal and newborn mouse fascia dentata to the hippocampus of newborn rats, we conclude that 1) the survival of the mouse xenografts improves from less than 10% to 60–70% by decreasing the donor age from newborn to embryonic days 13–16; 2) the surviving xenografts develop an organotypic organization (Fig. 9), including a mouse-specific CCK immunoreactivity of the hilodentate associational system and dentate mossy fibers; 3) the xenografts receive an AChE-positive cholinergic host projection when located in normal cholinoreceptive areas of the rat host brain; 4) xenografts encroaching on the trajectories of the host rat commissural

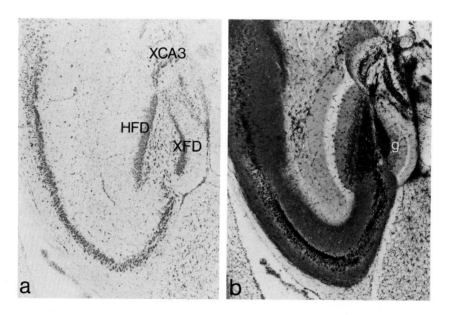

Fig. 9. Xenograft of mouse fascia dentata (FD) and CA3 (CA3) encroaching on host rat fascia dentata (HFD). Donor, E16 C67 mouse; recipient, newborn Kyoto rat; survival, 4 months. The xenograft is well-integrated as seen in both cell (a) and Timm staining (b). Xenograft granule cell bodies are unstained or lightly stained (g) in contrast to the densely Timm-stained Kyoto granule cells. Note the normal laminar, rat host perforant pathway innervation of the *outer* parts of the xenograft molecular layer. Host commissural innervation of the *inner* zone of the graft molecular layer was demonstrated by antero-grade axonal degeneration (data not shown). ×31.

or perforant path systems or their terminations in the host rat fascia dentata receive a laminar- and also neuropeptide-specific host innervation of the dentate molecular layer (Fig. 9b); and 5) CCK-reactive mouse mossy fibers with proper xenograft location can project into the mossy fiber layer of the host rat CA3.

Heterotopic Grafts Outside the Hippocampal Region

Most studies of hippocampal grafts have intended to place the grafts within or next to the recipient hippocampus or its major afferent input routes. The anatomical connections of these grafts have been dealt with above. Hippocampal and dentate tissue have, however, also been placed in other brain areas, as well as in the spinal cord (Bregman and Reier, 1986) and the anterior eye chamber (Olson et al., 1977, 1980; Goldowitz et al., 1982, 1984a,b; Jensen et al., 1984; Sørensen and Zimmer, 1988a,b). From what has been reported, the intrinsic cellular organization of heterotopic hippocampal and dentate grafts does not appear to differ from homotopic ones, although some abnormal, immature traits have been observed in intraocular dentate grafts (Sørensen and Zimmer, 1988a,b).

Regarding host–graft interconnections it is natural to distinguish between grafts placed in the brain and spinal cord and grafts placed in the anterior eye chamber. In the brain, dense host projections have been demonstrated to the "perforant path zones" in the outer part of the molecular layer of dentate grafts placed in the neocortex or corpus callosum of newborn rats (Fig. 2, cell 6) (Sunde and Zimmer, 1983; Zimmer et al., 1983). These afferents were presumably of contralateral, host neocortical origin, as they were traced by degeneration following corpus callosum transections. From other brain areas, such as cerebellum, basal ganglia, thalamus, and brain stem, information is sparse and mainly consists of observations of exchange of nerve fibers observed in silver staining (Sunde and Zimmer, 1983; our unpublished observations). One exception is the consistent AChE staining of hippocampal and dentate grafts placed in areas of the brain or spinal cord with normal AChE staining. Such graft AChE staining suggests that host cholinergic afferents present in the respective recipient brain areas, such as neocortex, thalamus, habenula, and brain stem, and spinal cord can invade these heterotopically located grafts. The ingrowth, expressed by the extent and density of the AChE staining, has, however, not yet been systematically investigated and compared between the different areas and between recipients of different maturity. It is clear, however, that dentate grafts in the neocortex show consistent and dense AChE staining (Sunde and Zimmer, 1983; Zimmer et al., 1983) compared with, for example, grafts in the basal ganglia, which in particular in adult recipients can appear almost blank (our unpublished data). This difference most likely reflects a difference between basal forebrain and intrinsic striatal cholinergic neurons in the growth ability or affinity for dentate target tissue, as also recently demonstrated by intrahippocampal grafting of these neurons (Nilsson et al., 1988b).

Host projections to intracortical hippocampal grafts have also been studied by Woodruff et al. (1987), who placed grafts of embryonic tissue from the hippocampal region in large bilateral, neocortical, and hippocampal lesion cavities in adult rats, primarily to study behavioral effects of the grafts. After graft injection by the fluorescent retrograde tracer Fast Blue, labeled neurons were found in the adjacent parts of the ipsilateral host neocortex, cingulate cortex, and host hippocampus. Some of the labeled neocortical cells were reported to be up to 4 mm away from the graft injection site. It is presently not clear whether this host neocortical innervation of the grafts is representative for grafting to adult rats or brought about by the extensive bilateral lesioning of the cortex.

Regarding connections of hippocampal grafts in the spinal cord, Bregman and Reier (1986) observed that rat hippocampal grafts placed in lesions of the newborn rat spinal cord did not rescue rubrospinal cells from retrograde death in contrast to homotypic spinal graft. This implies that hippocampal grafts do not serve as a target for rubrospinal fibers.

Following grafting to the anterior eye chamber, hippocampal and dentate tissues have been observed both anatomically and physiologically to be innervated by cholinergic and adrenergic nerves from the autonomic ground plexus of the iris (Olson et al., 1977, 1980; Hoffer et al., 1977a,b; Woodward et al., 1977; Taylor et al., 1978).

ELECTROPHYSIOLOGICAL STUDIES OF HIPPOCAMPAL GRAFTS

At the time of this writing, the available literature contained reports of electrophysiological recordings from 1) rat hippocampal allografts placed in the cerebellum of adult rats (Hounsgaard and Yarom, 1985a,b); 2) rat hippocampal allografts placed in lesion cavities at the septal pole of the hippocampus of adult rats (Segal et al., 1981; Buzsáki et al., 1987a,b) or as cell suspensions within the adult recipient hippocampus (Buzsáki and Gage, 1987); 3) human hippocampal xenografts placed in lesion cavities at the septal pole of the hippocampus of adult rats (Buzsáki and Gage, 1988); 4) rat hippocampal allo- and xenografts placed in the parietal cortex and/or the adjacent dorsal hippocampus of adult rats and adult rabbits (Vinogradova et al., 1985); and 5) rat hippocampal allografts in the anterior eye chamber of adult rats, placed either as single hippocampal grafts or in combination with brain stem catecholamine-containing grafts (Hoffer et al., 1977a,b; Taylor et al., 1978, 1980; Freedman et al., 1979).

The results of these and more recent electrophysiological studies of hippocampal grafts are dealt with in detail by Gage and Buzsáki (Chapter 16, this volume). Here we conclude, in accordance with the anatomical findings presented earlier, 1) that the grafted hippocampal neurons retain their basic cell type-specific electroresponsive properties, 2) that the grafts may be more prone to epileptic activity than is the normal hippocampus because of less inhibitory activity or a shift in balance between inhibitory and excitatory circuits, and 3) that both cholinergic host septal connections and host hippocampal and (direct or indirect) entorhinal connections can elicit distinct electrophysiological synaptic reactions within the grafts, modifying the firing patterns and activity of the graft neurons, for instance in relation to different behavioral activities (Buzsáki et al., 1987b).

BEHAVIORAL EFFECTS

The study of behavioral effects of hippocampal grafts is in its beginning unlike the study of other grafts, such as, for instance, grafts of cholinergic neurons *into* the hippocampus (see Gage and Buzsáki, Chapter 16, this volume). In two studies in which fetal hippocampal tissue was grafted into aspiration lesions of the septodorsal hippocampus and the overlying neocortex of adult rats, some improvements were reported in spatial maze performance (Kimble et al., 1986) and in an operant bar-press paradigm (Woodruff et al., 1987). Several other experimental paradigms using more refined lesion methods and other behavioral tests for hippocampal function are, however, available and should be used.

The demonstration of the structural and connective integration of grafts placed in irradiation-damaged developing fascia dentata, in ibotenic acid-lesioned fascia dentata, and in ischemic lesions of the adult CA1 should encourage the use of these lesion models for grafting and behavioral testing. From initial studies of rats subjected to bilateral hippocampal X-irradiation at birth and tested in the Morris water-maze as adults we know that the irradiation causes behavioral impairment (Zimmer, Sunde, and Gage, unpublished results). Similar rats with dentate grafts restoring dentate connections for up to one-third of the septotemporal extent of the hippocampus *on one side* did not, however, show any improvement. In future studies we have therefore chosen to limit the damage and use only unilateral X-irradiation and grafting.

As stated above, the study of behavioral effects of hippocampal grafts is in its beginning. With the ongoing anatomical and electrophysiological studies as a basis and many well-documented behavioral tests at hand, this will, however, undoubtedly change within the next few years.

CONCLUDING REMARKS

A general theme in neural grafting today is the search for techniques for lesioning selected populations of neurons and preparation of pure cell lines for subsequent grafting. This approach is also of great importance for the study of the structural (developmental and connective) and functional interaction of hippocampal and dentate neurons. By virtue of their pattern of development, differential susceptibility to various noxious stimuli and treatments, and unique cellular and structural organization, the hippocampus and fascia dentata are, however, for many purposes ready for use almost as they are.

REFERENCES

Azmitia, E.C., M.J. Perlow, M.J. Brennan, and J.M. Lauder (1981) Fetal raphe and hippocampal transplants into adult and aged C57BL/6N mice: A preliminary immunocytochemical study. Brain Res. Bull. *7:*703–710.

Bayer, S.A. (1980) Development of the hippocampal region in the rat. I. Neurogenesis examined with [^{3}H]-thymidine autoradiography. J. Comp. Neurol. *190:*87–114.

Bayer, S.A., and J. Altman (1975) The effects of X-irradiation on the postnatally-forming granule cell population in the olfactory bulb, hippocampus, and cerebellum of the rat. Exp. Neurol. *48:*167–174.

Benveniste, H., J. Drejer, A. Schousboe, and N.H. Diemer (1984) Elevation of the extracellular concentrations of glutamate and aspartate in rat hippocampus during transient cerebral ischemia monitored by intracerebral microdialysis. J. Neurochem. 43:1369–1974.

Björklund, A., U. Stenevi, R.H. Schmidt, S.B. Dunnett, and F.H. Gage (1983) Intracerebral grafting of neuronal cell suspensions. I. Introduction and general methods of preparation. Acta Physiol. Scand. [Suppl.] 522:1–7.

Bregman, B.S., and P.J. Reier (1986) Neural tissue transplants rescue axotomized rubrospinal cells from retrograde death. J. Comp. Neurol. 244:86–95.

Brundin, P., O.G. Nilsson, H.F. Gage, and A. Björklund (1985) Cyclosporin A increases survival of cross-species intrastriatal grafts of embryonic dopamine-containing neurons. Exp. Brain Res. 60:204–208.

Buzsáki, G., J. Czopf I. Kondàkor, A. Björklund, and F.H. Gage (1987a) Cellular activity of intracerebrally transplanted fetal hippocampus during behavior. Neuroscience 22:871–883.

Buzsáki, G., T. Freund, A. Björklund, and F.H. Gage (1988) Restoration and deterioration of function by brain grafts in the septohippocampal system. Prog. Brain Res. 78:69–77.

Buzsáki, G., and F.H. Gage (1987) Neural grafts: Possible mechanisms of action. In: T.L. Petit and G.O. Ivy (eds): Neural Plasticity: A lifespan Approach. New York: Alan R. Liss, Inc., pp. 171–199.

Buzsáki, G., F.H. Gage, L. Kellényi, and A. Björklund, (1987b) Behavioral dependence of the electrical activity of intracerebrally transplanted fetal hippocampus. Brain Res. 400:321–333.

Cotman, C.W. (1978) Neuronal Plasticity. New York: Raven Press.

Cotman, C.W. (1985) Synaptic Plasticity. London: Guilford Press.

Coyle, J.T., and R. Schwarcz (1983) The use of excitatory amino acids as selective neurotoxins. In: A. Björklund and T. Hökfelt (eds): Handbook of Chemical Neuroanatomy, Vol. 1: Methods in Chemical Neuroanatomy. Amsterdam: Elsevier, pp. 508–527.

Daniloff, J.K., W.C. Low, R.P. Bodony, and J. Wells (1985) Cross-species neural transplants of embryonic septal nuclei to the hippocampal formation of adult rats. Exp. Brain Res. 59:73–82.

Daniloff, J.K., J. Wells, and J. Ellis (1984) Cross-species septal transplants: A recovery of choline acetyltransferase activity. Brain Res. 324:151–154.

Das, G.D. (1974) Transplantation of embryonic neural tissue in the mammalian brain. I. Growth and differentiation of neuroblasts from various regions of the embryonic brain in the cerebellum of neonatate rats. TIT. J. Life Sci. 4:93–124.

Das, G.D. (1983) Neural transplantation in mammalian brain: Some conceptual and technical considerations. In R.B. Wallace and G.D. Das (eds): Neural Tissue Transplantation Research. New York: Springer Verlag, pp. 1–64.

Das, G.D., J.D. Houle, J. Brasko, and K.G. Das (1983) Freezing of neural tissues and their transplantation in the brain of rats: Technical details and histological observations. J. Neurosci. Methods 8:1–15.

Finsen, B., F. Oteruelo, and J. Zimmer (1987) Immunological reactions to brain grafts. Characterization of lymphocytic and astroglial reactions. Neuroscience [Suppl.] 22:S258.

Finsen, B., F. Oteruelo, and J. Zimmer (1988a) Immunocytochemical characterization of the cellular immune response to intracerebral xenografts of brain tissue. Prog. Brain Res. 78:261–270.

Finsen, B., P.H. Poulsen, and J. Zimmer (1988b) Xenografting of fetal mouse hippocampal tissue to the brain of adult rats: Effects of cyclosporin A treatment. Exp. Brain Res. 70:117–133.

Finsen, B., and J. Zimmer (1986) Timm staining of hippocampal nerve cell bodies in the Kyoto rat. A cell marker in allo- and xenografting of rat and mouse brain tissue, revealing neuronal migration. Dev. Brain Res. *29*:51–59.

Freedman, R., D. Taylor, A. Seiger, L. Olson, and B. Hoffer (1979) Seizures and related epileptiform activity in hippocampus transplanted to the anterior chamber of the eye. II. Modulation by cholinergic and adrenergic input. Ann. Neurol. *6*:281–295.

Frotscher, M., and J. Zimmer (1986) Intracerebral transplants of the rat fascia dentata: A Golgi/electron microscope study of dentate granule cells. J. Comp. Neurol. *246*:181–190.

Frotscher, M., and J. Zimmer (1987) GABAergic nonpyramidal neurons in intracerebral transplants of the rat hippocampus and fascia dentata: A combined light and electron microscopic immunocytochemical study. J. Comp. Neurol. *259*:266–276.

Gibbs, R.B., E.W. Harris, and C.W. Cotman (1985) Replacement of damaged cortical projections by homotypic transplants of entorhinal cortex. J. Comp. Neurol. *237*:47–64.

Goldowitz, D., Å. Seiger, and L. Olson (1982) Anatomy of the isolated area dentata grown in the rat anterior eye chamber. J. Comp. Neurol. *208*:382–400.

Goldowitz, D., Å. Seiger, and L. Olson (1984a) Regulation of axonal ingrowth into area dentata as studied by sequential, double intraocular brain tissue transplantation. J. Comp. Neurol. *227*:50–62.

Goldowitz, D., Å. Seiger, and L. Olson (1984b) Degree of hyperinnervation of area dentata by locus coeruleus in the presence of septum or entorhinal cortex as studied by sequential intraocular triple transplantation. Exp. Brain Res. *56*:351–360.

Hoffer, B., Å. Seiger, R. Freedman, L. Olson, and D. Taylor (1977a) Electrophysiology and cytology of hippocampal formation transplants in the anterior chamber of the eye. II. Cholinergic mechanisms. Brain Res. *119*:107–132.

Hoffer, B., Å. Seiger, D. Taylor, L. Olson, and R. Freedman (1977b) Seizures and related epileptiform activity in hippocampus transplanted to the anterior chamber of the eye. I. Characterization of seizures, interictal spikes, and synchronous activity. Exp. Neurol. *54*:233–250.

Hounsgaard, J., and Y. Yarom (1985a) Cellular physiology of transplanted neurons. In A. Björklund and U. Stenevi (eds): Neural Grafting in the Mammalian CNS. Amsterdam: Elsevier, pp. 401–408.

Hounsgaard, J., and Y. Yarom (1985b) Intrinsic control of electroresponsive properties of transplanted mammalian brain neurons. Brain Res. *335*:372–376.

Jensen, S., T. Sørensen, A.G. Møller, and J. Zimmer (1984) Intraocular grafts of fresh and freeze-stored rat hippocampal tissue: A comparison of survivability and histological and connective organization. J. Comp. Neurol. *227*:558–568.

Jensen, S., T. Sørensen, and J. Zimmer (1987) Cryopreservation of fetal rat brain tissue later used for intracerebral transplantation. Cryobiology *24*:120–134.

Johansen, F.F., M.B. Jøgensen, and N.H. Diemer (1983) Resistance of hippocampal CA-1 interneurons to 20 min of transient cerebral ischemia in the rat. Acta Neuropathol. [Berl.] *61*:135–140.

Johansen, F.F., M.B. Jørgensen, D.K.J. Ekström von Lubitz, and N.H. Diemer (1984) Selective dendrite damage in hippocampal CA1 stratum radiatum with unchanged axon ultrastructure and glutamate uptake after transient cerebral ischaemia in the rat. Brain Res. *291*:373–377.

Johansen, F.F., J. Zimmer, and N.H. Diemer (1987) Early loss of somatostatin neurons in dentate hilus after cerebral ischemia in the rat precedes CA-1 pyramidal cell loss. Acta Neuropathol. [Berl.] *73*:110–114.

Kimble, D.P., R. Bremiller, and G. Stickrod (1986) Fetal brain implants improve maze performance in hippocampal-lesioned rats. Brain Res. *363*:358–363.

Kromer, L.F., and A. Björklund (1980) Embryonic neural transplants provide model systems for studying development and regeneration in the mammalian CNS. In C. Di Bernadetta, R. Balázc, G. Gombos, and G. Porcellati (eds): Multidisciplinary Approach to Brain Development. pp. Amsterdam: Elsevier, pp. 409–426.

Kromer, L.F., A. Björklund, and U. Stenevi (1981a) Innervation of embryonic hippocampal implants by regenerating axons of cholinergic septal neurons in the adult rat. Brain Res. 210:153–171.

Kromer, L.F., A. Björklund, and U. Stenevi (1981b) Regeneration of the septohippocampal pathways in adult rats is promoted by utilizing embryonic hippocampal implants as bridges. Brain Res. 210:173–200.

Laurberg, S., and A. Hjorth-Simonsen (1977) Growing central axons deprived of normal target neurons by neonatal X-ray irradiation still terminate in a precisely laminated fashion. Nature 269:158–160.

Lindsay, R.M., and G. Raisman (1984) An autoradiographic study of neuronal development, vascularization and glial cell migration from hippocampal transplants labelled in intermediate explant culture. Neuroscience 12:513–530.

Lindsay, R.M., G. Raisman, and P.J. Seeley (1987) Neural tissue transplants: Studies using tissue culture manipulations, cell marking techniques and a plasma clot method to follow development of grafted neurons and glia. In H.H. Althaus, and W. Seifert (eds): NATO ASI Series H. Vol. 2: Glial-Neuronal Communication in Development and Regeneration. Heidelberg: Springer-Verlag, pp. 587–603.

Lund, R.D., F.-L.F. Chang, M.H. Hankin, and C.F. Lagenaur (1985) Use of a species-specific antibody for demonstrating mouse neurons transplanted to rat brains. Neurosci. Lett. 61:221–226.

Mason, D.W., H.M. Charlton, A. Jones, D.M. Parry, and S.J. Simmonds (1985) Immunology of allograft rejection im mammals. In A. Björklund and U. Stenevi (eds): Neural Grafting in the Mammalian CNS. Amsterdam: Elsevier, pp. 91–98.

Medawar, P.B. (1948) Immunity to homologous grafted skin. III. The fate of skin homografts transplanted to the brain, to subcutaneous tissue, and to the anterior chamber of the eye. Br. J. Exp. Pathol. 29:58–69.

Mudrick, L.A., K.G. Baimbridge, and J.J. Miller (1987) Fetal hippocampal cells transplanted into the ischemically damaged CA1 region demonstrate normal characteristics of adult CA1 cells. Am Soc Neurosci Abstr. 13:514.

Nieto-Sampedro, M., J.P. Kesslak, R. Gibbs, and C.W. Cotman (1987) Effects of conditioning lesions on transplant survival, connectivity, and function. In E.C. Azmitia and A. Björklund (eds): Cell and Tissue Transplantation into the Adult Brain. New York: The New York Academy of Sciences, pp. 108–118.

Nieto-Sampedro, M., M. Manthorpe, G. Barbin, S. Varon, and C.W. Cotman (1983) Injury-induced neuronotrophic activity in adult rat brain: Correlation with survival of delayed implants in the wound cavity. J. Neurosci. 3:2219–2229.

Nilsson, O.G., P. Brundin, H. Widner, R.E. Strecker, and A. Björklund (1988a) Human fetal basal forebrain neurons grafted to the denervated rat hippocampus produce an organotypic cholinergic reinnervation pattern. Brain Res. 456:193–198.

Nilsson, O.G., D.J. Clarke, P. Brundin, and A. Björklund (1988b) Comparison of growth and reinnervation properties of cholinergic neurons from different brain regions grafted to the hippocampus. J. Comp. Neurol. 268:204–222.

Olson, L., R. Freedman, Å. Seiger, and B. Hoffer (1977) Electrophysiology and cytology of hippocampal formation transplants in the anterior chamber of the eye. I. Intrinsic organization. Brain Res. 119:87–106.

Olson, L., Å. Seiger, and I. Strömberg (1983) Intraocular transplantation in rodents. A detailed account of the procedure and examples of its use in neurobiology with special reference to brain tissue grafting. In S. Fedoroff (ed): Advances in Cellular Neurobiology, Vol. 4. New York: Academic Press, pp. 407–442.

Olson, L., Å. Seiger, D. Tayler, R. Freedman, and B.J. Hoffer (1980) Conditions for adrenergic hyperinnervation in hippocampus: I. Histochemical evidence from intraocular double grafts. Exp. Brain Res. *39*:277–288.

Pulsinelli, W.A., and J.B. Brierley (1979) A new model of bilateral hemispheric ischemia in unanesthetized rat. Stroke *10*:267–272.

Raisman, G., and F.F. Ebner (1983) Mossy fibre projections into and out of hippocampal transplants. Neuroscience *9*:783–801.

Robain, O., G. Barbin, Y. Ben-Ari, F. Rozenberg, and A. Prochiantz (1987) GABAergic neurons of the hippocampus: Development in homotopic grafts and in dissociated cell cultures. Neuroscience *23*:73–86.

Segal, M., U. Stenevi, and A. Björklund (1981) Reformation in adult rats of functional septo-hippocampal connections by septal neurons regenerating across an embryonic hippocampal tissue bridge. Neurosci. Lett. *27*:7–12.

Sørensen, T., B. Finsen, and J. Zimmer (1987) Nerve connections between mouse and rat hippocampal brain tissue: Ultrastructural observations after intracerebral xenografting. Brain Res. *413*:392–397.

Sørensen, T., S. Jensen, A. Møller, and J. Zimmer (1986) Intracephalic transplants of freeze-stored rat hippocampal tissue. J. Comp. Neurol. *252*:468–482.

Sørensen, T., and J. Zimmer (1988a) Ultrastructural organization of normal and transplanted rat fascia dentata: I. A qualitative analysis of intracerebral and intraocular grafts. J. Comp. Neurol. *267*:15–42.

Sørensen, T., and J. Zimmer (1988b) Ultrastructural organization of normal and transplanted rat fascia dentata: II. A quantitative analysis of the synaptic organization of intracerebral and intraocular grafts. J. Comp. Neurol. *267*:43–54.

Stenevi, U., A. Björklund, and N.-A. Svendgaard (1976) Transplantation of central and peripheral monoamine neurons to the adult rat brain: Techniques and conditions for survival. Brain Res. *114*:1–20.

Sunde, N., S. Laurberg, and J. Zimmer (1984) Brain grafts can restore irradiation-damaged neuronal connections in newborn rats. Nature *310*:51–53.

Sunde, N., and J. Zimmer (1981a) Transplantation of central nervous tissue. An introduction with results and implications. Acta Neurol. Scand. *63*:323–335.

Sunde, N., and J. Zimmer (1981b) Dentate granule cells transplanted to hippocampal field CA1 form aberrant mossy fiber projection in rats. Neurosci. Lett. [Suppl.] *7*:S33.

Sunde, N.A., and J. Zimmer (1983) Cellular, histochemical and connective organization of the hippocampus and fascia dentata transplanted to different regions of immature and adult rat brains. Dev. Brain Res. *8*:165–191.

Sunde, N., J. Zimmer, and S. Laurberg (1985) Repair of neonatal irradiation-induced damage to the rat fascia dentata. Effects of delayed intracerebral transplantation. In A. Björklund, and V. Stenevi (eds): Neural Grafting in the Mammalian CNS. Amsterdam: Elsevier, pp. 301–308.

Taylor, D., R. Freedman, Å. Seiger, L. Olson, and B.J. Hoffer (1980) Conditions for adrenergic hyperinnervation in hippocampus: II. Electrophysiological evidence from intraocular double grafts. Exp. Brain Res. *39*:289–299.

Taylor, D., Å. Seiger, R. Freedman, L. Olson, and B. Hoffer (1978) Electrophysiological analysis of reinnervation of transplants in the anterior chamber of the eye by the autonomic ground plexus of the iris. Proc. Natl. Acad. Sci. U.S.A. *75*:1009–1012.

Tønder, N., F.B. Gaarskjaer, N.A. Sunde, and J. Zimmer (1986) Neonatal hippocampal neurons, retrogradely labeled with Granular Blue, survive intracerebral grafting and explantation to tissue culture. Exp. Brain Res. *65*:213–218.

Tønder, N., J.C. Sørensen, E. Bakkum, E. Danielsen, and J. Zimmer (1988) Hippocampal neurons grafted to newborn rats estalish efferent commissural connections. Exp. Brain Res. 72:577–583.

Tønder, N., T. Sørensen, and J. Zimmer (1989) Enhanced host perforant path innervation of neonatal dentate tissue after grafting to axon sparing, ibotenic acid lesions in adult rats. Exp. Brain Res. (in press).

Tønder, N., J. Zimmer, M.B. Jørgensen, F.F. Johansen, and N.H. Diemer (1987) Neuronal transplantation to ischemic lesions in the adult rat hippocampus. Neuroscience [Suppl.] 22:S263.

Vinogradova, O.S., A.G. Bragin, and V.F. Kitchigina (1985) Spontaneous and evoked activity of neurons in intrabrain allo- and xenografts of the hippocampus and septum. In: A. Björklund and U. Stenevi (eds): Neural Grafting in the Mammalian CNS. Amsterdam Elsevier, pp. 409–419.

Wendt, J.S., G.E. Fagg, and C.W. Cotman (1983) Regeneration of rat hippocampal fimbria fibers after fimbria transection and peripheral nerve or fetal hippocampal implantation. Exp. Neurol 79:452–461.

Woodruff, M.L., R.H. Baisden, D.L. Whittington, and A.E. Benson (1987) Embryonic hippocampal grafts ameliorate the deficit in DRL acquisition produced by hippocampectomy. Brain Res. 408:97–117.

Woodward, D., B. Hoffer, L. Olson, and Å. Seiger (1977) Intrinsic and extrinsic determinants of dendritic development as revealed by Golgi studies of cerebellar and hippocampal transplants in oculo. Exp. Neurol. 57:984–998.

Zhou, C.-F., G. Raisman, and R.J. Morris (1985) Specific patterns of fibre outgrowth from transplants to host mice hippocampi, shown immunohistochemically by the use of allelic forms of Thy-1. Neuroscience 16:819–833.

Zimmer, J. (1978) Development of the hippocampus and fascia dentata: Morphological and histochemical aspects. Prog. Brain Res. 48:289–304.

Zimmer, J., B. Finsen, T. Sørensen, and P.H. Poulsen (1988a) Xenografts of mouse hippocampal tissue. Exchange of laminar and neuropeptide specific nerve connections with the host rat brain. Brain Res. Bull. 20:369–379.

Zimmer, J., B. Finsen, T. Sørensen, and P.H. Poulsen (1988b) Xenografts of mouse hippocampal tissue. Formation of nerve connections between the graft fascia dentata and the host rat brain. Prog. Brain Res. 78:271–280.

Zimmer, J., B. Finsen, T. Sørensen, and N. Sunde (1987) Hippocampal transplants: Synaptic organization, their use in repair of neuronal circuits and mouse to rat xenografting. In H.H. Althaus and W. Seifert (eds): NATO ASI Series H, Vol. 2: Glial-Neuronal Communication in Development and Regeneration. Heidelberg: Springer-Verlag, pp. 547–564.

Zimmer, J., B. Finsen, T. Sørensen, N.A. Sunde, and P.H. Poulsen (1988c) Brain grafts: A survey with examples of repair and xenografting of hippocampal tissue. In F. Cohadon and J. Lobo Antunes (eds): Recovery of Function in the Nervous System. Fidia Research Series, 13:161–184.

Zimmer, J., S. Laurberg, and N. Sunde (1986) Non-cholinergic afferents determine the distribution of the cholinergic septohippocampal projection: A study of the AChE staining pattern in the rat fascia dentata and hippocampus after lesions, X-irradiation, and intracerebral grafting. Exp. Brain Res. 64:158–168.

Zimmer, J., and N. Sunde (1984) Neuropeptides and astroglia in intracerebral hippocampal transplants: An immunohistochemical study in the rat. J. Comp. Neurol. 227:331–347.

Zimmer, J., N. Sunde, and S. Laurberg (1983) Neuroanatomical aspects of normal and transplanted hippocampal tissue. In Seifert, W. (ed): Neurobiology of the Hippocampus. London: Academic Press, pp. 39–64.

Zimmer, J., N. Sunde, and T. Sørensen (1985a) Reorganization and restoration of central nervous connections after injury: A lesion and transplant study of the rat hippocampus. In B.E. Will, P. Schmitt, and J.C. Dalrymple-Alford (eds): Brain Plasticity, Learning, and Memory. New York: Plenum Publishing Corporation, pp. 505–518.

Zimmer, J., N. Sunde, T. Sørensen, S. Jensen, A.G. Møller, and B.H. Gähwiler (1985b) The hippocampus and fascia dentata. An anatomical study of intracerebral transplants and intraocular and in vitro cultures. In A. Björklund and U. Stenevi (eds): Neural Grafting in the Mammalian CNS. Amsterdam: Elsevier, pp. 285–299.

The Hippocampus—New Vistas, pages 287–305

18
Electrophysiological and Morphological Characterization of Hippocampal Interneurons

JEAN-CLAUDE LACAILLE, DENNIS D. KUNKEL, AND
PHILIP A. SCHWARTZKROIN

*Centre de Recherche en Sciences Neurologiques, Département de
Physiologie, Université de Montréal, Montréal, Québec, Canada (J.-C.L.);
Departments of Neurological Surgery (D.D.K., P.A.S.) and Physiology &
Biophysics (P.A.S.), University of Washington, Seattle, Washington*

INTRODUCTION

The trisynaptic circuit of the dentate gyrus and hippocampus is composed of three principal cell types: dentate granule cells, large pyramidal cells of the CA3 region, and smaller pyramidal cells of the CA1 region (Ramón y Cajal, 1911; Lorente de Nó, 1934). Their circuitry, arranged in a lamellar orientation transverse to the septotemporal axis, has been studied in detail by many investigators (Ramón y Cajal, 1911; Lorente de Nó, 1934; Andersen and Lømo, 1966; Andersen et al., 1971, 1973). In addition to these principal cells, many other cell types have been described morphologically in the dentate gyrus and hippocampus (Ramón y Cajal, 1911; Lorente de Nó, 1934; Amaral, 1978; Somogyi et al., 1983). Most of these neurons have axons that arborize locally and are called *local circuit neurons* or *interneurons*. Recent studies have indicated that the axons of some "interneurons" also project to extrahippocampal areas (e.g. CA1 interneuron projections to septal areas, Chronister and DeFrance, 1979; Schwerdtfeger and Buhl, 1986; nucleus accumbens, Totterdell and Hayes, 1987; retrosplenial cortex, van Groen and Wyss, personal communication; and contralateral hippocampus, Schwerdtfeger and Buhl, 1986).

Although hippocampal interneurons have been well described anatomically (see, e.g. Köhler and Chan-Palay, Chapter 12, and Sloviter, Chapter 28, both this volume), until recently very little was known of their physiology and of

Abbreviations: AHP, afterhyperpolarization; B cell, basket cell; CA1, pyramidal cell region CA (cornu Ammonis) 1 of hippocampus; CA3, pyramidal cell region CA (cornu Ammonis) 3 of hippocampus; EM, electron microscopy; EPSP, excitatory postsynaptic potential; G cell, granule cell; GABA, γ-aminobutyric acid; GAD, glutamic acid decarboxylase; HRP, horseradish peroxidase; IPSP, inhibitory postsynaptic potential; L-M cell, lacunosum-moleculare interneuron; O/A cell, oriens/alveus interneuron; P cell, pyramidal cell; SRIF, somatotropin release inhibiting factor (somatostatin).

their influence on principal cells. With the hippocampal slice preparation, it has been possible to obtain intracellular recordings from hippocampal interneurons and to label them with intracellular markers. Using this combined approach, we have identified three types of interneurons in the CA1 region: basket (B) cells, oriens/alveus (O/A) interneurons, and lacunosum-moleculare (L-M) interneurons. In this chapter, we will review our studies and suggest possible roles for these interneurons in hippocampal function. As summarized in the simplified diagram of Figure 1, our results indicate that these cells are all inhibitory interneurons. Basket cells and O/A interneurons mediate feed-forward *and* feedback inhibition onto CA1 pyramidal cells, whereas L-M interneurons appear to mediate *only* feed-forward inhibition (Fig. 1).

BASKET CELLS
Anatomical and Physiological Characterization

Many types of basket cells—so called because of the "basket-like" appearance of their axonal plexus around the pyramidal cell somata in stratum pyramidale—have been previously described (Ramón y Cajal, 1911; Lorente de Nó, 1934). Intracellular recordings and subsequent labeling have been obtained from interneurons situated near the border of strata pyramidale and oriens (Schwartzkroin and Mathers, 1978; Knowles and Schwartzkroin, 1980;

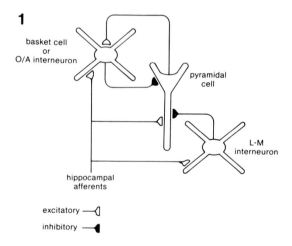

Fig. 1. Simplified local circuit diagram. Hippocampal afferents make excitatory synapses on pyramidal *and* nonpyramidal cell types, resulting in feed-forward inhibition of pyramidal cells. Pyramidal cells make excitatory synapses on basket and O/A interneurons, but not on L-M interneurons. In turn, basket cells and O/A interneurons make inhibitory connections on pyramidal cells, completing a recurrent (feedback) inhibitory loop. L-M interneurons also form inhibitory synapses on pyramidal cells. Basket cells and O/A interneurons mediate feed-forward *and* feedback inhibition; L-M interneurons mediate *solely* feed-forward inhibition of pyramidal cells.

Schwartzkroin and Kunkel, 1985). As illustrated in Figure 2, these interneurons resemble the "pyramidal basket cells" of Ramón y Cajal (1911) and Lorente de Nó (1934). From the large soma (approximately 45 μm in diameter), basal dendrites descend into s. oriens and apical dendrites ascend through pyramidale and branch within strata radiatum and lacunosum-moleculare. Their axons, seen in HRP-injected cells or in Golgi preparations, project laterally for several hundred micra, giving off many collaterals that enter s. pyramidale and form basket-like plexes around pyramidal cell somata (Ramón y Cajal, 1911; Lorente de Nó, 1934; Schwartzkroin and Mathers, 1978; Schwartzkroin and Kunkel, 1985). At the electron microscopic level, the basket cell soma contains a convoluted nucleus, dense endoplasmic reticulum, and numerous organelles (Tömböl et al., 1979; Schwartzkroin and Kunkel, 1985; Schlander and Frotscher, 1986). Their dendrites are aspinous (or sparsely spiny), appear beaded (have periodic swellings), and receive many synaptic contacts (primarily asymmetric). The axonal processes also display periodic enlargements (varicosities) and terminate in symmetric synaptic contacts. Most of these interneurons are thought to be GABAergic, since they appear similar to neurons that are immunoreactive for GABA (Gamrani et al., 1986) or glutamic acid decarboxylase (GAD) (Ribak et al., 1978; Kunkel et al., 1986).

In intracellular recordings, basket cells display properties that clearly distinguish them from pyramidal cells (Schwartzkroin and Mathers, 1978; Knowles and Schwartzkroin, 1980; Ashwood et al., 1984; Schwartzkroin and Kunkel, 1985; Kawaguchi and Hama, 1987a). As illustrated in Figure 3, these interneurons have very brief action potentials (0.8 ms), a short time constant (approximately 3 ms), and a large spike afterhyperpolarization (5–10 mV, 10–30 ms). They respond to somatic depolarization with a nondecrementing train of action potentials, which is followed by a large, long-lasting afterhyperpolarization (100–800 msec). At resting potential, basket cells spontaneously fire action potentials at a high rate and display a constant barrage of excitatory postsynaptic potentials (EPSPs).

Afferents

Basket cells are under synaptic control from many sources. In intracellular recordings (Fig. 3), stimulation of s. radiatum (Schaffer collaterals and commissural fibers) evokes an EPSP followed by an inhibitory postsynaptic potential (IPSP) (Schwartzkroin and Mathers, 1978; Ashwood et al., 1984). Interneuron EPSPs have a faster rise time than pyramidal cell EPSPs evoked from the same stimulation sites. With increasing stimulus intensity, the EPSP usually triggers a burst of action potentials. Similar synaptic responses, but no antidromic spike, can be evoked from stimulation of the alveus. Degeneration/EM studies have shown that basket cells receive synaptic contacts from commissural fibers originating in contralateral hippocampus (Frotscher and Zimmer, 1983; Schwartzkroin and Kunkel, 1985) and that these contacts are of the asymmetic type. These results support the view that basket cells can be activated by Schaffer collaterals and by commissural fibers, as previously suggested from extracellular studies (Ashwood et al., 1984; Buzsáki and Ei-

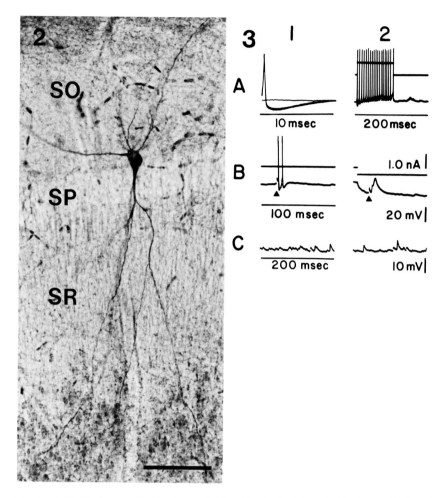

Fig. 2. HRP-filled pyramidal basket cell. Physiologically identified basket cell labeled with HRP. Soma is located at the strata oriens–pyramidale border; basal dendrites extend into stratum oriens (SO) and apical dendrites into s. radiatum (SR). SP, stratum pyramidale. Scale bar = 100 μm. (Reproduced from Schwartzkroin and Kunkel, 1985, with permission of the publisher.)

Fig. 3. Basket cell physiological properties. **A:** 1, short duration action potential and large afterhyperpolarization; 2, nonaccommodating train of action potentials evoked by a depolarizing pulse. **B:** 1, spikes evoked by orthodromic stimulation (triangle); 2, hyperpolarization uncovers the underlying EPSP. **C:** Examples of spontaneous synaptic potentials. (Reproduced from Schwartzkroin and Mathers, 1978, with permission of the publisher.)

delberg, 1982). Since basket cells are excited by these inputs at a shorter latency than are pyramidal cells, they must be activated in a "feed-forward" manner with respect to pyramidal cells.

Local Circuit Synaptic Interactions

Physiological and anatomical approaches have been used to show local synaptic connections of basket cells. In simultaneous intracellular recordings obtained from interneuron–pyramidal cells pairs, synaptic interactions were examined by stimulating one cell (intracellularly) and examining the presence of synaptic potentials in the other (Knowles and Schwartzkroin, 1980). Pyramidal cells were found to excite basket cells and basket cells to inhibit pyramidal cells: During a spike train evoked intracellularly in the interneuron, the pyramidal cell membrane gradually hyperpolarized; when a burst of spikes was evoked in the pyramidal cell, EPSPs were elicited in the interneuron. Occasionally, reciprocal synaptic connections were found between pyramidal and basket cells of a given pair, with the pyramidal cell always exciting the basket cell and the basket cell always inhibiting the pyramidal cell. These results demonstrate directly a pathway for feedback (recurrent) inhibition of interneurons onto pyramidal cells.

Individual basket cells, which had been physiologically identified, were injected with HRP for further morphological characterization at the EM level (Schwartzkroin and Kunkel, 1985). HRP-filled processes were found making synaptic contacts primarily with pyramidal cell somata, but also on proximal and basal pyramidal cell dendrites. HRP-filled terminals were also found in contact with interneuron-like dendritic processes. These synapses, although partly obscured by HRP dense reaction product in the presynaptic bouton, consistently appeared to be of the symmetric type. These findings further support the view that basket cells mediate inhibition onto pyramidal cells and that interneurons may inhibit other interneurons.

O/A INTERNEURONS
Anatomical and Physiological Characterization

Intracellular recordings and subsequent intracellular labeling have been obtained from interneurons at the s. oriens–alveus border (Lacaille et al., 1987). Although cells with different morphologies were occasionally seen, the majority were similar to Ramón y Cajal's cells (1911) with horizontal axon. Somata were multipolar, 20–30 μm in diameter, and located at the oriens–alveus border (Fig. 4). Most dendrites coursed parallel to the alveus; in many cells, one or two dendrites turned abruptly and ascended through strata oriens, pyramidale, and radiatum. The axon branched profusely in s. oriens and pyramidale. At the electron microscopic level, O/A interneurons have an ultrastructure similar to that of basket cells (Tombӧl et al., 1979; Schlander and Frotscher, 1986; Totterdell and Hayes, 1987; Kunkel and Schwartzkroin, 1988). Like those of the basket cell, their dendrites lack spines, show periodic swellings, and receive many synaptic contacts; their axons are varicose and end in symmetric synaptic contacts. O/A interneurons have a morphology and distribution similar to those

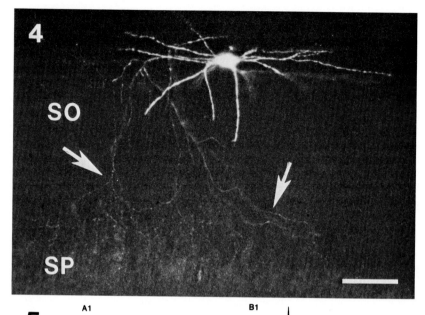

4

SO

SP

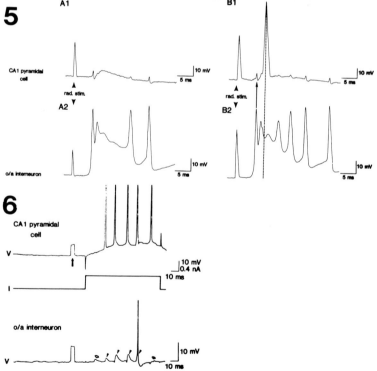

5

A1

CA1 pyramidal
cell

rad. stim.

A2

o/a interneuron

10 mV
5 ms

10 mV
5 ms

B1

rad. stim.

B2

10 mV
5 ms

10 mV
5 ms

6

CA1 pyramidal
cell

V

I

10 mV
0.4 nA

10 ms

o/a interneuron

V

10 mV
10 ms

of nonpyramidal cells which show GABA-like immunoreactivity (Gamrani et al., 1986) or SRIF (somatotropin release inhibiting factor)-like immunoreactivity (Köhler and Chan-Palay, 1982; Morrison et al., 1982; Roberts et al., 1984; Bakst et al., 1985; Obata-Tsuto, 1987); these cells appear to colocalize GABA and SRIF (Somogyi et al., 1984).

O/A interneuron electrophysiological properties are quite similar to those of basket cells (Lacaille et al., 1987): The action potentials are brief (approx. 1 ms) and of relatively small amplitude (43 mV); input resistance is high (42 megohms); the time constant is fast (5.6 ms); a large afterhyperpolarization (AHP) follows individual spikes; spontaneous firing rate is high (27 Hz); the cells receive a constant barrage of EPSPs; and they fire in nonaccommodating trains of action potentials in response to intracellular depolarizing current pulses. In some O/A interneurons, a slow AHP is seen following a burst of action potentials.

Afferents

Electrical stimulation of s. radiatum or of the alveus evokes large-amplitude EPSPs in O/A interneurons, which usually trigger a burst of action potentials (Lacaille et al., 1987). The source of the alvear fibers that excite O/A (and basket) interneurons is unknown. Since commissural fibers and Schaffer collaterals course in s. radiatum, it is likely that O/A interneurons receive excitatory synapses from ipsilateral and contralateral CA3 pyramidal cells. As shown in Figure 5, these excitatory synaptic responses are more powerful in O/A inter-

---

Fig. 4. Physiologically identified O/A interneuron subsequently labeled with Lucifer yellow. Soma is at the s. oriens–alveus border. Most dendrites are oriented parallel to the alveus, but three large dendrites ascend through s. pyramidale (SP) toward s. lacunosum-moleculare. Thin axon (arrows) can be seen in the background, arborizing extensively in s. oriens (SO) and pyramidale. Scale bar = 100 μm. (Reproduced from Lacaille et al., 1987, with permission of the publisher.)

Fig. 5. Feed-forward synaptic activation. Simultaneous intracellular recordings from CA1 pyramidal cell and O/A interneuron. Stimulation of s. radiatum (arrowheads) elicited an EPSP–IPSP in the pyramidal cell (A1) and a large EPSP with multiple spikes in the interneuron (A2). Higher intensity stimulation triggered an action potential in the pyramidal cell (B1) and more action potentials in the interneuron (B2). Initial action potential discharge in the interneuron preceded the pyramidal cell action potential by 2.0 ms (cf. B1 and B2). (Reproduced from Lacaille et al., 1987, with permission of the publisher.)

Fig. 6. Excitation of O/A interneuron by pyramidal cell. Simultaneous intracellular recordings were obtained from a CA1 pyramidal cell and an O/A interneuron. A train of action potentials was evoked in the pyramidal cell by an intracellular depolarizing pulse. In the interneuron, unitary EPSPs (arrowheads) were elicited by the first four pyramidal cell action potentials. The fourth EPSP reached threshold and evoked an action potential, but the fifth pyramidal action potential failed to evoke a response (black arrow) in the interneuron. A spontaneous EPSP (open arrow) preceded this activity. (Reproduced from Lacaille et al., 1987, with permission of the publisher.)

neurons than in pyramidal cells (i.e., O/A interneurons have a lower threshold) and trigger action potential discharge at shorter latency. This result indicates that O/A interneurons are excited in a feed-forward manner with respect to pyramidal cells.

Local Circuit Synaptic Interactions

Simultaneous intracellular recordings and HRP injection with EM analysis were used to uncover the local synaptic interactions of O/A interneurons (Lacaille et al., 1987). In paired recordings, intracellular stimulation of CA1 pyramidal cells evoked unitary EPSPs in O/A interneurons (Fig. 6). These EPSPs were of sufficient amplitude (2.16 mV mean peak amplitude) to evoke action potentials in the O/A interneuron (with a probability of 0.66). Mean latency from the presynaptic action potential to unitary EPSP peak was 3.8 ms, sufficiently short to be consistent with monosynaptic transmission.

Synaptic connections from O/A interneurons to pyramidal cells were seen infrequently, but when present, O/A interneurons were found to inhibit pyramidal cells. The inhibition was similar to the slowly developing hyperpolarization characteristic of basket cell-evoked inhibition of pyramidal cells. Although this inhibition contrasts markedly with the sharply rising inhibitory events found in the CA3 region (Miles and Wong, 1984), the hyperpolarization was sufficient to delay or block CA1 pyramidal cell action potentials evoked at rheobase. Reciprocal interaction within a pair—the pyramidal cell exciting the interneuron and the interneuron inhibiting the pyramidal cell—has shown directly the existence of a recurrent (feedback) inhibitory loop. O/A interneurons were also found to inhibit presumed basket cell interneurons located in s. pyramidale.

Ultrastructural evidence suggested that O/A interneurons inhibit pyramidal and nonpyramidal cells (Lacaille et al., 1987). Following HRP injection in a physiologically identified O/A interneuron and EM processing, O/A interneuron synaptic contacts (of the symmetric type) were seen onto both pyramidal and nonpyramidal cells. Symmetric contacts (characteristic of inhibitory synapses) were found on pyramidal cell proximal dendrites (most often basal but also apical), somata, and initial segments. An HRP-filled O/A interneuron axon also made symmetric synaptic contacts with aspinous dendritic processes, presumably of other interneurons.

L-M INTERNEURONS
Anatomical and Physiological Characterization

Interneurons at the border between s. lacunosum-moleculare and s. radiatum were penetrated intracellularly, characterized physiologically, and subsequently labeled (Kawaguchi and Hama, 1987a; Lacaille and Schwartzkroin, 1988a,b; for labeling in the CA3 region, see Misgeld and Frotscher, 1986). From the morphology of their somata (fusiform and multipolar) and dendrites, L-M interneurons appear generally similar to stellate cells of s. lacunosum described by Ramón y Cajal (1911) and Lorente de Nó (1934) (Fig. 7). Extensive dendritic and axonal projections have been found (Lacaille and Schwartzkroin, 1988a;

Kunkel et al., 1988), with dendritic trees spanning two-thirds of the CA1 region and part of the dentate gyrus. The dendrites were mostly smooth and beaded, and radiated out from the soma along s. lacunosum-moleculare. Some dendrites projected into s. radiatum, where they branched, or, occasionally, continued across s. pyramidale and into s. oriens. Other dendrites ascended into s. lacunosum-moleculare and crossed the hippocampal fissure into the dentate gyrus molecular layer. The axon usually emerged from a primary dendrite in s. lacunosum-moleculare. It was varicose and often projected millimeters along the L-M layer. The axon also branched almost immediately and ramified in s. radiatum; some axonal processes reached as far as s. pyramidale and s. oriens. Axonal projections were not restricted to the CA1 region, for some axon collaterals ascended into s. lacunosum-moleculare, crossed the hippocampal fissure, and coursed into the molecular layer of the dentate gyrus. At the ultrastructural level, L-M interneurons appeared similar to other nonpyramidal cells (Kunkel et al., 1988) (convoluted nucleus, dense cytoplasmic organelles); many synaptic contacts were found on their aspinous dendrites.

Intracellular recordings from L-M interneurons revealed distinctive membrane properties (Kawaguchi and Hama, 1987a; Lacaille and Schwartzkroin, 1988a,b). Similar to other interneurons and in contrast to pyramidal cells, their input resistance was high (64 megohms), a prominent afterhyperpolarization followed each action potential, and there was little frequency accommodation during depolarizing current pulses. Like pyramidal cells, action potential amplitude was large (60 mV), action potential duration long (2.0 ms), time constant relatively slow (8.6 ms), spontaneous firing absent or very low, and little spontaneous synaptic activity. In contrast to CA1 pyramidal cells, basket cells, and O/A interneurons, anodal break excitation was prominent in L-M interneurons and their mode of firing changed from "sustained" to "burst" type with hyperpolarization of the membrane.

Afferents

Both excitatory and inhibitory afferents impinge on L-M interneurons, with EPSPs and IPSPs evoked from stimulation of major hippocampal fiber pathways (Lacaille and Schwartzkroin, 1988a,b). As with basket and O/A interneurons, the synaptic excitation of L-M interneurons is more rapid than the excitation of pyramidal cells, resulting in feed-forward activation (Lacaille and Schwartzkroin, 1988b). Additionally, and consistent with anatomical observations of L-M interneuron dendrites in the dentate gyrus, stimulation of the dentate gyrus molecular layer evokes an EPSP in L-M interneurons. The projections of excitatory and inhibitory afferent fibers have, however, different orientations. Excitatory afferent fibers run transverse to the septotemporal axis of the hippocampus, whereas inhibitory afferents run primarily in a longitudinal orientation (Lacaille and Schwartzkroin, 1988a). Thus, excitatory afferents appear to have a lamellar, and inhibitory afferents an interlamellar, trajectory.

The origin of afferent fibers onto L-M interneurons was assessed with selective lesions and subsequent EM examination of degenerating synaptic contacts (Kunkel et al., 1988). Degenerating synaptic contacts were found on L-

M interneuron somata and primary dendrites (Fig. 8) following selective lesions of ipsilateral Schaffer collaterals, commissural fibers, or ipsilateral entorhinal cortex. Ultrastructurally, these degenerating synaptic contacts were of the asymmetric type, typical of excitatory synapses. The origin of the inhibitory afferents remains unclear. However, since interneuron-to-interneuron inhibition has been observed in CA1 (Lacaille et al., 1987; Lacaille and Schwartzkroin, 1988b), and since GAD-positive symmetric synaptic contacts have been observed on GAD-positive CA3 L-M interneurons (Misgeld and Frotscher, 1986), the inhibition onto CA1 L-M interneurons is likely to arise from other CA1 inhibitory interneurons.

It is also interesting to note that three other groups of extrahippocampal afferents innervate s. lacunosum-moleculare densely: cholinergic afferents from septum (Matthews et al., 1987), serotonergic afferents from raphe (Zhou and Azmitia, 1986), and noradrenergic afferents from locus coeruleus (Loy et al., 1980). Although it has not yet been demonstrated at the ultrastructural level whether these afferents make contact specifically with L-M interneurons, they are strategically placed to do so.

Local Circuit Synaptic Interactions

In simultaneous intracellular recordings of L-M interneurons and CA1 pyramidal cells, synaptic connections between these cells were demonstrated (Lacaille and Schwartzkroin, 1988b). Pyramidal cells were never seen to excite or inhibit L-M interneurons, but L-M interneurons were found to inhibit pyramidal cells. The hyperpolarizing inhibition appeared similar in both intrasomatic and intradendritic penetrations of pyramidal cells and was sufficient to block postsynaptic spikes evoked at rheobase in the pyramidal cell (Fig. 9). The IPSPs evoked in pyramidal cell dendrites by L-M stimulation were sensitive to variations in membrane potential, with IPSP amplitude increasing with depolarization of the pyramidal cell membrane. The hyperpolarization decreased with membrane hyperpolarization, and it was flat at a mean membrane potential of -74 mV; further hyperpolarization did not reverse the response. In simultaneous recordings of L-M interneurons and s. pyramidale "basket cell" interneurons, L-M interneurons inhibited s. pyramidale interneurons, but no synaptic connections were found in the reverse direction.

Morphological observations also suggested an inhibitory function for L-M interneurons (Kunkel et al., 1988). Following HRP injection into physiologically identified L-M interneuron and EM analysis, the L-M interneuron axon was seen making synaptic contacts with pyramidal cells (Fig. 10) and interneurons (Fig. 11) of the CA1 region. These axodendritic synaptic contacts were found in strata lacunosum-moleculare and radiatum and were of the symmetric type. The HRP-filled axon also crossed the hippocampal fissure, coursed in s. moleculare of the dentate gyrus, and made axodendritic symmetric synapses onto granule cells and interneurons in the middle and outer thirds of s. moleculare. These anatomical results suggest that L-M interneurons mediate inhibition in the dentate gyrus as well as in CA1 neurons.

LOCAL CIRCUITRY

Our current knowledge of hippocampal CA1 local circuitry is summarized in Figure 12. Since L-M interneuron processes also penetrate the dentate gyrus, a granule cell and part of the dentate gyrus are included in the diagram. A pyramidal cell (P), a pyramidal basket cell (B), an oriens/alveus interneuron (O/A), a lacunosum-moleculare interneuron (L-M), and a granule cell (G) are illustrated. For simplicity, the origin of individual afferents is not identified.

Afferent fibers make excitatory synapses with O/A, P, B, and L-M cells in strata lacunosum-moleculare (synapses t, u, v, w, respectively), radiatum (synapses g, a, f, l), and oriens (synapses m, n, o, p). The greater efficacy of these synapses on interneurons results in earlier excitation of O/A, B, and L-M interneurons with respect to pyramidal cells. Afferents from the alveus make excitatory synapses on O/A, B, and L-M cells (synapses i, h, r, respectively). Afferents in s. moleculare of dentate gyrus make excitatory synapses on G cells and L-M interneurons (synapses aa and bb).

Pyramidal cells make excitatory synapses on B and O/A interneurons (synapses b and c). In turn, basket cells make inhibitory synapses on pyramidal cell somata (synapse d) and possibly on O/A and L-M interneurons (synapses e and s). O/A interneurons make inhibitory synapses onto P cell somata and B cells (synapses j and k, respectively) and possibly on L-M interneurons (synapse q). L-M interneurons make inhibitory synapses on P cell dendrites (synapse x), on s. pyramidale interneurons (possibly B cells, synapse y), and possibly on O/A interneurons (synapse z). L-M interneurons also make inhibitory synapses on G cells (synapse cc) and interneurons (data not shown) of dentate gyrus.

DISCUSSION AND PERSPECTIVES

It is evident from our summary diagram that the local circuitry of the hippocampus is quite complex, with numerous interactions between interneurons and pyramidal cells and between interneurons and interneurons. The circuitry is, in reality, much more complex than represented here, since many types of interneurons, which have been described morphologically (e.g. "chandelier" cells of Somogyi et al., 1983), have not been included.

For the specific types of interneurons that have been identified, and their connections within the local circuitry described, there appear to be two classes: those mediating feed-forward *and* feedback inhibition of pyramidal cells (O/A interneurons and basket cells) and those mediating *solely* feed-forward inhibition (L-M interneurons). Intrinsic membrane properties of these interneurons segregate them in the same way; O/A interneurons and basket cells have similar intrinsic properties, whereas L-M interneurons have quite distinctive membrane properties. The time course of the interneuron-mediated IPSPs in pyramidal cells also suggests such a division; O/A interneuron- and basket cell-evoked IPSPs decay more rapidly than L-M interneuron-evoked IPSPs (25–40 ms vs. 40–150 ms, respectively). O/A and basket cell activation by pyramidal cells, the more rapid decay of their IPSPs, and the predominance of their ax-

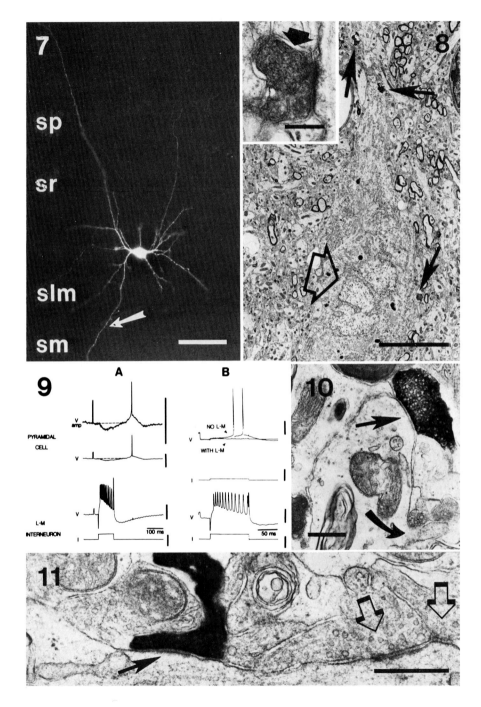

7

sp

sr

slm

sm

8

9

A   B

PYRAMIDAL
CELL

NO L-M

WITH L-M

L-M
INTERNEURON

100 ms   50 ms

10

11

osomatic synapses suggest that these interneurons mediate the early IPSP component seen in pyramidal cells (Kandel et al., 1961; Andersen et al., 1964a,b; Newberry and Nicoll, 1985), associated most closely with recurrent inhibition. Characteristics of L-M interneuron IPSPs (slow kinetics and negative equilibrium potential resistant to current manipulation) and the predominance of L-M synapses on pyramidal cell dendrites suggest that L-M interneurons mediate the late IPSP of CA1 pyramidal cells (Alger and Nicoll, 1982a,b; Alger, 1984; Newberry and Nicoll, 1985). Finally, the extent of their cellular processes set apart basket and O/A interneurons from L-M interneurons. Basket cell and O/A interneuron processes are confined to the CA1 region, but L-M interneuron dendrites and axons ramify in both CA1 and dentate gyrus. Thus, whereas the inhibitory influence of basket and O/A interneurons is confined to the CA1 region, L-M interneuron influence is widespread, perhaps helping to synchronize or phase lock different cell populations.

Additional levels of complexity in these local circuits appear when one considers the variety of putative neurotransmitters in identified interneurons (e.g.

Fig. 7. Physiologically identified L-M interneuron filled with Lucifer yellow. Soma is located in s. lacunosum-moleculare (slm) near s. radiatum (sr). Dendrites extend into s. radiatum and even sometimes into strata pyramidale (sp) and oriens. Other dendrites ascend into lacunosum-moleculare, cross the hippocampal fissure, and project (arrow) into s. moleculare (sm) of the dentate gyrus. The axon emerged from a dendrite and projected into strata lacunosum-moleculare and radiatum. Scale bar = 100 μm. (Reproduced from Lacaille and Schwartzkroin, 1988a, with permission of the publisher.)

Fig. 8. Low-power electron micrograph of L-M interneuron with degenerating synaptic contacts (black arrows) on its soma and primary dendrite following lesion of commissural fibers. This interneuron is in s. lacunosum-moleculare near the s. radiatum border. Its nucleus (open arrow) is convoluted, and numerous organelles fill the cytoplasm. Bar = 10 μm. Inset: Higher power micrograph of one of the degenerating synaptic contacts showing typical asymmetric profile. Bar = 0.25 μm. (Reproduced from Kunkel et al., 1988, with permission of the publisher.)

Fig. 9. Inhibition of a pyramidal cell by an L-M interneuron. **A:** Stimulation of the interneuron (bottom traces) evoked a hyperpolarization of the pyramidal cell (high gain, top trace; low gain, bottom trace). **B:** Rheobasic stimulation of the pyramidal cell alone evoked two spikes. The same rheobasic stimulation did not evoke spikes when given concurrently with L-M interneuron stimulation. (Reproduced from Lacaille and Schwartzkroin, 1988b, with permission of the publisher.)

Fig. 10. Synaptic contact of HRP-filled L-M interneuron axon on a presumed pyramidal cell dendrite (straight arrow) in s. lacunosum-moleculare (a spine can be seen emerging from the dendrite at the curved arrow). A thin, even postsynaptic membrane specialization indicates this contact is of the symmetric type. Bar = 0.5 μm. (Reproduced from Kunkel et al., 1988, with permission of the publisher.)

Fig. 11. HRP-filled L-M interneuron synaptic contact (black arrow) on a nonpyramidal dendrite in s. radiatum. Typical of nonpyramidal dendrites, this dendrite received numerous shaft synapses (open arrows) and was aspinous. Bar = 0.5 μm. (Reproduced from Kunkel et al., 1988, with permission of the publisher.)

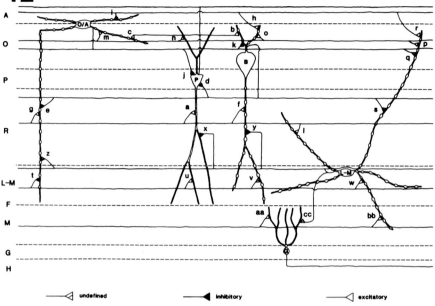

Fig. 12. Summary local circuit diagram of the CA1 region. A, alveus; O, oriens; P, pyramidale; R, radiatum; L-M, lacunosum-moleculare; F, hippocampal fissure. Dentate gyrus upper blade: M, moleculare; G, granular layer; H, hilus. Excitatory (open) and inhibitory (filled) synapses have been demonstrated physiologically; undefined synapses (striped) have not been demonstrated physiologically but have been identified morphologically. See text for further details. (Reproduced from Lacaille and Schwartzkroin, 1988b, with permission of the publisher.)

see Sloviter, Chapter 28, this volume) and the special effects of afferents on interneurons; for example 1) although most of the interneurons in CA1 are GABAergic (and presumably mediate inhibition by GABA release), a number of these cells colocalize other substances, particularly peptides (Somogyi et al., 1984). We know little about conditions under which these peptides are released, about their effects on pyramidal cells, or about their interactions with GABA. 2) Afferent fibers synapsing in CA1 may have quite different effects on interneurons and pyramidal cells. Enkephalin-induced excitation in the CA1 region is due to inhibition of interneurons (Madison and Nicoll, 1988), not excitation of pyramidal cells. Early inhibitory effects of ACh application to CA1 is mediated by fast ACh excitation of interneurons (Benardo and Prince, 1982).

Interneuron features and local circuit connectivities in other hippocampal subregions may be significantly different from the features described here for

CA1. For example, the interneuron–pyramidal cell inhibitory interaction described by Miles and Wong (1984) is much more potent than any interaction recorded in CA1. However, Misgeld and Frotscher (1986) and Kawaguchi and Hama (1987b) have described CA3 interneuron types that are parallel to the L-M and basket cell–O/A interneurons of CA1, suggesting some "conservation" of local circuit interactions in the pyramidal cell regions of hippocampus. The dentate gyrus presents an entirely new array of local circuit neurons—mossy cells, SRIF neurons—whose interactions with the granule cells are still to be investigated.

The goal of our studies of local circuitry in hippocampus is twofold: to understand how the interneuronal connections are involved in information processing in normal hippocampus and to assess their sensitivities to noxious insult that might lead to pathological discharge from hippocampus. Studies of GABA inhibition on hippocampal pyramidal cells suggest that these cells may be under the constant control of tonic inhibitory bombardment. Blockade of $GABA_A$ and/or $GABA_B$ receptors leaves the tissue pathologically hyperexcitable. We do not know, however, which interneurons are critical to this tonic inhibitory control, whether particular interneuron populations are associated selectively with $GABA_A$ or $GABA_B$ receptors, or whether all interneurons have preferential terminal domains on the pyramidal cells. Our studies, and those from other laboratories, suggest that basket cells and O/A interneurons have a high density of terminals around pyramidal cell bodies and initial segments and that L-M interneurons have a higher density of terminals on pyramidal cell dendrites, but these distributions are by no means absolute.

It is also unclear whether particular interneuron types are specifically activated by different afferent pathways. Some interneurons have been labeled "theta cells" (Fox et al., 1986), suggesting that they may be strongly activated by septal input phasing the theta activity of hippocampal pyramidal cells. However, the septal effect on interneurons remains unclear. The intrinsic features of L-M interneurons suggest that they are appropriate candidates for phasing theta activity of hippocampal pyramidal cells, but no studies have yet been carried out to examine this possibility.

Another important, and as yet unplowed, field of investigation is selective vulnerability of different interneuronal populations to noxious or traumatic stimulation. Although it has been widely assumed that interneurons are particularly vulnerable to CNS insult, that assumption has not been supported in hippocampus. For example, although IPSP activity is quite sensitive to hypoxic/anoxic insult, there is little evidence to show that interneurons are damaged at a lower threshold than are pyramidal cells by such treatments (Janigro and Schwartzkroin, 1986). A variety of experimental preparations that show hyperexcitability correlated with a loss of IPSP activity do *not* show a correlated loss of GABAergic interneurons. For example, CA1 GABAergic interneurons remain in hyperexcitable hippocampus following intraventricular kainic acid injections (which destroy the CA3 region) (Franck et al., 1988). Indeed, there is preliminary evidence from the kainate model that interneuronal ramifications hypertrophy (sprout) (Davenport and Babb, 1986) and may, in fact, increase the level of inhibition in a "hyperexcitable" neuronal system. GABAergic basket cells in the dentate region remain intact in hyperexcitable granule cell preparations following long-term stimulation of the perforant pathway (Sloviter, 1987). Even in human epileptic temporal lobe, where there is often a significant loss of neurons, the proportion of presumed inhibitory interneurons seems constant relative to pyramidal cells (Babb and Brown, 1986).

The fate of interneurons in neuropathological states, and their roles in normal hippocampus, remain unclear. However, given their powerful modulation of hippocampal input, it seems certain that the local circuitry is critical in maintaining appropriate hippocampal function.

ACKNOWLEDGMENTS

Studies were supported by NIH, NINCDS grants NS 18897 and NS 15317 (PAS). P.A.S. is an affiliate of the Child Development and Mental Retardation Center, University of Washington. J.-C.L. was partially supported by a NATO Science Fellowship from NSERC of Canada and by a Postdoctoral Fellowship and a Scholarship from FRSQ of Quebec.

REFERENCES

Alger, B.E. (1984) Characteristics of a slow hyperpolarizing synaptic potential in rat hippocampal pyramidal cells in vitro. J. Neurophysiol. 52:892–910.

Alger, B.E., and R.A. Nicoll (1982a) Feedforward dendritic inhibition in rat hippocampal pyramidal cells studied in vitro. J. Physiol. [Lond.] 328:105–123.

Alger, B.E., and R.A. Nicoll (1982b) Pharmacological evidence for two kinds of GABA receptors on rat hippocampal pyramidal cells studied in vitro. J. Physiol. [Lond.] 328:125–141.

Amaral, D.G. (1978) A Golgi study of cell types in the hilar region of the hippocampus of the rat. J. Comp. Neurol. 182:851–914.

Andersen, P., B.H. Bland, and J.D. Dudar (1973) Organization of the hippocampal output. Exp. Brain Res. 17:152–168.

Andersen, P., T.V.P. Bliss, and K.K. Skrede (1971) Lamellar organization of hippocampal excitatory pathways. Exp. Brain Res. 13:222–238.

Andersen, P., J.C. Eccles, and Y. Løyning (1964a) Location of postsynaptic inhibitory synapses on hippocampal pyramids. J. Neurophysiol. 27:592–607.

Andersen, P., J.C. Eccles, and Y. Løyning (1964b) Pathway of postsynaptic inhibition in the hippocampus. J. Neurophysiol. 27:608–619.

Andersen, P., and T. Lømo (1966) Mode of activation of hippocampal pyramidal cells by excitatory synapses on dendrites. Exp. Brain Res. 2:247–260.

Ashwood T.J., B. Lancaster, and H.V. Wheal (1984) In vivo and in vitro studies on putative interneurones in the rat hippocampus: Possible mediators of feed-forward inhibition. Brain Res. 293:279–291.

Babb, T.L., and W.J. Brown (1986) Neuronal, dendritic and vascular profiles of human temporal lobe epilepsy correlated with cellular physiology in vivo. In A.V. Delgado-Escueta, A.A. Ward, D.M. Woodbury, and R.J. Porter (eds): Basic Mechanisms of the Epilepsies: Molecular and Cellular Approaches. New York: Raven Press, pp. 949–966.

Bakst, I., J.H. Morrison, and D.G. Amaral (1985) The distribution of somatostatin-like immunoreactivity in the monkey hippocampal formation. J. Comp. Neurol. 236:423–442.

Benardo, L.S., and D.A. Prince (1982) Cholinergic excitation of mammalian hippocampal pyramidal cells. Brain Res. *249:*315–331.

Buzsáki, G., and E. Eidelberg (1982) Direct afferent excitation and long-term potentiation of hippocampal interneurons. J. Neurophysiol. *48:*597–607.

Chronister, R.B., and J.F. DeFrance (1979) Organization of projection neurons of the hippocampus. Exp. Neurol. *66:*509–523.

Davenport, C.J., and T.L. Babb (1986) Kainate induced sprouting of inhibitory (GAD) interneurons and mossy fiber recurrent collaterals in the ipsi- and contralateral hippocampus. Neurosci. Abstr. *12:*343.

Fox, S.E., S. Wolfson, and J.B. Ranck, Jr. (1986) Hippocampal theta rhythm and the firing of neurons in walking and urethane anesthetized rats. Exp. Brain Res. *62:*495–508.

Franck, J.E., D.D. Kunkel, D.G. Baskin, and P.A. Schwartzkroin (1988) Inhibition in kainate-lesioned epileptogenic hippocampi: Physiologic, autoradiographic and immunocytochemical observations. J. Neurosci. *8:*1991–2002.

Frotscher, M., and J. Zimmer (1983) Commissural fibers terminate on non-pyramidal neurons in the guinea pig hippocampus—A combined Golgi/EM degeneration study. Brain Res. *265:*289–293.

Gamrani, H., B. Ontoniente, P. Seguela, M. Geffard, and A. Calas (1986) Gamma-aminobutyric acid-immunoreactivity in the rat hippocampus. A light and electron microscopic study with anti-GABA antibodies. Brain Res. *364:*30–38.

Janigro, D., and P.A. Schwartzkroin (1986) Dissociation of the IPSP and response to GABA during spreading depression-like depolarizations in hippocampal slices. Brain Res. *404:*189–200.

Kandel, E.R., W.A. Spencer, and F.J. Brinley (1961) Electrophysiology of hippocampal neurons. I. Sequential invasion and synaptic organization. J. Neurophysiol. *24:*225–242.

Kawaguchi, Y., and K. Hama (1987a) Two subtypes of non-pyramidal cells in rat hippocampal formation identified by intracellular recording and HRP injection. Brain Res. *411:*190–195.

Kawaguchi, Y., and K. Hama (1987b) Fast-spiking non-pyramidal cells in the hippocampal CA3 region, dentate gyrus and subiculum of rats. Brain Res. *425:*351–355.

Knowles, W.D., and P.A. Schwartzkroin (1980) Local circuit synaptic interactions in hippocampal brain slices. J. Neurosci. *1:*318–322.

Köhler, C., and V. Chan-Palay (1982) Somatostatin-like immunoreactive neurons in the hippocampus: An immunocytochemical study in the rat. Neurosci. Lett. *34:*259–264.

Kunkel, D.D., A.E. Hendrickson, J.Y. Wu, and P.A. Schwartzkroin (1986) Glutamic acid decarboxylase (GAD) immunocytochemistry of developing rabbit hippocampus. J. Neurosci. *6:*541–552.

Kunkel, D.D., J.-C Lacaille, and P.A. Schwartzkroin (1988) Ultrastructure of stratum lacunosum-moleculare interneurons of hippocampal CA1 region. Synapse *2:*382–394.

Kunkel, D.D., and P.A. Schwartzkroin (1988) Ultrastructural characterization and GAD co-localization of somatostatin-like immunoreactive neurons in CA1 of rabbit hippocampus. Synapse *2:*371–381.

Lacaille, J.-C., A.L. Mueller, D.D. Kunkel, and P.A. Schwartzkroin (1987) Local circuit interactions between oriens/alveus interneurons and CA1 pyramidal cells in hippocampal slices: Electrophysiology and morphology. J. Neurosci. *7:*1979–1993.

Lacaille, J.-C., and P.A. Schwartzkroin (1988a) Stratum lacunosum-moleculare interneurons of hippocampal CA1 region: I. Intracellular response characteristics, synaptic responses, and morphology. J. Neurosci. *8:*1400–1410.

Lacaille, J.-C., and P.A. Schwartzkroin (1988b) Stratum lacunosum-moleculare interneurons of hippocampal CA1 region: II. Intrasomatic and intradendritic recordings of local circuit synaptic interactions. J. Neurosci. *8*:1411–1424.

Lorente de Nó, R. (1934) Studies on the structure of the cerebral cortex. II. Continuation of the study on the ammonic system. J. Physchol. Neurol. [Lpz.] *46*:113–117.

Loy, R., D.A. Koziell, J.D. Lindsey, and R.Y. Moore (1980) Noradrenergic innervation of the adult rat hippocampal formation. J. Comp. Neurol. *189*:699–710.

Madison, D.V., and R.A. Nicoll (1988) Enkephalin hyperpolarizes interneurones in the rat hippocampus. J. Physiol. [Lond.] *398*:123–130.

Matthews, D.A., P.M. Salvaterra, G.D. Crawford, C.R. Houser, and J.E. Vaughn (1987) An immunocytochemical study of choline acetyltransferase-containing neurons and axon terminals in normal and partially deafferented hippocampal formation. Brain Res. *402*:30–43.

Miles, R., and R.K.S. Wong (1984) Unitary inhibitory synaptic potentials in the guinea-pig hippocampus in vitro. J. Physiol. *356*:97–113.

Misgeld, U., and M. Frotscher (1986) Postsynaptic-GABAergic inhibition of non-pyramidal neurons in the guinea-pig hippocampus. Neuroscience *19*:193–206.

Morrison, J.H., R. Benoit, P.J. Magistretti, N. Ling, and F.E. Bloom (1982) Immunocytochemical distribution of pro-somatostatin-related peptides in hippocampus. Neurosci. Lett. *34*:137–142.

Newberry, N.R., and R.A. Nicoll (1985) Comparison of the action of baclofen with gamma-aminobutyric acid on rat hippocampal pyramidal cells in vitro. J. Physiol. [Lond.] *360*:161–185.

Obata-Tsuto, H.L. (1987) Light and electron microscopic study of somatostatin-like immunoreactive neurons in rat hippocampus. Brain Res. Bull. *18*:613–620.

Ramón y Cajal, S. (1911) Histologie du Systeme Nerveux de l'Homme et des Vertebres. Paris: A. Maloine.

Ribak, C.E., J.E. Vaughn, and K. Saito (1978) Immunocytochemical localization of glutamic acid decarboxylase in neuronal somata following cochicine inhibition of axonal transport. Brain Res. *140*:321–332.

Roberts, G.W., P.L. Woodhams, J.M. Polak, and T.J. Crow (1984) Distribution of neuropeptides in the limbic system of the rat: The hippocampus. Neuroscience *11*:35–77.

Schlander, M, and M. Frotscher (1986) Non-pyramidal neurons in the guinea pig hippocampus. A combined Golgi-electron microscope study. Anat. Embryol. *174*:35–47.

Schwartzkroin, P.A., and D.D. Kunkel (1985) Morphology of identified interneurons in the CA1 regions of guinea pig hippocampus. J. Comp. Neurol. *232*:205–218.

Schwartzkroin, P.A., and L.H. Mathers (1978) Physiological and morphological indentification of a nonpyramidal hippocampal cell type. Brain Res. *157*:1–10.

Schwerdtfeger, W.K., and E. Buhl (1986) Various types of non-pyramidal hippocampal neurons project to the septum and contralateral hippocampus. Brain Res. *386*:146–154.

Sloviter, R.S. (1987) Decreased hippocampal inhibition and a selective loss of interneurons in experimental epilepsy. Science *235*:73–76.

Somogyi, P., A.J. Hodgson, A.D. Smith, M.G. Nunzi, A. Gorio, and J.Y. Wu (1984) Different populations of GABAergic neurons in the visual cortex and hippocampus of cat contain somatostatin- or cholescystokinin-immunoreactive material. J. Neurosci. *4*:2590–2603.

Somogyi, P., M.G. Nunzi, A. Gorio, and A.D. Smith (1983) A new type of specific interneuron in the monkey hippocampus forming synapses exclusively with the axon initial segment of pyramidal cells. Brain Res. *259*:137–142.

Tomböl, T., M. Babosa, F. Hajdu, and G. Somogyi (1979) Interneurons: An electron microscopic study of the cat's hipocampal formation, II. Acta Morphol. Acad. Sci. Hung. *27*:297–313.

Totterdell, S., and L. Hayes (1987) Non-pyramidal hippocampal projection neurons: A light and electron-microscopic study. J. Neurocytol. *16*:477–485.

Zhou, F.C., and E.C. Azmitia (1986) Induced homotypic sprouting of serotonergic fibers in hippocampus. II. An immunocytochemistry study. Brain Res. *373*:337–348.

The Hippocampus—New Vistas, pages 307–315
© 1989 Alan R. Liss, Inc.

19
Serotonin Modulation of Hippocampal Activity

MENAHEM SEGAL

The Center for Neuroscience, The Weizmann Institute of Science, Rehovot, Israel

INTRODUCTION

The serotoninergic innervation of the hippocampus (HPC) has been of particular interest in view of the multitude of functions ascribed to serotonin (5-hydroxytryptamine [5-HT]) in the brain. These functions include regulation of sleep wakefulness cycles, feeding, drinking, sex, hormone secretion, pain, mood, and cognitive functions (Calas, 1981; Haber et al., 1981; Jacobs and Gelperin, 1981; Soubrie, 1986). The hippocampus, a major component of the limbic system, has been associated with at least some of these functions. Serotonin-containing fibers originate in the dorsal and median raphe nuclei and innervate the entire forebrain in a seemingly diffuse manner (Azmitia and Segal, 1978). Within the hippocampal system this innervation is not entirely random; a dense network of 5-HT–containing fibers is seen in the dentate hilus, with more diffuse patterns elsewhere. There is a gradient of fiber density from the temporal (highest) to the septal (lowest) poles of the hippocampus. These fibers make distinct synaptic contacts with postsynaptic hippocampal neurons, as described elsewhere (Azmitia, 1978).

The hippocampus is among the richest regions in the brain in serotonin receptors (Biegon et al., 1982). The availability of various selective 5-HT ligands facilitated the classification of 5-HT receptors into at least seven subtypes: 5-HT1a,b,c, 5-HT2, and 5-HT3a,b,c (Richardson and Engel, 1986; Peroutka, 1986). The hippocampus is especially rich in 5-HT1a binding sites, whereas the other receptors are less abundant there. The 5-HT1a receptors estimated by the specific binding of $[^3H]5\text{-HT}$ exhibit an uneven distribution in the hippocampus; large amount of 5-HT binding sites are found in the dentate gyrus and region CA1 of the hippocampus proper. By comparison, the CA3 region contains relatively few 5-HT binding sites. There seems to be no gradient of 5-HT binding sites along the dorsal-ventral axis, unlike the case of the serotoninergic innervation (Biegon et al., 1982; Segal, 1981a).

IN VITRO EXPERIMENTS

Initial experiments illustrated that 5-HT hyperpolarizes pyramidal neurons of region CA1 and the dentate gyrus (Segal, 1980; Jahnsen, 1980). This hyperpolarization is associated with an increase in conductance (Fig. 1). The reversal potential as well as the sensitivity of the response to changes in $[K]_{out}$ indicated that 5-HT activates a K current (Segal, 1980; Andrade and Nicoll, 1987), although there was a suggestion that it may activate a Cl conductance in dentate granular cells (Assaf et al., 1981). Later experiments indicated that 5-HT increases $[K]_{out}$ in accordance with its action to increase K outflow of the cells (Segal and Gutnick, 1980). A regional selectivity of the response to 5-HT was recorded; CA1 cells were much more responsive to 5-HT than were CA3 cells (Segal, 1981b).

Recently, several other effects of 5-HT were described. One is a blockade of a slow Ca-dependent K current underlying the slow afterhyperpolarization (AHP) that follows a burst discharge (Baskys et al., 1987; Colino and Halliwell, 1987; Andrade and Nicoll, 1987). This effect of 5-HT is similar to that seen in response to isoproterenol (Madison and Nicoll, 1982; Haas and Konnerth, 1983) but is not mediated by the same receptor types. Interestingly, the 5-HT–mediated blockade of AHP is shorter lasting than the blockade produced by isoproterenol or acetylcholine. While the 5-HT–induced blockade of AHP might be a genuine response, it might result from shunting of the dendritic Ca spike resulting from an increase in K conductance. Some experiments indicate that the increase in K conductance and the blockade of AHP can be dissociated pharmacologically (Andrade and Nicoll, 1987) or by aging (Baskys et al., 1987).

Another effect of 5-HT is a slow depolarization that follows the initial increase in K conductance. This slow depolarization is generated more in ventral HPC than in dorsal HPC neurons (Colino and Halliwell, 1987). It involves an increase in input resistance of the recorded cells much like the response to ACh, but is not mediated by the same receptor. The depolarizing response to 5-HT is not blocked by spiperone, indicating that it is not mediated by 5-HT1a or 5-HT2 receptor types (Andrade and Nicoll, 1987; Colino and Halliwell, 1987).

In response to afferent stimulation, CA1 neurons typically respond with a short latency fast excitatory postsynaptic potential (EPSP) followed by a fast inhibitory response (IPSP) lasting 10–20 ms. The latter response is mediated by an increase in Cl^- conductance. The fast IPSP (fIPSP) is followed by a slow IPSP (sIPSP) mediated probably by γ-aminobutyric acid (GABA) acting at a $GABA_B$ receptor and activating a K conductance (Hablitz and Thalman, 1987). Topical application of 5-HT reduces primarily the sIPSP and on occasion also the fIPSP (Fig. 1). The reduction of the sIPSP can be seen with a 5-HT concentration that does not produce an appreciable potential change in the recorded neurons. The reduction in the IPSPs probably underlies the increase in EPSPs seen elsewhere (Mauk et al., 1988). The reduced IPSPs are mediated by the same receptor type that mediates the increase in K conductance, as indicated by its sensitivity to spiperone (Segal, unpublished observations).

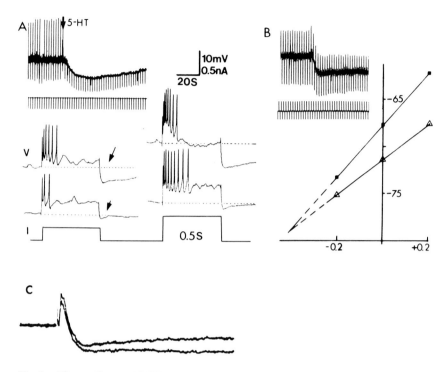

Fig. 1.   Three effects of 5-HT on CA1 hippocampal neurons. **A:** A dual action of 5-HT in the same neuron. Top is a continuous chart record of responses to topical application of a microdrop containing 1 mM 5-HT (arrow). The cell hyperpolarizes, and this is associated with a decrease in input resistance estimated by the voltage deflections in response to constant current pulses (bottom record) applied at a rate of 0.5 Hz. Below are two specimen responses to 0.5 s depolarizing current pulses applied before (top) and after (bottom) exposure of the cell to 5-HT. On the left is a response to a small, and on the right is a response to a large, current pulse. Dotted lines indicate resting membrane potential. Note the nearly total disappearance of the hyperpolarization that follows the response to the depolarizing current pulse. The response to the higher pulse is also associated with a larger number of spikes following 5-HT. Resting membrane potential is − 70 mV. **B:** The hyperpolarization has an apparent reversal potential of about − 80 mV. The insert is a continuous chart record of another cell from A, where depolarizating and hyperpolarizing current pulses are applied alternatively at a rate of 0.5 Hz. 5-HT hyperpolarizes the cell and causes a decrease in its input resistance. An analysis of the current-voltage relations indicates an apparent reversal potential of − 80 mV. Resting membrane potential is − 67 mV. **C:** Effects of 5-HT on an EPSP–IPSP sequence: 200 ms traces taken before (bottom) and after (top) application of 5-HT. Traces are taken from the same membrane potential. The application of 5-HT resulted in an increased EPSP and a reduction of the long IPSP.

PHARMACOLOGY OF THE SEROTONINERGIC RESPONSE IN THE HIPPOCAMPUS

The lack of selective 5-HT antagonists has hampered a clear classification of the receptor types underlying the responses to 5-HT seen in the hippocampus. Initial experiments performed in the intact hippocampus, employing iontophoresis of several 5-HT–related compounds, did not yield a clear and selective antagonistic action, as most drugs used also had a partial agonistic action (Segal, 1976). Further experiments in a slice preparation indicated that metergoline or methysergide partially antagonized the K conductance increase evoked by 5-HT (Segal, 1980). More recently, a long exposure to spiperone was found to antagonize selectively this inhibitory effect of 5-HT (Andrade and Nicoll, 1987) Extracellular studies in the hippocampus indicated that ketanserin, a 5-HT2 antagonist, blocked the inhibitory effect of 5-HT on a population spike in a slice without affecting the transient facilitatory effect of the drug (Rowan and Anwyl, 1985).

A number of 5-HT analogs are said to bind selectively to 5-HT1a or 5-HT1b receptor sites (Richardson and Engel, 1986; Peroutka, 1986). When tested in the dorsal raphe, the 5-HT1a ligands (e.g. 8-OHDPAT) do indeed mimic the effects of 5-HT to hyperpolarize raphe neurons (Sprouse and Aghajanian, 1987). In the hippocampus, though, these ligands act more as partial agonists while having also a potent antagonistic action toward effects of 5-HT measured intracellularly (Andrade and Nicoll, 1987; Segal, unpublished observations). Thus it is likely that the 5-HT1a receptor residing in the raphe is of a different nature from the hippocampal 5-HT1a receptor type.

POSTSYNAPTIC MECHANISMS ACTIVATED BY 5-HT

The possible mediation of 5-HT effects by the activation of a second messenger-generating system was studied by a number of research groups. Initial observations suggested the presence of a high-affinity 5-HT–stimulated adenylate cyclase that is active in developing brain and has different characteristics from the common 5-HT binding site (Enjalbert et al., 1978) Later studies indicate that 5-HT can cause a reduction of cyclic adenosine monophosphate (cAMP) generated by other ligands (Clarke et al., 1987). This would imply that the 5-HT receptor is linked to a guanosine triphosphate (GTP) binding protein (G protein) of the Gi type. In other systems, Gi action is blocked by the drug pertussis toxin. Indeed, hippocampal slices taken from brains injected with pertussis toxin lose their ability to exhibit the effects of 5-HT on cyclic AMP generation (Clarke et al., 1987) and the effects of 5-HT on membrane potential (Andrade and Nicoll, 1987).

The relevance of 5-HT to the cyclic AMP generating system remained unclear in view of the activation by 5-HT of a physiological response (blockade of the AHP) that is similar to that produced by activation of β receptor and assumed to be mediated by cyclic AMP generation (Madison and Nicoll, 1982).

IN VIVO STUDIES

While considerable effort has been devoted to the elucidation of the membrane mechanisms underlying the action of 5-HT, the in vitro preparation has not been used for the investigation of 5-HT released from its terminals and acting at a receptor site that normally sees 5-HT in situ. The issue of identity of action is of major importance in view of the increasing number of cases in which there seems to be a mismatch between the preterminal fiber and receptor distribution and the diversity of putative nonsynaptic receptors (for example, the cholinergic receptor subtype distributions in the forebrain). Initial studies employing electrical stimulation of the raphe nuclei indicated the presence of a potent nonserotoninergic component in hippocampal responses to raphe stimulation (Segal, 1975). This observation is consistent with the heterogeneous composition of the nucleus raphe medianus (Crunelli and Segal, 1985). An alternative way to electrical stimulation of the raphe as a means of activation of a serotoninergic synapse takes advantage of the ability of some drugs to release 5-HT from its terminals. Fenfluramine (FFA) and P-chloroamphetamine (PCA) have been reported to release 5-HT (Invernizzi et al., 1986). Parenteral injection of FFA causes a marked enhancement of reactivity of the dentate gyrus to afferent stimulation (Fig. 2). This is expressed in an increase in population spike that is not accompanied by a parallel change in the population EPSP, indicating that 5-HT released by FFA is enhancing the excitability of dentate granular cells (Richter-Levin and Segal, 1988). The site of action of FFA or PCA to produce these effects is currently being investigated (Richter-Levin and Segal, unpublished observations). These experiments partially confirm earlier ones done with the freely moving rat in which 5-HT of raphe origin

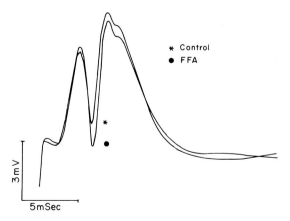

* Control
● FFA

3 m V

5 m Sec

Fig. 2.   Responses of dentate gyrus to stimulation of the perforant pathway before (control) and after parenteral injection of 4 mg/kg fenfluramine (FFA) into a chloral hydrate-anesthetized rat. Fenfluramine caused an increase in population spike with no effect on the slope of the EPSP (initial rising slope). (Reproduced from Richter-Levin and Segal, 1988, with permission of the publisher.)

was assumed to underly excitability changes in the hippocampus (Winson, 1980). The relations of these to the more general suggestions of the role of 5-HT in generation of hippocampal theta rhythms (Vanderwolf, 1987) remains to be elucidated.

RAPHE GRAFT IN THE HIPPOCAMPUS

One approach to the above-mentioned inability to study a serotoninergic pathway in vitro is to transplant serotoninergic neurons of the raphe into the hippocampus. This has been attempted successfully; grafted raphe neurons were found to extend 5-HT–containing fibers into the host hippocampus (Azmitia et al., 1981). These fibers possess the ability to take up [^{3}H]5-HT much the same as normal serotoninergic fibers do. Grafted 5-HT–containing neurons share the same physiological properties with normal 5-HT neurons that grow in their normal site in the brain. These properties include high input resistance, broad action potentials that contain a Ca component, a fast and large afterhyperpolarization following each action potential discharge, a prominent transient outward rectification that is deinactivated by polarization of the cell to potentials below rest, and a lack of anomalous inward rectification at hyperpolarized potentials. These properties are absent in the grafted neurons on the day of grafting but develop in the host brain (Segal, 1987). Electrical stimulation of the grafted dorsal raphe produces a slow hyperpolarization of host hippocampal neurons (Segal, 1987). This response is enhanced by preloading the slice with a 5-HT precursor, 5-hydroxytryptophane (5-HTP), indicating that it is dependent on activation of 5-HT synapses. In addition, stimulation of the graft causes a reduction of the AHP as seen following topical application of 5-HT (Fig. 3). It thus appears that the raphe graft makes a connection with

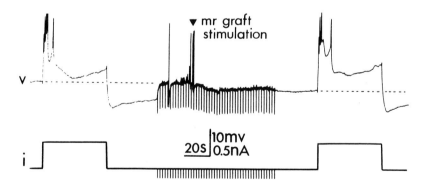

Fig. 3. Electrical stimulation of a raphe graft causes a slow hyperpolarization and a reduction in a slow afterhyperpolarization, which follows a 0.5 s depolarizing current pulse (left and right). Center: The chart speed was slowed and a hyperpolarizing current pulse applied every 2 s to assess input resistance of the recorded cell. Tetanic stimulation of the graft produced a 3–4 mV hyperpolarization and a reduction of input resistance of the recorded cell.

host hippocampal neurons that is likely to use 5-HT as a neurotransmitter. This short serotoninergic pathway lends itself to a more extensive pharmacological and physiological analysis of the raphe–hippocampal connection.

DISCUSSION

A renewed interest in serotonin neurotransmission in the brain followed the synthesis of selective 5-HT receptor ligands and classification of several 5-HT receptor types in the brain and elsewhere (Peroutka, 1986). While these ligands express selective action in binding studies, they still fail to resolve the complex physiological action of 5-HT in the brain. Thus, presumably selective 5-HT1a agonists have only a weak agonistic action while having a potent antagonistic action on presumably 5-HT1a receptors in the hippocampus. This picture is different for hindbrain receptors (Sprouse and Aghajanian, 1987). Likewise, spiperone is commonly used as a 5HT1a antagonist, but it also has a potent 5-HT2 antagonistic action (Peroutka, 1986). The long list of presently available 5-HT antagonists is clearly not satisfactory for the study of the physiology of central 5-HT neurotransmission. This situation markedly contrasts that seen with the central modulatory neurotransmitters acetylcholine and noradrenaline, in which the selectivities of agonist and antagonist actions are distinct. It is likely that this situation reflects the unique nature of the serotoninergic receptor, which may have different arrangements of agonist and antagonist binding sites than other neurotransmitter receptor types.

Recent studies that employ molecular biological approaches to the isolation and characterization of the serotoninergic receptor population may help in resolving the complexity of this receptor.

Another issue of recent interest involves the roles of 5-HT in regulation of hippocampal activity. While the ionic mechanisms underlying the actions of 5-HT are being unraveled, it is still not clear which if any roles 5-HT neurons play in regulating hippocampal activity in the intact, freely moving rat. There has been a suggestion that 5-HT of raphe origin regulates hippocampal theta rhythm and is involved in cognitive functions of the hippocampus (Vanderwolf, 1987). The mechanisms underlying these functions are still unclear. The complex action of 5-HT in the hippocampus, which involves an increase in K conductance of pyramidal neurons while at the same time reducing substantially an inhibitory drive impinging on these same neurons, allows an increase in their reactivity to excitatory afferent without them being excessively excitable.

SUMMARY

Serotonin hyperpolarizes pyramidal neurons of the rat hippocampus by activating a K conductance. This action results in cessation of spontaneous activity of neurons recorded extracellularly in the intact brain. In addition to this inhibitory action, 5-HT blocks the slow afterhyperpolarization that follows a burst firing and causes a marked supression of inhibitory postsynaptic potentials in the recorded neurons.

In the intact rat brain, parenteral application of 5-HT–releasing drugs caused an increase in dentate gyrus population spike response to perforant pathway stimulation without a concomitant change in the EPSP, indicating that the released 5-HT modifies postsynaptic dentate granular cell reactivity to afferent stimulation.

A short 5-HT pathway was reconstructed by grafting 5-HT–containing raphe neurons into the hippocampus of the adult rat. This preparation is suitable for the in vitro analysis of a central serotoninergic synapse.

REFERENCES

Andrade, R., and R.A. Nicoll (1987) Pharmacologically distinct actions of serotonin on single pyramidal neurones of the rat hippocampus recorded in vitro. J. Physiol. 394:99–124.

Assaf, S.Y., V. Crunelli, and J.S. Kelly (1981) Action of 5-hydroxytryptamine on granule cells in the rat hippocampal slice. J. Physiol. [Paris] 77:377–380.

Azmitia, E.C. (1978) The serotonin producing neurons of the dorsal and median raphe nuclei. In L.L. Iversen and S.H. Snyder (eds): The Handbook of Psychopharmacology. New York: Plenum Press, pp. 233–314.

Azmitia, E.C., M.J. Perlow, M.J. Brennan, and J.M. Lauder (1981) Fetal raphe and hippocampal transplants into adult and aged C57BL/6N mice: A preliminary immunocytochemical study. Brain Res. Bull. 7:703–710.

Azmitia, E., and M. Segal (1978) The efferent connections of the dorsal and median raphe nuclei in the rat brain. J. Comp. Neurol. 179:641–668.

Baskys, A., N.E. Niesen, and P.L. Carlen (1987) Altered modulatory action of serotonin on dentate granular cells of aged rats. Brain Res. 419:112–116.

Biegon, A., T.C. Rainbow, and B.S. McEwen (1982) Quantitative autoradiography of serotonin receptors in the rat brain. Brain Res. 242:197–204.

Calas, A. (1981) The serotonergic neuron. J. Physiol. [Paris] 77:147–524.

Clarke, W.P., M. DeVivo, S.G. Beck, S. Maayani, and J. Goldfarb (1987) Serotonin decreases population spike amplitude in hippocampal cells through a pertussis toxin substrate. Brain Res. 410:357–361.

Colino, A., and J.V. Halliwell (1987) Differential modulation of three separate K conductances in hippocampal CA1 neurons by serotonin. Nature 328:73–76.

Crunelli, V., and M. Segal (1985) An electrophysiological study of neurons in the median raphe and their projections to septum and hippocampus. Neuroscience 15:47–60.

Enjalbert, A., S. Bourgoin, M. Hamon, J. Adrien, and J. Bockaert (1978) Postsynaptic serotonin-sensitive adenylate cyclase in the central nervous system. I. Development and distribution of serotonin and dopamine-sensitive adenylate cyclase in rat and guinea pig brain. Mol. Pharmacol. 14:2–10.

Haas, H.L., and A. Konnerth (1983) Histamine and noradrenaline decrease calcium activated potassium conductance in hippocampal pyramidal cells. Nature 302:432–434.

Haber, B., S. Gabay, M.R. Issidorides, and S.G.A. Alivisatos (1981) Serotonin, current aspects of neurochemistry and function. New York: Plenum Press.

Hablitz, J.J., and R.H. Thalman (1987) Conductance changes underlying a late synaptic hyperpolarization in hippocampal CA3 neurons. J. Neurophysiol. 58:160–179.

Invernizzi, R., C. Berettera, S. Garattini, and R. Samanin (1986) Isomers of fenfluramine differ markedly in their interaction with brain serotonin and catecholamine in the rat. Eur. J. Pharmacol. 120:9–15.

Jacobs, B.L., and A. Gelperin (1981) Serotonin Neurotransmission and Behaviour. Cambridge: MIT Press.

Jahnsen, H. (1980) The action of 5-hydroxytryptamine on neuronal membranes and synaptic transmission in area CA1 of the hippocampus in vitro. Brain Res., 197:83–94.

Madison, D.V., and R.A. Nicoll (1982) Noradrenaline blocks accommodation of pyramidal cell discharge in the hippocampus. Nature *299:*636–638.

Mauk, M.D., S.J. Peroutka, and J.D. Cocsis (1988) Buspirone attenuates synaptic activation of hippocampal pyramidal cells. J. Neurosci. *8:*1–11.

Peroutka, S.J. (1986) Pharmacological differentiation and characterization of 5-HT1a, 5-HT1b and 5-HT1c binding sites in rat frontal cortex. J. Neurochem. *47:*529–539.

Richardson, B.P., and G. Engel (1986) The pharmacology and function of 5-HT3 receptors. Trends Neurosci. *9:*424–428.

Richter-Levin, G. and M. Segal (1988) Serotonin releasers modulate reactivity of the rat hippocampus to afferent stimulation. Neuroscience Lett. *94:*173–176.

Rowan, M.J., and R. Anwyl (1985) The effect of prolonged treatment with tricyclic antidepressants on the actions of 5-HT in the hippocampal slice of the rat. Neuropharmacology *24:*131–137.

Segal, M. (1975) Physiological and pharmacological evidence for a serotonergic projection to the hippocampus. Brain Res. *94:*115–131.

Segal, M. (1976) 5-HT antagonists in the rat hippocampus. Brain Res. *103:*161–166.

Segal, M. (1980) The action of serotonin in the hippocampal slice preparation. J. Physiol. *303:*423–439.

Segal, M. (1981a) The action of serotonin in the rat hippocampus. In B. Haber, et al. (eds): Serotonin Current Aspects of Neurochemistry and Function. New York: Plenum Press, pp. 375–390.

Segal, M. (1981b) Regional differences in neuronal responses to 5-HT: Intracellular studies in hippocampal slices. J. Physiol. [Paris] *77:*373–375.

Segal, M. (1987) Interactions between grafted serotonin neurons and adult host rat hippocampus. Proc. N.Y. Acad. Sci. U.S.A. *495:*285–295.

Segal, M. and M.J. Gutnick (1980) Effects of serotonin on extracellular potassium concentration in the rat hippocampal slice. Brain Res. *195:*389–401.

Soubrie, P. (1986) Reconciling the role of central serotonin neurons in human and animal behavior. Behav. Brain Sci. *9:*319–364.

Sprouse, J.S., and G.K. Aghajanian (1987) Electrophysiological responses of serotonergic dorsal raphe neurons to 5HT1a and 5HT1b agonists. Synapse *1:*3–9.

Winson, J. (1980) Influence of raphe nuclei on neuronal transmission from perforant pathway through dentate gyrus. J. Neurophysiol. *44:*937–950.

Vanderwolf, C.H. (1987) Near-total loss of "learning" and "memory" as a result of combined cholinergic and serotonergic blockade in the rat. Behav. Brain Res. *23:*43–57.

The Hippocampus—New Vistas, pages 317–327
© 1989 Alan R. Liss, Inc.

20
Actions of Excitatory Amino Acid Agonists and Antagonists in the Hippocampus

H. McLENNAN

Department of Physiology, University of British Columbia, Vancouver, British Columbia, Canada

INTRODUCTION

Since the first demonstration by Yamamoto and McIlwain (1966) that synaptic field potentials could be obtained from slices of nervous tissue maintained in vitro and the subsequent report that stable intracellular recordings were possible in slices of mammalian hippocampus (Yamamoto, 1972), this latter preparation has sustained much physiological and pharmacological experimentation. It combines four most useful and interesting features: 1) the neurons and their dendritic processes are arranged in a highly ordered fashion, permitting the precise placement of stimulating and recording electrodes under visual control; 2) three anatomically distinct synaptic pathways are contained within the slice; 3) the plastic change in synaptic efficacy, known as long-term potentiation (LTP) (Bliss and Lømo, 1973) is strikingly obvious; and 4) certain cell types in the hippocampal formation are very sensitive to cytolysis following excessive excitation. These features are extensively considered throughout this volume; the present chapter will deal with the actions of the excitatory amino acids upon hippocampal neurons in relation to the features mentioned above.

EXCITATION

The ability of L-glutamate to excite neurons in all of the subfields of the cornu Ammonis (CA) in vivo was first described by Biscoe and Straughan (1966), and later work on the slice additionally showed that localized spots of particular sensitivity existed on the apical dendrites of pyramidal cells in the region of synaptic terminations (Dudar, 1974; Schwartzkroin and Andersen, 1975; Spencer et al., 1978). Subsequent experiments (Collingridge et al., 1983b) employing extracellular recording indicated that hippocampal neurons, like other nerve cells of the central nervous system, are excited by all three of the amino acids N-methyl-D-aspartate (NMDA), kainate, and quisqualate, which define the currently recognized receptor types for this class of compounds (McLennan, 1983, 1987; Watkins, 1986).

A combination of intracellular recording coupled with the use of selective antagonists has permitted an unequivocal definition of the electrophysiological effects induced by the eponymous amino acids in pyramidal neurons of area CA1. The results are illustrated in Figure 1 and may be summarized as follows.

Depolarization of the cell membrane rises rapidly following the commencement of ionophoretic administration of quisqualate in stratum radiatum and achieves a plateau that does not further increase if larger currents ejecting the excitant are used. At levels of depolarization larger then ca. 15 mV, action potentials that are tetrodotoxin (TTX) sensitive are superimposed on the depolarization, and, following termination of the ejecting current, repolarization is relatively rapid (7.8 ± 0.6 s, S.E.M., (N = 28).

The response to kainate resembles that to quisqualate except that the depolarization rises more slowly and continues throughout the period of application rather than reaching a plateau and can persist beyond the cessation of the ionophoretic current. The threshold for generation of action potentials again is ca. 15 mV; however, repolarization is considerably slowed, as might be expected from the persistent action observed (19.9 ± 1.9 s, N = 10).

A qualitatively quite distinct pattern of response is evoked by NMDA. The

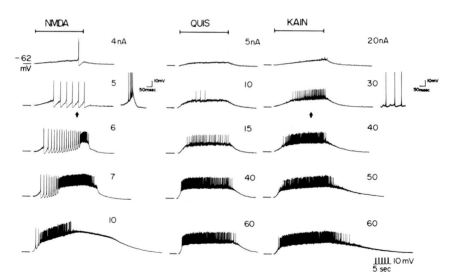

Fig. 1. Intracellular records from a pyramidal neuron of the CA1 region of the hippocampus during the ionophoretic application of N-methyl-D-aspartate (NMDA), quisqualate (QUIS), and kainate (KAIN) in stratum radiatum, using increasing ejecting currents. Sample oscilloscope enlargements (amplitudes truncated) of spike profiles taken at times indicated by arrows are shown to the right of corresponding chart records. (Reproduced from Peet et al., 1987a, with permission of the publisher.)

depolarization again is slowly rising, but when a level of ca. 5 mV is reached brief depolarizing shifts of the membrane potential appear superimposed on which are two to five action potentials. These bursting episodes can occur regularly (as in Fig. 1; NMDA 5 nA), and each is followed by a period of hyperpolarization. In the presence of TTX the depolarizing shifts can be seen to reach amplitudes of 40–50 mV, and it is now well recognized that they are calcium dependent (Dingledine, 1983; Peet et al., 1986). NMDA-induced depolarizations also increase with continuing application of the excitant, and at levels above 15 mV the bursting pattern is supplanted by simple action potentials (Fig. 1; NMDA 6, 7, and 10 nA). Repolarization times resemble those following quisqualate (8.0 ± 0.6 s, N = 35).

Figure 2 shows that differentiation of the actions of the three excitants can be achieved also by the use of antagonists. For the three excitants the effects only of NMDA are blocked by D-2-amino-5-phosphonovalerate (DAPV) (Davies et al., 1981), while kynurenate (KYNU) (Perkins and Stone, 1982; Ganong et

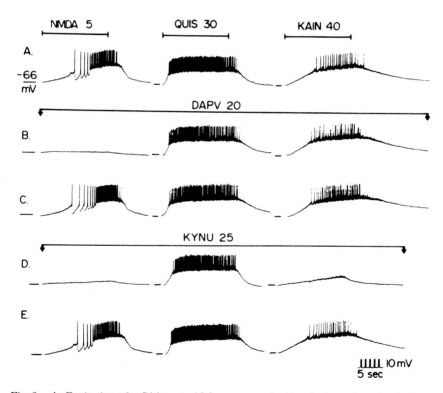

Fig. 2. **A:** Excitation of a CA1 pyramidal neuron evoked by the ionophoretic ejection of NMDA, quisqualate and kainate into striatum radiatum. **B:** During the concurrent ejection of 20 nA of DAPV. **C:** 4 min after DAPV ejection terminated. **D:** During the ejection of kynurenate, 25 nA. **E:** 2 min after kynurenate. (Unpublished observations.)

al., 1983) eliminates the actions of both NMDA and kainate, completely sparing quisqualate-induced effects unless very large "doses" are used. With the dual criteria of the patterns of excitation and of blockade, it is possible with assurance to assign the majority of the excitatory amino acids as reacting only with one of the three receptor types, as indicated in Table I. Only D-glutamate and D-aspartate exhibit equivocal results, since although their evoked pattern of firing generally resembled that of quisqualate the responses were readily blocked by both DAPV and KYNU (Peet et al., 1987b). It is important to note that all of these effects were obtained under conditions in which the cells were exposed to physiological concentrations of magnesium ions, which have been shown to possess a selective blocking action against NMDA responses (Ault et al., 1980).

It should be emphasized that these results, clear-cut as they appear, can only be accepted for hippocampal neurons and perhaps even then only for CA1 pyramidal cells, since comparable studies have not been executed in other subfields. It is becoming increasingly evident that the actions of the amino acids, and their antagonism, are not the same throughout the central nervous system: To adduce some examples, Do et al. (1986) in the striatum and Knöpfel et al. (1987) in the neocortex reported that L-homocysteate (but not the D-isomer) was completely NMDA-like in its ability to induce bursting and in its pattern of antagonism, which is not the case in the hippocampus; while in the spinal cord, where bursting does not occur, the endogenous tryptophan metabolite quinolinate and NMDA do not behave identically as they do in the hippocampal CA1 region (Magnuson et al., 1987).

Recent reports have indicated a fascinating new facet of the inter-relationships among the amino acids, initially through the description by Johnson and Ascher (1987) that glycine greatly potentiates the conductance change induced by NMDA. The effect appears to be an allosteric one, affecting the ion channels (Bonhaus et al., 1987), and Johnson and Ascher reported that the response to glutamate also was enhanced while those to quisqualate and kainate were not. The experiments were conducted with cortical and diencephalic neurons and have not been repeated with cells derived from the hippocampus, where the

TABLE I. Classification of Excitatory Amino Acids Acting On CA1 Hippocampal Neurons[a]

Quisqualate-like	Kainate-like	NMDA-like
L-glutamate	L-cis-ACPD	N-methyl-L-aspartate
L-aspartate	L-trans-ACPD	Quinolinate
D-homocysteate	D-trans-ACPD	D-cis-ACPD
L-homocysteate		Ibotenate
L-cysteate		Phthalate
		Itaconate

[a]ACPD, 1-amino-1,3-cyclopentane dicarboxylate. Data are from Curry et al. (1987) and Peet et al. (1987b).

action of glutamate is wholly quisqualate-like. The possible physiological importance of the glycine effect remains unclear.

EXCITATORY AMINO ACIDS AND SYNAPTIC EVENTS

There have been a number of reports of measurements of reversal potentials for the excitatory actions of the amino acids and for monosynaptic EPSPs evoked in hippocampal neurons. Some data are summarized in Table II.

Although the most complete results are those obtained from the dentate gyrus, it seems probable that the electrophysiological changes produced are similar at least in area CA1, namely, that all reversal potentials are near 0mV, indicating that ionic channels permeable to sodium and potassium are opened. Crunelli et al. (1984) emphasize, however, that the reversal potential measured for NMDA is significantly different from those of the other amino acids tested and from the EPSP, implying that, if the excitatory transmitter released upon granule cells from the terminals of the perforant pathway is an amino acid, NMDA receptors are not involved.

A similar conclusion has been derived from observing the effects of antagonists. On CA1 pyramidal cells activation of the monosynaptic Schaffer collateral input is largely unaffected by specific NMDA antagonists such as DAPV, but is reduced by such less selective agents as γ-D-glutamylglycine (Collingridge et al., 1983c; Crunelli et al., 1983; but see Hablitz and Langmoen, 1986) or KYNU (Peet et al., 1986). The evidence that the excitatory transmitter is glutamate acting on non-NMDA receptors thus is reasonably convincing.

The situation is quite different for the phenomenon known as *long-term potentiation* (LTP), the prolonged and considerable augmentation of response following brief high-frequency stimulation of afferent pathways (Bliss and Lømo, 1973) and other types of intense postsynaptic depolarization, including that

TABLE II. Reversal Potentials for Amino Acid Effects and EPSPs in Hippocampus

Cell type	Reversal potentials (mV ± S.D.)[a]		Reference
CA1 pyramidal	Glutamate	−1.5 ± 6.7 (11)	Hablitz and
	EPSP	−2.8 ± 9.6 (3)	Langmoen (1982)
	Quisqualate	+5.7 ± 9.0 (5)	Hablitz (1985)
	NMDA	ca. 0	
CA3 pyramidal	Glutamate		
	D-homocysteate	−13 to −19	Sawada et al.
	DL-homocysteate		(1982)
Dentate granule	Glutamate	−5.6 ± 1.3 (11)	
	Quisqualate	−3.9 ± 3.8 (4)	
	Kainate	−4.6 ± 4.0 (4)	Crunelli et al.
	NMDA	+1.8 ± 6.0 (10)	(1984)
	EPSP	−5.9 ± 4.1 (14)	

[a]Numbers of determinations in parentheses.

produced by the application of glutamate (Hvalby et al., 1987). Once again there is evidence for the involvement of glutamate in the process, since the release of this substance is increased during LTP (Bliss et al., 1986); but this time NMDA receptors are implicated, since the development of LTP is prevented by DAPV and other NMDA receptor antagonists (Collingridge et al., 1983c; Harris et al., 1984; Wigström et al., 1986; Errington et al., 1987). It is now known that at *trans*-membrane potentials near the resting level the ion channels activated by NMDA-like compounds are blocked by the magnesium of the extracellular fluid, and that depolarization displaces this block and allows the action of NMDA to become manifest. In the absence of magnesium a DAPV-sensitive component of the monosynaptic EPSP can be observed (Coan and Collingridge, 1985), although whether this is of any physiological significance is not known.

The conductance change elicited by NMDA has a large calcium component (Peet et al., 1986), and the bursting induced in hippocampal neurons by this substance similarly is calcium dependent. What the endogenous compound giving rise to these various types of NMDA-induced responses may be is problematical. As noted in Table I, neither L-glutamate, L-aspartate, nor L-homocysteate have ever been found to evoke bursting patterns of excitation in the hippocampus, and even with removal of magnesium from the extracellular medium there is no evidence that these compounds can activate NMDA receptors there. Thus, although maintenance of LTP may well be associated with the increased release of glutamate alluded to earlier (Bliss et al., 1986; Errington et al., 1987), its induction seems unlikely to be. An endogenous NMDA receptor activator that might be implicated is of course quinolinate, but its involvement with this or any other synaptic event has not been established.

Long-lasting increases in the synaptic responses evoked in all subregions of the hippocampus are enhanced by certain amino acids, particularly kainate (Collingridge and McLennan, 1981; Collingridge et al., 1983a), and this action is shared also by folate, which is only a very weak neuronal excitant. These phenomena may be more related to the cytotoxic actions of these two substances than to the development of LTP per se, as will be further discussed below.

The considerations above are based on the known characteristics of postsynaptic amino acid receptors. However, the fact that such NMDA antagonists as DAPV block the increased release of glutamate associated with LTP (Errington et al., 1987) implies a significant presynaptic locus of action, and, although it is permissible to assume that the pharmacological characteristics of such presynaptic receptors are the same as those postsynaptically located, no direct evidence for the correctness of the assumption exists.

TOXICOLOGY

The cytotoxic action of glutamate was first described by Lucas and Newhouse (1957), but much of the pioneering work in this field with this and other related excitatory amino acids is due to Olney and his colleagues (for a review of the earlier literature, see Olney, 1983); and the great sensitivity of certain hippocampal neurons to this action is well recognized. The various amino acids can be classified into three categories on the basis of the pattern of their toxic effects, and this classification is not in complete accord with that derived from the pharmacological evidence discussed earlier. One group, which includes NMDA, quinolinate, glutamate, and homocysteate, causes only local necrosis upon intracerebral injection; a second, which contains quisqualate and, most notably, kainate, produces not only local cellular destruction but also seizure-related distant lesions, while folate, which is only a very weak neuronal excitant, causes the "distant" damage but is without local effect.

Certain established pharmacological rules do apply; thus the toxic effects of NMDA and quinolinate are prevented by DAPV or KYNU (Olney et al., 1981; Foster et al., 1984), and there is reasonably general agreement that local cytotoxic and excitatory potencies run in parallel. Nevertheless, there are some perplexing aspects to the whole process. That deafferentation of a target area markedly reduces the sensitivity of the neurons therein to destruction was initially reported for the striatum (Biziere and Coyle, 1978; McGeer et al., 1978) but is equally true in the CA3 region of the hippocampus (Nadler and Cuthbertson, 1980), where the cells are exquisitely sensitive to kainate, and this may indicate that in the normal condition the toxic effect of the amino acids is a presynaptic one (de Montigny et al., 1987). Equally puzzling is the unequal sensitivity of the various types of hippocampal neurons to damage, with the granule cells of the dentate gyrus being particularly resistant.

The mechanism(s) underlying the toxicity remain somewhat in doubt. Local effects clearly require that neuronal depolarization take place, but whether prolonged depolarization per se can evoke cell damage is debated. Thus Rothman (1985) reported that high concentrations of potassium were toxic to cultured hippocampal cells, while Garthwaite et al. (1986a) using cerebellum, have stated the contrary. Some have claimed that the presence of calcium, and thus presumably its uptake, is essential (Garthwaite et al., 1986b), but this too has been denied at least for the acute phase of toxicity (Rothman, 1985; Rothman et al., 1987). A similar uncertainty surrounds the possible role of chloride ions (Rothman, 1985; Garthwaite et al., 1986b). The "distant" effects of certain of the amino acids are similarly mysterious, where both the powerfully excitatory kainate and the very weak folate induce similar (but apparently not identical [Tremblay et al., 1983]) patterns of damage. These actions seem to be related to the ability of both of these substances to induce seizure activity, which in turn may be due in part to a reduction in γ-aminobutyric acid (GABA)-mediated inhibitions (for references, see Kehl et al., 1984). These questions are all considered in greater detail elsewhere in this book.

EPILEPTIFORM ACTIVITY

The ability of NMDA-like compounds to evoke rhythmic bursting in hippocampal neurons has been described earlier, and the probability that a mechanism based on those processes is involved in certain forms of epileptiform and convulsive activity is heightened by the demonstration that NMDA receptor antagonists are effective in preventing them (Croucher et al., 1982; Meldrum et al., 1983; Peterson et al., 1983; Dingledine et al., 1986; Ashwood and Wheal, 1987). The development of seizure-like discharges in the hippocampus, which are prevented by NMDA receptor antagonists, can also be induced by alkalosis (J. Church and H. McLennan, unpublished observations; cf. Aram and Lodge, 1987), and this is associated also with a reduced level of inhibition (Kehl et al., 1984; Lancaster and Wheal, 1984; Dingledine et al., 1986; J. Church and H. McLennan unpublished observations). There is additional evidence that non-NMDA amino acid receptors are also likely to be involved in the genesis of seizure activity (Croucher et al., 1984; Schwarz and Freed, 1986; Turski et al., 1987), and thus it is conceivable that a balance between the levels of endogenous excitatory amino acids of both NMDA and non-NMDA types and GABA-mediated processes may regulate the overall levels of neuronal excitability in vivo.

ACKNOWLEDGMENTS

The author's work has been supported by the Medical Research Council of Canada and the British Columbia Health Care Research Foundation.

REFERENCES

Aram, J.A., and D. Lodge (1987) Epileptiform activity in rat neocortical slices: Block by antagonists of N-methyl-D-aspartate. Neurosci. Lett. 83:345–350.

Ashwood, T.J., and H.V. Wheal (1987) The expression of N-methyl-D-aspartate-receptor-mediated component during epileptiform synaptic activity in the hippocampus. Br. J. Pharmacol. 91:815–822.

Ault, B., R.H. Evans, A.A. Francis, D.J. Oakes, and J.C. Watkins (1980) Selective depression of excitatory amino acid induced depolarizations by magnesium ions in isolated spinal cord preparations. J. Physiol. 307:413–428.

Biscoe, T.J., and D.W. Straughan (1966) Micro-electrophoretic studies of neurones in the cat hippocampus. J. Physiol. 183:341–359.

Biziere, K., and J.T. Coyle (1978) Influence of cortico-striatal afferents on striatal kainic acid neurotoxicity. Neurosci. Lett. 8:303–310.

Bliss, T.V.P., R.M. Douglas, M.L. Errington, and M.A. Lynch (1986) Correlation between long-term potentiation and release of endogenous amino acids from dentate gyrus of anaesthetized rats. J. Physiol. 377:391–408.

Bliss, T.V.P., and T. Lømo (1973) Long-lasting potentiation of synaptic transmission in the dentate area of the anaesthetized rabbit following stimulation of the perforant path. J. Physiol 232:331–356.

Bonhaus, D.W., B.C. Burge, and J.O. McNamara (1987) Biochemical evidence that glycine allosterically regulates an NMDA receptor-coupled ion channel. Eur. J. Pharmacol. 142:489–490.

Coan, E.J., and G.L. Collingridge (1985) Magnesium ions block an N-methyl-D-aspartate receptor-mediated component of synaptic transmission in rat hippocampus. Neurosci. Lett. 53:21–26.

Collingridge, G.L., S.J. Kehl, R. Loo, and H. McLennan (1983a) Effects of kainic and other amino acids on synaptic excitation in rat hippocampal slices: 1. Extracellular analysis. Exp. Brain Res. 52:170–178.

Collingridge, G.L., S.J. Kehl, and H. McLennan (1983b) The antagonism of amino acid-induced excitations of rat hippocampal CA1 neurones in vitro. J. Physiol. 334:19–31.

Collingridge, G.L., S.J. Kehl, and H. McLennan (1983c) Excitatory amino acids in synaptic transmission in the Schaffer collateral-commissural pathway of the rat hippocampus. J. Physiol. *334*:33–46.

Collingridge, G.L., and H. McLennan (1981) The effect of kainic acid on excitatory synaptic activity in the rat hippocampal slice preparation. Neurosci. Lett *27*:31–36.

Croucher, M.J., J.F. Collins, and B.S. Meldrum (1982) Anticonvulsant action of excitatory amino acid antagonists. Science *215*:899–901.

Croucher, M.J., B.S. Meldrum, A.W. Jones, and J.C. Watkins (1984) γ-D-glutamylaminomethylsulfonic acid (GAMS), a kainate and quisqualate antagonist, prevents sound-induced seizures in DBA/2 mice. Brain. Res. *322*:111–114.

Crunelli, V., S. Forda, and J.S. Kelly (1983) Blockade of amino acid-induced depolarizations and inhibition of excitatory post-synaptic potentials in rat dentate gyrus. J. Physiol. *341*:627–640.

Crunelli, V., S. Forda, and J.S. Kelly (1984) The reversal potential of excitatory amino acid action on granule cells of the rat dentate gyrus. J. Physiol. *351*:327–342.

Curry, K., D.S.K. Magnuson, H. McLennan, and M.J. Peet (1987) Excitation of rat hippocampal neurones by the stereoisomers of *cis*- and *trans*-1-amino-1,3-cyclopentane dicarboxylate. Can. J. Physiol. Pharmacol. *65*:2196–2201.

Davies, J., A.A. Francis, A.W. Jones, and J.C. Watkins (1981) 2-Amino-5-phosphonovalerate (2APV), a potent and selective antagonist of amino acid-induced and synaptic excitation. Neurosci. Lett. *21*:77–81.

de Montigny, C., M. Weiss, and J. Ouellette (1987) Reduced excitatory effect of kainic acid on rat CA3 hippocampal neurons following destruction of the mossy projection with colchicine. Exp. Brain. Res. *65*:605–613.

Dingledine, R. (1983) *N*-methyl aspartate activates voltage-dependent calcium conductance in rat hippocampal pyramidal cells. J. Physiol. *343*:385–405.

Dingledine, R., M.A. Hynes, and G.L. King (1986) Involvement of *N*-methyl-D-aspartate receptors in epileptiform bursting in the rat hippocampal slice. J. Physiol. *380*:175–189.

Do, K.Q., P.L. Herrling, P. Streit, W.A. Turski, and M. Cuénod (1986) In vitro release and electrophysiological effects in situ of homocysteic acid, an endogenous *N*-methyl-(D)-aspartic acid agonist, in the mammalian striatum. J. Neurosci. *6*:2226–2234.

Dudar, J.D. (1974) In vitro excitation of hippocampal pyramidal cell dendrites by glutamic acid. Neuropharmacology *13*:1083–1089.

Errington, M.L., M.A. Lynch, and T.V.P. Bliss (1987) Long-term potentiation in the dentate gyrus: Induction and increased glutamate release are blocked by D(-)aminophosphonovalerate. Neuroscience *20*:279–284.

Foster, A.C., A. Vezzani, A.D. French, and R. Schwarcz (1984) Kynurenic acid blocks neurotoxicity and seizures induced in rats by the related brain metabolite quinolinic acid. Neurosci. Lett *48*:273–278.

Ganong, A.H., T.H. Lanthorn, and C.W. Cotman (1983) Kynurenic acid inhibits synaptic and acidic amino acid-induced responses in the rat hippocampus and spinal cord. Brain Res. *273*:170–174.

Garthwaite, J., G. Garthwaite, and F. Hajos (1986a) Amino acid neurotoxicity: Relationship to neuronal depolarization in rat cerebellar slices. Neuroscience *18*:449–460.

Garthwaite, G., F. Hajos, and J. Garthwaite (1986b) Ionic requirements for neurotoxic effects of excitatory amino acid analogues in rat cerebellar slices. Neuroscience *18*:437–446.

Hablitz, J.J. (1985) Action of excitatory amino acids and their antagonists on hippocampal neurons. Cell. Mol. Neurobiol. *5*:389–405.

Hablitz, J.J., and I.A. Langmoen (1982) Excitation of hippocampal pyramidal cells by glutamate in the guinea-pig and rat. J. Physiol. *325*:317–331.

Hablitz, J.J., and I.A. Langmoen (1986) N-methyl-D-aspartate receptor antagonists reduce synaptic excitation in the hippocampus. J. Neurosci. *6*:102–106.

Harris, E.W., A.H. Ganong, and C.W. Cotman (1984) Long-term potentiation in the hippocampus involves activation of N-methyl-D-aspartate receptors. Brain Res. *323*:132–137.

Hvalby, Ø., J.C. Lacaille, G.Y. Hu, and P. Andersen (1987) Postsynaptic long-term potentiation follows coupling of dendritic glutamate application and synaptic activation. Experientia *43*:599–601.

Johnson, J.W., and P. Ascher (1987) Glycine potentiates the NMDA response in cultured mouse brain neurons. Nature *325*:529–531.

Kehl, S.J., H. McLennan, and G.L. Collingridge (1984) Effects of folic and kainic acids on synaptic responses of hippocampal neurones. Neuroscience *11*:111–124.

Knöpfel, T., M.L. Zeise, M. Cuénod, and W. Zieglgänsberger (1987) L-homocysteic acid but not L-glutamate is an endogenous *N*-methyl-D-aspartic acid receptor preferring agonist in rat neocortical neurons in vitro. Neurosci. Lett *81*:188–192.

Lancaster, B., and H.V. Wheal (1984) Chronic failure of inhibition of the CA1 area of the hippocampus following kainic acid lesions of the CA3/4 area. Brain Res. *295*:317–324.

Lucas, D.R., and J.P. Newhouse (1957) The toxic effect of L-glutamate on the inner layers of the retina. Arch. Ophthalmol. *58*:193–201.

Magnuson, D.S.K., M.J. Peet, K. Curry, and H. McLennan (1987) The action of quinolinate in the rat spinal cord in vitro. Can. J. Physiol. Pharmacol. *65*:2483–2487.

McGeer, E.G., P.L. McGeer, and K. Singh (1978) Kainate-induced degeneration of neostriatal neurons: Dependency upon cortico-striatal tract. Brain Res. *139*:381–383.

McLennan, H. (1983) Receptors for the excitatory amino acids in the mammalian central nervous system. Prog. Neurobiol. *20*:251–271.

McLennan, H. (1987) Setting the scene: The excitatory amino acids—30 years on. In T.P. Hicks, D. Lodge, and H. McLennan (eds): Excitatory Amino Acid Transmission. New York: Alan R. Liss., pp. 1–18.

Meldrum, B., M. Wardley-Smith, and J.-C. Rostain (1983) 2-Amino-phosphonoheptanoic acid protects against high pressure neurological syndrome. Eur. J. Pharmacol. *87*:501–502.

Nadler, J.V., and G.J. Cuthbertson (1980) Kainic acid neurotoxicity toward hippocampal formation: Dependence on specific excitatory pathways. Brain Res. *195*:47–56.

Olney, J.W. (1983) Excitotoxins: An overview. In K. Fuxe, P. Roberts, and R. Schwarcz (eds): Excitotoxins. London: Macmillan Press, pp. 82–96.

Olney, J.W., J. Labruyere, J.F. Collins, and K. Curry (1981) D-Aminophosphonovalerate is 100-fold more powerful than D-alpha-aminoadipate in blocking N-methylaspartate toxicity. Brain Res. *221*:207–210.

Peet, M.J., K. Curry, D.S. Magnuson, and H. McLennan (1986) Ca^{2+}-dependent depolarization and burst firing of rat CA1 pyramidal neurones induced by *N*-methyl-D-aspartic acid and quinolinic acid: Antagonism by 2-amino-5-phosphonovaleric and kynurenic acids. Can. J. Physiol. Pharmacol. *64*:163–168.

Peet, M.J., K. Curry, D.S.K. Magnuson, and H. McLennan (1987a) Structural requirements for antagonism of burst firing of rat CA1 hippocampal neurones. In N. Chalazonitis and M. Gola (eds): Inactivation of Hypersensitive Neurons. New York: Alan R. Liss, pp. 105–112.

Peet, M.J., K. Curry, D.S.K. Magnuson, and H. McLennan (1987b) The N-methyl-D-aspartate receptor and burst firing of CA1 hippocampal pyramidal neurons. Neuroscience *22*:563–571.

Perkins, M.N., and T.W. Stone (1982) An iontophoretic investigation of the actions of convulsant kynurenines and their interaction with the endogenous excitant quinolinic acid. Brain Res. *247*:184–187.

Peterson, D.W., J.F. Collins, and H.F. Bradford (1983) The kindled amygdala model of epilepsy: Anticonvulsant action of amino acid antagonists. Brain Res. *275*:169–172.

Rothman, S.M. (1985) The neurotoxicity of excitatory amino acids is produced by passive chloride influx. J. Neurosci. *5*:1483–1489.

Rothman, S.M., J.H. Thurston, and R.E. Hauhart (1987) Delayed neurotoxicity of excitatory amino acids in vitro. Neuroscience *22*:471–480.

Sawada, S., S. Takada and C. Yamamoto (1982) Excitatory actions of homocysteic acid on hippocampal neurons. Brain Res. *238*:282–285.

Schwartzkroin, P.A., and P. Andersen (1975) Glutamic acid sensitivity of dendrites in hippocampal slices in vitro. Adv. Neurol. *12*:45–51.

Schwarz, S.S., and W.J. Freed (1986) Inhibition of quisqualate-induced seizures by glutamic acid diethyl ester and anti-epileptic drugs. J. Neural Transm. *67*:191–203.

Spencer, H.J., V.K. Gribkoff, and G.S. Lynch (1978) Distribution of acetylcholine, glutamate and aspartate sensitivity over the dendritic fields of hippocampal CA1 neurones. In R.W. Ryall and J.S. Kelly (eds): Iontophoresis and Transmitter Mechanisms in the Mammalian Central Nervous System. Amsterdam: Elsevier/North Holland Biomedical Press, pp. 194–196.

Tremblay, E., E. Cavalheiro, and Y. Ben-Ari (1983) Are convulsant and toxic properties of folates of the kainate type? Eur. J. Pharmacol. *93*:283–286.

Turski, L., B.S. Meldrum, W.A. Turski, and J.C. Watkins (1987) Evidence that antagonism at non-NMDA receptors results in anticonvulsant action. Eur J. Pharmacol. *136*:69–73.

Watkins, J.C. (1986) Twenty-five years of excitatory amino acid research. In P.J. Roberts, J. Storm-Mathisen, and H.F. Bradford (eds): Excitatory Amino Acids. London: Macmillan Press, pp. 1–39.

Wigström, H., B. Gustafsson, and Y.-Y. Huang (1986) Mode of action of excitatory amino acid receptor antagonists on hippocampal long-lasting potentiation. Neuroscience *17*:1105–1115.

Yamamoto, C. (1972) Intracellular study of seizure-like afterdischarges in thin hippocampal sections in vitro. Exp. Neurol. *35*:154–164.

Yamamoto, C. and H. McIlwain (1966) Electrical activities in thin sections from the mammalian brain maintained in chemically defined media in vitro. J. Neurochem. *13*:1333–1343.

The Hippocampus—New Vistas, pages 329–345

21
Synaptic Function of N-Methyl-D-Aspartate Receptors in the Hippocampus

GRAHAM L. COLLINGRIDGE

Department of Pharmacology, The School of Medical Sciences, The University of Bristol, Bristol, England

INTRODUCTION

The principal excitatory neurotransmitters in the vertebrate nervous system seem to be the acidic amino acids L-glutamate (Glu) and L-aspartate (ASP) and perhaps certain analogs such as L-homocysteate. These endogenous excitants interact with several types of excitatory amino acid receptors, which are generally named after the potent exogenous agonists N-methyl-D-aspartate (NMDA), kainate, and quisqualate (Watkins and Evans, 1981).

The development of selective NMDA antagonists has led to considerable information about these receptors (for references, see Cotman and Iversen, 1987). Areas of particular interest include their role in forms of synaptic plasticity in the adult and developing nervous systems (Collingridge, 1987) and their implication in neuropathologies, such as epilepsy and neurodegeneration (Meldrum, 1985). NMDA receptors are distributed heterogeneously throughout the central nervous system of vertebrates, with the highest levels in cortical structures, particularly the hippocampus.

The purpose of the present chapter is to describe the role of NMDA receptors in synaptic mechanisms in the hippocampus. This is preceded with a brief description of pertinent aspects of the pharmacology of acidic amino acids (for further details, see McLennan, Chapter 20, this volume), NMDA gated conductance mechanisms, and hippocampal NMDA receptor distribution.

Abbreviations: ACh, acetylcholine; AMPA, α-amino-3-hydroxy-5-methyl-4-isoxazole-propionic acid; APV, D-2-amino-5-phosphonovalerate; ASP, L-aspartate; CNQX, 6-cyano-7-nitroquinoxaline-2,3-dione; CPP, 3-([+]-2-carboxypiperazin-4-yl)-propyl-1-phosphonic acid; EPSP, excitatory postsynaptic potential; GABA, γ-aminobutyric acid; Glu, L-glutamate; IPSP, inhibitory postsynaptic potential; LTP, long-term potentiation; MK-801, (+)-5-methyl-10,11-dihydro-5H-dibenzo(a,d)cyclo hepten-5,10-imine maleate; NA, noradrenaline; NMDA, N-methyl-D-aspartate; PCP, phencyclidine; TCP, thienylcyclohexylpiperidine.

Excitatory Amino Acid Pharmacology

Responses to NMDA can be blocked by a wide range of compounds of diverse structure: 1) organic competitive antagonists, such as D-2-amino-5-phosphonovalerate (APV); 2) "noncompetitive" antagonists, including ketamine, phencyclidine (PCP), thienylcyclohexylpiperidine (TCP), and MK-801; and 3) certain divalent cations, most notably Mg^{2+}. Thus NMDA receptor-mediated processes can be identified on the basis of their sensitivity to three distinct classes of drugs. APV is a particularly useful compound, since, in addition to being selective for the NMDA class of excitatory amino acid receptor, it has not been found to interefere with any other neurotransmitter system.

Excitatory amino acids, such as kainate, quisqualate, and α-amino-3-hydroxy-5-methyl-4-isoxazole-propionic acid (AMPA), that act on non-NMDA receptor subtypes can be blocked by quinoxalinediones, such as 6-cyano-7-nitroquinoxaline-2,3-dione (CNQX) (Honoré et al., 1988). There are, however, no antagonists currently available that distinguish well between the non-NMDA receptor subtypes.

NMDA Conductance Mechanisms

Mg^{2+} exerts a voltage-dependent block of the channels that are directly linked to NMDA receptors (Nowak et al., 1984). The block is large at the normal resting membrane potentials of neurons but decreases as they are depolarized. NMDA channels are permeable to the monovalent cations Na^+ and K^+, and, significantly, they also have an appreciable permeability to Ca^{2+} (Mayer et al., 1987).

Distribution of NMDA Receptors in the Hippocampus

The distribution of NMDA receptors within the hippocampal formation has been determined using quantitative autoradiographic techniques at the light microscopic level (Cotman et al., 1987). A similar pattern of binding is seen irrespective of the means of labeling: NMDA-sensitive Glu binding, the binding of competitive (APV or CPP) or noncompetitive (TCP) NMDA antagonists, or the binding of glycine, an allosteric potentiator of NMDA at strychnine-insensitive sites. With the notable exception of the mossy fiber termination zone, there is a high density of NMDA receptors throughout the hippocampal formation. Especially high levels are found in the middle molecular layer of the dentate gyrus (corresponding to the termination zone of the medial perforant pathway) and, particularly, in strata oriens and radiatum of CA1 (where the Schaffer collateral-commissural fibers, which originate respectively from ipsi- and contralateral CA3 neurons, terminate).

INVOLVEMENT OF NMDA RECEPTORS IN SYNAPTIC TRANSMISSION

The extent to which NMDA receptors contribute to synaptic responses in the hippocampus is highly dependent on the experimental conditions employed. Important factors include the extracellular Mg^{2+} concentration, membrane potential, state of synaptic inhibition, and frequency of activation of excitatory pathways.

Low-Frequency Transmission

"Normal" conditions. In view of the marked plasticity displayed by hippocampal pathways, rates of stimulation are usually kept to 0.1 Hz or less. In hippocampal slices, using a standard perfusate (i.e. 1–4 mM Mg^{2+} and no convulsants) low-frequency-evoked synaptic potentials recorded extracellularly or intracellularly (at potentials of around -50 mV or more negative) are largely, if not totally, insensitive to APV and other NMDA antagonists (Fig. 1A i). The pathways that have been examined include the Schaffer collateral-commissural innervation of CA1 (Collingridge et al., 1983a), the lateral and medial perforant pathway inputs to dentate (Crunelli et al., 1982; Collingridge et al., 1984), and the perforant, commissural, and mossy fiber inputs to CA3 (Collingridge et al., 1987). Similar findings have generally been reported for in vivo recordings (Morris et al., 1986; Errington et al., 1987), indicating that the standard perfusate approximates physiological conditions. The synaptic connections that form between dissociated embryonic hippocampal neurons maintained in culture are also insensitive to NMDA antagonists under these conditions (Rothman and Samaie, 1985).

In contrast to the lack of effect of selective NMDA antagonists, drugs that also block non-NMDA type acidic amino acid receptors, such as γ-D-glutamylglycine and kynurenic acid, are synaptic depressants on those pathways tested (Crunelli et al., 1982; Collingridge et al., 1983a; Ganong et al., 1983; Sawada and Yamamoto, 1984). CNQX in doses that block kainate, quisqualate, and AMPA but are without effect on NMDA can totally depress the synaptic potential in CA1 (Blake et al., 1988) (Fig. 2A). Thus the receptor that mediates the synaptic potential under these "normal" low-frequency conditions is likely to be an acidic amino acid receptor of the non-NMDA type.

Mg^{2+}-free perfusate. In area CA1, if Mg^{2+} is omitted from the perfusate the synaptic response increases in amplitude and duration. A large proportion of the additional component is sensitive to Mg^{2+} in a dose-dependent manner over the low micromolar range (10–100 μM) and is blocked by competitive (Coan and Collingridge, 1987a) and noncompetitive (Coan and Collingridge, 1987b) NMDA antagonists (Fig. 1A ii). NMDA receptors, in the absence of Mg^{2+}, also contribute to synaptic transmission in the medial and lateral perforant pathways (Coan et al., 1987a) and in area CA3 (Anderson et al., 1986).

In Mg^{2+}-free perfusates, the evoked response appears epileptiform. In addition, synchronized spontaneous discharges often appear, generated by paroxysmal depolarizing shifts, that may be equated with interictal-like activity (Mody et al., 1987) and also full-blown ictal-like events (Anderson et al., 1986). The "interictals" originate in CA3 and entorhinal cortex where they can propagate to CA1 and dentate, respectively (Coan and Collingridge, 1987a; Mody et al., 1987; Walther et al., 1986). All these epileptiform events can be blocked by NMDA antagonists. There are also episodes of spreading depression. Thus,

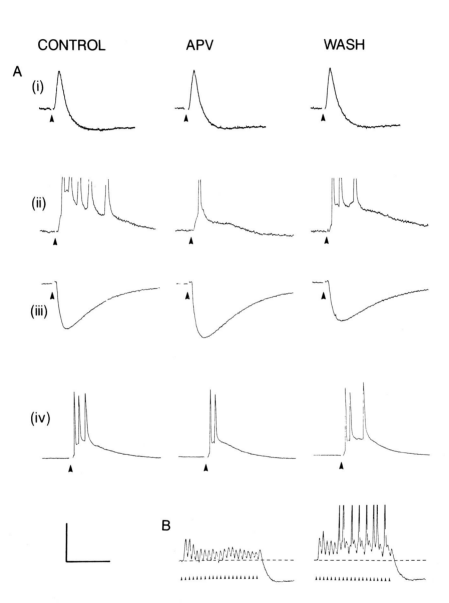

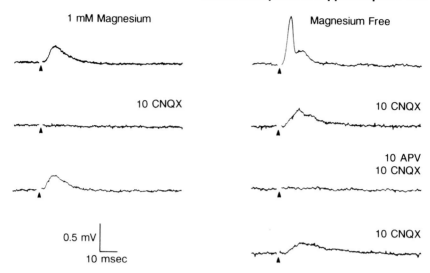

Fig. 2.   Synaptic antagonism by CNQX. The response to low-frequency Schaffer collateral commissural stimulation is blocked by CNQX in 1 mM Mg^{2+}-containing medium (left) but is only reduced by CNQX in Mg^{2+}-free medium (right). The CNQX-resistant component is blocked by APV. All traces are grease-gap recordings from the same slice in response to a constant stimulus intensity. Drugs were applied at 10 μM. (Reproduced from Blake et al., 1988, with permission of the publisher.)

the electrophysiological properties of hippocampal slice in Mg^{2+}-free medium are quite distinct from those of the normal hippocampus recorded in vivo.

Depolarized cells. In Mg^{2+}-containing medium an APV-sensitive synaptic component of the responses of CA1 neurones to Schaffer collateral-commissural stimulation can be recorded when cells are strongly depolarized by current injection (Collingridge et al., 1988b) (Fig. 1A iii).

Reduced synaptic inhibition. In Mg^{2+}-containing medium, an APV-sensitive synaptic component can be recorded when synaptic inhibition has been

---

Fig. 1.   Effects of APV (20 or 50 μM) on intracellularly recorded potentials evoked by Schaffer collateral commissural stimulation in rat hippocampal slices. **A:** Low-frequency (0.033 Hz) stimulation in i) "normal conditions" (i.e. 1 mM Mg^{2+}, no convulsant, cell at its resting membrane potential) or following the manipulation of *one* of these conditions: ii) Mg^{2+}-free medium, iii) a cell depolarized by current injection to −10 mV (prestimulus), or iv) in the presence of 2 μM bicuculline. **B:** High-frequency (100 Hz, 200 ms) stimulation under "normal conditions." Note that APV has an effect, corresponding to depression of a slow depolarizing potential, in all cells except that illustrated in A i. In this and subsequent figures, arrowheads mark the time of blanked stimulus artifacts. Calibration (mV/ms): A i, 8/40; ii, 20/30; iii, 20/40; iv, 40/30; B, 16/120. Parts A i and B were modified from Herron et al. (1986), with permission of Macmillan Magazines Ltd. Part A ii was modified from Herron et al. (1985a), part A iii from Collingridge et al. (1988c) and part A iv from Herron et al. (1985b), with permission of the publishers.

reduced or abolished by, for example, application of a $GABA_A$ antagonist such as picrotoxin or bicuculline (Herron et al., 1985b) (Fig. 1A iv). The size of the APV-sensitive component increases with membrane depolarization (Dingledine et al., 1986), as expected for an NMDA receptor-mediated event in the presence of Mg^{2+}.

It seems likely that synaptic inhibition limits NMDA receptor activation during an EPSP by rapidly hyperpolarizing the cell into a region (-70 to -90 mV) where the Mg^{2+} block of NMDA channels is substantial. In support of this idea, an NMDA receptor component has been demonstrated at potentials near rest when the hyperpolarizing aspect of the IPSP has been greatly reduced using voltage-clamp techniques (Collingridge et al., 1988b).

Other treatments that have resulted in a reduction of synaptic inhibition and the appearance of an NMDA receptor synaptic component include the addition of kainate or folate (Herron et al., 1987), the repeated application of periods of high-frequency stimulation in vitro (Slater et al., 1985; Anderson et al., 1987) or in vivo (Mody and Heinemann, 1987), and chronic injections of kainic acid into the hippocampus (Ashwood and Wheal, 1987). Activation of the NMDA receptor system in these models may also be due to a reduction in $GABA_A$ (and/or $GABA_B$)-mediated inhibition. Conversely, the reduction in inhibition may be secondary to activation of the NMDA receptor system (Stelzer et al., 1987).

Characteristics of the NMDA Receptor Component

From the studies described above and from work in which combinations of treatments (e.g. Mg^{2+}-free and convulsants) have been used (Forsythe and Westbrook, 1988; Wigström and Gustafsson, 1988), a number of interesting features of the NMDA receptor system have emerged, which are probably fundamental to its function. The NMDA receptor component has a similar threshold and latency to onset as does the non-NMDA receptor component, suggesting that this component is monosynaptic and may be mediated by the same neurotransmitter(s) released from the same fibers as the non-NMDA receptor component. In support of its monosynaptic origin, the NMDA receptor component can be recorded in isolation following blockade of non-NMDA receptors with CNQX in Mg^{2+}-free (Blake et al., 1988) (Fig. 2B) and, under certain conditions, in Mg^{2+}-containing (Collingridge et al., 1988b; Andreasen et al., 1988) medium.

The NMDA receptor component has a longer time to peak and duration (~100–200 ms) than the non-NMDA receptor component. The reasons for its slow time course are not known, but may relate to channel kinetics and to the high affinity of NMDA receptors for the neurotransmitter. The time course of the synaptic response, particularly the rise time, is likely to be affected by the Mg^{2+} concentration, and the duration is regulated by synaptic inhibition. Thus, in response to a single synchronized volley in "normal" solutions, the NMDA receptor component may be turned off before it has significantly begun.

Both NMDA and non-NMDA receptor-mediated synaptic components have reversal potentials close to 0 mV. The major charge carriers are Na^+ and K^+

for both events. Additionally, it has been shown, using cultured hippocampal cells, that the NMDA receptor component has, like responses to NMDA, a dependence on Ca^{2+}.

High-Frequency Transmission

As described above, NMDA receptors contribute little, if at all, toward the EPSP evoked by a single shock in the presence of Mg^{2+} and synaptic inhibition at membrane potentials at and around rest. However, under these experimental conditions an APV-sensitive component can be recorded during high-frequency stimulation (Collingridge et al., 1988c) (Fig. 1B).

This component comprises a slow depolarizing potential that starts after the first, and greatly outlasts the last, non-NMDA receptor EPSP. The faster non NMDA receptor EPSPs themselves are not directly affected by APV. The APV-sensitive component increases with membrane depolarization in the manner expected for an NMDA receptor-mediated event in the presence of Mg^{2+}. It has a similar threshold to that of the non-NMDA receptor EPSP. It can be detected at frequencies of around 10 Hz and increases with frequency of stimulation over the range 10–100 Hz. These properties are as expected on the basis of the behavior of the synaptic responses during single-shock stimulation, as described above.

The nature of the synaptic activation of the NMDA receptor system has several implications for synaptic transmission and its interpretation. For example, NMDA receptors could help a cell to fire in a repetitive or burst discharge in response to a high-frequency input. This may have implications both physiologically and pathologically. In the latter case, for example, NMDA receptors could help to propogate a burst discharge originating from an epileptiform focus through normal tissue (Herron et al., 1986). In cases in which activation of NMDA receptors is necessary to enable a neuron to fire, the action of APV to inhibit firing could be misinterpreted, on the basis of the extracellular recording of firing rates, as indicating the existence of a pure NMDA receptor-mediated synapse.

High-frequency homosynaptic trains provide one means of activating NMDA receptors under "normal" conditions. Theoretically, however, the activation requirement of an NMDA receptor agonist and sufficient membrane depolarization could be provided in other ways, for instance, by converging heterosynaptic inputs. Indeed, only one input need release an NMDA ligand; the other could release a different neurotransmitter/modulator, such as ACh or NA to provide the appropriate membrane potential conditions.

INVOLVEMENT OF NMDA RECEPTORS IN LONG-TERM POTENTIATION
Properties of LTP

High-frequency stimulation of excitatory pathways in the hippocampus often results in a potentiation of the synaptic response, which can last for many hours (in vitro) or weeks (in vivo) (Bliss and Lømo, 1973). This phenomenon is commonly termed long-term potentiation (LTP) (for details, see Lynch, Chapter 23, this volume).

There are a number of properties that make LTP an attractive model with which to study mechanisms that may be involved in learning and memory: 1) it can be induced by frequencies of stimulation (of approximately 10 Hz or greater, optimally presented at the theta frequency) that closely mimic firing patterns of hippocampal neurons; 2) the potentiation can be very long-lasting but is not irreversible; 3) LTP is specific to the tetanized pathway, other inputs onto the neurons are not normally potentiated; 4) there is the property of cooperativity, i.e. an intensity threshold, such that strong homosynaptic tetanizing shocks are required to induce LTP; 5) there is the property of associativity: a weak tetanus that will not itself induce LTP will do so if presented with, or shortly after, a strong tetanus to a converging heterosynaptic pathway (this latter property has been equated with pavlovian conditioning); and 6) the induction of LTP has "Hebbian-like" properties in that it requires conjoint pre-synaptic activity and sufficient postsynaptic membrane depolarization. As will be described below, the activation properties of the NMDA receptor system can account for most of these features.

NMDA Receptors Antagonists Block LTP

It is now firmly established that NMDA receptor activation is essential for LTP to be generated in several pathways in the hippocampus. Thus it has been shown that APV blocks the induction of LTP in the Schaffer collateral-commissural pathway (Collingridge et al., 1983a) (Fig. 3), the perforant pathway inputs to dentate (Morris et al., 1986; Errington et al., 1987), and the commissural innervation of CA3 (Harris and Cotman, 1986). All of these pathways innervate NMDA receptor-rich regions of the hippocampus.

In CA1, the induction of LTP is blocked by APV and a series of its homologs in parallel with the ability of these agents to depress responses to NMDA (Harris et al., 1984). The induction of LTP is also prevented by noncompetitive NMDA antagonists such as ketamine, PCP, (Stringer and Guyenet, 1983), and MK-801 (Coan et al., 1987b). Indeed, all substances tested that depress responses to NMDA also block LTP when applied appropriately.

The mossy fiber pathway is an interesting exception, since it innervates a region sparse in NMDA receptors and since LTP in this pathway neither shows associative properties nor is blocked by APV (Harris and Cotman, 1986; Kauer and Nicoll, 1988).

Since two fundamentally distinct types of LTP can occur within the hippocampus (even in the same CA3 pyramidal neurons) and since the early phase of LTP overlaps in time with other forms of post-tetanic potentiation, it is appropriate to distinguish potentiation resulting from NMDA receptor activation (irrespective of its duration) from other forms of potentiation. It is the former type of LTP that is most well known and will be specifically referred to here.

In contrast to the ability of NMDA antagonists to block the induction of LTP, these drugs have no effect on the potentiated response (Collingridge et al., 1983a; Errington et al., 1987). Thus NMDA receptors are only involved transiently in the induction phase, not in the maintenance phase, of LTP.

Pre-tetanus   Post 1st tetanus   Post 2nd tetanus

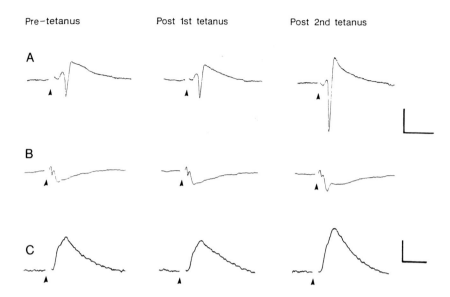

Fig. 3.   APV blocks the induction of LTP. Extracellular recordings in CA1 from the cell body **(A)** or dendritic **(B)** regions or intracellular recordings **(C)** in response to low-frequency stimulation of the Schaffer collateral-commissural pathway before (left) or 15 min following a period of high-frequency stimulation (100 Hz, 1 s) given in the presence (center) or washout (right) of APV (20 or 50 μM). Calibration (mV/ms): A, B, 4/10; C, 10/10. (A and B modified from Collingridge and Bliss [1987]; C modified from Collingridge [1985], with permission of the publisher.)

NMDA Receptor Involvement in "Kindling"

Repeated application of high-frequency stimulation induces interictal-like discharges in vitro (Slater et al., 1985; Anderson et al., 1987) and kindled seizures in vivo (McNamara et al., 1988) which are prevented if the stimulation is given in the presence of an NMDA antagonist. Thus kindling appears to be an extension of LTP. Unlike in LTP, NMDA antagonists can have a small effect on the "potentiated" response (Peterson et al., 1983), presumably because the synaptic potential is sufficiently long-lasting for activation of the NMDA receptor system to occur.

The Mechanism of Induction of LTP

It has been hypothesized (see Collingridge, 1985; Collingridge and Bliss, 1987) that during low-frequency transmission the neurotransmitter (e.g. Glu) binds to both NMDA and non-NMDA receptors. The binding of Glu to the non-

NMDA receptor gates a channel permeable to Na^+ and K^+, and this generates the EPSP. There is little or no contribution to the EPSP from the NMDA receptor, since the channels open more slowly (and may be blocked by Mg^{2+}) and conjointly activated IPSPs rapidly hyperpolarize the cell into a region of substantial Mg^{2+} block. Nevertheless, the NMDA receptor component retains the potential of contributing for up to ~100–200 ms after the initiation of the synaptic response, since a depolarizing step applied during this time can elicit LTP (Wigström and Gustafsson, 1988). Presumably, the binding of Glu to NMDA receptors increases channel opening probability for ~100–200 ms (perhaps because it remains bound throughout this time).

During high-frequency stimulation the cell is maintained much longer at a level at which the Mg^{2+} block of NMDA channels is considerably reduced. Thus the NMDA receptor component is observed and summates at frequencies of 5–10 Hz (because a single response lasts 100–200 ms). The NMDA component may increase nonlinearly, since each response becomes more effective as the cell is further depolarized. Factors that could contribute to the depolarization that alleviates the Mg^{2+} block include the fade of IPSPs, summation of non-NMDA receptor-mediated EPSPs, and an elevation of extracellular K^+.

The next stage in the induction process is believed to involve the entry of Ca^{2+} through NMDA channels (see Collingridge and Bliss, 1987). This aspect, the biochemical processes activated by NMDA-gated Ca^{2+}, and the mechanisms of maintenance of LTP are described in Chapter 23 (see Lynch, this volume).

Agonist-Induced LTP

On the assumption that activation of excitatory amino acid receptors, particularly the NMDA receptor, may induce LTP, studies have been performed to attempt to induce LTP by the application of agonists. With iontophoretic application to soma regions or brief perfusion, a lasting potentiation of the population spike can be elicited with kainate but not with either quisqualate or, perhaps surprisingly, NMDA (Collingridge and McLennan, 1981; Collingridge et al., 1983b). The mechanism of the kainate potentiation, which is seen in all regions of the hippocampus, is not known.

NMDA, when applied by brief perfusion or somatic application, leads to a fairly long-lasting depression of synaptic transmission (Collingridge et al., 1983b). However, a potentiating effect has been reported with perfusion of NMDA providing K^+ is elevated and quisqualate is first applied (Izumi et al., 1987).

More simply, a potentiating effect, which is prevented by APV, can be induced by local dendritic application of NMDA in area CA1 (Collingridge et al., 1983a; Kauer et al., 1988) and the dentate gyrus (Collingridge et al., 1984). The extent to which this potentiation utilizes the same mechanisms as LTP is presently not known.

Agonist-Induced Changes in Synaptic Antagonism

With prolonged application of L-glutamate some intriguing changes in the susceptibility of the Schaffer collateral-commissural pathway to antagonists occur. Thus, the synaptic response is initially depressed but then recovers to a state now sensitive to NMDA antagonists. This response then disappears and is replaced by a state insensitive to all antagonists (Krishtal et al., 1988).

Mg^{2+} Concentration and LTP

Since perfusion with Mg^{2+}-free medium results in activation of the NMDA receptor system during low-frequency transmission, it is of interest to know whether this treatment alone is sufficient to induce LTP, i.e. is high-frequency stimulation required solely to activate the NMDA receptor system or for other purposes as well? In area CA1, perfusion with Mg^{2+}-free medium for periods of approximately 30 min, while stimulating at 0.1 Hz, can induce LTP, as determined after reintroduction of Mg^{2+} (Coan and Collingridge, 1985). This effect is not seen if the Mg^{2+}-free perfusate contains APV (Avoli et al., 1988). It has been suggested that to induce LTP in this manner it is a requirement to have the CA3 region of the slice in synaptic contact with CA1 and that the propogation of epileptiform discharges from the CA3 region is necessary for Mg^{2+} free-induced LTP (Harris and Cotman, 1985; Neuman et al., 1987).

Other studies have investigated the effect of Mg^{2+} concentration on the tetanus-induced induction of LTP. As would be expected, the ease of induction is related to the concentration of this ion in the bathing medium. It has been shown that LTP is greatly facilitated in 100 μM Mg^{2+} compared with 500 μM to 2 mM (control) medium (Huang et al., 1987). LTP in low Mg^{2+} solutions is, as would be expected, blocked by APV.

Paradoxically, however, if slices are perfused with nominally Mg^{2+}-free medium, then it becomes very difficult to induce LTP (Coan and Collingridge, 1988) irrespective of the intensity of high-frequency stimulation that is used. In some of these experiments (using slices where the CA3 region had been removed to eliminate complications that might arise from propagated epileptiform activity) Mg^{2+} was re-added to the perfusate. In these instances, the slices were able to support LTP. Thus, saturation of the LTP process is unlikely to have occurred (Fig. 4).

One possibility is that a constant low level activation of the NMDA receptor system, afforded by low-frequency shocks in Mg^{2+}-free medium, turns off the induction mechanism. Thus, to induce LTP it is necessary to elevate intracellular free Ca^{2+} to a required level and for an appropriate time. In support of this idea, LTP *can* be produced in Mg^{2+}-free medium containing sufficient APV (e.g. 20 μM) to block NMDA receptor activation during low (but not high) frequency transmission (Coan et al., 1988).

PROSPECTIVES
NMDA Receptors and Synaptic Transmission

The current understanding of the involvement of NMDA receptors in synaptic transmission in the hippocampus has, for the most part, been based on studies that have used the regular synchronous activation of pathways by electrical stimulation. It now seems appropriate to determine the excitatory amino acid pharmacology of "unitary synapses" made between identified hippocampal neurons, to study transmission using physiologically more relevant patterns

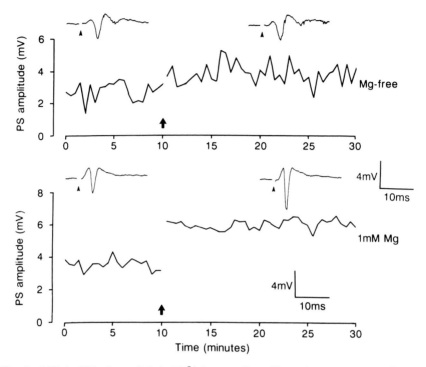

Fig. 4.   LTP is difficult to elicit in Mg^{2+}-free medium. Plots of successive population spike amplitudes before and after high-frequency stimulation (100 Hz, 1 s; at time marked by arrow) in Mg^{2+}-free medium (upper) and following reintroduction of 1 mM Mg^{2+}-containing medium (lower). Records were obtained 5 min before and 15 min following the high-frequency train (Coan and Collingridge, unpublished data).

of neuronal activity (Larson and Lynch, 1986; Rose et al., 1988), and to return to in vivo models (Abraham and Kairiss, 1988).

The modulation of NMDA receptor-mediated transmission by GABA-mediated inhibition is well documented. Logical predictions on its regulation by ACh, monoamine, and peptidergic transmitter candidates can now be tested.

Patch clamp and microfluorimetric techniques, mainly applicable at present to use with acutely dissociated cells and cultures, when applied to more organized preparations, such as slices (Gray and Johnston, 1987; Kudo et al., 1987) would be expected to provide important new information. Alternatively, cell cultures may be developed that retain the essential neuroanatomy to study LTP with these techniques (Gähwiler, 1981).

NMDA Receptors and LTP

It is well established that NMDA receptors are involved in the induction of associative forms of LTP in the hippocampus, and the mechanism of initiation of this process is beginning to be understood. Major advances will most likely now be made in the understanding of the maintenance of LTP. Although NMDA receptors are not thought to play an important role in maintenance per se, it is likely that NMDA agonists and antagonists will become increasingly useful tools in the study of this aspect of LTP (see Lynch, Chapter 23, this volume). For example, tetanus-induced biochemical changes should be APV sensitive if they are to be related specifically to associative LTP.

Certain details of the induction process remain to be worked out: 1) Is NMDA receptor activation alone sufficient to induce LTP? 2) Does the synaptic activation of non-NMDA type excitatory amino acid receptors play any role, directly or indirectly, in LTP? 3) Are NMDA receptors also localized presynaptically, or are they solely postsynaptic on hippocampal neurones? 4) What is the time course of NMDA receptor-mediated potentiation? With currently available drugs and techniques, these and many other questions concerning LTP should soon be answered.

REFERENCES

Abraham, W.C., and E.W. Kairiss (1988) NMDA receptor control of spontaneous complex spike discharge in hippocampal pyramidal cells. In H.L. Haas and G. Buzsáki (eds): Synaptic Plasticity in the Hippocampus. Berlin: Springer-Verlag, 35–37.

Anderson, W.W., D.A. Lewis, H.S. Swartzwelder, and W.A. Wilson (1986) Magnesium-free medium activates seizure-like events in the rat hippocampal slice. Brain Res. *398:*215–219.

Anderson, W.W., H.S. Swartzwelder, and W.A. Wilson (1987) The NMDA receptor antagonist 2-amino-5-phosphonovalerate blocks stimulus train-induced epileptogenesis but not epileptiform bursting in rat hippocampal slice. J. Neurophysiol. *57:*1–21.

Andreasen, M., J.D.C. Lambert, and M. Skovgaard Jensen (1988) Effects of new non-NMDA antagonists in the rat in vitro hippocampus. J. Physiol. [Lond.] *403:*57P.

Ashwood, T.J., and H.V. Wheal (1987) The expression of N-methyl-D-aspartate-receptor-mediated component during epileptiform synaptic activity in the hippocampus. Br. J. Pharmacol. *91:*815–822.

Avoli, M., C. Drapeau, and G. Kostopoulos (1988) Changes in synaptic transmission evoked in the "in vitro" hippocampal slice by a brief decrease in Mg^{++}. A correlate of long term potentiation? In H.L. Haas and G. Buzsáki (eds): Synaptic Plasticity in the Hippocampus. Berlin: Springer-Verlag, pp. 9–11.

Blake, J.F., M.W. Brown, and G.L. Collingridge (1988) CNQX blocks acidic amino acid induced depolarisations and synaptic components mediated by non-NMDA receptors in rat hippocampal slices. Neurosci. Lett. *89:*182–186.

Bliss, T.V.P., and T. Lømo (1973) Long-lasting potentiation of synaptic transmission in the dentate area of the anaesthetised rabbit following stimulation of the perforant path. J. Physiol. [Lond.] *232:*331–356.

Coan, E.J., and G.L. Collingridge (1985) Magnesium ions block an N-methyl-D-aspartate receptor-mediated component of synaptic transmission in rat hippocampal slices. Neurosci. Lett. *53:*21–26.

Coan, E.J., and G.L. Collingridge (1987a) Characterization of an N-methyl-D-aspartate receptor component of synaptic transmission in rat hippocampal slices. Neuroscience *22:*1–8.

Coan, E.J., and G.L. Collingridge (1987b) Effects of phencyclidine, SKF 10,047 and related psychotomimetic agents on N-methyl-D-aspartate receptor mediated synaptic responses in rat hippocampal slices. Br. J. Pharmacol. *91:*547–556.

Coan, E.J., and G.L. Collingridge (1988) Perfusion with Mg^{2+}-free medium can reversibly prevent the induction of LTP in rat hippocampus in vitro. J. Physiol. [Lond.] *401:* 71P.

Coan, E.J., G.L. Collingridge, and A.J. Irving (1988) APV facilitates the induction of long-term potentiation in Mg^{2+}-free medium in rat hippocampus in vitro. J. Physiol. [Lond.] *406:*178P.

Coan, E.J., C.F. Newland, and G.L. Collingridge (1987a) Synaptic activation of NMDA receptors in medial and lateral perforant pathways in the absence of magnesium ions. Neurol. Neurobiol. *24:*353–356.

Coan, E.J., W. Saywood, and G.L. Collingridge (1987b) MK-801 blocks NMDA receptor-mediated synaptic transmission and long term potentiation in rat hippocampal slices. Neurosci. Lett. *80:*111–114.

Collingridge, G.L. (1985) Long term potentiation in the hippocampus: Mechanisms of initiation and modulation by neurotransmitters. Trends Pharmacol. Sci. *6:*407–411.

Collingridge, G.L. (1987) The role of NMDA receptors in learning and memory. Nature *330:*604–605.

Collingridge, G.L., and T.V.P. Bliss (1987) NMDA receptors—Their role in long-term potentiation. Trends Neurosci. *10:*288–293.

Collingridge, G.L., E.J. Coan, C.E. Herron, and R.A.J. Lester (1987) Role of excitatory amino acid receptors in synaptic transmission and plasticity in hippocampal pathways. Neurol. Neurobiol. *24:*317–324.

Collingridge, G.L., C. Davies, and S.N. Davies (1988a) Actions of APV and CNQX on synaptic responses in rat hippocampal slices. Neurol. Neurobiol. *46:*171–178.

Collingridge, G.L., C.E. Herron, and R.A.J. Lester (1988b) Frequency-dependent N-methyl-D-aspartate receptor-mediated synaptic transmission in rat hippocampus. J. Physiol. [Lond.] *399:*301–312.

Collingridge, G.L., C.E. Herron, and R.A.J. Lester (1988c) Synaptic activation of N-methyl-D-aspartate receptors in the Schaffer collateral-commissural pathway of rat hippocampus. J. Physiol. [Lond.] *399:*283–300.

Collingridge, G.L., S.J. Kehl, R. Loo, and H. McLennan (1983a) Effects of kainic and other amino acids on synaptic excitation in rat hippocampal slices: 1. Extracellular analysis. Exp. Brain Res. *52:*170–178.

Collingridge, G.L., S.J. Kehl, and H. McLennan (1983b) Excitatory amino acids in synaptic transmission in the Schaffer-collateral commissural pathway of the rat hippocampus. J. Physiol. [Lond.] *334:*33–46.

Collingridge, G.L., S.J. Kehl, and H. McLennan (1984) The action of some analogues of the excitatory amino acids in the dentate gyrus of the rat. Can. J. Physiol. Pharmacol. *62:*424–429.

Collingridge, G.L., and H. McLennan (1981) The effect of kainic acid on excitatory synaptic activity in the rat hippocampal slice preparation. Neurosci. Lett. *27:*31–36.

Cotman, C.W., and L.L. Iversen (1987) Excitatory amino acids in the brain—Focus on NMDA receptors. Trends Neurosci. *10:*263–302.

Cotman, C.W., D.T. Monaghan, O.P. Ottersen, and J. Storm-Mathisen (1987) Anatomical organization of excitatory amino acid receptors and their pathways. Trends Neurosci. *7:*273–280.

Crunelli, V., S. Forda, G.L. Collingridge, and J.S. Kelly (1982) Intracellular recorded synaptic antagonism in the rat dentate gyrus. Nature *300*:450–452.

Dingledine, R., M.A. Hynes, and G.L. King (1986) Involvement of N-methyl-D-aspartate receptors in epileptiform bursting in the rat hippocampal slice. J. Physiol. [Lond.] *380*:175–189.

Errington, M.L., M.A. Lynch, and T.V.P. Bliss (1987) Long-term potentiation in the dentate gyrus: Induction and increased glutamate release are blocked by D(-)aminophosphonovalerate. Neuroscience *20*:279–284.

Forsythe, I.D., and G.l. Westbrook (1988) Slow excitatory postsynaptic currents mediated by N-methyl-D-aspartate receptors on cultured mouse central neurones. J. Physiol. [Lond.] *396*:515–534.

Gähwiler, B.H. (1981) Organotypic monolayer cultures of nervous tissue. J. Neurosci. Methods *4*:329–342.

Ganong, A.H., T.H. Lanthorn, and C.W. Cotman (1983) Kynurenic acid inhibits synaptic and acidic amino acid-induced responses in the rat hippocampus and spinal cord. Brain Res. *273*:170–174.

Gray, R., and D. Johnston (1987) Noradrenaline and α-adrenoceptor agonists increase activity of voltage-dependent calcium channels in hippocampal neurons. Nature *327*:620–622.

Harris, E.W., and C.W. Cotman (1985) Removal of magnesium induces NMDA receptor mediated LTP by triggering epileptiform activity. Soc. Neurosci. Abstr. *11*:845.

Harris, E.W., and C.W. Cotman (1986) Long-term potentiation of guinea pig mossy fiber responses is not blocked by N-methyl-D-aspartate antagonists. Neurosci. Lett. *70*:132–137.

Harris, E.W., A.H. Ganong, and C.W. Cotman (1984) Long-term potentiation in the hippocampus involves activation of N-methyl-D-aspartate receptors. Brain Res. *323*:132–137.

Herron, C.E., R.A.J. Lester, E.J. Coan, and G.L. Collingridge (1985a) Intracellular demonstration of an N-methyl-D-aspartate receptor mediated component of synaptic transmission in the rat hippocampus. Neurosci. Lett. *60*:19–23.

Herron, C.E., R.A.J. Lester, E.J. Coan, and G.L. Collingridge (1986) Frequency-dependent involvement of NMDA receptors in the hippocampus: A novel synaptic mechanism. Nature *322*:265–268.

Herron, C.E., S. McGuirk, R.A.J. Lester, and G.L. Collingridge (1987) NMDA receptor involvement in kainate and folate induced epileptiform activity in rat hippocampal slices. Neurol. Neurobiol. *24*:345–348.

Herron, C.E., R. Williamson, and G.L. Collingridge (1985b) A selective N-methyl-D-aspartate antagonist depresses epileptiform activity in rat hippocampal slices. Neurosci. Lett. *61*:255–260.

Honoré, T., S.N. Davies, J. Drejer, E.J. Fletcher, P. Jacobsen, D. Lodge, and F.E. Nielsen (1988) Quinoxalinediones: Potent competitive non-NMDA glutamate receptor antagonists. Science *241*:701–703.

Huang, Y.-Y., H. Wigström, and B. Gustafsson (1987) Facilitated induction of hippocampal long-term potentiation in slices perfused with low concentrations of magnesium. Neuroscience *22*:9–16.

Izumi, Y., H. Miyakawa, K. Ito, and H. Kato (1987) Quisqualate and N-methyl-D-aspartate (NMDA) receptors in induction of hippocampal long-term facilitation using conditioning solution. Neurosci. Lett. *83*:201–206.

Kauer, J.A., R.C. Malenka, and R.A. Nicoll (1988) NMDA ionophoresis or synaptic stimulation causes long-term potentiation (LTP) when paired with postsynaptic depolarization in hippocampal pyramidal cells. J. Physiol. [Lond.] *398*:23P.

Kauer, J.A., and R.A. Nicoll (1988) An APV-resistant non-associative form of long term potentiation in the rat hippocampus. In H.L. Haas and G. Buzsáki (eds): Synaptic Plasticity in the Hippocampus. Berlin: Springer-Verlag, pp. 65–66.

Krishtal, O.A., S.V. Smirnov, and Y.V. Osipchuk (1988) Changes in the state of the excitatory synaptic system in the hippocampus on prolonged exposure to excitatory amino acids and antagonists. Neurosci. Lett. 85:82–88.

Kudo, Y., K. Ito, H. Miyakawa, Y. Izumi, A. Ogura, and H. Kato (1987) Cytoplasmic calcium elevation in hippocampal granule cells induced by perforant path stimulation and L-glutamate application. Brain Res. 407:168–172.

Larson, J., and G. Lynch (1986) Induction of synaptic potentiation in hippocampus by patterned stimulation involves two events. Science 232:985–990.

Mayer, M.L., A.B. MacDermott, G.L. Westbrook, S.J. Smith, and J.L. Barker (1987) Agonist- and voltage-gated calcium entry in cultured mouse spinal cord neurons under voltage clamp measured using arsenazo III. J. Neurosci. 7:3230–3244.

McNamara, J.O., R.D. Russell, L.C. Rigsbee, and D.W. Bonhaus (1988) Anticonvulsant and antiepileptogenic actions of MK-801 in the kindling and electroshock models. Neuropharmacology 27:563–568.

Meldrum, B. (1985) Possible therapeutic applications of antagonists of excitatory amino acid neurotransmitters. Clin. Sci. 68:113–122.

Mody, I., and U. Heinemann (1987) NMDA receptors of dentate gyrus granule cells participate in synaptic transmission following kindling. Nature 326:701–704.

Mody, I., J.D.C. Lambert, and U. Heinemann (1987) Low extracellular magnesium induces epileptiform activity and spreading depression in rat hippocampal slices. J. Neurophysiol. 57:869–888.

Morris, R.G.M., E. Anderson, G.S. Lynch, and M. Baudry (1986) Selective impairment of learning and blockade of long-term potentiation by an N-methyl-D-aspartate receptor antagonist, AP5. Nature 319:774–776.

Neuman, R., E. Cherubini, and Y. Ben-Ari (1987) Is activation of N-methyl-D-aspartate receptor gated channels sufficient to induce long term potentiation? Neurosci. Lett. 80:283–288.

Nowak, L., P. Bregestovski, P. Ascher, A. Herbet, and A. Prochiantz (1984) Magnesium gates glutamate-activated channels in mouse central neurones. Nature 307:462–465.

Peterson, D.W., J.F. Collins, and H.F. Bradford (1983) The kindled amygdala model of epilepsy: Anticonvulsant action of amino acid antagonists. Brain Res. 275:169–172.

Rose, G.M., D.M. Diamond, K. Pang, and T.V. Dunwiddie (1988) Primed burst potentiation: Lasting synaptic plasticity invoked by physiologically patterned stimulation. In H.L. Haas and G. Buzsáki (eds): Synaptic Plasticity in the Hippocampus. Berlin: Springer-Verlag, pp. 96–98.

Rothman, S.M., and M. Samaie (1985) Physiology of excitatory synaptic transmission in cultures of dissociated rat hippocampus. J. Neurophysiol. 54:701–713.

Sawada, S., and C. Yamamoto (1984) Gamma-D-glutamylglycine and cis-2,3-piperidine dicarboxylate as antagonists of excitatory amino acids in the hippocampus. Exp. Brain Res. 55:351–358.

Slater, N.T., A. Stelzer, and M. Galvan (1985) Kindling-like stimulus patterns induce epileptiform discharges in the guinea pig in vitro hippocampus. Neurosci. Lett. 60:25–31.

Stelzer, A., N.T. Slater, and G. ten Bruggencate (1987) Activation of NMDA receptors blocks GABAergic inhibition in an in vitro model of epilepsy. Nature 326:698–701.

Stringer, J.L., and P.G. Guyenet (1983) Elimination of long-term potentiation in the hippocampus by phencyclidine and ketamine. Brain Res. 258:159–164.

Walther, H., J.D.C. Lambert, R.S.G. Jones, U. Heinemann, and B. Hamon (1986) Epileptiform activity in combined slices of the hippocampus, subiculum and entorhinal cortex during perfusion with low magnesium medium. Neurosci. Lett. *69:*156–161.

Watkins, J.C., and R.H. Evans (1981) Excitatory amino acid transmitters. Annu. Rev. Pharmacol. Toxicol. *21:*165–204.

Wigström, H., and B. Gustafsson (1988) Presynaptic and postsynaptic interactions in the control of hippocampal long term potentiation. Neurol. Neurobiol. *35:*73–107.

The Hippocampus—New Vistas, pages 347–362
© 1989 Alan R. Liss, Inc.

22
Electrophysiological Action of Adenosine in Rat and Human Hippocampus

R.W. GREENE AND H.L. HAAS

Harvard Medical School and Veterans Administration Medical Center, Brockton, Massachusetts (R.W.G.); II. Physiologisches Institut, Johannes Gutenberg-Universität, Mainz, Federal Republic of Germany (H.L.H.)

INTRODUCTION

Adenosine (AD) and its nucleotide derivatives have a universal role in energy metabolism. In the vertebrate nervous system additional role(s) for AD are suggested by the ubiquitous but uneven distribution of the following extracellular membrane receptors with high affinity for AD (Bruns et al., 1980), high affinity uptake and catabolic enzyme systems (Geiger and Nagy, 1984), and evoked release of AD (Wojcik and Neff, 1982). In particular, during pathophysiological conditions that increase metabolite demand relative to metabolite availability such as hypoxia, hypoglycemia, prolonged extracellular depolarization, exposure to convulsants, or electrically evoked seizure-like activity, an increase in the neuronal extracellular concentration of AD was observed (Pull and McIlwain, 1972; Berne et al., 1982). Exogenously administered AD has widespread depressant effects on neuronal activity (Phillis et al., 1975), which would presumably lower metabolic demand. Thus, it is conceivable that AD mediates a negative feedback mechanism to aid in homeostasis between metabolic and electrophysiological states of nervous tissue. However, until the last 10 years little has been known about the character of the depressant action of adenosine: if it is consistent with this neuromodulatory role or if endogenous adenosine exerts similar effects.

Brain slice preparations have been the source for major advances in our understanding of the depressant actions of AD on neuronal activity (Kuroda et al., 1976; Scholfield, 1978; Schubert and Mitzdorf, 1979; Okada and Ozawa, 1980; Dunwiddie and Hoffer, 1980). We have investigated these actions in detail in the hippocampal slice preparation and have shown adenosine to increase a calcium-dependent potassium conductance and a calcium- and voltage-independent potassium conductance. We have also observed a steady-state inhibitory tone exerted by endogenous AD in the absence of synaptic activity and controlled by an AD uptake system. In this chapter we summarize our published observations of AD action in the hippocampus (Hood et al., 1983; Haas et al., 1984; Haas and Greene, 1984, 1986, 1988; Greene et al., 1985; Greene and Haas, 1985) and some recent unpublished observations.

METHODS

Transverse, 450 μm thick slices from the hippocampi of young adult Wistar rats were used with essentially the techniques described previously for extracellular (Greene et al., 1985; Haas and Greene, 1988) and intracellular (Greene and Haas, 1985) studies of AD and caffeine actions on CA1 pyramidal neurons. Human hippocampal slices were prepared immediately after removal from patients suffering from temporal lobe epilepsy (M.G. Yasargil, unpublished data) and investigated in an in vitro perfusion chamber (Haas et al., 1979) for periods of up to 15 h. Field potentials, in particular the population spikes following electrical stimulation of afferent fibers to the CA1 and dentate regions, were similar to those described in hippocampal slices of the rat. Paired pulses revealed excitation and, more prominently, inhibition of the test pulse (this may be attributable to the antiepileptic treatment of the patients). Spontaneous epileptiform discharges were never observed. Tetanization (100–400 Hz for 40 to 1,000 ms) was followed by a comparatively small post-tetanic potentiation and occasionally by long-term potentiation (LTP) or a long-lasting depression of the synaptically evoked population spikes.

ELECTROPHYSIOLOGY OF ADENOSINE
Increase of Steady-State Potassium Conductance

Adenosine (10—100 μM) evokes a hyperpolarization and a decrease in input resistance in CA1 neurones (Okada and Ozawa, 1980; Segal, 1982). This effect is probably mediated by an increase in potassium conductance. It was not affected by intracellular chloride injection sufficient to reverse the polarity of inhibitory postsynaptic potentials (IPSPs) mediated by increases in chloride conductance. More importantly, under voltage-clamp control, the current evoked by AD varied with the extracellular potassium concentration as predicted by the Nernst equation for a change in potassium permeability (Fig. 1), similar to observations from cultured striatal neurons (Trussel and Jackson, 1985).

This steady-state increase appears to be neither calcium nor voltage sensitive (unlike striatal neurones; Trussel and Jackson, 1985). The addition of tetraethylammonium (10 mM), a calcium-dependent potassium current antagonist, or cadmium chloride (300 μM), a calcium current antagonist, to the extracellular media had no effect on the AD-evoked hyperpolarization. To determine whether the release of intracellular calcium was responsible, CA1 neurons were intracellularly injected with the calcium buffer EGTA (1 M in the recording pipette) and then exposed to AD. However, the AD-evoked hyperpolarization was unaltered (Fig. 2).

The voltage sensitivity of this response was tested both directly (under voltage-clamp control) and with pharmacological antagonists of voltage-sensitive

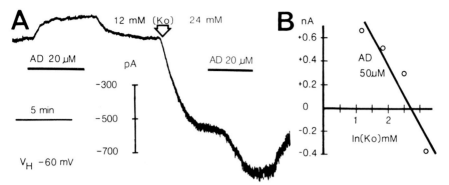

Fig. 1. Current evoked by adenosine (AD) varies inversely with the log of the extra-cellular potassium concentration. **A:** A chart record of current during voltage-clamp at a membrane potential (V_H) of −60 mV. Extracellular potassium concentration was 12 mM during the first exposure to adenosine (10 μM). At the time indicated by the arrow, the extracellular potassium concentration (Ko) was increased to 24 mM, with a resulting reversal of polarity in response to the second exposure to adenosine (20 μM). **B:** A graph of the change in current evoked by adenosine (in nA; ordinate) with respect to the natural log of the extracellular potassium concentration (in mM; abscissa).

currents. When the membrane potential is rapidly altered from a holding potential negative to −75 mV to a command potential positive to −55 mV, an early outward transient current, sensitive to 4-aminopyridine (4-AP), I_A, (Gustafsson et al., 1982) was observed (Fig. 3). Exposure to AD did not increase the A current, and the AD-evoked hyperpolarization was not reduced by 4-AP (the latter was examined because it is likely that some steady-state I_A is present at resting membrane potential). Hyperpolarizing shifts of the membrane potential from magnitudes positive to −60 mV to negative to −80 mV result in a slow inward current relaxation sensitive to external CsCl, termed "I_Q" (Halliwell and Adams, 1982). The amplitude of the slow relaxation (the current measured at the end of a 400 ms duration hyperpolarizing shift subtracted from the initial current measured 40 ms after the shift) was not increased during exposure to AD (Fig. 3). In the presence of CsCl (5 mM) this inward relaxation was completely abolished; however, the AD-evoked current was unaffected.

The only agent we found capable of antagonizing the AD-evoked current (not to be confused with antagonism at the AD receptor, discussed below) is the nonspecific potassium channel antagonist BaCl (2 mM; Fig. 2). A similar potassium current, I_S, has been described in invertebrates with characteristics that include 1) absence of inactivation, 2) absence of calcium sensitivity, 3) absence of voltage sensitivity, 4) ionic specificity primarily for potassium, and 5) modulation by putative neurotransmitters (Siegelbaum et al., 1982; Pollock et al., 1985).

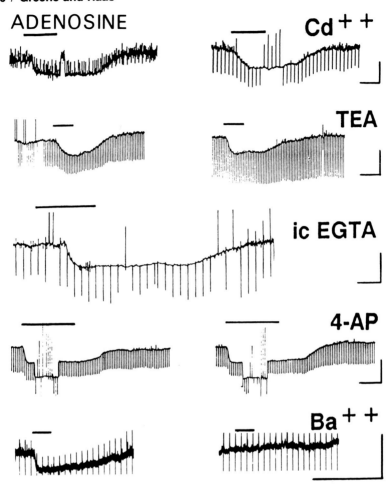

Fig. 2. Membrane hyperpolarizations by adenosine (100 μM, present in the perfusion fluid during time indicated by bars above traces) in five different CA1 pyramidal cells are unaffected by exposure to cadmium (100 μM, Cd), tetraethylammonium (10 mM, TEA), 4-aminopyridine (100 μM, 4-AP) but abolished by barium (2mM, Ba). Controls are on the left side. Intracellular EGTA (1 M in the recording pipette) left the adenosine action unaltered. Tetrodotoxin (TTX) was in the medium for the experiments with TEA, 4-AP, and Ba. Calibration: 2 min, 10 mV.

Increase of Calcium-Dependent Potassium Current

Calcium-dependent potassium current is composed of 2 parts: 1) a fast-activating, voltage-sensitive component (I_C) (Brown and Griffith, 1983) that affects spike repolarization and the fast afterhyperpolarization (AHP) (Storm, 1987) and 2) a slow, voltage-insensitive component (I_{AHP}) (Lancaster and Adams,

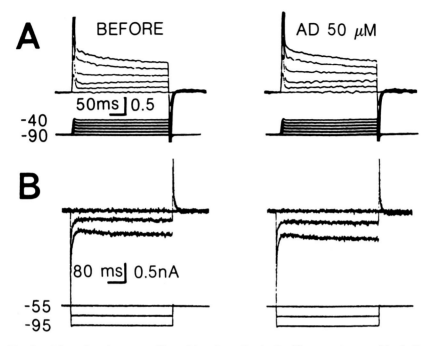

Fig. 3. Adenosine does not affect either I_A or I_Q. **A:** Oscilloscope traces of both the current (upper row) and membrane potential (bottom row) of a neuron voltage-clamped to -90 mV. The membrane potential was shifted to -40 mV in 10 mV steps of 300 ms duration before and during adenosine (50 μM) exposure. Note that the early, transient, outward component of the current traces did not change. **B:** Same as A except the membrane potential was shifted from -55 mV to more hyperpolarized levels, and the slowly developing inward relaxation of I_Q was examined. Note the lack of tail current because of a holding potential near the reversal potential of I_Q.

1986) responsible for accommodation and the long-duration AHP (Madison and Nicoll, 1984). AD (5–50 μM) enhanced both accommodation and the long-duration AHP. Under voltage-clamp control, both I_C and I_{AHP} were increased in the presence of AD (Fig. 4). Exposure to higher concentrations of AD often resulted in a decrease of the long-duration AHP in association with a decrease in input resistance. This decrease was probably due to the AD-evoked increase in the steady-state potassium conductance, which shunted both the calcium influx and the I_{AHP}.

The enhancement of the long-duration AHP can be attributed primarily to a decrease in the rate at which the AHP decayed to resting membrane potential (best described by a single exponential with a shorter time constant for control than in the presence of AD) (Greene and Haas, 1985). Because this decay was likely to reflect the return of intracellular calcium concentration to control levels (Thomas and Gorman, 1977; Smith et al., 1983) we suggest that AD acted by decreasing calcium reuptake, perhaps by reducing the calcium affinity of

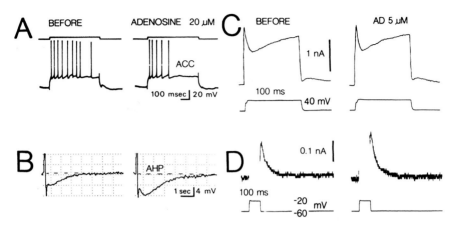

Fig. 4. Adenosine (AD) increases accommodation (ACC) of firing and afterhyperpolarizations (AHP). **A:** The response of a CA1 pyramidal cell to depolarizing current injection (+0.4 nA for 600 ms; upper trace is current) before and during adenosine 20 μM. **B:** Amplitude and time course of afterhyperpolarizations following a burst of action potentials are enhanced by adenosine. **C,D:** Adenosine increases the delayed outward currents (D) without altering the slow inward current (C). Single electrode voltage-clamp records before and during adenosine exposure. Records in C are identical to those in D except that a slower time course and greater current amplification are illustrated in D.

calcium binding proteins regulated by cyclic adenosine monophosphate (cAMP) protein phosphorylation: Histamine, norepinephrine (both via a cAMP-dependent mechanism) (Haas, 1984; Madison and Nicoll, 1984), and cAMP reduce accommodation and increase the rate of AHP repolarization (Madison and Nicoll, 1982; Haas and Konnerth, 1983; Haas and Greene, 1986). AD activation of the A_1 receptor decreases cAMP (Fredholm et al., 1986).

Decrease of Calcium Current

AD has been shown to antagonize calcium currents in the peripheral nervous system (I_{Ca} (Henon and McAfee, 1983; Dolphin et al., 1986; MacDonald et al., 1986). In hippocampal neurons a similar mechanism was suggested based on AD-evoked inhibition of the Ca-dependent action potential observed in the presence of tetrodotoxin (Proctor and Dunwiddie, 1983; Haas and Greene, 1984). However, this inhibition may have resulted from a shunt of the I_{Ca} secondary to the AD-evoked increase in potassium currents. Under voltage-clamp control and in the presence of barium (Ba), which antagonized the potassium currents, an AD-induced inhibition of I_{Ca} was not observed (Halliwell and Schofield, 1984). It is important to note the holding potential of −40 to −35 mV employed in this study. At this potential, I_{Ca} was activated, increasing intracellular Ba and, probably, intracellular Ca concentrations, which may have significantly reduced the observed I_{Ca} (Eckert and Chad, 1984). Further, at this holding potential only one of three kinds of I_{Ca}, the L current, can be activated, because both the T and the N currents are inactivated (Fox et al., 1987). Thus the status of the action of AD on I_{Ca} is presently unclear.

Presynaptic Actions

The regular anatomical organization of the hippocampus results in large extracellular potentials caused by an almost synchronized population synaptic response to a single stimulation of an afferent tract (e.g. population excitatory postsynaptic potentials [EPSP] can be recorded from the CA1 dendritic region following stratum radiatum stimulation). Adenosine has a powerful inhibitory action on the population EPSP as well as on the intracellular recorded EPSP (Proctor and Dunwiddie, 1983). However, a postsynaptic action on distal dendritic sites is very difficult to differentiate from a presynaptic action on nerve terminals. The presynaptic sites are not amenable to direct electrophysiological analysis, but indirect methods allow an estimation of transmitter release. Although hippocampal circuitry is more complex than a simple excitatory junction, paired pulse facilitation occurs in much the same way as has been described at the neuromuscular junction (Katz and Miledi, 1968; Rahamimoff, 1968; Andersen, 1960; Dunwiddie and Lynch, 1978; Buckle and Haas, 1982). Facilitation of a test response by a preceding conditioning response is believed to depend on residual calcium in nerve terminals. Under conditions of high transmitter release a depression of the test response occurs, presumably because of exhaustion of the immediately releasable transmitter (Betz, 1970; McNaugton et al., 1981). A reduction in the paired pulse facilitation would indicate an increase in release, while an enhancement would suggest less transmitter depletion and thus decreased release. This indirect approach has

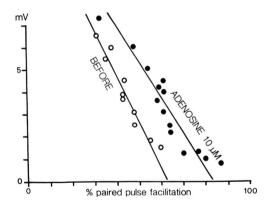

Fig. 5. Paired pulse facilitation is increased by adenosine (10 μM). Extracellularly recorded EPSP were evoked in stratum radiatum at 60 ms intervals. Facilitation of the test response (abscissa) is plotted against the amplitude of the conditioning response (ordinate). As facilitation depends on the response amplitude, it is necessary to compare responses at several stimulation intensities before and during adenosine action. Therefore, facilitation is shown here as a function of the conditioning response.

been used to ascribe a presynaptic action to 4-aminopyridine (Buckle and Haas, 1982), which blocks a transient potassium current (Thompson, 1977) and increases transmitter release. Adenosine had an opposite effect on the paired pulse paradigm: It increased synaptic facilitation (Fig. 5). This effect was enhanced in media containing higher calcium concentrations when release is high (Dunwiddie and Haas, 1985). These findings were explained by a presynaptic action of adenosine on nerve terminals, resulting in reduced transmitter release. Although the preceding paragraphs show that adenosine has marked postsynaptic actions, it seems likely that a presynaptic action contributes to its depressant effects in the CNS, perhaps mediated by a mechanism similar to that observed postsynaptically.

Antiepileptic Activity

It is well established that epileptiform activity can be induced in the hippocampus in vitro with convulsants such as bicuculline or penicillin. More recently, such activity was evoked in the absence of synaptic activity by exposure of the hippocampus to perfusate containing low calcium and high magnesium (Haas and Jefferys, 1984). Adenosine was shown to be effective in the antagonism of both the convulsant (Dunwiddie et al., 1981) and low Ca^{2+}/high Mg^{2+} types of epileptiform activities (Fig. 6) (Haas et al., 1984) as well as in antagonizing induced epilepsy in vivo (Maitre et al., 1974).

The inhibition exerted by AD was well suited for specific antagonism of epileptic discharge. The AD-evoked increase in calcium dependent potassium currents did not alter short-duration excitatory input, but did reduce the effect of long-duration excitatory input, as illustrated by the observed enhancement

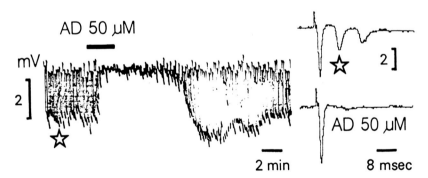

Fig. 6. Adenosine (AD) blocks epileptiform activity in low-calcium (0.2 mM) high-magnesium (4mM) medium. Averaged records on the right show the multiple discharge of pyramids following alveus stimulation (antidromic activation) before and during adenosine. The trace on the left displays the size of the second population spike (star) through a sample and hold amplifier. Note the larger antidromic spike during adenosine (cells are hyperpolarized) and the rebound increase in the second population spike after washout.

of accommodation and the long-duration AHP (Fig. 4). Presynaptic inhibition mediated by AD may obtain specificity of action by the localization and density of the presynaptic AD receptors. With neuronal exposure to concentrations of AD in excess of 50 μM, the most prominent effect was a concentration-dependent increase in potassium conductance (Greene and Haas, unpublished observations). This was a more powerful inhibitory effect than the enhancement of the calcium-dependent potassium currents but less specific in that all excitatory input was reduced. These effects are all consistent with the antiepileptic actions of AD, which suggests an antiepileptic role for endogenous AD.

ACTION OF ENDOGENOUS ADENOSINE

The extracellular adenosine levels are about 1 μM, with little variation throughout the CNS (for review, see Dunwiddie, 1985); however, these concentrations vary by at least two orders of magnitude in hyperactive tissue. Such variations have been measured despite the presence of high-affinity uptake systems, which might require saturation before AD levels appreciably alter, raising the possibility that AD levels at the receptor site vary to a higher degree with less physiological perturbation than has been measured. Although the concept of a purinergic tone is not new, we present, in the following, some new evidence for an electrophysiological tonic action of endogenous adenosine.

Antagonists

The methylxanthine caffeine (100 μM) not only antagonized the adenosine actions on hippocampal neurons but also produced the opposite effect, a blockade of a nonvoltage, noncalcium-dependent potassium conductance and accommodation with the associated long-lasting calcium-dependent AHP (Greene et al., 1985). Caffeine increased EPSPs (measured extra- and intracellularly) and population spikes. The plot of the AD concentration-response graph was shifted in parallel to the right in the presence of caffeine, and the efficacy of caffeine was increased in the presence of exogenous adenosine consistent with the action of a competitive inhibitor (Fig. 7). Although other effects of caffeine such as a reduction of action potential amplitude and a reduction of the depolarizing plateau following slow spikes in the presence of barium and TTX (probably a persistent Ca/Ba current) were also observed, these occurred usually with higher concentrations and prolonged applications. These effects are all distinct from those resulting from the intracellular action of caffeine (i.e. release of intracellular calcium and inhibition of phosphodiesterase) because of the latter's comparative lack of potency (ED_{50} in the mM range) (Neering and McBurney, 1984).

Uptake Inhibition

Uptake of AD can be inhibited in olfactory cortical slices in the absence of an effect at the adenosine receptor site by nitrobenzylthioinosine (NBTI) (Sanderson and Scholfield, 1986). NBTI produced a hyperpolarization and activation of potassium currents similar to those seen with adenosine (see also Motley and Collins, 1983; Sebastiao and Ribeiro, 1985). The efficacy of caffeine

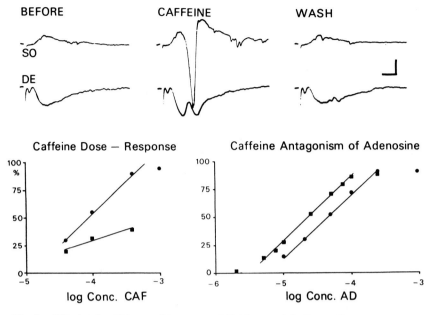

Fig. 7. Effects of caffeine on hippocampal field potentials. Recordings in stratum py-ramidale (upper traces; SO, somatic) and stratum radiatum (lower traces; DE, dendritic) taken before, during, and after the application of caffeine. In the presence of caffeine (middle record, 300 μM) the dendritic EPSP was increased in amplitude and a large somatic population spike appeared. Bottom diagrams: The interaction between caffeine (CAF) and adenosine (AD) on extracellularly recorded hippocampal EPSP. Each point in the two graphs represents 20 averaged EPSP. Left graph shows the concentration-response curve for caffeine before (squares) and after (circles) the addition of adenosine (40 μM) to the bathing medium. The response was measured as the percentage of increase from baseline of the extracellularly recorded EPSP. The graph on the right illustrates a parallel shift to the right of the adenosine concentration-response curve by caffeine (before, squares; during 50 μM caffeine, circles). The response was measured as the percentage of reduction of the baseline extracellularly recorded EPSP.

in increasing synaptic potentials was significantly enhanced in the presence of NBTI, similar to the effect of adding exogenous AD to the perfusate (Fig. 8).

Catabolism

The catabolic enzyme of adenosine, adenosine deaminase, mimicked the effects of caffeine. In the presence of adenosine deaminase, application of caffeine was no longer effective in increasing the evoked EPSP, presumably because the electrophysiologically active endogenous AD was catabolized (Fig 9). Notably, during perfusion with media containing low Ca, high Mg, which blocks synaptic activity (Haas and Jefferys, 1984), adenosine deaminase was effective, as was NBTI (Fig. 8).

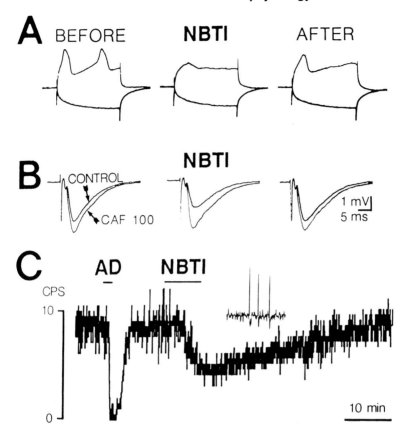

Fig. 8. Antagonism of the adenosine uptake system by nitrobenzylthioinosine (NBTI).
A: Intracellular recording from a CA1 pyramid in a tetrodotoxin-poisoned slice. NBTI
(20 μM) caused a slow and long-lasting hyperpolarization (3 mV; data not shown) and
a block of the slow calcium spikes. Superimposed responses to ± 0.5 nA, 120 ms pulses;
spike amplitude, 45 mV. **B:** Inhibition of evoked field EPSP by NBTI is antagonized by
caffeine (CAF). Three sets of oscilloscope traces (two traces per set) of the extracellular
EPSP evoked by stratum radiatum stimulation and recorded in the CA1 apical dendritic
layer. They were taken before, during, and after exposure to NBTI (1 μM). In each set,
the larger potential was taken in the presence of caffeine (100 μM). **C:** NBTI inhibits
neuronal firing in the absence of synaptic activity. Extracellular records of action potentials (illustrated in inset) were obtained in low-calcium, high-magnesium medium
and used to generate the chart record of firing rate (counts per second [CPS]) with
respect to time. The rate was decreased during application of adenosine (AD, first horizontal bar; 20 μM) and NBTI (second horizontal bar; 10 μM).

HUMAN HIPPOCAMPUS

Adenosine (10–100 μM) hyperpolarized human hippocampal neurons by 6–
10 mV associated with a decrease in input resistance. Under voltage-clamp,
an outward current evoked by AD was observed. Long-lasting afterhyperpo-

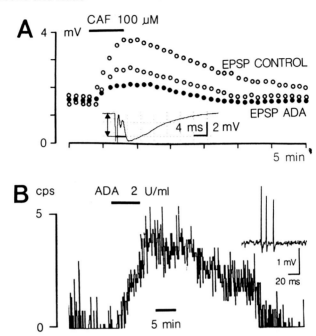

Fig. 9. Adenosine deaminase (ADA) reduces the effect of caffeine (CAF) and increases cell firing. **A:** Graph of the field EPSP magnitude measured as indicated by the inset at a fixed time from the stimulus for the ordinate and time for the abscissa. Filled circles represent measurements taken during exposure to adenosine deaminase, 0.5 units/ml. Control and partial recovery are illustrated by open circles. The time of caffeine exposure is indicated by the horizontal bar. Stimulus intensity was reduced during perfusion with adenosine deaminase (but prior to exposure to caffeine) so that the EPSP amplitude was equal to that of the control. **B:** Extracellularly recorded action potential firing rate (ordinate, counts per second) versus time (abscissa) in low-calcium, high-magnesium medium, which abolished synaptic activity. The time of addition of adenosine deaminase to the medium is indicated by the horizontal bar. A typical oscilloscope trace is shown in the inset.

larizations, accommodation of firing, and an outward tail current after depolarizing voltage jumps were enhanced (Fig. 10). In conclusion, human hippocampal neurons display properties very similar to the respective rodent cells. Increased activation of CNS AD receptors may be an effective antiepileptic maneuver, although peripheral effects preclude the simple administration of AD. Perhaps agonists targeted specifically for the CNS or similarly targeted uptake inhibitors may eventually find a place in the antiepileptic pharmacy.

SUMMARY AND CONCLUSIONS

Endogenous adenosine was shown to exert an inhibitory tone on neurons in the in vitro hippocampal slice controlled in part by an uptake system. Further, the inhibitory tone was present even when the synaptic activity was blocked, thus implicating a nonsynaptic source for this extracellular AD.

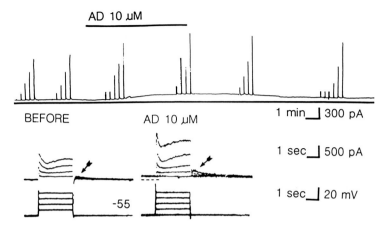

AD 10 μM

BEFORE   AD 10 μM   1 min⌐| 300 pA

1 sec⌐| 500 pA

1 sec⌐| 20 mV

-55

Fig. 10.   Adenosine induces outward current and increases outward tail (arrows) current. Single electrode voltage-clamp record from CA1 pyramid in a slice prepared from a human hippocampus removed for treatment of epilepsy. Upper trace: current record, adenosine 10 μM present in medium during time indicated by horizontal bar; lower traces: current responses to voltage jumps from −55 to −45, −35, −25, and −15 mV before and during adenosine action.

Based on the effects exerted by exogenous AD, we conclude that the inhibitory tone is mediated by at least two mechanisms: an increase in a voltage- and calcium-insensitive potassium current and an increase in calcium-dependent potassium currents (both I_C and I_{AHP}). There is good evidence for a presynaptic site of action, but the mechanism is unknown. A third mechanism of action present in the peripheral nervous system, a decrease in calcium currents, cannot be ruled out on the available evidence. These mechanisms are probably responsible for the antiepileptic activity of AD and are consistent with a possible role for AD as a mediator of homeostasis between metabolic state and electrophysiological activity in the vertebrate CNS.

REFERENCES

Andersen, P. (1960) Interhippocampal impulses. II. Apical dendritic activation of CA1 neurons. Acta Physiol. Scand. *48:*178–208.

Berne, M., H.R. Winn, and R. Rubio (1982) The effect of inadequate oxygen supply to the brain on cerebral adenosine levels. In F.C. Rose and W.K. Amery (eds): Cerebral Hypoxia in the Pathogenesis of Migraine. London: Pitman, pp. 82–91.

Betz, W.J. (1970) Depression of transmitter release at the neuromuscular junction of the frog. J. Physiol. [Lond.] *206:*629–644.

Brown, D.A, and W.H. Griffith (1983) Calcium-activated outward current in voltage-clamped hippocampal neurones of the guinea-pig. J. Physiol. [Lond.] *337:*297–301.

Bruns, R.F., J.W. Daly, and S.H. Snyder (1980) Adenosine receptors in brain membranes: Binding of N^6- cyclohexyl[^{3}H]adenosine and 1,3-diethyl-8-[3H]phenylxanthine. Proc. Natl. Acad. Sci. U.S.A. *77:*5547–5551.

Buckle, P.J., and H.L. Haas (1982) Enhancement of synaptic transmission by 4-aminopyridine in hippocampal slices of the rat. J. Physiol. *326:*109–122.

Dolphin, A.C., S.R. Forda, and R.H. Scott (1986) Calcium-dependent currents in cultured rat dorsal root ganglion neurons are inhibited by an adenosine analogue. J. Physiol. *373*:47–61.

Dunwiddie, T.V. (1985) The physiological role of adenosine in the central nervous system. Int. Rev. Neurobiol. *27*:63–139.

Dunwiddie, T.V., and H.L. Haas (1985) Adenosine increases synaptic facilitation in the in vitro rat hippocampus: Evidence for a presynaptic site of action. J. Physiol. *369*:365–377.

Dunwiddie, T.V., and B.J. Hoffer (1980) Adenine nucleotides and synaptic transmission in the in vitro rat hippocampus. Br. J. Pharmacol. *69*:59–68.

Dunwiddie, T.V., B.J. Hoffer, and B.B. Fredholm (1981) Alkylxanthines elevate hippocampal excitability evidence for a role of endogenous adenosine. Naunyn Schmiedebergs Arch. Pharmacol. *316*:326–330.

Dunwiddie, T.V., and G.S. Lynch (1978) Long-term potentiation and depression of synaptic responses in the rat hippocampus: Localization and frequency dependency. J. Physiol. [Lond.] *276*:353–367.

Eckert, R., and J.E. Chad (1984) Inactivation of Ca channels. Prog. Biophys. Mol. Biol. *44*:215–267.

Fox, A.P., M.C. Nowycky, and R.W. Tsien (1987) Kinetic and pharmacological properties distinguishing three types of calcium currents in chick sensory neurones. J. Physiol. [Lond.] *394*:149–172.

Fredholm, B.B., B. Jonzon, and K. Lindstom (1986) Effect of adenosine receptor agonists and other compounds on cyclic AMP accumulation in forskolin-treated hippocampal slices. Arch. Pharmacol. *332*:173–178.

Geiger, J.D., and J.I. Nagy (1984) Brain Res. Bull. *13*:657–666.

Greene, R.W., and H.L. Haas (1985) Adenosine actions on CA1 pyramidal neurones in rat hippocampal slices. J. Physiol. *366*:119–127.

Greene, R.W., H.L. Haas, and A. Hermann (1985) Effects of caffeine on hippocampal pyramidal cells in vitro. Br. J. Pharmacol. *85*:163–169.

Gustafsson, B., M. Galvan, P. Grafe, and H. Wigström (1982) A transient outward current in a mammalian central neurone blocked by 4-aminopyridine. Nature *299*:252–254.

Haas, H.L. (1984) Histamine potentiates neuronal excitation by blocking a calcium dependent potassium conductance. Agents Actions *14*:534–537.

Haas, H.L., and R.W. Greene (1984) Adenosine enhances afterhyperpolarization and accomodation in hippocampal pyramidal cells. Pflugers Arch. *402*:244–247.

Haas, H.L., and R.W. Greene (1986) Effects of histamine on hippocampal pyramidal cells of the rat in vitro. Exp. Brain Res. *62*:123–130.

Haas, H.L., and R.W. Greene (1988) Endogenous adenosine inhibits hippocampal CA1 neurones. Naunyn Schmiedebergs Arch. Pharmacol. *337*:561–565.

Haas, H., and J.G.R. Jefferys (1984) Low-calcium field burst discharges of CA1 pyramidal neurones in rat hippocampal slices. J. Physiol. *354*:185–201.

Haas, H., J.G.R. Jefferys, N.T. Slater, and D.O. Carpenter (1984) Modulation of low calcium induced field bursts in the hippocampus by monoamines and cholinomimetrics. Pflugers Arch. *400*:28–33.

Haas, H.L., and A. Konnerth (1983) Histamine and noradrenaline decrease calcium-activated potassium conductance in hippocampal pyramidal cells. Nature *302*:432–434.

Haas, H.L., B. Schaerer, and M.T. Vomansky (1979) A simple perfusion chamber for the study of nervous tissue slices in vitro. J. Neurosci. Methods *1*:323–325.

Halliwell, J.V., and P.R. Adams (1982) Voltage-clamp analysis of muscarinic excitation in hippocampal neurons. Brain Res. *250*:71–92.

Halliwell, J.V., and C.N. Scholfield (1984) Somatically recorded ca-currents in guinea-pig hippocampal and olfactory cortex neurons are resistant to adenosine action. Neurosci. Lett 50:13–18.

Henon, B.K., and D.A. McAfee (1983) The ionic basis of adenosine receptor actions on post-ganglionic neurones in the rat. J. Physiol. [Lond.] 336:607–620.

Hood, T.W., J. Siegfried, and H.L. Haas (1983) Analysis of carbamazepine actions in hippocampal slices of the rat. Cell. Mol. Neurobiol. 3(3):213–222.

Katz, B., and R. Miledi (1968) The role of calcium in neuromuscular facilitation. J. Physiol. [Lond.] 195:481–492.

Kuroda, Y., M. Saito, and K. Kobayashi (1976) Concomitant changes in cyclic AMP level and postsynaptic potentials of olfactory cortex induced by adenosine derivatives. Brain Res. 109:196–201.

Lancaster, B., and P.R. Adams (1986) Calcium-dependent current generating the after-hyperpolarization of hippocampal neurons. J. Neurophysiol. 55:1268–1282.

MacDonald, R.L., J.H. Skerritt, and M. Werz (1986) Adenosine agonists reduce voltage-dependent calcium conductance of mouse sensory neurons in cell culture. J. Physiol. 370:75–90.

Madison, D.V., and R.A. Nicoll (1982) Noradrenaline blocks accommodation of pyramidal cell discharge in the hippocampus. Nature 299:636–638.

Madison, D.V., and R.A. Nicoll (1984) Control of the repetitive discharge of rat CA1 pyramidal neurones in vitro. J. Physiol. [Lond.] 354:319–331.

Maitre, M., L. Cielsielski, A. Lehmann, E. Kempf, and P. Mandel (1974) Protective effect of adenosine and nicotinamide against audiogenic seizure. Biochem. Pharmacol. 23:2807–2816.

McNaughton, B.L., C.A. Barnes, and P. Andersen (1981) Synaptic efficacy and e.p.s.p. summation in granule cells of rat fascia dentata studied in vitro. J. Neurophysiol. 46:952–966.

Motley, S.J., and G.G.S. Collins (1983) Endogenous adenosine inhibits excitatory transmission in the rat olfactory cortex slice. Neuropharmacology 22:1081–1086.

Neering, I.R., and R.N. McBurney (1984) Role for microsomal Ca storage in mammalian neurones? Nature 309:158–160.

Okada, Y., and S. Ozawa (1980) Inhibitory action of adenosine on synaptic transmission in the hippocampus of the guinea pig in vitro. Eur. J. Pharmacol. 68:483–492.

Phillis, J.W., G.K. Kostopoulos, and J.J. Limacher (1975) A potent depressant action of adenine derivatives on cerebral cortical neurons. Eur. J. Pharmacol. 30:125–129.

Pollock, J.D., L. Bernier, and J.S. Camardo (1985) Serotonin and cyclic adenosine 3':5'-monophosphate modulate the potassium current in tail sensory neurons in the pleural ganglion of Aplysia. J. Neurosci. 5:1862–1871.

Proctor, W.R., and T.V. Dunwiddie (1983) Adenosine inhibits calcium spikes in hippocampal pyramidal neurons in vitro. Neurosci. Lett. 35:197–201.

Pull, I., and H. McIlwain (1972) Adenine derivatives as neurohumoral agents in the brain. Biochem. J. 130:975–981.

Rahamimoff, R. (1968) A dual action of calcium ions on neuromuscular facilitation. J. Physiol. 195:471–480.

Sanderson, G., and C.N. Scholfield (1986) Effects of adenosine uptake blockers and adenosine on evoked potentials of guinea-pig olfactory cortex. Pflugers Arch. 406(1):25–30.

Scholfield, C.N. (1978) Depression of evoked potentials in brain slices by adenosine compounds. Br. J. Pharmacol. 63:239–244.

Schubert, P., and U. Mitzdorf (1979) Analysis and quantitative evaluation of the depressive effect of adenosine on evoked potentials in hippocampal slices. Brain Res. *172:*186–190.

Sebastiao, A.M., and J.A. Ribeiro (1985) Enhancement of transmission at the frog neuromuscular junction by adenosine deaminase: Evidence for an inhibitory role of endogenous adenosine on neuromuscular transmission. Neurosci. Lett. *62:*267–270.

Segal, M. (1982) Intracellular analysis of a post-synaptic action of adenosine in the rat hippocampus. Eur. J. Pharmacol. *79:*193–199.

Siegelbaum, S.A., J.S. Camardo, and E.R. Kandel (1982) Serotonin and cyclic AMP close single K^+ channels in Aplysia sensory neurones. Nature *299:*413–417.

Smith, S.J., A.B. MacDermott, and F.F. Weight (1983) Detection of intracellular Ca^{2+} transients in sympathetic neurones using arsenazo III. Nature *304:*350–352.

Storm, J.F. (1987) Action potential repolarization and a fast after-hyperpolarization in rat hippocampal pyramidal cells. J. Physiol. [Lond.] *385:*733–759.

Thomas, M.V., and A.L.F. Gorman (1977) Internal calcium changes in a bursting pacemaker neuron measured with arsenazo III. Science *196:*531–533.

Thompson, S.H. (1977) Three pharmacologically distinct potassium channels in molluscan neurones. J. Physiol. [Lond.] *265:*465–488.

Trussell, L.O., and M.B. Jackson (1985) Adenosine-activated potassium conductance in cultured striatal neurons. Proc. Natl. Acad. Sci. U.S.A. *82:*4857–4861.

Trussell, L.O., and M.B. Jackson (1987) Dependence of an adenosine-activated potassium current on a GTP-binding protein in mammalian central neurons. J. Neurosci. *7:*3306–3316.

Wojcik, W.J., and N.H. Neff (1982) Adenosine measurement by a rapid HPLC-fluorometric method: Induced changes of adenosine content in regions of rat brain. J. Neurochem. *39:*280–282.

23
Biochemical Correlates of Long-Term Potentiation

M.A. LYNCH

National Institute for Medical Research, Mill Hill, London, England

INTRODUCTION

Long-term potentiation (LTP) in the hippocampus is a remarkable example of synaptic plasticity which has been the focus of attention as a biological correlate of learning and memory for the past decade or longer. It was first described by Bliss and Lømo (1973) in the perforant path–granule cell synapses of the rabbit and has been shown to occur in other monosynaptic pathways in the hippocampus since that time, both in anesthetized animals and in hippocampal slices (Schwartzkroin and Wester, 1975). The phenomenon describes an enduring increase in synaptic efficacy following a brief train of high-frequency stimulation to the afferent input to dentate gyrus (perforant pathway), area CA3 (commissural input and mossy fibers), or area CA1 (commissural input and Schaffer collaterals). LTP has been shown to persist for days or even weeks (Bliss and Gardner-Medwin, 1973) and it is this persistence, resulting from a relatively modest train of stimuli, that suggests that LTP may provide a useful model for learning and memory.

Two specific features of LTP combine to make it a relatively strong candidate for a biological substrate of learning and memory: input specificity and associativity. Since LTP was first described, the question of specificity has been a subject of great interest. It was suggested by Bliss and Lømo (1973) that LTP was confined to the pathway that had received the tetanus (i.e. perforant pathway–granule cell synapses): these investigators found no evidence of heterosynaptic facilitation. Later, direct evidence was obtained for input specificity in CA1 pyramidal cell synapses (Andersen et al., 1977; Lynch et al., 1977) and perforant pathway–granule cell synapses (Lovinger and Routtenberg, 1988). Although there are isolated reports of heterosynaptic facilitation, the generally accepted view is that it is only pathways that are active during tetanization which will sustain L.T.P.

The associative nature of LTP, investigated by using two stimulating electrodes, has been studied in detail by McNaughton et al. (1978) and by Levy's group (Levy and Steward, 1979, 1983; Levy et al., 1983). Two "weak" pathways, converging on the one population of cells and unable to sustain LTP when stimulated separately, were found to be capable of sustaining LTP when tetanized simultaneously (McNaughton et al., 1978). It was further shown that a "weak" pathway could also sustain LTP if stimulated in conjunction with a "strong" pathway converging on the same population of cells (Levy and Steward, 1979). The property of associativity has been widely studied, and the temporal parameters required to produce the effect are now well characterized (see Bliss and Lynch, 1987). Associativity is exactly the kind of feature that is required to explain certain forms of classical conditioning, and the fact that it has been ascribed to LTP strengthens the suggestion that LTP may be a biological substrate for learning and/or memory.

INDUCTION OF LTP
Tetanus-Induced LTP

To induce LTP, strong depolarization of the postsynaptic region is required; the stimulation given must therefore be of sufficient strength and duration. It was observed in the earliest studies that a threshold for the induction of LTP existed (Bliss and Gardner-Medwin, 1973), and this was later studied systematically by McNaughton et al. (1978). It was shown that weak shocks that did not evoke a population spike also failed to induce LTP, although it had already been noted that firing of target cells was not a prerequisite for the induction of the effect (Bliss and Lømo, 1973). However, it is generally considered that the threshold for the induction of LTP is approximately that which will evoke a population spike. The term *cooperativity* had been used to describe this property of LTP; a strong shock is necessary to stimulate a sufficiently large number of afferents, and it is the convergent activity in these fibers that results in strong depolarization of the postsynaptic region and the consequent induction of LTP.

Induction of LTP by Exposure to Elevated Calcium

Although early experiments were confined to tetanus-induced LTP, it is now clear that LTP or an LTP-like condition can be induced in different ways. Exposure of hippocampal slices to elevated calcium or perfusion of the hippocampus in vivo with a high concentration of calcium induces a condition strikingly similar to LTP. This was first described in area CA1 of the hippocampal slice by Turner et al. (1982). These observations have been extended to the dentate gyrus, both in vitro (Williams and Bliss, 1988) and in vivo (Bliss et al., 1987b), and to area CA3 in vivo (Bliss et al., 1984). In the dentate gyrus, at least, calcium-induced LTP seems to share a common mechanism with tetanus-induced LTP (Bliss et al., 1987b).

Induction of LTP by Phorbol Esters

The significant finding that activators of protein kinase C (phorbol diacetate and phorbol dibutyrate) can induce a long-lasting potentiation was recently reported (Malenka et al., 1986). The effect, which was observed in CA1 cells of the hippocampal slice, was considered to resemble LTP closely, since induction of LTP by tetanization was blocked if slices were pretreated with phorbol esters, suggesting that the two types of potentiation shared a common mechanism. Essentially similar results were obtained by Gustafsson et al. (1988): Application of phorbol ester (phorbol diacetate) induced an LTP-like change in area CA1 of the hippocampus. However, on the basis of results obtained in their occlusion experiments, Gustafsson et al. concluded that blockade of tetanus-induced LTP was partly independent of protein kinase C (PKC) activation. This finding contrasts to some degree with the result of Malenka et al. (1986), whose results suggest near-total occlusion of tetanus-induced LTP with PKC pretreatment. Oleoylacetylglycerol (OAG), a synthetic analog of diacylglycerol, also induced an LTP-like response in area CA1 and dentate gyrus of the hippocampal slice (Williams et al., 1988), although the degree of potentiation induced by OAG was somewhat less than with phorbol esters. It appears that activation of PKC alone is sufficient to induce an LTP-like condition (Hu et al., 1987). Moreover, oleic acid, a putative activator of PKC (Murakami and Routtenberg, 1985), has been shown to inhibit the decay of potentiation but induced LTP only when paired with a tetanus (Linden et al., 1987). Taken together, these results strongly implicate activation of PKC in the induction of LTP.

MECHANISMS INVOLVED IN LTP

To consider the mechanisms involved, it is convenient to separate LTP into two components, its induction and its maintenance. The induction of LTP describes the changes that occur during tetanization that allow the effect to be established, while the maintenance is concerned with the mechanisms underlying the expression of the effect.

Mechanisms Underlying the Induction of LTP

Requirement for pre- and postsynaptic elements. Much progress has been made in defining mechanisms underlying the induction of LTP. The evidence implicating postsynaptic involvement has been accumulating for some time: Lynch and his coworkers (1983) found that injection of EGTA, a calcium chelator, into CA1 cells prevented the induction of LTP. A postsynaptic role in induction was later confirmed when Malinow and Miller (1986) showed that hyperpolarization of target cells also blocked the induction of LTP. However, in a number of recent papers, reported almost simultaneously, the requirement for both pre- and postsynaptic elements in the induction of LTP was clearly demonstrated. Kelso et al. (1986), Sastry et al. (1986), and Wigström et al. (1986) showed that if CA1 cells were strongly depolarized at a time when single test shocks were applied to the afferent input, the response to test shocks was potentiated. A long-lasting potentiation could be obtained by repeating this pattern of stimulation, and maximum potentiation was observed after 20–30 pairings. The role played by both sides of the synapse was further emphasized by the finding that dendritic application of glutamate together with single afferent shocks also induced LTP; neither procedure alone was sufficient (Hvalby et al., 1987). These reports provide the strongest evidence that conjoint activity pre- and postsynaptically are essential for the induction of LTP.

The role of the NMDA receptor. In the past 5 years or so, the pivotal role played by the NMDA receptor in the induction of LTP has been clarified. The interest was stimulated by the observation of Collingridge et al. (1983) that D-amino phosphorovalerate (APV), an antagonist at the NMDA subtype of glutamate receptor, blocked the induction of LTP without significantly affecting normal transmission. It was subsequently established that the channel associated with this receptor is subject to a voltage-dependent magnesium block (Nowak et al., 1984; Mayer et al., 1984), which is lifted under conditions of strong depolarization, and that in its open state the channel is permeable to calcium ions (Mayer and Westbrook, 1985; Ascher and Nowak, 1986).

The NMDA model. On the basis of these experiments, a scheme has been formulated suggesting a plausible sequence of events leading to the induction of LTP: Strong depolarization following the high-frequency train relieves the magnesium block on the NMDA receptor, and this relief, plus the coincident occupation of the NMDA receptor, allows calcium influx into the postsynaptic region. The entry of calcium ions is the critical inductive step which triggers a biochemical cascade leading to the expression of LTP. If this scheme is to be acceptable, then it must be possible to accommodate the properties of associativity, input specificity, and cooperativity within the scheme. It must also be possible, if the same mechanism is shared, to suggest how LTP is induced by calcium or phorbol esters. The three properties of LTP listed can all be incorporated into the NMDA scheme without difficulty. With respect to calcium-induced LTP, which in the dentate gyrus is APV-sensitive (Bliss et al., 1986), the necessary depolarization may be achieved by an increase in glutamate release from terminals which the imposed calcium gradient has loaded with an elevated cytosolic calcium concentration. With respect to phorbol ester-induced LTP, PKC activation is downstream of calcium entry, and activation of the NMDA receptor and the associated entry of calcium ions through the NMDA-coupled channel are by-passed. It appears then that the NMDA model can plausibly account for the experimental data relating to the induction of LTP.

Maintenance of LTP

Progress in defining the mechanisms underlying the maintenance of LTP has been relatively slow. The original hypothesis proposed by Hebb (1949) to explain an increase in synaptic efficacy was that a "growth process" or "metabolic change" occurred in one or both of the cells involved in the activity. Consistent with the idea that a "growth process" was responsible, several workers have reported that protein synthesis was an absolute requirement for the maintenance of the longer-lasting components of LTP. In addition, there is a wealth of evidence indicating that morphological changes occur following the induction of LTP, and the persistence of these changes has implicated them in the maintenance of the effect. Consistent with the idea that a "metabolic change" was responsible, workers from several laboratories have reported a variety of biochemical and neurochemical changes that could be classified as "metabolic changes" and that may contribute to the maintenance of LTP; among these are changes in transmitter release, receptor binding, uptake and storage of calcium, protein phosphorylation, and phospholipid turnover.

Protein synthesis. Although early reports suggested that either the induction (Stanton and Sarvey, 1984) or the maintenance (Fifkova et al., 1982; Krug et al., 1984) of LTP was blocked by protein synthesis inhibitors, the literature was confused and there was no clear consensus of which protein synthesis inhibitors were effective or what conditions were required to establish an effect. Recent results from two groups have helped to clarify some of these points. Anisomycin, present before or immediately after the induction of LTP, blocked the longer-lasting component of LTP in both CA1 in vitro (Frey et al., 1988) and the dentate gyrus in vivo (Otani et al., 1989). It was concluded that the initial phase of the maintenance of LTP is probably independent of protein synthesis, while the later phase requires the synthesis of new proteins.

Morphological changes. Since the first report that LTP in the perforant pathway was accompanied by an increase in the area of boutons and spines in the terminal zone (Fifkova and van Harreveld, 1977), several reports suggesting changes in morphology have followed. Changes have been reported in the number of spines and boutons, in the width of the spine neck, the length of the spine shaft, and the number of shaft synapses (see Bliss and Lynch, 1987). Evidence supporting the idea that both pre- and postsynaptic elements are involved in the maintenance of LTP has been obtained from morphological studies; there is an increase in the number of synaptic vesicles in potentiated tissue (Desmond and Levy, 1986), and LTP was also found to be associated with morphological changes in postsynaptic densities (Greenough et al., 1986).

Neurochemical changes. During the past year or so the debate concerning the locus of control of LTP has been resolved by the incontrovertible evidence indicating the involvement of both pre- and postsynaptic elements at least in the induction process (Wigström et al., 1986; Hvalby et al., 1987). One theory, which suggested that postsynaptic mechanisms were primarily responsible for the maintenance of the effect, was the so-called receptor theory, which proposed that there was an increase in the number of postsynaptic glutamate receptors following the induction of LTP (Baudry and Lynch, 1980). Although this provided an attractive hypothesis, others have failed to confirm these findings (Sastry and Goh, 1984; Lynch et al., 1985), and it now seems likely that the original experiments on which the theory was based examined not just binding sites but also uptake sites (Foster and Fagg, 1984; Mena et al., 1987).

The first evidence suggesting that a presynaptic mechanism plays a role in the maintenance of LTP was provided by the results of Skrede and Malthe-Sørenssen (1981), who demonstrated that unstimulated release of radiolabeled D-aspartate, a marker for glutamate, was significantly increased following tetanic stimulation. Over the past few years we have used a technique that combines push–pull cannulation and electrophysiological recording (Errington et al., 1983), to show that there is an increase in the release of newly synthesized glutamate (Dolphin et al., 1982) and endogenous glutamate (Bliss et al., 1986a) associated with LTP. Figure 1B shows a typical electrophysiological response to test stimuli delivered to the perforant pathway before and after induction

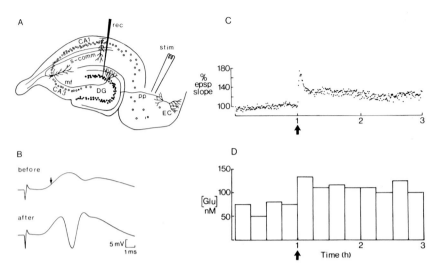

Fig. 1. **A:** Diagram showing a cross section through the hippocampus with stimulating electrode (stim) in perforant pathway (pp) and recording electrode (rec) in the cell body layer of the dentate gyrus (DG). For clarity, the push–pull cannula, to which the recording electrode is glued, is not included in the diagram. Artificial cerebrospinal fluid is perfused through the push part of the cannula, and the pull part of the cannula samples the extracellular fluid in the region of the perforant pathway–granule cell synapses. After an initial period of perfusion to allow equilibration to occur within the pump, samples of perfusate are collected over dry ice at 15 min intervals for 1 h before a high-frequency train (250 Hz, 200 ms) of stimuli is delivered to the perforant pathway in the LTP group. Sampling continues for a further 2 h and responses evoked by test stimuli delivered at 30 s intervals are monitored throughout the 3 h. In the control group the same number of stimuli are delivered to the perforant pathway, but no high-frequency train is given. **B:** Sample recordings obtained before and after the high-frequency train of stimuli. **C:** The changes in EPSP slope with time, expressed as a percentage of the slope during the 10 min immediately before the tetanus is delivered (arrow). **D:** The change in glutamate release, measured by HPLC, over the 3 h experimental period. The arrow marks the time at which the tetanus was given. Note the sustained increase in release of glutamate after the tetanus compared with before.

of LTP (but see Aniksztejn et al., 1988); the change in excitatory postsynaptic potential (EPSP) slope with time, computed from these records, is shown in Figure 1C. We have found that a long-lasting increase in EPSP slope, the best measure of LTP, is associated with an increase in glutamate release: Results from a typical release experiment are shown in Figure 1D.

LTP appears to be tightly coupled to an increase in glutamate release: If the induction of LTP is blocked by stimulation of the commissural input to the dentate gyrus immediately prior to high-frequency stimulation of the per-forant pathway (Douglas et al., 1983), or by perfusion with the NMDA antagonist APV (Collingridge et al., 1983), the increase in transmitter release is inhibited

(Bliss et al., 1986; Errington et al., 1987). Furthermore, using an ex vivo method in which slices or synaptosomes were prepared from control tissue or tissue in which LTP had been induced in vivo, we found that potentiation was associated with an increase in K^+-induced, Ca^{2+}-dependent release of [^{3}H]glutamate (Feasey et al., 1986; Lynch and Bliss, 1986; Lynch et al., 1985). In addition, we found that the increase in transmitter release was still evident in a group of animals in which LTP persisted for 3 days compared with a control group, while in another group in which LTP was no longer present 10 days after tetanization, release was comparable to that in a control group (Bliss et al., 1987a). It is clear, therefore, that the maintenance of LTP is closely associated with an increase in transmitter release, and we propose that this may be at least in part responsible for the maintenance of LTP.

As a first step in examining the mechanism responsible for the maintained increase in transmitter release, we measured calcium concentration in synaptosomes prepared from control and potentiated tissue and found that LTP was associated with an increase in intrasynaptosomal calcium (Lynch et al., 1987). We also found, in accord with findings in other systems (Knight and Baker, 1983; Nichols et al., 1985) that stimulation of PKC resulted in increased transmitter release (Lynch and Bliss, 1986). An increase in phosphatidylinositol (PI) turnover could conceivably give rise to increased intrasynaptosomal calcium concentration and increased activation of PKC. Investigating this possibility, we found that there was an increase in PI turnover in slices and synaptosomes prepared from potentiated tissue compared with control tissue in both area CA3 (Lynch et al., 1988b) and dentate gyrus (Fig. 2A); also, there was an increase in the concentration of inositol-1,4,5-trisphosphate (InsP$_3$), one of the consequences of an increase in PI turnover, in synaptosomes obtained from potentiated tissue (Lynch et al., 1988b). As in the case of many preparations, our results suggested that InsP$_3$ stimulates release of calcium from some intracellular store (Fig. 2B). There was an increase in the concentration of calcium in InsP$_3$-treated synaptosomes obtained from control tissue, but the effect was lost in potentiated tissue: Thus InsP$_3$ may contribute to the increase in the concentration of calcium in synaptosomes. Baimbridge and Miller (1981) reported that the influx of calcium into potentiated hippocampal slices was significantly greater than into control slices. This observation was later confirmed and extended to show that calcium influx into synaptosomes prepared from potentiated tissue was enhanced (Agoston and Kuhnt, 1986). Therefore, the increase in intrasynaptosomal calcium associated with LTP may result in part from an InsP$_3$-induced release of calcium from intracellular stores, secondary to an increase in PI turnover, and in part from an increase in calcium influx into synaptosomes. Since release of transmitter is calcium dependent, these mechanisms, which modulate free calcium concentration in synaptosomes, may play a crucial role in controlling glutamate release.

The second consequence of an increase in PI turnover in synaptosomes is an increase in diacylglycerol, which activates PKC, which in turn stimulates phosphorylation of proteins and also possibly release of glutamate. Protein F1 or B50, a presynaptically located substrate for PKC, has been shown to be

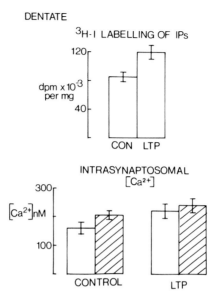

DENTATE

^{3}H-I LABELLING OF IPs

Fig. 2. The top panel shows the labeling of inositol phosphates (IPs) by [^{3}H]inositol in synaptosomes prepared from control and potentiated tissue. There was a significant increase in labeling associated with LTP, suggesting that PI turnover was increased. Separation of inositol phosphates into InsP, InsP$_2$, and InsP$_3$ showed that there was an increase in concentration of InsP$_3$ in potentiated tissue. The bottom panel shows the effect of InsP$_3$ on the concentration of calcium in synaptosomes prepared from control tissue and tissue that had been potentiated in vivo. The concentration of calcium in potentiated synaptosomes (open histogram, LTP) was significantly increased compared to the concentration in control synaptosomes (open histograms, control). Addition of InsP$_3$ (hatched histograms, control and LTP) during preparation of synaptosomes resulted in increased calcium concentration in control tissue but no significant change in potentiated tissue.

phosphorylated following the induction of LTP: Changes in the phosphorylation of the protein were directly related to the magnitude and persistence of LTP (Lovinger et al., 1986; see Routtenberg, 1985). Since protein F1 or B50 is identical to the growth cone protein pp1 and the growth-related protein GAP43 (Snipes et al., 1987), it has been suggested that phosphorylation of this protein may be associated with some of the morphological changes described following potentiation (Desmond and Levy, 1983). However, the role of PKC in LTP is not confined to presynaptic changes; Hu et al. (1987) have shown that injection of purified PKC into CA1 pyramidal cells produces LTP-like changes in cell excitability, pinpointing a postsynaptic role.

Since induction of LTP requires the occupation of NMDA receptors by glutamate with a consequent increase in calcium influx postsynaptically, and the maintenance of LTP appears to involve presynaptic changes leading to increased glutamate release, it follows that there should be some factor produced postsynaptically that can act as a retrograde signal and turn on a presynaptic switch. Possible candidates for this messenger are arachidonic acid or lipoxygenase metabolites of arachidonic acid, since they are small, lipid-soluble compounds that could cross membranes with ease. The suggestion that these compounds could fulfill such a role in the hippocampus was originally made by Piomelli et al. (1987).

As a first step in examining the possible role of arachidonic acid in LTP, perfusate collected during experiments was examined for arachidonic acid content. There was a significant increase in arachidonic acid content in samples

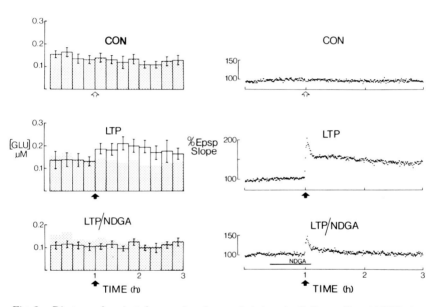

Fig. 3. Diagram showing changes in release of glutamate (left panel) and EPSP slope (right panel) in three groups of animals: control (top), LTP (middle), and LTP/NDGA (bottom). Rats were anesthetized with urethane, placed in a head holder, and the stimulating electrode and recording electrode, with attached push–pull cannula, were stereotaxically lowered into the perforant pathway and granule cell synapses, respectively. Test shocks were delivered to the perforant pathway at 30 s intervals, and after 1 h (arrow) a high-frequency train of stimuli (250 Hz for 200 ms) was given in the LTP and the LTP/NDGA groups. The control groups received the same total number of stimuli but no tetanus. Artificial cerebrospinal fluid was perfused through the cannula and samples collected over dry ice at 15 min intervals in all groups. NDGA (200 μM) was added to the medium for 30 min before and 5 min after the tetanus in the LTP/NDGA group as indicated by the bar. Perfusate was analyzed for glutamate concentration by HPLC as previously described (Bliss et al., 1986). The results demonstrate that LTP was associated with an increase in release of glutamate and that both the induction of LTP and the associated increase in glutamate release were blocked by perfusion with NDGA.

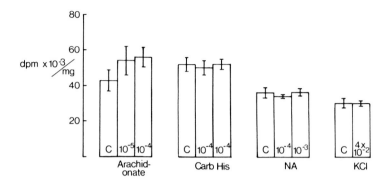

Fig. 4. The effect of several agents on [³H]inositol labeling of inositol phosphates was examined in synaptosomes prepared from dentate gyrus. The method is as described in the legend to Figure 2. Carbachol (Carb, 10^{-4} M), histamine (His, 10^{-4} M), noradrenaline (NA, 10^{-4} and 10^{-3} M), and KCl (4×10^{-2} M) had no significant effect on labeling compared with control (C). Arachidonate (10^{-4} and 10^{-5} M) significantly increased labeling compared to the corresponding controls (C; $P < 0.05$; Student's t test for paired data).

collected after the tetanus compared to before (Bliss et al., 1988). The drug nordihydroguaiaretic acid (NDGA), an inhibitor of lipoxygenase (the enzyme responsible for metabolism of arachidonic acid to hydroperoxyeicosatetraenoic acid and hydroxyeicosatetraenoic acid and then to leukotrienes) and, at higher concentrations phospholipase A_2, was investigated for its effect on the induction of LTP, release of glutamate, and on arachidonic acid content in perfusates. NDGA blocked the induction of LTP and the associated increase in release of glutamate (Fig. 3), and it also blocked the increase in arachidonic acid that we found to accompany LTP (Bliss et al., 1988). The increase in the release of arachidonic acid was consistent with the retrograde messenger hypothesis, providing it could be established that it was released from postsynaptic rather than presynaptic regions. To test this, slices and synaptosomes were prepared from control and potentiated tissue and release assessed. There was an increase in arachidonic acid release from potentiated slices—no increase was observed in synaptosomes (Clements, and Lynch, 1989). If synaptosomes represent a preparation that is relatively free of postsynaptic elements, we can conclude that arachidonic acid release associated with LTP is not likely to arise from presynaptic sources. On the other hand, if slices contain both pre- and post-synaptic elements and if presynaptic elements do not contribute significantly to the release of arachidonic acid in LTP, then it follows that the origin of arachidonic acid is largely postsynaptic or glial. This result lends some weight to the hypothesis that arachidonic acid may play the role of a retrograde messenger in LTP. We have recently obtained further evidence consistent with the hypothesis. As suggested above, an increase in PI turnover in synaptosomes

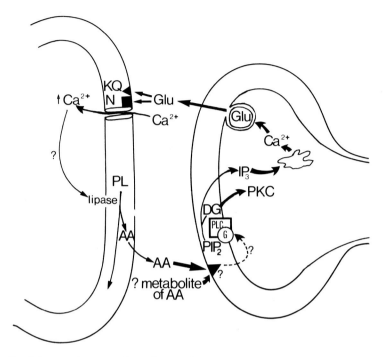

Fig. 5. Scheme of proposed mechanism leading to sustained increase of transmitter release LTP. The induction of LTP results from the occupation of NMDA receptors (N) by glutamate (Glu) and the subsequent entry of calcium (Ca^{2+}) into the postsynaptic region, depolarization having relieved the magnesium block on the channel. The elevated calcium postsynaptically triggers a number of events, including activation of calcium-dependent lipases, that stimulate the liberation of free arachidonic acid (AA). Arachidonic acid (or a metabolite of arachidonic acid) is then released into the synaptic area and stimulates the phospholipase C–G protein complex (PLC/G) on the presynaptic terminal, leading to increased hydrolysis of phosphatidylinositol bisphosphate (PIP_2) and production of $InsP_3$ (IP_3) and diacylglycerol (DG). These second messengers stimulate release of calcium (Ca) from some intrasynaptosomal site and activation of PKC, respectively. Either or both of these changes may contribute to the increase in release of glutamate associated with LTP.

may be responsible for increasing the concentration of calcium in synaptosomes through the action of $InsP_3$ and increasing PKC activity through the action of diacylglycerol, either of which could underlie the LTP-associated increase in glutamate release. Of the several agents tested, only arachidonic acid increased PI turnover in synaptosomes (Lynch et al., 1988a) (see Fig. 4), implying that some of the presynaptic changes leading to the increase in the glutamate release may be arachidonic acid induced.

SUMMARY AND CONCLUSIONS

A working hypothesis based on established data and on some of our recent findings is described in Figure 5. It is likely that the induction of LTP results from the occupation of the NMDA receptor by glutamate, the concurrent strong depolarization, allowing the postsynaptic influx of calcium through the voltage-dependent ionophore linked to the NMDA receptor. The entry of calcium is likely to trigger a number of events, including the activation of proteases, that may result in cytoskeletal and subsequent morphological changes. Another function of calcium may be to increase the activity of lipases, e.g. PLA_2, with a consequent liberation of arachidonic acid that would then be available for release into the perfusate. The stimulation by arachidonic acid of PI turnover and the consequent production of the two second messengers, $InsP_3$ and dia-cylglycerol, in synaptosomes may be the trigger to stimulate release of calcium from intrasynaptosomal stores and to activate PKC. These two effects working in tandem could stimulate the increase in release of glutamate which is associated with, and is at least in part responsible for the maintenance of LTP.

I thank Dr. T.V.P. Bliss for discussions and comments on an earlier version of this chapter.

REFERENCES

Agoston, D.V. and U. Kuhnt (1986) Increased Ca-uptake of presynaptic terminals during long-term potentiation in hippocampal slices. Exp. Brain Res. *62*:663–668.

Andersen, P., S.H. Sundberg, O. Sveen, and H. Wigström (1977) Specific long-lasting potentiation of synaptic transmission in hippocampal slices. Nature *266*:736–737.

Aniksztejn, L., Y. Ben-Ari, and M.P. Roisin (1988) Release of endogenous excitatory amino acids and long-term potentiation of synaptic transmission in the hippocampus of the anaesthetized rat. J. Physiol. *398*:21P.

Ascher, P., and L. Nowak (1986) Calcium permeability of the channels activated by N-methyl-D-aspartate (NMDA) in mouse central neurones. J. Physiol. *377*:35P.

Baimbridge, K.G., and J.J. Miller (1981) Calcium uptake and retention during long-term potentiation of neuronal activity in the rat hippocampal slice preparation. Brain Res. *221*:299–305.

Baudry, M., and G. Lynch (1980) An hypothesis regarding the cellular mechanisms responsible for long-term synaptic potentiation in the hippocampus. Exp. Neurol. *68*:202–204.

Bliss, T.V.P., A.C. Dolphin, and K.J. Feasey (1984) Elevated calcium induces a long-lasting potentiation of commissural responses in hippocampal CA3 cells of the rat in vivo. J. Physiol. *350*:65P.

Bliss, T.V.P., R.M. Douglas, M.L. Errington, and M.A. Lynch (1986) Correlation between long-term potentiation and release of endogenous amino acids from dentate gyrus of anaesthetized rats. J. Physiol. *377*:391–408.

Bliss, T.V.P., M.L. Errington, S. Laroche, and M.A. Lynch (1987a) Increase in K^+-stimulated Ca^{2+}-dependent release of ^3H glutamate from rat dentate gyrus three days after induction of long-term potentiation. Neurosci. Lett. *83*:107–112.

Bliss, T.V.P., M.L. Errington, and M.A. Lynch (1987b) Calcium-induced long-term potentiation in the dentate gyrus is accompanied by a sustained increase in glutamate release. In T.P. Hicks, D. Lodge, and H. McLennan (eds): Excitatory Amino Acid Transmission New York: Alan R. Liss, pp. 337–340.

Bliss, T.V.P., M.L. Errington, M.A. Lynch, and J.H. Williams (1988) The lipoxygenase inhibitor nordihydroguaiaretic acid (NDGA) blocks the induction of both tetanus-induced and calcium-induced long-term potentiation in the hippocampus of the rat. Pflugers Arch. *441*:R120.

Bliss, T.V.P., and A.R. Gardner-Medwin (1973) Long-lasting potentiation of synaptic transmission in the dentate area of the unanaesthetized rabbit following stimulation of the perforant path. J. Physiol. *232*:357–374.

Bliss, T.V.P., and T. Lømo (1973) Long-lasting potentiation of synaptic transmission in the dentate area of the anaesthetized rabbit following stimulation of the perforant path. J. Physiol. *232*:331–356.

Bliss, T.V.P., and M.A. Lynch (1987) Long-term potentiation of synaptic transmission in the hippocampus. Properties and mechanisms. In P.W. Landfield and S.A. Deadwyler (eds): Long-term Potentiation: From Biophysics to Behavior. New York: Alan R. Liss, pp. 3–72.

Clements, M.P., and M.A. Lynch (1989) LTP is associated with increased liberation of arachidonic acid from postsynaptic but not presynaptic elements Neurosci. Lett. (in press).

Collingridge, G.L., S.J. Kehl, and H. McLennan (1983) Excitatory amino acids in synaptic transmission in the Schaffer collateral-commissural pathway of the rat hippocampus. J. Physiol. *334*:33–46.

Desmond, N.L., and W.B. Levy (1983) Synaptic correlates of associative potentiation/depression: An ultrastructural study in the hippocampus. Brain Res. *265*:21–30.

Desmond, N.L., and W.B. Levy (1986) More front-line synaptic vesicles with long-term synaptic potentiation in the hippocampal dentate gyrus. Soc. Neurosci. Abstr. *12*:504.

Dolphin, A.C., M.L. Errington, and T.V.P. Bliss (1982) Long-term potentiation of the perforant path in vivo is associated with increased glutamate release. Nature *297*:496–498.

Douglas, R.M., B.L. McNaughton, and G.V. Goddard (1983) Commissural inhibition and facilitation of granule cell discharge in fascia dentata. J. Comp. Neurol. *219*:285–294.

Errington, M.L., A.C. Dolphin, and T.V.P. Bliss (1983) A method for combining field potential recording with local perfusion in the hippocampus of the anaesthetized rat. J. Neurosci. Methods *7*:353–357.

Errington, M.L., M.A. Lynch, T.V.P. Bliss (1987) Long-term potentiation in the dentate gyrus: Induction and increased glutamate release are blocked by D(-)aminophosphonovalerate. Neuroscience *20*:279–284.

Feasey, K.J., M.A. Lynch, and T.V.P. Bliss (1986) Long-term potentiation is associated with an increase in calcium-dependent, potassium-stimulated release of [^{14}C]glutamate from hippocampal slices: An ex vivo study in the rat. Brain Res. *364*:39–44.

Fifkova, E., C.L. Anderson, S.J. Young, and A. van Harreveld (1982) Effect of anisomycin on stimulation-induced changes in dendritic spines of dentate granular cells following stimulation of the entorhinal area. J. Neurocytol. *6*:699–721.

Fifkova, E., and A. van Harreveld (1977) Long-lasting morphological changes in dendritic spines of dentate granular cells following stimulation of the entorhinal area. J. Neurocytol. *6*:211–230.

Foster, A.C., and G.E. Fagg (1984) Acidic amino acid binding sites in mammalian neuronal membranes: Their characteristics and relationship to synaptic receptors. Brain Res. Rev. *7*:103–164.

Frey, U., M. Krug, K. Reymann, and H.-J. Matthies (1988) Anisomycin, an inhibitor of protein synthesis, blocks late phases of LTP phenomena in the hippocampal CA1 region. Brain Res. *452*:57–65.

Greenough, W.T., H.-M. Hwang, F.-L.F. Chang, C. Wallace, and B. Anderson (1986) Changes in intramembranous particle aggregrates in neuronal membranes of CA1 pyramidal cells following induction of LTP in hippocampal slices. Soc. Neurosci. Abstr. *12*:505.

Gustafsson, B., Y.-Y. Huang, and H. Wigström (1988) Phorbol ester-induced synaptic potentiation differs from long-term potentiation in the guinea pig hippocampus in vitro. Neurosci. Lett. *85*:77–81.

Hebb, D.O. (1949) The organization of behavior. Soc. Neurosci. Abstr. *12*:505.

Hu, G.-Y., O. Hvalby, S.I. Waalas, K.A. Albert, P. Skjeflo, P. Andersen, and P. Greengard (1987) Protein kinase C injection into hippocampal pyramidal cells elicits features of long-term potentiation. Nature *328*:426–429.

Hvalby, O., J.-C. Lacaille, G.-Y. Hu, and P. Andersen (1987): Postsynaptic long-term potentiation follows coupling of dendritic glutamate application and synaptic activation. Experientia *43*:599–601.

Kelso, S.R., A.H. Ganong, and T.H. Brown (1986) Hebbian synapses in hippocampus. Proc. Natl. Acad. Sci. USA *83*:5326–5330.

Knight, D.E., and P.F. Baker (1983) The phorbol ester TPA increases the affinity of exocytosis for calcium in leaky adrenal medullary cells. FEBS Lett. *160*:98–100.

Krug, M., B. Lossner, and T. Ott (1984) Anisomycin blocks the late phase of long-term potentiation in the dentate gyrus of freely moving rats. Brain Res. Bull. *13*:39–42.

Levy, W.B., S.E. Brassel, and S.D. Moore (1983) Partial quantification of the associative synaptic learning rule of the dentate gyrus. Neuroscience *8*:799–803.

Levy, W.B., and O. Steward (1979) Synapses as associative memory elements in the hippocampal formation. Brain Res. *175*:233–245.

Levy, W.B., and O. Steward (1983) Temporal contiguity requirements for long-term associative potentiation/depression in the hippocampus. Neuroscience *8*:791–797.

Linden, D.J., F.-S. Sheu, K. Murakami, and A. Routtenberg (1987) Enhancement of long-term potentiation by *cis*-unsaturated fatty acid: Relation to protein kinase C and phospholipase A$_2$. J. Neurosci. *7*:3783–3792.

Lovinger, D.M., P.A. Colley, R.F. Akers, R.B. Nelson, and A. Routtenberg (1986) Direct relation of long-term synaptic potentiation to phosphorylation of membrane protein F1, a substrate for membrane protein kinase C. Brain Res. *399*:205–211.

Lovinger, D., and A. Routtenberg (1988) Synapse-specific protein kinase C activation enhances maintenance of long-term potentiation in rat hippocampus. J. Physiol. *400*:321–335.

Lynch, G., T. Dunwiddie, and V. Gribkoff (1977) Heterosynaptic depression: A postsynaptic correlate of long-term potentiation. Nature *266*:737–739.

Lynch, G., J. Larson, S. Kelso, G. Barrionuevo, and F. Schottler (1983) Intracellular injections of EGTA block induction of hippocampal long-term potentiation. Nature *305*:719–721.

Lynch, M.A., and T.V.P. Bliss (1986) Long-term potentiation of synaptic transmission in the hippocampus: Effect of calmodulin and oleoyl-acetyl-glycerol (OAG) on release of ^{3}H glutamate. Neurosci. Lett. *65*:171–176.

Lynch, M.A., M.P. Clements, and T.V.P. Bliss (1988a) Increased hydrolysis of phosphatidylinositol-4,5-bidphosphate in long-term potentiation. Neurosci. Lett. *84*:291–296.

Lynch, M.A., M.P. Clements, M.L. Errington, and T.V.P. Bliss (1987) Increase in intrasynaptosomal calcium in long-term potentiation. Neurosci. Lett. [Suppl.] *22*:S511.

Lynch, M.A., M.P. Clements, M.L. Errington, and T.V.P. Bliss (1988b) Neurochemical changes associated with long-term potentiation in the hippocampus. Neurochem. Int. [Suppl.] *13*:17.

Lynch, M.A., M.L. Errington, and T.V.P. Bliss (1985) Long-term potentiation of synaptic transmission in the dentate gyrus: Increased release of [^{14}C] glutamate without increase in receptor binding. Neurosci. Lett. *62:*123–129.

Malenka, R.C., D.V. Madison, and R.A. Nicoll (1986) Potentiation of synaptic transmission in the hippocampus by phorbol esters. Nature *319:*774–776.

Malinow, R., and J.P. Miller (1986) Postsynaptic hyperpolarization during conditioning reversibly blocks induction of long-term potentiation. Nature *320:*529–530.

Mayer, M.L., and G.L. Westbrook (1985) Divalent cation permeability of N-methyl-D-aspartate channels. Soc. Neurosci. Abstr. *11:*785.

Mayer, M.L., G.L. Westbrook, and P.B. Guthrie (1984) Voltage-dependent block by Mg^{2+} of NMDA responses in spinal cord neurones. Nature *309:*261–263.

McNaughton, B.L., R.M. Douglas, G.V. Goddard (1978) Synaptic enhancement in fascia dentata: Cooperativity among coactive afferents. Brain Res. *157:*277–293.

Mena, E.E., M.F. Gullak, and M.J. Pagozzi (1987) Effect of chaotropic series ions on anion-dependent L-glutamate binding sites. In T.P. Hicks, D. Lodge, and H. McLennan (eds): Excitatory Amino Acid Transmission. New York: Alan R. Liss, pp. 55–58.

Murakami, K., and A. Routtenberg (1985) Direct activation of purified protein kinase C by unsaturated fatty acids (oleate and arachidonate) in the absence of phospholipids and calcium. FEBS Lett. *192:*189–193.

Nichols, R.A., J.W. Haycock, J.K.-T. Wang, and P. Greengard (1985) Phorbol ester enhances calcium-dependent neurotransmitter release from rat brain synaptosomes. Soc. Neurosci. Abstr. *11:*846.

Nowak, L., P. Bregestovski, P. Ascher, A. Herbet, and A. Prochiantz (1984) Magnesium gates glutamate-activated channels in mouse central neurones. Nature *307:*462–465.

Otani, S., C.J. Marshall, W.P. Tate, G.V. Goddard, and W.C. Abrahams (1989) Maintenance of long-term potentiation in rat dentate gyrus requires protein synthesis but not messenger RNA synthesis immediately post-tetanization. Neuroscience *28:*519–526.

Piomelli, D., A. Volterra, N. Dale, S.A. Siegelbaum, E.R. Kandel, J.H. Schwartz, and F. Belardetti (1987) Lipoxygenase metabolites of arachidonic acid are second messengers for presynaptic inhibition of *Aplysia* sensory cells. Nature *328:*38–43.

Routtenberg, A. (1985) Synaptic plasticity and protein kinase C. Prog. Brain Res. *69:*211–234.

Sastry, B.R., and J.W. Goh (1984) Long-lasting potentiation in the hippocampus is not due to an increase in glutamate receptors. Life Sci *34:*1497–1501.

Sastry, B.R., J.W. Goh, and A. Auyeung (1986) Associative induction of posttetanic and long-term potentiation in CA1 neurons of rat hippocampus. Science *232:*988–990.

Schwartzkroin, P., and K. Wester (1975) Long-lasting facilitation of a synaptic potential following tetanization in the in vitro hippocampal slice. Brain Res. *89:*107–119.

Skrede, K., and D. Malthe-Sørenssen (1981) Increased resting and evoked release of transmitter following repetitive electrical tetanization in hippocampus: A biochemical correlate to long-lasting synaptic potentiation. Brain Res. *208:* 436–441.

Snipes, G.J., S.Y. Chan, C.B. McGuire, B.R. Costello, J.J. Norden, J.A. Freeman, and A. Routtenberg (1987) Evidence for the coidentification of GAP-43, a growth-associated protein and F1, a plasticity-associated protein. J. Neurosci. *7:*4066–4075.

Stanton, P.K., and J.M. Sarvey (1984) Blockade of long-term potentiation in rat hippocampal CA1 region by inhibitors of protein synthesis. J. Neurosci. *4:*3080–3088.

Turner, R.W., K.G. Baimbridge, and J.J. Miller (1982) Calcium-induced long-term potentiation in the hippocampus. Neuroscience *7:*1411–1416.

Wigström, H., B. Gustafsson, Y.-Y. Huang, and W.C. Abraham (1986) Hippocampal long-lasting potentiation is induced by pairing single afferent volleys with intracellularly injected depolarizing current pulses. Acta Physiol. Scand. *126*:317–319.

Williams, J.H., and T.V.P. Bliss (1988) Induction but not maintenance of calcium-induced long-term potentiation in dentate gyrus and area CA1 of the hippocampal slice is blocked by nordihydroguaiaretic acid. Neurosci. Lett. *88*:81–85.

Williams, J.H., M.A. Lynch, and T.V.P. Bliss (1988) Oleoylacetyl-glycerol (OAG) produces long-lasting increases in synaptic transmission in hippocampal slices and an associated increase in release of radiolabelled amino acids. Abstr. Eur. Neurosci. Assn *1*:313.

The Hippocampus—New Vistas, pages 379–394
© 1989 Alan R. Liss, Inc.

24

Behavioral and Anatomical Studies of the Avian Hippocampus

VERNER P. BINGMAN, PAOLA BAGNOLI, PAOLO IOALÈ, AND
GIOVANNI CASINI

*Department of Psychology, University of Maryland, College Park,
Maryland (V.P.B.); Dipartimento di Fisiologia e Biochimica (P.B.) and
Dipartimento di Scienze del Comportamento Animale (P.I., G.C.),
Università di Pisa, Pisa and Centro di Studio per la Faunistica ed
Ecologia Tropicali de C.N.R., Firenze (P.I.), Italy*

INTRODUCTION

Functional analyses of the hippocampus and related areas have suggested a diversity of hypotheses to explain the role of this central forebrain structure in behavior (Isaacson, 1982). It has been in the investigation of mnemonic processes, however, that the vast majority of research effort has been expended. This emphasis on memory function, beginning with clinical studies of humans with presumed hippocampal damage (Scoville and Milner, 1957), followed by experimental studies with monkeys and rats (Gaffan, 1974; Mishkin, 1978; O'-Keefe and Nadel, 1978; Morris et al., 1982; Olton, 1983), has proven to be more than justified, having clearly demonstrated a critical role for the hippocampus in what appears to be a limited set of memory processes.

One research tactic that has only recently been exploited, however, has been an attempt to perform relatively controlled experimental animal studies in a "natural world" setting. Ideally, such studies should provide a better understanding of how hippocampal involvement in memory processes may manifest itself within the complexity of free-living conditions. It is here that studies on the avian hippocampus seem to have made their most important contribution, with investigations into the role of the hippocampus in naturally occurring spatial behavior. In particular, these studies have examined the importance of the hippocampus for memory processes in the context of spatial recognition and spatial navigation.

THE QUESTION OF HOMOLOGY

The primary goal of research on the mammalian hippocampus continues to be the hope of understanding the neural regulation of memory processes. If bird studies are to be of relevance to this central issue, therefore, it would appear necessary to demonstrate, within reason, that the avian and mammalian hippocampus are homologous, thus providing at least the basis of functional similarity. To address this question, we will first compare at various anatomical levels the avian and mammalian hippocampus.

Morphology and Pathway Connections

The avian hippocampal region, consisting of a medial hippocampus and dorsomedial parahippocampus (Karten and Hodos, 1967), shares with the mammalian hippocampus a similar topological relationship with respect to the lateral ventricle (Craigie, 1935), its three-layered organization, and a diversity of cell types (Mollá et al., 1986). Nonetheless, they are strikingly different in appearance, as the characteristic subdivisions of the mammalian hippocampus (the dentate gyrus, hilar region, Ammon's horn) are not discernible in birds (Fig. 1).

Pathway connections are another source of information to address the question of homology, as well as being central to any question of functional similarity, and, at this level, the hippocampal region of birds and mammals are strikingly similar (Benowitz and Karten, 1976; Krayniak and Siegel, 1978; for a comprehensive review, see Casini et al., 1986). The most important findings are that, as in mammals, the avian hippocampal region is in receipt of projections from monoaminergic brain stem nuclei (medial raphe, locus coeruleus), mammillary area of the hypothalamus, a region of the ventral medial telencephalon—the archistriatum (thought to be homologous with the mammalian amygdala [Zeier and Karten, 1971], and the diagonal band of the ventral septum. There is also a robust commissural system and efferent projections to the septum, mammillary region of the hypothalamus, and archistriatum.

One problem that has not been specifically addressed is the apparent absence of an entorhinal cortex in birds and thus the absence of a perforant pathway homolog. Beyond the question of homology, the absence of sensory input to the avian hippocampus would also raise serious doubts regarding functional similarity with the mammalian hippocampus. Casini et al. (1986), however, have demonstrated a reciprocal pathway connection between the avian hippocampal region and one layer of a multilaminated area of the anterior forebrain, the Wulst (Miceli et al., 1979). The Wulst is a recipient area of fibers originating from a number of distinct thalamic nuclei and is a telencephalic target of visual (Karten et al., 1973; Streit et al., 1980) and somatosensory (Delius and Bennetto, 1972) input. Indeed, the particular layer of the Wulst that connects with the hippocampal region, the hyperstriatum dorsale, has been reported to receive projections from both visual and nonvisual thalamic nuclei (Karten et al., 1973). The avian hyperstriatum dorsale, therefore, appears similar to the entorhinal cortex of mammals, receiving sensory input that may be further processed at the level of the hippocampus via a reciprocal pathway connection.

A B

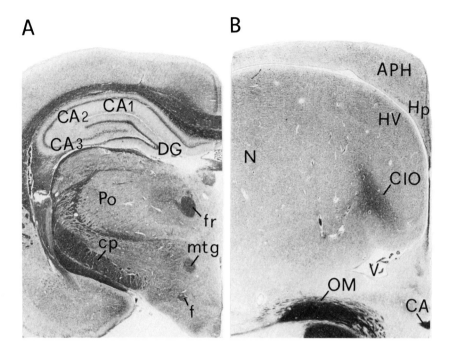

Fig. 1. **A:** Photomicrograph of a Kluver-Barrera–stained coronal section through rat brain showing the general morphology of the mammalian hippocampus and its major subdivisions (CA fields of Ammon's horn, dentate gyrus). CA1,2,3, fields of Ammon's horn; cp, posterior commissure; DG, dentate gyrus; f, fornix; fr, fasciculus retroflexus; mtg, mammillotegmental tract; Po, posterior thalamic nuclear group. (Abbreviations are derived from the atlas of Paxinos and Watson [1982].) **B:** Photomicrograph of a Kluver-Barrera–stained coronal section through pigeon brain. The avian dorsomedial forebrain, which includes hippocampus and area parahippocampalis, corresponds to the mammalian hippocampus. APH, area parahippocampalis; CA, commissura anterior; CIO, capsula interna occipitalis; Hp, hippocampus; HV, hyperstriatum ventrale; N, neostriatum; OM, tractus occipitomesencephalicus; V, ventriculus. (Abbreviations are derived from the atlas of Karten and Hodos [1967].)

Neurochemistry

Another source of information that can be brought to bear on the question of homology is an examination of the presence and distribution of neurotransmitter- and transmitter-related substances. Krebs et al. (1987) have employed immunohistochemical techniques in such an examination of the avian hippocampal region and have reported preliminary results. Similar to findings from mammalian studies (Davies and Köhler, 1985; Amaral and Campbell, 1986; Sloviter and Nilaver, 1987), the avian hippocampus was found to have somatostatin-, avian pancreatic polypeptide-, and vasoactive intestinal polypeptide-

like immunoreactivity in multipolar shaped cell bodies, as well as cholecys-
tokinin-, glutamic acid decarboxylase-, and substance P-like labeled terminals.
Combined with the pathway data, a robust serotoninergic projection from the
medial raphe nucleus and a smaller cholinergic projection from the diagonal
band of the ventral septum was also suggested. The immunohistochemical
results indicate the presence of transmitter and transmitter-related substances
similar to those found in mammals. Indeed, in some cases, transmitter immunoreactivity was found in similar cell types as in mammals, and, taken together, the results stand in further support of the hypothesis of homology.
Nonetheless, the immunohistochemical investigation also revealed some differences, most notable of which is the possible absence of a mossy fiber system
in birds, as suggested by the failure to identify any appropriate leu-enkephalin–
like immunoreactivity. Interestingly, the origin of mossy fibers (the dentate
gyrus) is among the last of the mammalian hippocampal subdivisions to differentiate during development (Bayer and Altman, 1974). Perhaps the mossy
fiber system is a uniquely mammalian variant of hippocampal structural organization, evolving subsequent to the separation of the reptilian ancestors
that led to birds and mammals, respectively.

The previous anatomical account emphasizes the similarity in the organization of the hippocampal region of birds and mammals. As such, the results
indicate these structures to be homologous. Although differences are apparent,
not at all surprising given the approximate 250 million years of independent
evolution, the striking anatomical similarity would suggest that the avian hippocampus also bears a similar functional relationship with the mammalian
hippocampus, perhaps differing only in the details and sophistication of its
operation (differences have also been suggested between humans and nonhuman mammals; Horel, 1978). As such, studies of the avian hippocampus
would seem to be of important relevance in the general discussion of hippocampal function in behavior and memory.

BEHAVIOR

In our discussion of the avian hippocampus and behavior, we will focus on
work that has taken place under natural or simulated natural conditions. We
are thus reglecting important recent operant studies, which are more concerned
with generating strict behavioral comparisons with similarly studied mammals
(Sahgal, 1984; Good, 1987; Reilly and Good, 1987). The work we will describe
almost exclusively involves investigations of behavioral performance following
hippocampal ablation in two diverse natural settings: the homing behavior of
pigeons and food-storing among the Paridae (tits and chickadees) and Corvidae
(crows, jays, and nutcrackers). We will emphasize what we perceive to be two
components of spatial performance: 1) spatial recognition or recall of places
previously visited and behavior associated with such recall (e.g. recovering a
stored seed) and 2) spatial navigation or locating a goal area relying on external
cues or landmarks (e.g. flying in the direction of the home loft in homing pigeons).

In the experiments performed with hippocampal ablated homing pigeons, controls were generally represented by Wulst-ablated birds, as Wulst removal was found not to affect generally homing behavior (Bingman et al., 1984).

Spatial Recognition: Retrograde Effects of Hippocampal Ablation

In their initial work on homing pigeons, Bingman et al. (1984, 1985) reported that following hippocampal ablation, experimental birds generally failed to return home whether they were released 50 km or just 500 m from and in full view of their loft. Several birds released from long distances were nevertheless observed to return to the vicinity of the loft. The pigeons did not appear to suffer any sensory or motor impairment, and the fact that they flew off in the direction of home when released from distant locations suggested that they were still motivated to return home. The most plausible explanation for the birds' behavior was that, as a result of hippocampal ablation, they were unable to recognize their loft. To test the extent of possible retrograde memory losses, an additional experiment was performed to examine the effect of hippocampal ablation on the ability of homing pigeons to use information gathered prior to surgery to recognize a location (a previous training site) and recall the appropriate direction home (Bingman et al., 1987a).

When one transports a homing pigeon to a location where it has never been before, say 50 km from home, and then releases it, the bird will generally fly in an approximate homeward direction. We are unable to give a detailed account of the mechanisms thought to be employed for homeward orientation (for a review of the various positions, see Papi and Wallraff, 1982). Briefly, however, a pigeon is thought first to rely on a navigational mapping system to determine its position relative to home and then to employ an independent compass mechanism to take up a homeward bearing. The best available evidence indicates that olfactory cues play an important (Papi, 1986), but perhaps not exclusive (Wiltschko et al., 1987), role for the navigational map. Pigeons from the loft used by Bingman et al. (1987a), however, were invariably impaired in their ability to orient homeward when rendered anosmic and released from locations never visited before (Papi, 1986). Importantly, when similarly treated anosmic pigeons from the same loft were released from a location where they had been on a number of previous occasions, they succeeded in orienting homeward (Benvenuti et al., 1973; Hartwick et al., 1977). With repeated exposure to the same release site, therefore, these homing pigeons acquire the ability to rely on cues around the release site to orient homeward even when their navigational map is rendered disfunctional (during the previous visits, the birds would not have been made anosmic).

In the experiment currently being described, Bingman et al. (1987a) exploited the fact that, from familiar locations, homing pigeons can rely on local cues to orient homeward. They first trained a group of pigeons with repeated releases from two locations to enable them to acquire the use of cues around those sites to orient homeward in the event their navigational map was rendered disfunctional. Subsequent to training, some of the birds were then subjected to hippocampal ablation. Postoperatively, the birds were again released from the training locations, but under anosmic conditions. For the experimental releases, therefore, the birds were limited to using familiar cues around the release site if they were to orient homeward successfully. In the experimental releases, control birds oriented homeward, indicating that they had acquired and retained the use of cues around the release sites. The hippocampal ablated birds, however, failed to orient homeward, behaving in a manner consistent with a retrograde memory loss. In contrast to controls, they apparently failed to recognize the release sites and/or recall the direction home.

The failure of hippocampal-ablated homing pigeons to recognize their loft or a previous training location following surgery suggests that retrograde memory losses are a regular feature of hippocampal ablation in birds. However, hippocampal ablation does not result in total amnesia. For example, as we previously mentioned, hippocampal-ablated homing pigeons were successful in orienting homeward from a distant, unknown release site immediately following surgery (Bingman et al., 1984), indicating that memories associated with their navigational map and compass mechanisms were unaffected by such treatment. Finally, similar retrograde losses have been reported in mammals (Walker and Olton, 1984; Salmon et al., 1987), suggesting similarities between birds and mammals at this functional level.

Spatial Recognition: Anterograde Effects of Hippocampal Ablation

It is important to emphasize that in the experiments that revealed retrograde memory losses, the hippocampal-ablated pigeons had no postoperative exposure to relevant stimuli, i.e. the home loft (the birds recovered from surgery at a different location and were then tested for loft recognition without first being returned home) and the preoperative training site (Bingman et al., 1984, 1985, 1987a). Interestingly, when hippocampal-ablated pigeons were allowed to recover at their own loft or given postoperative training releases from a distant location, the birds behaved as controls, returning to their loft without difficulty and orienting homeward from the training sites when rendered anosmic and thus unable to use their navigational map (Bingman et al., 1985, 1988). These results indicate that whatever recognition memory processes are involved in the control of these behaviors, hippocampal ablation leads to a robust retrograde loss, while postoperative acquisition is left unimpaired.

Although work on homing pigeons has yet to reveal a persistent anterograde spatial recognition deficit, such an impairment has been reported in food-storing birds such as nutcrackers (*Nucifraga caryoctatus;* Krushinskaya, 1966) and black-capped chickadees (*Parus atricapillus;* Sherry and Vaccarino, 1989) who have undergone hippocampal ablation. The essential finding that emerges from both of these studies is that birds that have undergone hippocampal ablation are strikingly impaired at recovering seeds that they themselves had cached in an experimental aviary only a few hours earlier. Hippocampal ablation seemingly disrupts the ability of food-storing birds to recognize the location of cache sites. The importance of the hippocampus in food-storing behavior is highlighted by the report that within families, food-storing species consistently have a larger hippocampus (Krebs et al., 1989).

An important question then is why does hippocampal ablation lead to anterograde deficits in cache site recognition but not in the recognition tasks described for homing pigeons, and what might this reveal about hippocampal memory function? The recognition tasks described for homing pigeons involve repeated exposure to the relevant stimuli (home loft or training site), and the appropriate behavior with respect to these stimuli is consistently associated with a reward (entering the loft or flying in the homeward direction is always coupled with access to food, water, mates, and so forth). Cache site recognition, in contrast, is based on one trial exposure to the relevant stimulus (the location of the cache site), and this exposure is not associated with any obvious reward (food reward occurs only after the cache site is relocated). Drawing from concepts developed from mammalian studies, the homing pigeon recognition tasks discussed would appear to involve mechanisms of reference memory (Olton et al., 1980; Olton, 1983) and/or associative memory (Gaffan, 1972, 1974). As described for homing pigeons, hippocampal-lesioned mammals are generally unimpaired in tasks that are thought to involve these memory processes. Recognizing the location of a cache site, however, would seem to involve mechanisms of recognition memory (Gaffan, 1972, 1974; Mishkin, 1978; Zola-Morgan and Squire, 1986), and, as described for food-storing birds, hippocampal-lesioned mammals are generally impaired in tasks that involve recognition memory as described by the investigators. Anterograde recognition deficits in birds and mammals appear similarly dependent on the conditions of the task under study.

Spatial Navigation

In contrast to spatial recognition, spatial navigation implies more than recall of locations previously visited when in sensory contact with them. Clearly, spatial recognition is a component of spatial navigation, but in navigation, spatial memories are further employed to permit the location of goal areas in the absence of sensory contact with them (the "cognitive mapping" model of O'-Keefe and Nadel [1978] would only be one possible mechanism underlying spatial navigation). In discussing spatial navigation, we will examine the performance of hippocampal-ablated homing pigeons with at least 6 months of postoperative experience. We wish to emphasize that such pigeons are able to recognize their loft or previous training sites in a manner that does not differ from controls. The behavior of such pigeons, therefore, offers an approximation of the chronic effects of hippocampal ablation on spatial performance.

The critical empirical result is that hippocampal-ablated homing pigeons consistently take more time to return home following release compared with control birds, regardless of whether they are released from a previous training site (Bingman et al., 1988a) or a site they have never been before (Bingman et al., 1988b). Sensory (Bingman and Hodos, manuscript in preparation) and motor or motivational (Bingman et al., 1987a,b) deficits have not been identified, and the impairment in homing performance on the part of hippocampal-ablated pigeons has been interpreted as reflecting a deficit in their ability to navigate a course homeward. Assuming a navigational impairment, it becomes important to specify the nature of the behavioral deficit, i.e. what it is that the hippo-campal-ablated birds are having difficulty doing, before beginning a discussion of spatial memory processes that may be disrupted as a result of hippocampal ablation. Unfortunately, a complete behavioral account is still lacking. None-theless, a number of lines of evidence suggest that hippocampal-ablated homing pigeons are impaired in their ability to utilize landmarks within a familiar en-vironment to direct goal-oriented responses efficiently.

Before examining this hypothesis, we wish to summarize for the reader the spatial tasks in which hippocampal-ablated homing pigeons are unimpaired. First, hippocampal-ablated homing pigeons are unimpaired in their ability to orient homeward from areas never before visited and thus from areas where they would need to rely on their navigational map and associated compass mechanisms (Bingman et al., 1984, 1988b). The hippocampus plays no necessary role in this type of navigation. Olfactory cues are a critical component of the navigational map used by the birds in these studies (Papi, 1986), and, given the anatomical connections between the hippocampus and recipient areas of olfactory bulb efferents (Reiner and Karten, 1985; Casini et al., 1986), this finding is somewhat surprising. Second, with limited postoperative training, hippo-campal-ablated homing pigeons rendered unable to use their navigational map behave as controls in being able to use local landmarks to orient homeward from a repeated release site (Bingman et al., 1988a). The complete mechanism through which homing pigeons use local landmarks to orient homeward from repeated release sites is unclear. However, use of landmarks not only for site recognition but also for guiding orientation has been suggested by Bingman and Ioalé (manuscript in preparation). Their results indicate that one component of a homeward orientation response based on landmark information may be something like "fly over the farm house," the farm house being one part of a proximate goal that directs a bird in an approximate homeward direction. The use of landmarks as orientation guides strikes us as being a task analogous to the guidance orientation of O'Keefe and Nadel (1978), empirically examined in rodents by the use of clustered cues to identify the location of a goal area (O'Keefe and Conway, 1980). Interestingly, the theoretical prediction of un-impaired performance in guidance orientation as a result of hippocampal lesion (O'Keefe and Nadel, 1978) is supported by both mammalian and avian exper-iments.

Whatever the navigational strategy employed at a release site, hippocampal-ablated birds fly off in an approximate homeward direction as controls, yet they take more time to return home. It appears that somewhere between the release site and the home loft the hippocampal-ablated pigeons begin to have difficulty finding their way home. It is generally believed that as a returning pigeon flies over increasingly familiar terrain, it begins to rely on familiar land-marks to navigate home (Michener and Walcott, 1967; Schmidt-Koenig and Walcott, 1978). Landmark use near the loft to navigate home, however, differs from landmark use to orient homeward from a repeated release site, and it is with landmark use near the loft that hippocampal-ablated pigeons have been hypothesized to have difficulty (Bingman et al., 1987b, 1988a,b).

One prediction of this hypothesis is that even when hippocampal-ablated homing pigeons are released near their loft, within 10 km or so, and thus within the area that would be familiar to them based on free flights from home, they should still take more time to return to their loft. Indeed, results from experiments performed with pigeons at the University of Maryland indicate that, even from short distances, hippocampal-ablated homing pigeons took more time to return home than did a group of Wulst-ablated control birds (Fig. 2) (Bingman and Mench, manuscript in preparation). In an additional study with the same pigeons, radio transmitters were attached to the backs of pigeons to record their movements to the loft (Bingman and Mench, manuscript in preparation). Difficulty on the part of hippocampal-ablated pigeons to navigate a course homeward would be expected to manifest itself in a less direct flight path home. Based on four radio-tracked hippocampal-ablated and four Wulst-ablated pigeons, hippocampal-ablated birds were generally found to take a considerably less direct path home, supporting the hypothesis that they are indeed impaired at navigating a course home when within the area of familiarity around their loft.

Behaviorally, hippocampal-ablated homing pigeons appear impaired in their ability to use landmarks in the vicinity of their loft to navigate home. At an empirical level, this result is similar to the impairment of hippocampal-lesioned rodents to locate a hidden escape platform in the aversive Morris waterbath (Morris et al., 1982). Again, birds and mammals were found to suffer similar behavioral impairments as a result of hippocampal ablation.

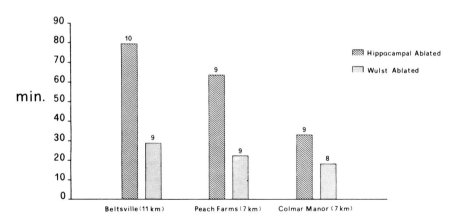

Fig. 2. Mean homing times of hippocampal-ablated (dashed columns) and Wulst-ablated (dotted columns) pigeons obtained in three short-distance releases. Numbers of birds released are indicated on the top of each column.

The previous behavioral account provides a reasonable estimation of what hippocampal-ablated homing pigeons do, but offers little unambiguous information regarding the spatial memory mechanisms involved in navigation that may be disrupted as a result of hippocampal ablation. At this juncture, therefore, any discussion of mechanism is necessarily speculative and certainly controversial. However, we think it revealing to consider the difference between the use of landmarks at a repeated release site, where hippocampal-ablated birds have no difficulty, and the use of landmarks in the familiar area that surrounds the loft, where hippocampal-ablated birds appear impaired. With respect to the landmark environment around a repeated release site, there is one, invariant homeward orientation response, as a bird is always released from the same point (Fig. 3A). In contrast, landmarks in the vicinity of the home loft can be perceived from effectively an infinite number of locations within the area of familiarity, depending on, among other things, the approach direction of the bird (Fig. 3B). That means that with respect to any one landmark or group of landmarks, there is an infinite number of position-specific orientation responses that would direct a bird to its loft. Based on these considerations, we would hypothesize further that the hippocampus plays a specific role in spatial navigation in which variable or flexible orientation responses based on landmarks are involved, but no necessary role in the case of invariant responses. Support

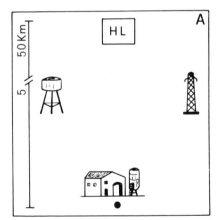 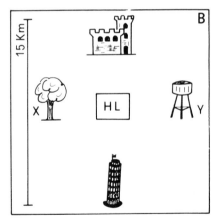

Fig. 3. From a repeated release site (in **A** the release site is identified by filled circle), invariant orientation response based on local landmarks is sufficient to direct a bird toward home. The position of the loft is identified by HL. The loft always lies beyond the farm house in a direction between the water tower and the electric tower. In contrast, within the familiar area around the home loft (in **B**), there is an infinite number of position-specific orientation responses based on local landmarks that would direct a bird home. For example, from position X, the loft lies beyond the tree, to the right of the castle, to the left of the leaning tower, and in front of the water tower. Approaching from point Y, however, the spatial relationship of bird and loft with respect to local landmarks would be exactly opposite.

for this hypothesis is also given by Sherry and Vaccarino (1989), who reported a deficit on the part of hippocampal-ablated chickadees in a task that may involve flexible use of landmarks, where no deficit was found in a task based on invariant responses.

This emphasis on flexible orientation responses with respect to landmarks is reminiscent of O'Keefe and Nadel's "cognitive mapping" model (1978), and indeed the long-term behavior, i.e. nonretrograde effects, of hippocampal-ablated birds is generally consistent with predictions from their model. In our opinion, however, the critical test of a functioning cognitive map is the ability of organisms to generate an appropriate orientation response with respect to goal areas from locations within a familiar environment. We would like to describe the results of one set of experimental releases that bear on the question of whether homing pigeons do indeed have a "cognitive map" and what effect hippocampal ablation may have on such a map. We need to emphasize that the results are from one set of releases and amount to little more than an anecdote. It is presented as a basis for discussion and a guide for future experiments.

The experiment involved two groups of pigeons, a hippocampal-ablated and a control, Wulst-ablated group. In the first phase of the experiment, the pigeons were transported and released from a location south and within sight of the city of Volterra in the mountains of Tuscany, 49 km from the loft. Birds were released singly, and the vanishing bearing and time taken to return home were recorded. No additional experimental manipulations were performed. As a result of this release, we assumed that the pigeons had gained some familiarity with the landmarks around Volterra. Ten days later, the birds were again released within sight of Volterra, but this time north of the city, about 10 km from the first release site and 45 km from home. The treatment of the birds was identical to that during the first release, except that they were now rendered anosmic by a combined procedure of being transported to and maintained at the release site with their nostrils plugged and, just prior to release, having their nostrils sprayed with the local anesthetic xylocaine. As a result of this treatment (Ioalé, 1983), they could not use their navigational map to orient homeward on the second release. If the pigeons were to orient homeward on the second release, therefore, they would have needed to rely on information gathered during the first release, perhaps using landmarks in the vicinity of Volterra that they were able to perceive from both release sites (we were able to see several of the same surrounding villages and geographical features from both sites). However, successful orientation based on landmarks would have required the birds to adjust their orientation for the second release (e.g. for the first release the city of Volterra was to their right when flying homeward, while for the second release it would have been to their left). An examination of the vanishing bearings of the control birds from the second release site (Fig. 4) reveals that they were successful in orienting homeward. This result suggests that these birds were able to generate a goal-directed orientation response from a novel location within a familiar environment. As such, their behavior is at least consistent with expectations based on the existence of a "cognitive map." In contrast,

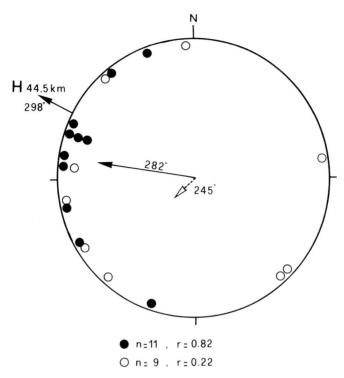

Fig. 4.   Initial orientation of hippocampal-ablated (○) and Wulst-ablated (●) pigeons from a location within a familiar environment. For this release the birds were rendered anosmic (see text). Each dot on the periphery of the circle indicates the vanishing bearing of one bird, and the home direction is indicated by H. The inner arrows represent the mean vectors for hippocampal (open arrow)- and Wulst (filled arrow)-ablated pigeons. n, number of vanishing bearings; r, length of the mean vector; N, north.

the hippocampal-ablated birds failed to give any indication that they were able to determine the home direction (Fig. 4). Assuming the existence of a "cognitive map" to explain the behavior of the controls, hippocampal ablation appears to disrupt the functioning of at least some of the neural processes that would be associated with it.

Before going too far, we wish to emphasize that this experiment does not prove the existence of a "cognitive map" or hippocampal involvement in it. Indeed, alternative explanations for the reported results are not difficult to imagine. For example, the angular difference in homeward direction between the two release sites is only about 10°. Thus the difference in behavior between the two groups could be explained by the ability of the control bird to recall the homeward direction from the first release, i.e. west northwest, then flying off more or less in that same direction for the second release relying solely on a compass mechanism without even considering local landmarks. Although such an interpretation would identify a memory function for the hippocampus, it would not indicate a working "cognitive map." This and other explanations notwithstanding, the different behavior of the groups is at least an indication supporting the possible existence of a cognitive map and hippocampal involvement in such a map, and replication and extension of this experiment to test alternative interpretations is needed.

SUMMARY AND PERSPECTIVES

In summarizing recent work on the avian hippocampus, we have intentionally attempted to draw comparisons with mammalian studies. The picture that emerges is that, with respect to both anatomy and role in memory processes as suggested by lesion studies, the avian and mammalian hippocampus appear to be quite similar. Given this similarity, the challenge now is to identify in what way birds may be uniquely suited to address unanswered questions regarding the role of the hippocampus in behavior.

Birds have traditionally been focal organisms for ethological studies, and there is a vast literature describing both their behavior and associated mechanisms under natural conditions (the homing behavior of pigeons has been studied for about 40 years). Birds are ideally suited, therefore, to examine behavioral changes following hippocampal manipulation (e.g. lesion, pharmacological) as they occur under free-living conditions. Relying on behavioral observations from field studies, avian researchers are in a particularly strong position to design relevant, controlled laboratory studies to test carefully alternative hypotheses regarding specific behavioral-memory processes involving the hippocampus (e.g. working memory, "cognitive mapping," and so forth). Indeed, given the inherent difficulty in defining all the relevant variables in a field study, companion laboratory experiments such as those of Sherry and Vaccarino (1989) are inevitable.

Nonetheless, field studies remain at the heart of investigations examining the role of the avian hippocampus in behavior. For example, we are currently involved in an ontogenetic study examining the spatial performance of homing pigeons that had undergone hippocampal ablation at 4 weeks of age, before they began to fly spontaneously from their loft. Preliminary results indicate a devasting effect of hippocampal ablation on their ability to return to their loft following free flights. This result suggests that spatial performance deficits following hippocampal ablation may be much more severe in young animals. Additionally, we will shortly begin an examination of homing pigeon spatial performance following disruption of cholinergic and serotoninergic inputs to the hippocampus. Again, our emphasis will be on behavioral changes under "real world" conditions in the hope of revealing the importance of these transmitter inputs for proper hippocampal function.

Finally, we appeal to researchers in neurophysiology to consider examining the avian hippocampus for the presence of such well-known mammalian electrophysiological characteristics as theta rhythm, long-term potentiation, and place cells. The existence of such phenomena in birds would add to our understanding from lesion studies, indicating functional similarity in birds and mammals at the finer level of cellular mechanisms.

ACKNOWLEDGMENTS

We are greatly indebted to Professor W. Hodos for comments on the manuscript. We thank Professor F. Papi for helpful suggestions in carrying out this study. The excellent technical assistance of A. Bertini, S. Carnasciali, B. Margheritti, and C. Pucci is gratefully acknowledged. This work was supported by Consiglio Nazionale delle Ricerche and Ministero della Pubblica Istruzione. Part of this work was also supported by a National Science Foundation grant to V.P.B.

REFERENCES

Amaral, D., and M. Campbell (1986) Transmitter systems in the primate dentate gyrus. Hum. Neurobiol. 5:169–180.

Bayer, S., and J. Altman (1974) Hippocampal development in the rat cytogenesis and morphogenesis examined with autoradiography and low-level X-irradiation. J. Comp. Neurol. 158:55–80.

Benowitz, L., and H. Karten (1976) The tractus infundiboli and other afferents to the parahippocampal region of the pigeon. Brain Res. 102:174–180.

Benvenuti, S., V. Fiaschi, L. Fiore, and F. Papi (1973) Homing performance of inexperienced and directionally trained pigeons subjected to olfactory nerve section. J. Comp. Physiol. 83:81–92.

Bingman, V., P. Bagnoli, P. Ioalè, and G. Casini (1984) Homing behavior of pigeons after telencephalic ablations. Brain Behav. Evol. 24:94–108.

Bingman, V., P. Ioalè, G. Casini, and P. Bagnoli (1985) Dorsomedial forebrain ablations and home loft association behavior in homing pigeons. Brain Behav. Evol. 26:1–9.

Bingman, V., P. Ioalè, G. Casini, and P. Bagnoli (1987a) Impaired retention of preoperatively acquired spatial reference memory in homing pigeons following hippocampal ablation. Behav. Brain Res. 24:147–115.

Bingman, V., P. Ioalè, G. Casini, and P. Bagnoli (1987b) Pigeon homing and the avian hippocampal complex: A complementary experimental paradigm. In P. Ellen and C. Thinus-Blanc (eds): Cognitive Processes and Spatial Orientation in Animal and Man. Dordrecht, The Netherlands: Nijhof, pp. 273–283.

Bingman, V., P. Ioalè, G. Casini, and P. Bagnoli (1988a) Unimpaired acquisition of spatial reference memory, but impaired homing performance in hippocampal ablated pigeons. Behav. Brain Res. 27:179–187.

Bingman, V., P. Ioalè, G. Casini, and P. Bagnoli (1988b) Hippocampal ablated homing pigeons show a persistant impairment in the time required to return home. J. Comp. Physiol. A 163:559–563.

Casini, G., V. Bingman, and P. Bagnoli (1986) Connections of the pigeon dorsomedial forebrain studied with WGA-HRP and ^{3}H proline. J. Comp. Neurol. 245:454–470.

Craigie, E. (1935) The hippocampal and parahippocampal cortex of the emu (Dromiceius). J. Comp. Neurol. 61:563–591.

Davies, S., and C. Köhler (1985) The substance P innervation of the rat hippocampal region. Anat. Embryol. 173:45–57.

Delius, J., and K. Bennetto (1972) Cutaneous sensory projections to the avian forebrain. Brain Res. 37:205–221.

Gaffan, D. (1972) Loss of recognition memory in rats with lesions of the fornix. Neuropsychologia 10:327–341.

Gaffan, D. (1974) Recognition impaired and association intact in the memory of monkeys after transection of the fornix. J. Comp. Physiol. Psychol. 86:1100–1109.

Good, M. (1987) The effects of hippocampal–area parahippocampalis lesions on discrimination learning in the pigeon. Behav. Brain Res. *26*:171–184.

Hartwick, R., A. Foá, and F. Papi (1977) The effect of olfactory deprivation by nasal tubes upon homing behavior in pigeons. Behav. Ecol. Sociobiol. *2*:81–89.

Horel, J. (1978) The neuroanatomy of amnesia. A critique of the hippocampal memory hypothesis. Brain *101*:403–445.

Ioalè, P. (1983) Effects of anaesthesia of the nasal mucosae on the homing behaviour of pigeons. Z. Tierpsychol. *61*:102–110.

Isaacson, R. (1982) The Limbic System. New York: Plenum.

Karten, H., and W. Hodos (1967) A Stereotaxic Atlas of the Brain of the Pigeon *(Columba livia)*. Baltimore: Johns Hopkins University Press.

Karten, H., W. Hodos, W. Nauta, and A. Revzin (1973) Neural connections of the visual Wulst of the avian telencephalon: Experimental studies in the pigeon *(Columba livia)* and owl *(Speotito cunicularia)*. J. Comp. Neurol. *150*:253–276.

Krayniak, P., and A. Siegel (1978) Efferent connections of the hippocampus and adjacent regions in the pigeon. Brain Behav. Evol. *15*:372–338.

Krebs, J., J. Erichsen, and V. Bingman (1987) The immunohistochemistry and cytoarchitecture of the avian hippocampus. Soc. Neurosci. Abstr. *13*:1125.

Krebs, J., D. Sherry, S. Healy, V.H. Perry, and A. Vaccarino (1989) Hippocampal specialization of food-storing birds. Proc. Natl. Acad. Sci. (in press).

Krushinskaya, N. (1966) Some complex forms of feeding behavior of nutcracker *Nucifraga caryocatactes*, after removal of old cortex. Zh. Evol. Biokim. Fisiol. *11*:563–568.

Miceli, D., H. Gioanni, J. Reperant, and J. Peyrichoux (1979) The avian visual Wulst: I. An anatomical study of afferent and efferent pathways. II. An electrophysiological study of the functional properties of single neurons. In A. Granda and J. Maxwell (eds): Neural Mechanisms of Behaviour in the Pigeon. New York: Plenum, pp. 223–254.

Michener, M., and C. Walcott (1967) Homing of single pigeons—An analysis of tracks. J. Exp. Biol. *47*:99–131.

Mishkin, M. (1978) Memory in monkeys severely impaired by combined but not separate removal of amygdala and hippocampus. Nature *273*:297–298.

Mollá, R., J. Rodriguez, S. Calvet, and J.M. Garcia-Verdugo (1986) Neuronal types of the cerebral cortex of the adult chicken *(Gallus gallus)*. A Golgi study. J. Hirnforsch. *27*:381–390.

Morris, M., R. Garrud, P. Rawlins, and J. O'Keefe (1982) Place navigation impaired in rats with hippocampal lesions. Nature *297*:681–683.

O'Keefe, J., and D. Conway (1980) On the trail of the hippocampal engram. Physiol. Psychol. *8*:229–238.

O'Keefe, J., and L. Nadel (1978) The Hippocampus as a Cognitive Map. Oxford: Clarendon Press.

Olton, D. (1983) Memory functions and the hippocampus. In W. Seifert (ed) Neurobiology of the Hippocampus. New York: Academic Press, pp. 335–373.

Olton, D., J. Becker, and G. Handelmann (1980) Hippocampal function: Working memory or cognitive mapping? Physiol. Psychol. *8*:239–246.

Papi, F. (1986) Pigeon navigation: Solved problems and open questions. Monitore Zool. Ital. *20*:471–517.

Papi, F., and H. Wallraff (1982) Avian Navigation. Berlin: Springer.

Paxinos, G., and C. Watson (1982) The Rat Brain in Stereotaxic Coordinates. New York: Academic Press.

Reilly, S., and M. Good (1987) Enhanced DRL and impaired force-choice alternation performance following hippocampal lesions in the pigeon. Behav. Brain Res. *26*:185–197.

Reiner, A., and H. Karten (1985) Comparisons of olfactory bulb projections in pigeons and turtles. Brain Behav. Evol. *27*:11–27.

Sahgal, A. (1984) Hippocampal lesions disrupt recognition memory in pigeons. Behav. Brain Res. *11*:47–58.

Salmon, D., S. Zola-Morgan, and L. Squire (1987) Retrograde amnesia following combined hippocampus–amygdala lesions in monkeys. Psychobiology *15*:37–47.

Schmidt-Koenig, K., and C. Walcott (1978) Tracks of pigeons homing with frosted lenses. Anim. Behav. *26*:480–486.

Scoville, W., and B. Milner (1957) Loss of recent memory after bilateral hippocampal lesions. J. Neurol. Neurosurg. Psychiatry *20*:11–21.

Sherry, D., and A. Vaccarino (1989) The hippocampus and memory for food caches in Black-capped chickadees. Behav. Neurosci. (in press).

Sloviter, R., and G. Nilaver (1987) Immunocytochemical localization of GABA-, cholecystokinin-, vasoactive intestinal polipeptide- and somatostatin-like immunoreactivity in the area dentata and hippocampus of the rat. J. Comp. Neurol. *256*:42–60.

Streit, P., M. Stella, and M. Cuénod (1980) Transneuronal labelling in the pigeon visual system. Neuroscience *5*:763–775.

Walker, J., and D. Olton (1984) Fimbria-fornix lesions impair spatial working memory but not cognitive mapping. Behav. Neurosci. *2*:226–242.

Wiltschko, W., R. Wiltschko, and M. Jahnel (1987) The orientation behavior of anosmic pigeons in Frankfurt a.M., Germany. Anim. Behav. *35*:1324–1333.

Zeier, H., and H. Karten (1971) The archistriatum of the pigeon. Organization of afferent and efferent connections. Brain Res., *31*:313–326.

Zola-Morgan, S., and L. Squire (1986) Memory impairment in monkeys following lesions limited to the hippocampus. Behav. Neurosci. *4*:155–160.

The Hippocampus—New Vistas, pages 395–410

25
Structural Variations of the Hippocampal Mossy Fiber System and Avoidance Learning

H.-P. LIPP AND H. SCHWEGLER

Institute of Anatomy, University of Zürich, Zürich, Switzerland (H.-P.L.); Zentrum für Morphologie, J.-W.-Goethe-Universität, Frankfurt, Federal Republic of Germany (H. S.)

INTRODUCTION

This chapter will review our studies on variations of the mossy fiber projection and their relations to two-way avoidance learning. Methodologically, it will give an example of how brain–behavior relationships can be analyzed without or with little intervention in the brain. The approach is conceptually related to neurophysiological recording, or studies using deoxyglucose, but differs from techniques based on brain lesions, which assess the capacities and interactions of the residual brain structures.

The first step is the *identification* of potential structural correlates of behavior by investigating the brains of strains selectively bred for extremes in a given behavior. This is followed by a *verification* using samples of animal strains known to differ in one or more of the variables suspected to be linked to behavioral variation. If correlations can be verified, they are tested for *robustness*. The final step involves *testing for causality* by manipulating the structural variables pre- or postnatally. Most of this can be achieved simply by investigating genetically defined rodent strains.

GENERAL METHODS

The studies reported here are based on the morphometric analysis of 840 mouse and rat brains from genetically defined strains. All morphometry was performed on frozen and Timm-stained sections. This now widely used stain visualizes the terminal fields of hippocampal projections in the form of colored bands or patches. Because of its content of zinc, the hippocampal mossy fiber projection is stained with particular clarity (Fig. 1) and is measured easily and reliably. In most cases we measured all of the hippocampal subfields of CA3 and CA4, but we shall concentrate here only on the mossy fiber projections that showed the majority of correlations. The laminated subfields of CA3/CA4

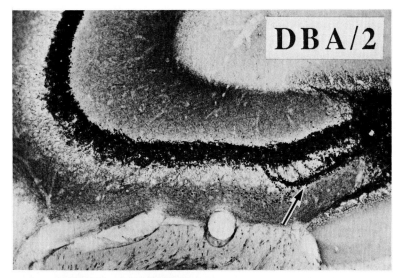

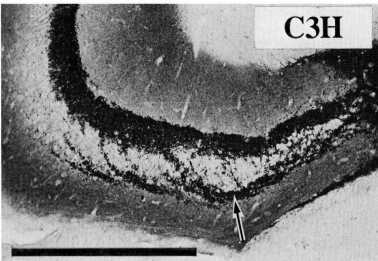

Fig. 1. Genetically determined extremes of the infrapyramidal mossy fiber projection (arrows) as seen in strains DBA/2 and C3H. For details of structures, see Figure 2. Timm's stain, horizontal sections from the midseptotemporal level. Bar = 0.5 mm.

and the partitioning of the mossy fiber projections are shown in Figure 2. The intra/infrapyramidal mossy fiber projection (IIP-MF) includes, in our definition, all darkly Timm-stainable patches that appear clearly separated from the suprapyramidal mossy fiber layer (the stratum lucidum). Morphometric analysis was done either manually on a graphic tablet (by means of measuring outlines

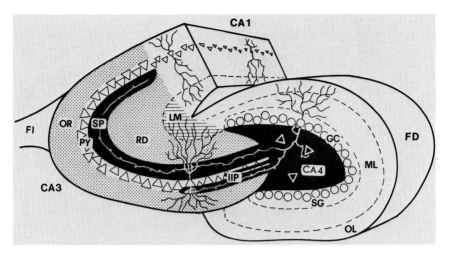

Fig. 2. Diagram of the Timm-stainable hippocampal fields in CA3/CA4 as revealed on hippocampal cross sections. Black areas, terminal fields of the mossy fiber projections; stippled areas, terminal fields of the intrinsic associational projections (Schaffer collaterals and commissural projections); hatched area, terminal field of entorhinal projection to CA3. CA1, regio superior; CA3, regio inferior; CA4, hilus of the fascia dentata; FD, fascia dentata (dentate gyrus); FI, fimbria hippocampi; GC, granule cell layer; IIP, intra- and infrapyramidal mossy fiber projection; LM, stratum lacunosum-moleculare; ML, medial molecular layers in fascia dentata; OL, outer molecular layer; OR, stratum oriens; RD, stratum pyramidale; RD, stratum radiatum; SG, supragranular dentate layer; SP, suprapyramidal mossy fiber projection.

and distribution of patches on drawings made with the aid of a microprojector) or else by means of a video image analyzer. The common measure is the mean area of mossy fibers from five horizontal sections from the midseptotemporal level of the hippocampus (or a corresponding volume). Data from the left and right hippocampi were pooled (although they were analyzed separately).

Because of some difficulties in comparing absolute values obtained by differential techniques (a given technique is highly reliable but has in most cases a systematic bias), the data points of the scatterplots are standardized, i.e. they are expressed in units of standard deviations from the mean of the sample (Edwards, 1979). Further details of histology, morphometry, and statistics can be found in two major papers (Schwegler and Lipp, 1983; Lipp et al., 1988b).

REVIEW OF PUBLISHED AND UNPUBLISHED STUDIES
Identification of Relevant Structural Traits

The key to our studies was a report by Barber et al. (1974), who described extensive genetic variability of the intra- and infrapyramidal mossy fiber projection (IIP-MF) in the mouse. To test whether the reported variability of the IIP-MF might be related to two-way avoidance, small samples of rats selectively bred for extremes in two-way avoidance were studied first in both the Roman high-avoidance (RHA) and Roman low-avoidance (RLA) rats (Bignami and

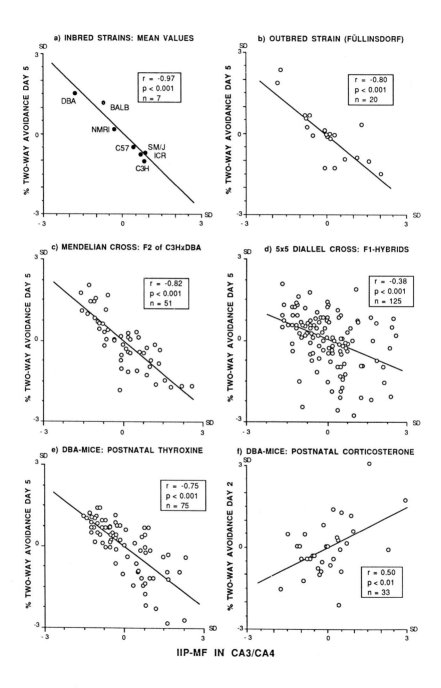

a) INBRED STRAINS: MEAN VALUES

r = -0.97
p < 0.001
n = 7

DBA
BALB
NMRI
C57
SM/J
ICR
C3H

b) OUTBRED STRAIN (FÜLLINSDORF)

r = -0.80
p < 0.001
n = 20

c) MENDELIAN CROSS: F2 of C3HxDBA

r = -0.82
p < 0.001
n = 51

d) 5x5 DIALLEL CROSS: F1-HYBRIDS

r = -0.38
p < 0.001
n = 125

e) DBA-MICE: POSTNATAL THYROXINE

r = -0.75
p < 0.001
n = 75

f) DBA-MICE: POSTNATAL CORTICOSTERONE

r = 0.50
p < 0.01
n = 33

% TWO-WAY AVOIDANCE DAY 5

% TWO-WAY AVOIDANCE DAY 2

IIP-MF IN CA3/CA4

Bovet, 1965). If the IIP-MF projection were involved in the mediation of two-way avoidance, then genetic selection must lead to a differentiation of that structural trait (together with a differentiation of all other genetically based variables influencing two-way avoidance). Indeed, the poorly avoiding RLA rats had an IIP-MF projection almost twice as large as the RHA rats. However, several other subfields in CA3/CA4 were significantly different in the two strains as well (Schwegler and Lipp, 1981, 1983). Thus, the data clearly indicated a *potential* involvement of the mossy fibers and other hippocampal subfields. However, it was not clear whether these multiple structural differences were behaviorally relevant, for they may have been caused also by genetic drift (Smith, 1985) or by corollary genetic selection of variables of little importance for the task.

The association between hippocampal traits and avoidance learning was then tested using a small sample of seven inbred mouse strains known to differ in their inborn ability for two-way avoidance (Buselmaier et al., 1981). The mossy fiber projections of these strains were measured in four animals per strain. A strong correlation ($r = -0.97$; Fig. 3a) between the strain means for two-way avoidance and the IIP-MF projections was observed (Schwegler and Lipp, 1981, 1983). *No* significant correlations were found with the other hippocampal subfields. In contrast to the Roman strains that were selected for acquisition (performance in the first 35 trials of training), the correlation in mice was with performance at day 5 of training (after about 350 trials). This score was chosen because of previous behavior genetic studies on two-way avoidance learning in mice (Buselmaier et al., 1978, 1981). This experiment was repeated in another shuttle-box using 23 mice from six strains only (Flühmann, 1980). Individual learning scores were obtained for each mouse. The correlation coefficient was again -0.81 ($P < 0.01$) and the direction of the regression largely determined by the anatomical and behavioral mean values of the strains (Fig. 4a).

Using the same experimental set-up, 20 male random-bred mice (outbred Füllinsdorf albino) were tested individually for their performance of two-way avoidance at day 5 of training, and their IIP-MF projections were measured afterwards (Schwegler et al., 1981). Such animals are characterized by a more or less random distribution of many genetic factors influencing morphology

---

Fig. 3. Standardized regression plots of the extent of the IIP-MF and performance of avoidance learning in several samples of mice. **a:** Negative correlation shown by the mean values of several inbred mouse strains. **b:** Negative correlation between the individual values of IIP-MF and avoidance learning in outbred mice. **c:** Genetic randomized IIP-MF projection (by means of an F_2 cross) and negative correlation with adult avoidance learning. **d:** Genetically varied IIP-MF projection (by means of a 5×5 diallel cross) and adult avoidance learning. **e:** Developmentally induced variation of the IIP-MF in isogenic animals (DBA/2 mice) and adult avoidance learning (after postnatal injections of saline and thyroxine; plot shows all animals). **f:** Same strain as in e, but postnatally treated with corticosterone. The resulting variability of the IIP-MF appears now positively correlated with two-way avoidance (for explanation, see text).

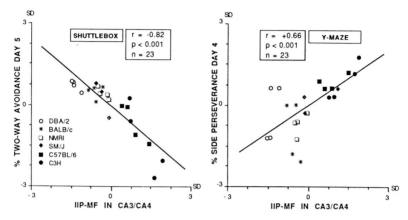

Fig. 4. Correlations between the extent of the IIP-MF projection (as measured in animals from six different mouse strains) and performance in two-way avoidance at day 5, the last day of training (left). The right plot shows the correlation of the IIP-MF of the same animals with the percentage of side perseverance during the last day of training. The worst mice in the shuttle-box were the most obstinate perseverants in the Y maze. Note the possibility of *within-strain* correlations, for example in the strains C57BL/6 and C3H.

and behavior, the randomness being maintained by systematic outbreeding within a large animal stock. Again, a strong negative correlation was observed (r = −0.80, P < 0.01; Fig. 3b). The variability of the other subfields of CA3/CA4 was not related to two-way avoidance, a finding similar to the results of the inbred strain study. Thus, the association of two-way avoidance as identified in the rat strains could be confirmed in mouse strains and appeared to be *robust*, since it persisted despite the potentially confounding influence of behaviorally relevant genetic factors randomly distributed across the mice.

Genetic and Developmental Manipulations

Subsequently, attempts were made to manipulate the IIP-MF projection during development and to observe whether the behavior of the adult animals (approximately 90 days later) might covary with the developmentally varied mossy fiber distribution. Because it seemed unrealistic to attempt a precise developmental control of the IIP-MF projection, we tried to randomize the size of the IIP-MF projection and to study whether behavior would follow the individual differences found in the brains of the animals. The reader may note that this is no longer a purely correlational study in which it is not possible to distinguish between causative and dependent variables, but a test for (statistical) causality. The structural traits were manipulated long before testing, without behavioral feedback, and the IIP-MF remained fairly stable over time (yet not the recurrent mossy fiber collaterals in the hilus of the fascia dentata) (Amaral, 1979; Claiborne et al., 1986; Laurberg and Zimmer, 1981; Wolfer et al., 1987b).

Postnatal Thyroxine Injections

In a series of experiments (Lipp et al., 1981, 1984, 1988b), the growth of the IIP-MF projection was disturbed by postnatal injections of thyroxine. It had been shown that such postnatal injections applied to rats produced a distinct yet rather variable hyperplasia of the IIP-MF projection (Lauder and Mugnaini, 1977, 1980), but only during the first 4 weeks after birth. Fifty-one RHA rat pups were injected with varying doses of thyroxine and 18 with saline during 18 days after birth—the period in which the mossy fibers develop. The Roman high-avoidance strain has a genetically minor IIP-MF projection and an excellent capacity for two-way avoidance learning. The thyroxine treatment enlarged the IIP-MF projection remarkably, but a considerable individual variability of the treatment effects was evident also. Saline did not induce a significant hyperplasia of the IIP-MF, but the treated control rats showed a much larger variability of the IIP-MF as compared with nontreated rats. Regardless of whether the animals had obtained thyroxine or saline, the individually varying IIP-MF projections were strongly correlated with the capacity of avoidance learning of the adult animals: The larger the IIP-MF projection was, the more trials were needed to reach a criterion of five consecutive correct avoidance responses ($r = 0.74$ for thyroxine, $P < 0.0001$; $r = 0.77$ for saline, $P < 0.01$).

To verify this result, the experiment was repeated in mice (Lipp et al., 1988b). Two inbred strains with small IIP-MF projections and good avoidance abilities were treated for 12 days postnatally with varying dosages of saline. One sample was small, 18 BALB/c mice; the other consisted of 75 DBA/2 mice, divided into five groups of 15 mice. Three of these groups received different doses of thyroxine, one saline, and one was left untreated. While the postnatal thyroxine injections had produced rather exuberant IIP-MF projections in the rats, it led to a more subtle yet still distinct hyperplasia of the IIP-MF in the mice.

In both strains, a strong correlation between the experimentally varied IIP-MF projection and two-way avoidance was found again: the larger the IIP-MF projection, the poorer the avoidance performance at day 5. In the BALB/c mice, the correlation coefficients were $r = -0.79$ ($P < 0.01$) and -0.75 ($P < 0.0001$) in the entire sample of the DBA/2 mice (Fig. 3e). All five subgroups of the DBA/2 mice showed negative correlations, not significant in the untreated mice, but highly significant in the saline-treated animals ($r = -0.95, P < 0.01$) and in animals having received the smallest doses of thyroxine ($r = -0.90, P < 0.01$). With higher dosages of thyroxine, the correlations were weaker but still significant. A multivariate analysis of dosage effects showed that the treatment had induced morphological changes with opposite effects on behavior: a reduction of brain weight that was associated with an improved performance of two-way avoidance and, concomitantly, variation of the IIP-MF that correlated negatively with the behavioral scores.

The analysis of the learning curves showed that the initial learning capacity of the animals was *not* affected: All groups acquired the task about equally fast (and correlations with the IIP-MF were barely apparent at these stages). Ongoing training, however, led to a behavioral differentiation among the animals that turned out to be strongly correlated with the IIP-MF. Other hippocampal subfields had a statistically negligible relation with the behavior scores. However, the average performance of the treated mice was still better as compared with most other mouse strains.

Genetically Induced Variations of the IIP-MF Projection

In parallel studies, the extent of the IIP-MF projection was randomized genetically (Heimrich, 1985; Heimrich et al., 1985; Schwegler et al., 1985). This was done by producing a mendelian F_2 generation from two progenitor strains, DBA/2 and C3H. DBA/2 mice have scanty IIP-MF projections (Fig. 1) and generally perform well in two-way avoidance. C3H mice are characterized by extensive IIP-MF projections (Fig. 1) and poor two-way avoidance learning, at least in our set-up. The F_2 generation (N = 51) had a large variability in the IIP-MF projection, which showed an approximately normal distribution (indicating a polygenic mode of inheritance), while the two-way avoidance performance at day 5 again was strongly and negatively correlated with the IIP-MF ($r = -0.82, P < 0.00001$), (Fig. 3c). In this case, the range of the avoidance scores was much larger than in the throxine-treated DBA/2 mice.

In another cross-breeding study, the IIP-MF distribution was varied by means of 5×5 diallel cross in which five mouse strains with differential IIP-MF projections were mated according to a scheme that resulted in 25 F_1 groups representing all possible combinations of the parental genotypes (Crusio and Schwegler, 1987). In the 125 mice investigated, the variability of the IIP-MF projection was again negatively correlated with the avoidance scores, albeit much weaker. Here, negative correlations were observed for days 2–5 of conditioning, the coefficients ranging from -0.25 to -0.38 (Fig. 3d). However, the correlation coefficients from day 2 and day 5 had a different data structure. In the early phases of training, the correlation was largely based on the means of the 25 groups (which probably reflects a correlation of the IIP-MF with the persistence of inborn [and thus mostly inappropriate] coping responses when faced with a shuttle-box). On the last day, however, mice from a given (isogenic) hybrid group had often developed diverging behavioral scores: The (unchanged) extent of the IIP-MF was apparently related to the degree of behavioral change induced by the training procedure itself. More IIP-MF appeared to be associated with an increased persistence of acquired but inappropriate responses.

Somatic Variations of the IIP-MF as a Result of Chimerism

The last example for randomization of the IIP-MF is a study on mouse chimeras representing a mosaic of cells from BALB/c and C57BL/6 (Bär, 1987). In 35 chimeras, this (somatic) variation of the IIP-MF was significantly but moderately correlated with two-way avoidance ($r = -0.36$), yet only with the score from day 2 of training.

Other Strain Comparisons

Further studies confirming a negative relationship between the extent of the IIP-MF and avoidance were based on a comparison of rat strains. Two strains selectively bred for differential exploratory activity in a square alley, the Naples high (NHE) and Naples Low Excitable (NLE) rats (Lipp et al., 1987), were found to have both comparatively minor IIP-MF projections and did not show differential two-way avoidance performance. However, the control strain, the Naples random-bred (NRB), showed an IIP-MF projection twice as large as NHE or NLE rats and a correspondingly poor avoidance performance (Schwegler, Lipp, and Sadile, unpublished data).

A similar observation was made in rats selected for differential hypothalamic self-stimulation (Lieblich et al., 1978). The progenitor stocks of the two HI and LO lines showed a strong difference of the IIP-MF, the strain with the larger IIP-MF projection again showing much poorer acquisition of two-way avoidance (Lieblich et al., 1987).

Lacking or Positive Correlations

Recent data, however, indicate that the correlation between IIP-MF and avoidance might also depend on some unknown technical parameter of shuttle-box conditioning. After establishing a new and computer-operated set of shuttle-boxes in the Zürich laboratory, we initially could not replicate the strain order found for mice we had found in Heidelberg (Schwegler and Lipp, 1983) and in Lausanne (Flühmann, 1980). Nor did we observe (Lipp, unpublished data) a correlation with the IIP-MF in a sample of random-bred mice, although these animals showed strong correlations with swimming navigation (see Discussion). On the other hand, the new set-up revealed *positive correlations* between two-way avoidance and magnitude of the IIP-MF after postnatal injections of corticosterone or oil as vehicle solution in 33 DBA/2 mice (Wolfer et al., 1987b). This treatment is known to impair avoidance learning of adult rats (Olton et al., 1975). The IIP-MF projections were not enlarged, but the treatment induced considerable variability of the IIP-MF and morphological asymmetries in both corticosterone- and oil-treated mice. Thus these morphological effects might reflect developmental instability rather than an effect of specific biochemical processes. The chief finding was that the variation of the IIP-MF was *positively* correlated with avoidance performance at day 2 ($r = 0.50$; Fig. 3f), while the size of the suprapyramidal mossy fiber projection was equally positively correlated with the avoidance scores of day 5. It must be noted that the average performance of all these mice was atypically poor for DBA/2 mice. Whether this was related to the new shuttle-box set-up or to a global effect of the treatment cannot be determined yet. Presently we are testing the strains DBA/2, BALB/c, and C57BL/6 under a variety of conditions in the shuttle-box. Preliminary data indicate that a strain rank order reflecting the strain-typical mossy fiber distribution can be established by using relatively low intensities of punishment.

DISCUSSION
1. Are Hippocampal Circuitry Variations Causative for Individual Behavioral Differences?

Taken together, the data show that mossy fiber variations appear to influence processes important for two-way avoidance learning. Moreover, the structural differences, or a closely related intrahippocampal factor, appear to be causative for the behavioral changes. Causation is defined here as the regression of a dependent variable on an independent one—there is no other way to define causality when using statistical methods. The alternative hypothesis would postulate a hidden extrahippocampal variable that covaries extremely well with the mossy fibers but is ultimately responsible for the behavioral changes, for example dopamine levels in the substantia nigra. We do not exclude that an *intrahippocampal* variable other than infrapyramidal mossy fibers might be responsible for the behavioral change; in fact, we believe that this is quite likely. However, the problem here is to demonstrate that structural (or associated) biochemical variability in a circumscribed brain region such as the hippocampus is causative for differential talents in given tasks; to our knowledge, this has not been demonstrated yet. The following argumentation will show that the alternative hypothesis of infrapyramidal mossy fibers as a marker for extrahippocampal variation in the brain is highly unlikely.

First, the likelihood of a nonfunctional correlation caused by genetic association is low. Such a correlation may be caused by linkage disequilibrium ("chromosomal linkage") or by genetic factors being tied in in other ways. Yet many of the correlations were seen after genetic randomization through meiotic crossing-over. The other evidence against any form of nonfunctional linkage comes from the thyroxine studies. There, the variation of the mossy fibers was produced in inbred (hence isogenic) animals. The thyroxine treatment would have to activate a tied genetic factor at the same time, and tó the same extent, as it did for the mossy fibers. Otherwise, it is impossible to explain correlation coefficients as strong as -0.95.

The second argument against a causative role of the mossy fibers is that the correlation may be based on unconditionally balanced brain systems. For instance, mossy fibers and nigral dopamine levels might share a common step in the synthesis of an enzyme, and developmental fluctuation of one system is thus inevitably reflected by the other system. This argument appears difficult to disprove. Fortunately, we were able to observe the odd findings of correlations with reversed sign, after postnatal disturbance of hippocampal maturation, by means of corticosterone and oil (or, more likely, by the associated handling stress). As shown below, it is possible to offer an explanation of how mossy fiber variations might also result in reverse correlations. However, the postulated extrahippocampal system ought then to share such and other functional peculiarities with hippocampal traits, and it must show also the same developmental properties (critical periods, lack of adult plasticity) as mossy fibers do. It would seem unlikely that remote brain systems are balanced even in capriciousness. Finally, the sometimes extremely high correlation coefficients make it difficult to invoke an additional intervening variable: Such strong correlations are indicative for a site of direct action.

Third, a series of studies (not discussed here for reasons of space) has shown correlations between mossy fibers and behavioral tasks known to be influenced by hippocampal lesions such as habituation (Crusio and Schwegler, 1987; Lipp et al., 1987), radial maze learning (Crusio et al., 1987), water maze learning (Schwegler et al., 1988), and swimming navigation (Lipp et al., 1988a;

Wolfer et al., 1987a). For swimming navigation and radial maze learning, the sign of the correlation is as one would expect from hippocampal lesion studies. These (generally) show that lesions *improve* two-way avoidance but impair performance in the two other tasks. Yet the extent of the IIP-MF projection covaries *positively* with performance in the radial maze and swimming navigation, at least in mice. It must be added, however, that habituation shows correlations that are strain-dependent in rats, positive in one strain and negative in another (Lipp et al., 1987), and that are rather weak in mice (Crusio and Schwegler, 1987; Schwegler, 1986). In addition, mice with randomized genotype showed a strong positive correlation between the extent of the IIP-MF projection and the ability of discrimination learning in an automatized Y maze (Lipp et al., 1985, 1986), large IIP-MF projections being associated with a superior capacity of choice optimization.

Based on this battery of arguments, we shall accept—in a probabilistic sense—that hippocampal circuitry variations, either of mossy fibers or of something else, are partially responsible for differential abilities of two-way avoidance learning.

2. Is There a Specific Behavioral Mechanism Associated With Variations of the Mossy Fibers?

The observation that the correlation coefficients ranged from 0.35 to 0.95 clearly indicates, not surprisingly, the presence of other factors influencing two-way avoidance learning. Note that the best correlations were observed after subtle interventions (postnatal injections of weak concentrations of thyroxine or saline) in isogenic mice. Here, the influence of other genetic factors weakening the correlation IIP-MF/avoidance is zero; they were all "held constant." Conversely, the low correlations in the hybrid mice from the diallel cross suggest a strong interference, perhaps from the high motor activity arising from hybridization (the heterosis effect). Hence, the mossy fiber factor represents certainly one of several processes influencing two-way avoidance. But which one?

This question can only be answered tentatively from the observations with the shuttle-box. In this apparatus, the animal has only one solution to solve the task: a fast move out of the compartment with the conditioning stimulus. Yet this response is in conflict with the majority of species-specific coping responses (Blanchard and Blanchard, 1969; Bolles, 1970, 1971) and also with a variety of acquired ones. For example, small rodents such as mice have an innate tendency for immobility in threatening situations. Another intefering factor is the acquisition of coping habits that minimize exposure to shock. Consequently, the analysis of shuttle-box learning must rely on additional information from other tests and on observation of the actual behavior in the apparatus.

Our interpretation of the behavioral factor associated with the IIP-MF projection (at least in mice) is based on observations made in the radial maze, Y maze, and swimming navigation and on occasional observations of individuals during two-way avoidance learning. Actually, the factor apparently fitting best with mossy fiber variations is *behavioral predictability*. The perhaps most telling example is given in Figure 4, which shows the relation between the extent of the IIP-MF in mice from six inbred strains and their performance in the shuttle-box or a tubular Y maze, respectively. The Y-maze task was also based on avoidance learning. While the IIP-MF correlated negatively with the capacity of two-way avoidance, they were positively correlated with side perseverance: Mice with larger IIP-MF projections had a much stronger tendency to repeat their former choice, irrespective of the position of the discriminative stimulus. This fits well with observations of the behavior in the shuttle-box. Poor performance in the late stages of conditioning was most often caused by repeating a behavioral cycle, resulting in minimal exposure to shock; mice were also inattentive to the stimulus light because they were grooming. In such cases, the next responses were usually correct, but afterwards the mice waited progressively longer with the avoidance response until they were punished. Also, the superior radial maze performance of the mouse strain C3H (with large IIP-MF projections; see Fig. 2) was clearly due to response chaining, that is, visiting monotonically one arm after the other (Crusio et al., 1987). Behavioral predictability is more than perseverance, however. Mice with extended IIP-MF projections and good Y-maze discrimination learning were not characterized by faster learning but by the regularity of their correct (and sometimes incorrect) responses. This apparently enabled them to evaluate the efficiency of a given choice strategy. The positive correlations of the IIP-MF with performance in swimming navigation may be interpreted similarly.

Such behavioral predictability or temporal orderliness of behavioral patterns may correspond to distractability, mice or rats with large IIP-MF projections being less distractable. There are certainly other hypotheses by which a behavioral factor can be attributed to mossy fiber variations. This one appears preferable, however, because it *is independent of the actual behavior*. This makes it possible to explain the phenomenon of correlations with reversed sign. For example, if a mouse placed in a shuttle-box has a high tendency for locomotor activity under stress, and a large IIP-MF projection, then this response pattern is more likely to prevail and to lead to superior acquisition of two-way avoidance. On the other hand, if a mouse who initially freezes has a large IIP-MF projection, the inappropriate reaction may be prolonged and the end result is poorer performance. In other words, the extent of the IIP-MF projection may influence the probability of any behavioral change; the more IIP-MF, the lesser the likelihood to interrupt an ongoing behavioral program, whatever it is.

3. Relation With the Hippocampus?

The interpretation of circuitry variations biasing the probability of behavioral change fits well with older theories of hippocampal function, notably with the ideas of Kimble (1968, 1975), Douglas (1975), Douglas and Pribram (1969), and (Isaacson and Kimble (1972), yet it does not exclude interpretation by more recent theories (Deadwyler et al., 1987; Gray, 1982; Meck et al., 1984; O'Keefe and Nadel, 1978; Olton et al., 1979; Rawlins, 1985; Teyler and DiScenna, 1984,

1986). The main problem of this interpretation is that not one of the prevailing hippocampal theories takes variability and individuality into account. We shall present elsewhere a theory of how to integrate our findings on structural and behavioral variability into the framework of lesion studies and hippocampal theories. One hint will be given, though. We believe that the array of "lamellar loops" building up the hippocampal formation is a set of parallel control loops, each with a reverberating activity level corresponding to the activity in connected subsystems in cortex and subcortical structures—the hippocampus as a cerebellum of the limbic system (Lipp, 1989a,b). The chief task of this array of control loops is to *stabilize parallel processing across the brain* by means of a double process: maintaining the status quo of multiple system activities under conditions of ongoing behavior and coordinating the simultaneous transition of activity states under conditions of excitement. Optimal stabilization is reflected behaviorally in predictability and temporal orderliness. Suboptimal stabilization has two outcomes that resemble the effects of hippocampal lesions: hyperactivity, irritability and unpredictable behavior at one end of the spectrum and stubbornness and sensory neglect at the other.

Smooth operation of stabilization requires two things: The degree of interference between activity levels in the lamellar loops must be controlled, and the ability of holding the reverberating activity must be granted. Either of these processes may be sensitive to variations in the extent of the mossy fiber projection: Large projections are likely to limit lamellar cross-talk, since the input of the associational systems is correspondingly reduced, and they may equally facilitate long-term potentiation, perhaps because of a stronger capacity of driving an ensemble of neurons in CA3 (Vinogradova, 1975). Mossy fiber variations are certainly only one among several mechanisms by which cross-talk and potentiation may be tuned. Given their structural invariance and commanding position in the circuitry of Ammon's horn, however, it would not seem surprising to find physiological covariates of their morphology directly responsible for the individual differences in behavior.

SUMMARY

Behaviorally relevant traits of neuronal circuitry traits can be identified in the intact brain of rodent strains with inherited differences of hippocampal circuitry and/or behavior. In rats and mice, the extent of the intra/infrapyramidal mossy fiber projection is often strongly correlated with two-way avoidance learning. Most correlations are negative, but infrequently none or positive correlations can be found as well. The most parsimonious explanation is that mossy fiber variations influence the probability of transitions between behavioral states.

ACKNOWLEDGMENTS

These studies were supported by the Swiss National Foundation for Scientific Research (NF 3.041) and the Deutsche Forschungsgemeinschaft (DFG Schw 252). We appreciate the invaluable help of many collaborators, in particular Isolde Bär, Bernd Heimrich, Wim E. Crusio, David P. Wolfer, Marie-

Claire Leisinger-Trigona, and Zafiro Hausheer-Zarmakupi. We thank Helga Weber for photographic artwork.

REFERENCES

Amaral, D.G. (1979) Synaptic extensions from the mossy fibers of the fascia dentata. Anat. Embryol 155:241–251.

Bär, I. (1987) Aggregationschimären zwischen zwei Mäuseinzuchtstämmen: Erzeugung und Konsequenzen für das Verhalten und die Hippocampusmorphologie. Ph D Thesis, Heidelberg: University of Heidelberg.

Barber, R.P., J.E. Vaughn, R.E. Wimer, and C.C. Wimer (1974) Genetically-associated variations in the distribution of dentate granule cell synapses upon the pyramidal cell dendrites in mouse hippocampus. J. Comp. Neurol. 156:417–434.

Bignami, G., and D. Bovet (1965) Experience de sélection par rapport à une réaction conditionnée d'évitement chez le rat. C.R. Acad. Sci. 260:1239–1244.

Blanchard, R.J., and D.C. Blanchard (1969) Crouching as an index of fear. J. Comp. Physiol. Psychol. 67:370–375.

Bolles, R.C. (1970) Species-specific defense reactions and avoidance learning. Psychol. Rev. 77:32–48.

Bolles, R.C. (1971) Species-specific defense reactions. In R. Brush (ed): Aversive Conditioning and Learning. New York: Academic Press, pp. 183–234.

Buselmaier, W., S. Geiger and W. Reichert (1978) Monogene inheritance of learning speed in DBA and C3H mice. Hum. Genet. 40:209–214.

Buselmaier, W., Th. Vierling, W. Balzereit, and H. Schwegler (1981) Genetic analysis of avoidance learning by means of different psychological testing systems with inbred mice as model organisms. Psychol. Res. 43:317–333.

Claiborne, B.J., D.G. Amaral, and W.M. Cowan (1986) A light and electron microscopic analysis of the mossy fibers of the rat dentate gyrus. J. Comp. Neurol. 246:435–458.

Crusio, W.E., and H. Schwegler (1987) Hippocampal mossy fiber distribution covaries with open-field habituation in the mouse. Behav. Brain Res. 26:153–158.

Crusio, W.E., H. Schwegler, and H.-P. Lipp (1987) Radial-maze performance and structural variation of the hippocampus in mice: A correlation with mossy fibre distribution. Brain Res. 425:182–185.

Deadwyler, S.A., R.E. Hampson, T.C. Foster, and G. Marlow (1987) The functional significance of long-term potentiation: Relation to sensory processing by hippocampal circuits. In P.W. Landfield and S.A. Deadwyler (eds): Long-Term Potentiation: From Biophysics to Behavior. New York: Alan R. Liss, pp. 499–534.

Douglas, R.J. (1975) The development of hippocampal function: Implications for theory and for therapy. In R.L. Isaacson and K.W. Pribram (eds): The Hippocampus, Vol. 2. Neurophysiology and Behavior. New York: Plenum Press, pp. 327–361.

Douglas, R.J., and K. H. Pribram (1969) Distraction and habituation in monkeys with limbic lesions. J. Comp. Physiol. Psychol. 69:473–480.

Edwards, A.L. (1979) Multiple Regression and the Analysis of Variance and Covariance. San Francisco: W.H. Freeman, pp. 1–212.

Flühmann, S. (1980) Covariations héréditaires entre la distribution des fibres moussues hippocampiques chez la souris et la capacité d'apprentissage d'évitement: Une comparaison entre deux appareils (shuttle-box et labyrinthe en forme d'Y). Geneva: University of Geneva, Masters Thesis, pp. 1–80.

Gray, J.A. (1982) The Neuropsychology of Anxiety: An Enquiry Into the Functions of the Septo-Hippocampal System. Oxford: Clarendon Press, pp. 1–548.

Heimrich, B. (1985) Genetische Grundlagen der Hippocampusverschaltungen bei Nagern. Heidelberg: University of Heidelberg, PhD Thesis.

Heimrich, B., H. Schwegler, and W.E. Crusio (1985) Hippocampal variation between the inbred mouse strains C3H/HeJ and DBA/2: A quantitative-genetic analysis. J. Neurogenet. 2:389–401.

Isaacson, R.L., and D.P. Kimble (1972) Lesions of the limbic system: Their effects upon hypotheses and frustration. Behav. Biol. 7:767–793.

Kimble, D.P. (1968) Hippocampus and internal inhibition. Psychol. Bull. 70:285–295.

Kimble, D.P. (1975) Choice behavior in rats with hippocampal lesions. In R.L. Isaacson and K.W. Pribram (eds): The Hippocampus, Vol.2. Neurophysiology and Behavior. New York: Plenum Press, pp. 309–326.

Lauder, J.M., and E. Mugnaini (1977) Early hyperthyroidism alters the distribution of mossy fibres in the rat hippocampus. Nature 268(5618):335–337.

Lauder, J.M., and E. Mugnaini (1980) Infrapyramidal mossy fibers in the hippocampus of the hyperthyroid rat. A light and electron microscopic study. Dev. Neurosci. 3(4–6):248–265.

Laurberg, S., and J. Zimmer (1981) Lesion-induced sprouting of hippocampal mossy fiber collaterals to the fascia dentata in developing and adult rats. J. Comp. Neurol. 200:433–459.

Lieblich, I., E. Cohen, and A. Beiles (1978) Selection for high and for low rates of self-stimulation in rats. Physiol. Behav. 21:843–849.

Lieblich, I., P. Driscoll, and H.-P. Lipp (1987) Genetic relation between the readiness to self-stimulate lateral hypothalamus, two-way avoidance learning and the proportions of hippocampal synaptic fields in regio inferior. Behav. Genet. 17:427–438.

Lipp, H.-P. (1989a) Die Individualität von Gehirn und Verhalten Ein Essay, eine Evolutionstheorie, und Experimente. Habilitationsschrift. Zürich: University of Zürich (in press).

Lipp, H.-P. (1989b) Is the hippocampus a cerebellum of the limbic system? Verh. Anat. Ges. (in press).

Lipp, H.-P., R. Schoepke, D.P. Wolfer, H. Schwegler, and M.-C. Leisinger-Trigona (1988a) Hippocampal mossy fiber variations and swimming navigation in mice. Abstr. 20th Ann. Meet. Eur. Brain Behav. Soc. 1988 (EBBS).

Lipp, H.-P., H. Schwegler, and P. Driscoll (1981) Early hyperthyroidism alters both genetically dependent mossy fiber distribution and acquisition of two-way avoidance in rats. Neurosci. Lett. Suppl. 7:S46.

Lipp, H.-P., H. Schwegler, and P. Driscoll (1984) Postnatal modification of hippocampal circuitry alters avoidance learning in adults rats. Science 225:80–82.

Lipp, H.-P. H. Schwegler, and Z. Hausheer-Zarmakupi (1986) The infrapyramidal mossy fiber projection in the hippocampus of the mouse: A positive correlation with Y-maze avoidance learning. Soc. Neurosci. Abstr. 12:751.

Lipp, H.-P., H. Schwegler, B. Heimrich, A. Cerbone, and A.G. Sadile (1987) Strain-specific correlations between hippocampal structural traits and habituation in a spatial novelty situation. Behav. Brain Res. 24:111–123.

Lipp, H.-P., H. Schwegler, B. Heimrich, and P. Driscoll (1988b) Infrapyramidal mossy fibers and two-way avoidance learning: Developmental modification of hippocampal circuitry and adult behavior of rats and mice. J. Neurosci. 8:1905–1921.

Lipp, H.-P., H. van der Loos, D. Anders, and P. Driscoll (1985) An automatized Y-maze for multimodal discrimination training of mice. Experientia 41:831.

Meck, W.H., R.M. Church, and D.S. Olton (1984) Hippocampus, time, and memory. Behav. Neurosci 98:3–22.

O'Keefe, J., and L. Nadel (1978) The Hippocampus as a Cognitive Map. Oxford: Clarendon Press.

Olton, D.S., J.T. Becker, and G.E. Handelmann (1979) Hippocampus, space, and memory. Behav. Brain Sci. 2:313–365.

Olton, D.S., C.G. Johnson, and E. Howard (1975) Impairment of conditioned active avoidance in adult rats given corticosterone in infancy. Dev. Psychobiol. 8:55–61.

Rawlins, J.N.P. (1985) Associations across time: The hippocampus as a temporary memory store. Behav. Brain Sci. 8:479–486.

Schwegler, H. (1986) Die Grundlagen des Lernens. Neurobiologische und genetische Ansätze. Habilitationsschrift, Heidelberg: University of Heidelberg.

Schwegler, H., W.E., Crusio, H.-P. Lipp, P. Lichter, and B. Heimrich (1988) Water-maze learning in the mouse correlates with variation in hippocampal morphology. Behav. Genet. 18:153–166.

Schwegler, H., B. Heimrich, W.E. Crusio, and H.-P. Lipp (1985) Hippocampal mossy fiber distribution and two-way avoidance learning in rats and mice. In B.E. Will, P. Schmitt, and J.C. Dalrymple-Alford (eds): Brain Plasticity, Learning, and Memory. London: Plenum Publishing Corporation, pp. 127–138.

Schwegler, H., and H.-P. Lipp (1981) Is there a correlation between hippocampal mossy fiber distribution and two-way avoidance performance in mice and rats?. Neurosci. Lett. 23:25–30.

Schwegler, H., and H.-P. Lipp (1983) Hereditary covariations of neuronal circuitry and behavior: Correlations between the proportions of hippocampal synaptic fields in the regio inferior and two-way avoidance in mice and rats. Behav. Brain Res. 7:1–39.

Schwegler, H., H.-P. Lipp, H. van der Loos, and W. Buselmaier (1981) Individual hippocampal mossy fiber distribution in mice correlates with two-way avoidance performance. Science 214:817–819.

Smith, R.H. (1985) Behavioral measures of drift in Mus musculus. Behav. Genet. 15(5):483–497.

Teyler, T.J., and P. DiScenna (1984) Long-term potentiation as a candidate mnemonic device. Brain Res. Rev. 7:15–28.

Teyler, T.J., and P. DiScenna (1986) The hippocampal memory indexing theory. Behav. Neurosci. 100:147–154.

Vinogradova, O.S. (1975) Functional organization of the limbic system in the process of registration of information: facts and hypotheses. In R.L. Isaacson, and K.H. Pribram (eds): The Hippocampus, Vol. 2. Neurophysiology and Behavior. New York: Plenum Press, pp. 3–70.

Wolfer, D.P., H.-P. Lipp, M.-C. Leisinger-Trigona, and Z. Hausheer-Zarmakupi (1987a) Correlations between hippocampal circuitry and behavior: Infrapyramidal mossy fibers and navigation in a Morris water maze. Acta Anat. 128:346.

Wolfer, D.P. H.-P. Lipp, H. Schwegler, and M. Brust (1987b) Hippocampal mossy fibers and avoidance learning in mice treated postnatally with corticosterone: Correlations with extent and left/right asymmetry. Soc. Neurosci. Abstr. 13:225.10.

The Hippocampus—New Vistas, pages 411–424
© 1989 Alan R. Liss, Inc.

26
Mnemonic Functions of the Hippocampus: Single Unit Analyses in Rats

DAVID S. OLTON

Department of Psychology, Johns Hopkins University, Baltimore, Maryland

INTRODUCTION

Although hippocampal function mediates memory of some kind, a great deal of information is still needed to identify both the types of mnemonic information processed by the hippocampus and the neural mechanisms that underlie this processing. In this context, an analysis of hippocampal function through single unit recording in nonspatial mnemonic tasks in rats can make three important contributions: It complements the extensive information obtained from experiments studying the memory impairments following hippocampal lesions, identifies the relationship between spatial and nonspatial mnemonic processes, and provides a bridge to relate many different neural descriptions of the hippocampus with behavioral descriptions. Each of these contributions will be reviewed in turn, indicating first the relevant background information and then how this new information can help to improve our knowledge of hippocampal function in memory.

1. Experiments describing the behavioral and cognitive changes that follow hippocampal lesions have provided strong evidence that the hippocampus and closely related structures are critical for normal processing of some kinds of memory. The reports about patient HM, who had bilateral removal of the temporal lobes, and extensive animal models with both rats and monkeys all consistently demonstrate that a profound amnesic syndrome follows damage to temporal lobe structures, especially the hippocampus (Corkin, 1984; Markowska et al., 1988; Mishkin, 1982; Olton, 1983; Rawlins, 1985; Squire and Zola-Morgan, 1983; Zola-Morgan and Squire, 1986; Zola-Morgan et al., 1986).

Although lesion analyses make the unique contribution of demonstrating the functions that require a certain structure, they have the disadvantage of studying an abnormal system (Olton, 1986). Recording analyses have complementary contributions and disadvantages. Although they cannot demonstrate that the recorded activity is necessary for the function with which it is correlated, they can obtain information from the normal (as well as the abnormal) brain. Together, these analyses provide converging operations, and a consistent answer from both approaches has a greater validity than an answer obtained from either one of them alone (Garner et al., 1956; Platt, 1964).

2. Spatial tasks have made two important contributions to our understanding of hippocampal function. Because they are often learned rapidly and performed well, they provide a means with which to assess many different cognitive processes in rats and other animals (Kesner and DiMattia, 1988; Morris, 1984; O'Keefe and Nadel, 1978; Olton, 1979). In addition, they have demonstrated an important function of the hippocampus. The activity of complex spike cells in the hippocampus is closely correlated with many different aspects of the rat's spatial behaviors: its position in the apparatus, direction of movement, and velocity of movement. These results have led to the suggestion that the hippocampus forms the neural basis of a spatial cognitive map (McNaughton et al., 1983; Muller and Kubie, 1987; Muller, et al., 1987; O'Keefe and Nadel, 1978; O'Keefe, 1979; Olton, 1988).

The relationship between spatial and nonspatial mnemonic interpretations of hippocampal function has many important implications. Spatial mnemonics (the method of loci, and so forth) have a long history of being used to remember nonspatial information, leading to the suggestion that the same cognitive module may have both spatial and nonspatial functions (Neisser, 1987). A comparison of the spatial and nonspatial correlates of an individual hippocampal unit can help to determine the extent to which the same neural module can have spatial and nonspatial mnemonic functions, which in turn has implications for our understanding of the relationship between the relevant cognitive modules. Neurally, of course, these data will also help to indicate the flexibility of single units in the hippocampus, and the extent to which an individual unit can respond to different cognitive demands, information that is necessary to determine the specificity of hippocampal function.

3. Because the hippocampus has such an elegant neuroanatomical, neurochemical, and electrophysiological organization, it has been used extensively for many different types of neurobiological investigations (see previous chapters in this volume). If reductionistic analyses are to incorporate data from the most molecular aspects of brain function and behavior, then links between different levels of analyses must be made throughout the entire range of possibilities. Single unit recording offers an excellent opportunity to bridge the electrophysiological and behavioral levels of analysis, and rats are likely to be the most effective animals to make this bridge. Because primates are so scarce and valuable, intensive neurobiological studies are not practical in them. Because the behavioral tasks for rats can measure many of the types of memory studied in humans, they also provide a strong link to the more cognitive approaches (Olton, 1985a,b; Olton and Wenk, 1987; Roitblat, 1987). Finally, many of the experiments making the electrophysiological–behavioral links must obtain all of the different measures in the same animal at the same in order to

be maximally effective. Currently, rats provide the model of choice for this approach.

EXPERIMENTAL STRATEGY

In reality, of course, no task is truly "nonspatial." Every activity occurs in both space and time, and consequently has both a spatial and temporal context (Olton, 1987a,b; Rawlins and Tsaltis, 1983; Solomon, 1979, 1980). Consequently, the term *nonspatial* is really a brief way of saying *spatially irrelevant.* Although the behavior takes place in a spatial context, spatial cues are not relevant to identify the correct response in the discrimination.

In some tasks, the opportunity to respond is given in only a single location, and the rat indicates its choice by either making the response ("go") or not making the response ("no go"). Because the response occurs in the same place, the location of the response is not relevant to correct performance in the task.

The relevant discriminative stimuli can also be presented in the same location. Thus, a light or a speaker can be used as the discriminative stimulus. If the light is illuminated, one response is correct; if the light is not illuminated, another response is correct.

Even tasks that have both stimuli and responses in different locations can incorporate procedures to make the spatial aspects of the stimuli and responses irrelevant to the correct performance of the discrimination. This point can be illustrated by comparing two types of delayed conditional discriminations conducted in a T maze. One arm has vertical stripes; the other has small circles. The spatial discrimination uses places as the relevant discriminative stimuli. At the beginning of each trial, the rat is forced to go to one arm of the T maze. The rat is removed from the maze for a delay interval and then returned to the maze to make a choice between both arms. Reinforcement is available only in the arm in the location that was entered immediately prior to the delay interval. During the delay interval, the two arms are interchanged during some trials and left in place during other trials so that the visual pattern in the arm entered at the beginning of the trial cannot be used to indicate the arm that is correct at the end of the trial. Consequently, to perform correctly at the end of the delay, the animal must have information about the location of the arm entered prior to the delay. With appropriate control procedures, the experiment can be conducted in such a way that the only relevant information to solve the discrimination is the set of stimuli that identify the spatial location of each arm.

A similar nonspatial delayed conditional discrimination uses the same general procedure, but arranges the testing conditions so that the discriminative stimuli are nonspatial. At the beginning of each trial, the rat is forced to enter the arm with the vertical stripes. After the delay interval, the rat is given a choice between both arms, and reinforcement is located only in the arm with the stripes, the same arm that was entered prior to the delay. Again, the arms are interchanged during the delay interval of some (but not all) trials so that the spatial location of the arm entered at the beginning of the trial cannot predict which arm is correct after the delay. Consequently, the visual patterns on the arms can be used as the discriminative stimuli. Control procedures can make the spatial stimuli irrelevant, and they require the animal to use the nonspatial, visual patterns in the arms as the discriminative stimuli.

The examples just given reflect only a few of the combinations of procedures that can be used in nonspatial discriminations. The taxonomy of both spatial and mnemonic processes is complicated, and by no means complete (Morris, 1984; O'Keefe and Nadel, 1978; Squire, 1987; Tulving, 1985). Thus, these examples are not meant to describe all the differences between nonspatial and spatial tasks, but to illustrate a few procedures similar to ones that have actually been used for recording.

Many of the experiments recording single unit activity during nonmnemonic spatial tasks have used variations of the delayed conditional discrimination, a procedure that emphasizes recent memory. The emphasis on this type of memory is appropriate because it is a major component of the amnesic syndrome following damage to the hippocampus. In many clinical screening tests, recent memory is assessed by presenting the patient some information, imposing a short delay interval, often filled with distracting information, and then asking for recall of that information (Folstein et al., 1975). For example, the examiner speaks three words to the patient and then immediately asks the patient to repeat those words. After a short period of conversation, the examiner asks the patient to recall the previously presented words. Typically, amnesic patients show impaired recall at this time, but normal recall of the words immediately after they were presented. This dissociation of choice accuracy before and after the delay interval is typically used to infer that the impairment after the delay is due to a failure of memory rather than of other more general cognitive processes (such as sensation, motivation, comprehension of speech, and so forth). In essence, the dissociation suggests that the impairment at the end of the delay interval is not due to impairments of cognitive processes required for both immediate recall and delayed recall, but due to cognitive processes selectively emphasized in the delayed recall, processes that are most likely associated with memory of some kind (Corkin, 1984; Kaushall et al., 1981.

Delayed conditional discriminations for animals use the same general testing procedure. At the beginning of each trial, a stimulus is presented and then removed. A delay interval follows. At the end of the delay, the animal is given at least two alternative choices. The correct choice at the end of the delay interval is conditional (depends) on the stimulus presented at the beginning of the interval. Consequently, to respond accurately at the end of the delay interval, the animal must have information about the stimulus that was presented at the beginning of the interval. Damage to the hippocampus in both rats and monkeys typically produces a significant impairment in the performance of delayed conditional discriminations with both spatial and nonspatial stimuli. The results from the animal models are very similar to those from human patients with damage to the hippocampus (Eichenbaum et al., 1988;

Morris, 1985; Olton, 1983; Olton and Feustle, 1981; Raffaele and Olton, 1988; Squire and Zola-Morgan, 1983; Zola-Morgan and Squire, 1986).

Spatial versions of delayed conditional discriminations have been used for many years. Rats learn them quickly, perform them well, and use well-documented mnemonic processes to solve them. These advantages have led to a substantial use of spatial tasks to investigate the neurobiological bases of memory (Kesner and DiMattia, 1988; Olton, 1987a,b; Morris, 1983; O'Keefe and Nadel, 1978).

However, spatial tasks have some inherent difficulties when used in conjunction with the recording of single units to examine the neural bases of memory. This point can be made most clearly by considering the differences between a *behavioral* and a *mnemonic correlate* of unit activity. A behavioral correlate is the empirically defined and readily observed description of the animal's behavior during the relevant electrophysiological activity. In contrast, the mnemonic correlate is the cognitive process (registration of information, retrieval of information, comparison of stimuli, and so forth) that takes place during that behavior (Eichenbaum et al., 1988; Wible et al., 1986). Analyses of spatial tasks are complicated by the fact that many different cognitive strategies can underlie the same type of behavior. Thus any single behavioral correlate may be associated with several different mnemonic correlates. Although considerable progress has been made to design experiments that dissociate different cognitive strategies underlying spatial behavior (Morris, 1984; O'Keefe and Nadel, 1978; Olton, 1979), and although similar problems persist in nonspatial tasks, nonspatial procedures have inherent advantages over spatial ones when the goal is to identify mnemonic correlates of single unit activity. As will become obvious in the subsequent discussion of particular experiments, both the precise control over the presentation and removal of the relevant stimuli and the opportunity to make a response are critical for appropriate interpretation of the results. Perievent histograms and independent manipulation of the time of each event are necessary to determine which event was responsible for the changes in neural activity. Nonspatial experiments can provide these manipulations, which in turn permit more accurate indentification of mnemonic correlates. For example, a unit might increase its activity when a stimulus is presented. This behavioral correlate might reflect at least three different psychological processes: perception of the stimulus (with no memory), registration of the stimulus so that it will be remembered, and recall of information associated with that stimulus. These different interpretations can be dissociated with an experimental procedure presenting this stimulus in a delayed conditional discrimination as described previously. If unit activity reflects perception, it should increase activity whenever the stimulus is presented, both as a sample and for a choice. If unit activity reflects only registration of information to be remembered, it should increase activity when the stimulus is presented as the sample, but not as the choice. If unit activity reflects only recall of information that has been remembered, it should increase when the stimulus is presented as the choice but not as the sample. Similar logic can be used for other types of analyses and will become apparent in the discussion of the experiments that follow. (Fuster and Jervey, 1983; Rolls, 1987).

BEHAVIORAL CORRELATES OF HIPPOCAMPAL UNIT ACTIVITY
Delayed-Match-to-Sample and Simultaneous Two-Choice Discriminations With Visual Stimuli

Hippocampal unit activity was significantly correlated with various aspects of performance in a delayed-match-to-sample (DMTS) task with visual stimuli and much less correlated in a visual discrimination task that used the same apparatus, but involved a different kind of memory (Wible et al., 1986). These data are important for two reasons. First, they show that delayed conditional discriminations for rats, like those for monkeys, elicit hippocampal unit correlates (Watanabe and Niki, 1985). Second, they provide a dissociation, showing that these correlates are more significantly associated with some types of memory rather than others.

The apparatus had a start box connected to two goal boxes. One goal box was painted white, the other black. The goal boxes were built so that they could be removed and interchanged with each other. A guillotine door separated the start box from the two goal boxes. Reinforcement was provided by a sucrose solution that could be injected into a small cup in each goal box.

The nonspatial DMTS task was conducted using a procedure similar to the one described previously. For the *sample phase*, sucrose was placed in the cup in one goal, and the other goal was blocked. The rat was placed in the start, allowed to enter the available goal, and drank the sucrose there. For the *choice phase*, the rat was returned to the start, and both goals were made available. If the rat made a correct choice and entered the same goal that was visited during the sample phase, sucrose was placed in the cup and the rat was allowed to drink. If the rat made an incorrect choice and entered the other goal, no reward was available. To force the rat to use the nonspatial discriminative stimuli (the brightness of the two goals), they were interchanged randomly between the sample phase and choice phase and during the intertrial interval. Consequently, the rat was unable to use the spatial location of the goal entered during the sample phase to indicate the correct response during the choice phase, but had to remember the visual characteristics of that goal.

Each rat was trained to a high level of choice accuracy. Microelectrodes were implanted to record from the CA1 layer of the hippocampus using the techniques described by Kubie (1984). The electrophysiological signal was led through a headstage containing field effect transistors and through additional amplifiers. A window discriminator was used to discriminate single units. The position of the rat in the maze was recorded on a video camera and registered as X–Y coordinates. Data analysis correlated the position of the rat in the maze, the discriminated unit activity, and other aspects of the procedure (the phase of the trial, correctness of response, location of each goal box, and so forth).

The data were analyzed while the rat was in the goal box during the sample phase and during the choice phase of correct trials. During this time, the rat's behavior was consistent, drinking out of the cup containing the sucrose. Consequently, artifacts caused by different types of behavior were minimized.

Two nonspatial aspects of the task had strong behavioral correlates with unit activity. The first was related to the discriminative stimuli, the goal boxes. Some units (10/27) had a significantly different rate of activity when the rat was in one goal as compared with the other. Most of the units had an increased rate of activity in the black goal relative to the white goal, but some had the opposite pattern.

Other units (5/27) had differential activity during the sample phase and choice phase. Some units had an increased rate during the sample phase relative to the choice phase, while others had the opposite pattern.

In addition to the main effects of a single variable (type of goal box, phase of task), interactions occurred from all variables. For example, some units (4/27) had an interaction between the type of goal box and the phase of the task. One unit had an increased rate of activity when the rat was in the black goal box during the sample phase, but not when the rat was in the other goal box during that phase, or in the same goal box during the choice phase. Consequently, the unit responded to the conjunction of the type of goal box and the phase of the task.

In addition to the two nonspatial variables (type of goal box, phase of task), the location of the goal box (on the left or right side of the apparatus) had an influence on unit activity. Some units (7/27) had a main effect on location. Others had an interaction of location with either the type of goal box (6/27) or the phase of the task (4/27).

The visual discrimination task used the same apparatus and same general recording procedures. However, the stimulus-response-reinforcement contingencies were changed to make two different two-choice simultaneous discriminations rather than a DMTS task. For the *cue task*, one goal was correct on every trial regardless of the spatial location of that goal. Thus, for example, for a given rat, the black goal might contain reinforcement, while the white goal might not. For the *spatial task*, the goal in the same spatial location was correct. During this task, for example, the goal on the right side of the apparatus might have reinforcement on every trial. This type of discrimination does not require recent memory, as in DMTS, because the response to each stimulus is the same for every trial. Consequently, the rat can use long-term memory, based on experience in many trials, to determine the correct response on any given trial.

Relatively few units had behavioral correlates during the cue task or the spatial task. Of 29 units, 14 showed no significant change in firing rate in any condition. Of the remaining units, behavioral correlates were associated with the type of task (cue or spatial) being performed (13/29), the location (left or right) of the goal (3/29), and the type (black or white) of goal (5/29). These variables also interacted to influence unit activity. Interactions occurred between the task (cue or spatial) and the type of goal (black or white), the task and the location of the goal box (left or right), and the type of goal and the location of the goal (a total of nine units).

In conjunction with the results from the DMTS task, these correlates provide two important conclusions. First, hippocampal unit activity was stimulated less by this visual discrimination than by the DMTS task, demonstrating that the type of memory requirement of a task significantly influences the involvement of hippocampal units. Second, the conjunction of significant variables (type of discriminative stimulus, phase of task, and so forth) had significant effects on hippocampal unit activity, suggesting that individual units responded to several relevant variables simultaneously.

Go–No Go Discriminations With Olfactory Stimuli

The activity of single units in the hippocampus was correlated with specific components of an olfactory discrimination task, showing that these nonspatial mnemonic components of this task activated the hippocampus (Eichenbaum et al., 1987). At one end of the testing arena was a small port through which an air stream was presented. A system of solenoid valves controlled the entrance of specific olfactory stimuli into this air stream when the rat placed its nose in the port. At the other end of the arena was a cup in which reward (0.05 ml water) could be delivered.

In each pair of olfactory stimuli, one was designated as the S + and the other as S −. When the rat placed its nose in the port, stimulus was presented. If the stimulus S +, the correct response for the rat was to hold its nose in the port for 2 s; following this response, reward was available in the cup at the other side of the arena, and the rat could obtain that reward by going to the cup. If the stimulus was S −, no reinforcement was available so that the optimal response for the rat was to withdraw from the port to wait for the next trial. The rats were trained to a stable level of choice accuracy. Recordings were made through a bundle of microwires, each of which was 25 μM in diameter. The rat's position in the apparatus was recorded by a video camera. The information about the behavior of the rat and the activity of the discriminated unit was analyzed by a computer to provide perievent histograms of the unit activity.

Some of the units showed substantial nonspatial mnemonic correlates. *Cue-sampling cells* responded maximally when the rat placed its nose in the port and sniffed the olfactory stimuli. Two characteristics of cue-sampling cells indicate that their activity was influenced by the memory of past experience. First, the activity of these cells was greater in the presence of S + than in the presence of S −. This differential activity increased as a function of experience with a given pair of odors. Furthermore, if the rat had several pairs of odors, activity in the presence of each S + odor was greater than activity in the presence of each S − odor. Together, these data demonstrate that the differential activity in the presence of S + and S − was due not to the sensory characteristics of the odors, but to the past reinforcement history associated with them.

The activity of cue-sampling cells on any given trial also reflected the stimulus that had been presented on the previous trial. Activity was greater when the stimulus on the preceding trial had been S − than if it had been S + (even though the stimulus on the preceding trial did not influence the events on the current trial). Consequently, these units also reflected recent memory for the events on the immediately preceding trial (see Deadwyler, 1985; Meck et al., 1987).

These cue-sampling cells were obviously not place cells. The activity of these cells while the rat was in the same place (at the port) changed as a function of the rat's past experience with the olfactory stimuli. In addition, these cue-sampling cells had very low rates of activity when the rat placed its nose in the port but no odor was available (which occurred during the intertrial interval).

Together, all of these data indicate that these hippocampal units responded to nonspatial, mnemonic characteristics of the task. The fact that an individual unit could respond to both long-term memory associated with an odor (the response-reinforcement contingenciess over many trials) and short-term memory (the stimulus, S+ or S−) on the preceding trial implies that the hippocampus is involved in processing both kinds of memory. This lack of dissociation is surprising in light of the differential responding of hippocampal units in other procedures (Wible et al., 1986) and the differential effects of lesions (Eichenbaum et al., 1987). The linkage of specific neural structures to specific mnemonic processes provides one of the most significant challenges in understanding the neurobiological bases of memory, and resolving apparent discrepancies such as these should help this neurocognitive classification and the interpretation of data from both lesion and recording studies (Eichenbaum et al., 1987; Olton, 1985b; Olton et al., 1986).

Go–No Go Responding to Auditory Stimuli

Single units in the granule cell layer of the dentate gyrus showed differential activity in response to auditory stimuli as a result of differential response-reinforcement contingencies associated with those stimuli (Deadwyler et al., 1979). The apparatus was a small chamber that contained a speaker, which could deliver auditory stimuli, and a response mechanism that detected a nose-poke and delivered reinforcement when the nose-poke was made at the correct time. Differential conditioning was established to tones of two different frequencies, which were presented in random order. Following a positive tone, a nose-poke produced reinforcement. Following a negative tone, no reinforcement was available. Each rat was trained to a stable level of criterion performance with the two tones. Then, the discrimination was reversed so that the previously positive tone became the negative one (and the correct response to this tone changed from making a nose-poke to not making a nose-poke), and the previously negative tone became the positive tone (and the correct response changed from not making a nose-poke to making a nose-poke).

Single units responded to the reinforcement contingencies associated with the tones rather than to the frequency of the tones themselves. Poststimulus histograms showed that unit activity was greater on trials presenting the positive stimulus than on trials presenting the negative stimulus. This differential relationship of unit activity and the positive/negative nature of the stimulus persisted even after the discrimination had been reversed. Consequently, greater activity was associated with the positive stimulus irrespective of its frequency, and lower activity was associated with the negative stimulus irrespective of its frequency. Consequently, these units reflected the memory of the response-reinforcement contingencies associated with each stimulus rather than the stimulus itself (cf. Deadwyler et al., 1985).

Auditory Continuous Nonmatch-to-Sample Discrimination

Single units in several parts of the hippocampal system responded to different components of an auditory continuous nonmatch-to-sample discrimination (Sakurai, 1988). For each trial a stimulus was presented. One second later a door was opened to expose a panel. If the stimulus for the current trial was different from that on the previous trial (nonmatch trial), the correct response was to press the panel (go response). If the stimulus for the current trial was the same as that on a previous trial (match trial), the correct response was to refrain from pressing the panel (no-go response). Entorhinal cortex had many units with sensory correlates; activity increased when one discriminative stimulus was presented, but not when the other one was presented. These sensory correlates of these entorhinal units suggest that they were involved in the detection/identification of the discriminative stimuli. CA1 and CA3 had units that responded to the interaction of a particular sequence of stimuli on two successive trials and the making of a go response. Activity in these units increased only on nonmatch trials when the rat made a go response. These units did not respond to just the motor response; activity did not increase when the rat made an incorrect go response on a match trial. These units did not respond to just a particular stimulus; activity increased on a nonmatch trial when the rat made go response with either stimulus present. Because neural activity in these units was different on correct nonmatch trials as compared to incorrect match trials (both of which had the same response), and was the same on all correct nonmatch trials irrespective of the stimulus presented during that trial, they must reflect some mnemonic comparison of the stimulus on the present trial with the stimulus on the previous trial. If that stimulus was different, these units increased activity. If that stimulus was the same, these units did not change their activity. Ironically, these units must have been more accurate at identifying the nature of the trial than the rat's response because their activity correctly indicated a match trial even on those match trials when the rat incorrectly made a go response.

Together, the results from all four unit studies described here (Deadwyler et al., 1979; Eichenbaum et al., 1987; Sakunai, 1988; Wible et al., 1986) demonstrate that hippocampal units reflect the memory of stimulus-response-reinforcement contingencies to a variety of nonspatial stimuli. These types of correlates occurred in two different areas of the hippocampus (CA1 pyramidal cell layer and the dentate gyrus) in response to three different modalities of stimulation (auditory, olfactory, visual), providing substantial generality to the conclusion that the hippocampus has a major role in nonspatial as well as spatial memory.

NEW VISTAS

Operant conditioning techniques were developed within a conceptual framework that repudiated links to both cognitive and neural analyses. A strong emphasis on purely empirical description, coupled with the cost of apparatus and the difficulty training animals, discouraged the use of these techniques to investigate the neurobiological bases of memory. However, the emphasis on comparative cognition (Hulse et al., 1978; Roitblat, 1987) has radically changed this situation. Sophisticated cognitive analyses have developed new techniques for controlling behavior, and powerful conceptual approaches can identify precisely the computational process underlying each aspect of performance. These developments provide the opportunity to pursue the three issues raised at the beginning of this chapter more effectively than in the past. The combination of these opportunities and the data summarized here should lead to significantly new views of hippocampal function.

First, new behavioral correlates of hippocampal unit activity can be identified in tasks that have well-described computational/cognitive analyses. Consequently, the empirically observed behavioral correlates can be used to infer mnemonic correlates, which are ultimately a prerequisite to link together the cognitive and neurobiological analyses of memory.

Second, the intensive investigation of spatial correlates of hippocampal unit activity can be combined with the investigation of nonspatial correlates to determine the relationship of these two. As pointed out previously, every event happens both in a particular place and at a particular time so that it can be placed in both a temporal and a spatial context. Although our experimental designs and interpretations have often considered spatial and temporal variables independently, they have many attributes in common. As the analysis of nonspatial, mnemonic, and temporal correlates of hippocampal unit activity catches up to the analysis of spatial correlates, these endeavors should have substantial influence on each other. Empirically, the extent to which an individual unit has behavioral correlates in different tasks can help to indicate the extent to which the hippocampus is flexible in the type of information that it processes. Procedurally, many of the experimental strategies used to design experiments in these different areas of endeavor can be effectively adopted by the other endeavors so that carefully controlled and meaningful comparisons can be made to identify the similarities and differences in the spatial and nonspatial interpretations of hippocampal function. Theoretically, these results should have a profound effect on the way in which we conceptualize the modularity of mind. Because neuronal processes and mental activity are different ramifications of the same underlying processes, and because the function of neuronal units can be studied more directly than the function of different cognitive units, neurocomputational analyses linking together behavioral and mnemonic correlates provide the most effective way to identify the ways in which different modules are interrelated. If, as suggested above, temporal and spatial analyses are fundamentally interrelated, then the same neural mechanisms are most likely involved in both of them. If, however, they represent different computational activities, then the neural systems involved in them should likewise be independent.

Third, other electrophysiological analyses can be linked to unit activity, and this link can be used to integrate endeavors that have proceeded somewhat independently for technical reasons. For example, long-term enhancement (LTE) of hippocampal activity has often been interpreted as a model of memory. Unfortunately, its relationship to the more cognitive analyses of memory that have resulted from investigations of animals and humans following damage to the hippocampus has been limited. With the demonstration of behavioral and mnemonic correlates of hippocampal unit activity in tasks similar to those used to establish our current conceptual framework for memory and amnesia, and the ability to study the interrelationship of single unit activity and LTE, the involvement of LTE in memory can be pursued more effectively. A similar strategy can be adopted for any neural and any cognitive approach that can be individually linked to single unit activity; although the relationship between the molecular and cognitive may be difficult to establish directly, the indirect link through single unit activity may provide an effective transition that cannot otherwise be obtained.

ACKNOWLEDGMENTS

I thank A. Markowska, G. Wenk, and C. Wible for comments on the manuscript and D. Harris and J. Thomassen for its preparation.

REFERENCES

Corkin, S. (1984) Lasting consequences of bilateral medial temporal lobectomy: Clinical course and experimental findings in H.M. Semin. Neurol. *4*:249–259.

Deadwyler, S.A. (1985) Involvement of hippocampal systems in learning and memory. In N.M. Weinberger, J.L. McGaugh, and G. Lynch (eds): Memory Systems of the Brain. New York: The Guilford Press, pp. 134–149.

Deadwyler, S.A., M.O. West, E. Christian, R.E. Hampson, and D.C. Foster (1985) Sequence related changes in sensory evoked potentials in the dentate gyrus: A mechanism for item-specific short-term information storage in the hippocampus. Behav. Neural Biol. *44*:201–212.

Deadwyler, S.A., M.O. West, and G. Lynch (1979) Activity of dentate granule cells during learning: Differentiation of perforant path input. Br. Res. *169*:29–43.

Eichenbaum, H., A. Fagan, P. Mathews, and N.J. Cohen (1988) Hippocampal system dysfunction and odor discrimination learning in rats: Impairment or facilitation depending on representational demands. Behav. Neurosci. *102(3)*:331–339.

Folstein, M.F., S.E. Folstein, and P.R. McHugh (1975) A practical method for grading the cognitive state of patients for the clinician. J. Psychiatry Res. *12*:189–198.

Fuster, J.M., and J.P. Jervey (1983) Inferotemporal neurons distinguish and retain behaviorally relevant features of visual stimuli. Science *212*:1175–1178.

Garner, W.R., H.W. Hake, and C.W. Eriksen (1956) Operationism and the concept of perception. Psychol. Rev. *63*:149–159.

Hulse, S.H., H. Fowler, and W.K. Honig (eds) (1978) Cognitive Processes in Animal Behavior. Hillsdale, NJ: Erlbaum.

Kaushall, P.I., M. Zetin, and L.R. Squire (1981) A psychosocial study of chronic, circumscribed amnesia. J. Nerv. Ment. Dis. *169*:383–389.

Kesner, R.P., and B.V. DiMattia (1988) Neurobiology of an attribute model of memory. In A.N. Epstein and A. Morrison (eds): Progress in Psychobiology and Physiological Psychology. New York: Academic Press (in press).

Kubie, J. (1984) A drivable bundle of microwires for collecting single unit data from freely moving rats. Physiol. Behav. *32:*115–118.

Markowska, A.L., D.S. Olton, E.A. Murray, and D. Gaffan (1988) A comparative analysis of the role of fornix and cingulate cortex in memory: Rats. Exp. Brain Res. 74:187–201.

McNaughton, B.L., C.A. Barnes, and J. O'Keefe (1983) The contributions of position, direction and velocity to single unit activity in the hippocampus of freely moving rats. Exp. Brain Res. *52:*41–49.

Meck, W.H., R.M. Church, G.L. Wenk, and D.S. Olton (1987) Nucleus basalis magnocellularis and medial septal area lesions differentially impair temporal memory. J. Neurosci. *7:*3505–3511.

Mishkin, M. (1982) A memory system in the monkey. Philos. Trans. R. Soc. Lond. *B298:*85–95.

Morris, R.G.M. (1983) An attempt to dissociate "spatial-mapping" and "working-memory" theories of hippocampal function. In W. Seifert (ed): Neurobiology of the Hippocampus. New York: Academic Press, pp. 405–432.

Morris, R.G.M. (1984) Developments of a water-maze procedure for studying spatial learning in the rat. J. Neurosci. Methods *11:*47–60.

Morris, R.G.M. (1985) Moving on from modeling amnesia. In N.M. Weinberger, J.L. McGaugh, and G. Lynch (eds): Memory Systems of the Brain. New York: Guilford Press, pp. 452–462.

Muller, R.U., and J.L. Kubie (1987) The effects of changes in the environment on the spatial firing of hippocampal complex-spike cells. J. Neurosci. *7:*1951–1968.

Muller, R.U., J.L. Kubie, and J. Rank (1987) Spatial firing patterns of hippocampal complex-spike cells in a fixed environment. J. Neurosci. *7:*1935–1950.

Neisser, U. (1987) A sense of where you are: Functions of the spatial module. In P. Ellen and C. Thinus-Blanc (eds): Cognitive Processes and Spatial Orientation in Animal and Man. Dordrecht, The Netherlands: Martinus Nijhoff Publishers, pp. 293–310.

O'Keefe, J. (1979) A review of the hippocampal place cells. Prog. Neurobiol. *13:*419–439.

O'Keefe, J., and L. Nadel (1978) The Hippocampus as a Cognitive Map. Oxford, UK: Clarendon Press.

Olton, D.S. (1979) Mazes, maps, and memory. Am. Psychol. *34:*583–596.

Olton, D.S. (1983) Memory functions and the hippocampus. In W. Seifert (ed): Neurobiology of the Hippocampus. London: Academic Press, pp. 335–373.

Olton, D.S. (1985a) Criteria for establishing and evaluating animal models. In D.S. Olton, E. Gamzu, and S. Corkin (eds): Memory Dysfunction: An Integration of Animal and Human Research from Preclinical and Clinical Perspectives, New York: The New York Academy of Sciences, pp. 113–121.

Olton, D.S. (1985b) Memory: Neuropsychological and ethopsychological approaches to its classification. In L. Nilson and T. Archer (eds): Perspectives On Learning and Memory. Hillsdale, NJ: Lawrence Erlbaum Associates, pp. 95–113.

Olton, D.S. (1986) Interventional approaches to memory: Lesions. In J.L. Martinez and R. Kesner (eds): Learning and Memory: A Biological View. New York: Academic Press, pp. 379–397.

Olton, D.S. (1987a) Temporally constant and temporally changing spatial memory: Single unit correlates in the hippocampus. In P. Ellen and C. Thinus-Blanc (eds): Cognitive Processes and Spatial Orientation in Animal and Man. Dordrecht, The Netherlands: Martinus Nijhoff, pp.16–27.

Olton, D.S. (1987b) The radial arm maze as a tool in neuropharmocology. Physiol. Behav. *40*:793–797.

Olton, D.S. (1988) Spatial perception: Behavioral and single unit analyses. In W.C. Stebbins and M.A. Berkley Comparative Perception. New York: Plenum Press (in press).

Olton, D.S., and W.A. Feustle (1981) Hippocampal function required for nonspatial working memory. Exp. Brain Res. *41*:380–389.

Olton, D.S., and G.L. Wenk (1987) Dementia: Animal models of the cognitive impairments produced by degeneration of the basal forebrain cholinergic system. In H.Y. Meltzer (ed): Psychopharmacology: A Third Generation of Progress. New York: Raven Press, pp. 941–953.

Olton, D.S., C. Wible, and M. Shapiro (1986) Mnemonic theories of hippocampal function. Behav. Neurosci. *100*:852–855.

Platt, J.R. (1964) Strong inference. Science *146*:347–353.

Raffaele, K., and D. Olton (1988) Hippocampal and amygdaloid involvement in working memory for nonspatial stimuli. Behav. Neurosci. *102(3)*:349–355.

Rawlins, J.N.P. (1985) Associations across time: The hippocampus as a temporal memory store. Behav. Brain Sci. *8*:479–497.

Rawlins, J.N.P., and E. Tsaltis (1983) The hippocampus, time, and working memory. Behav. Brain Res. *10*:233–262.

Roitblat, H.L. (1987) Introduction to Comparative Cognition. New York: W.H. Freeman and Company.

Rolls, E.T. (1987) Information representation, processing, and storage in the brain: Analysis at the single neuron level. In J.-P. Changeaux and M. Konishi (eds): The Neural and Molecular Bases of Learning. Berlin: Springer-Verlag, pp. 503–540.

Sakurai, Y. (1988) Thalamocortical, hippocampus, and auditory neuronal activity related to auditory working memory process in the rat. Society for Neuroscience Abstracts 14:862.

Solomon, R. (1979) Temporal versus spatial information processing theories of hippocampal function. Psychol. Bull. *86*:1272–1279.

Solomon, R. (1980) A time and a place for everything? Temporal processing views of hippocampal function with special reference to attention. Physiol. Psychol. *8*:254–261.

Squire, L.R. (1987) Memory and Brain. New York: Oxford University Press.

Squire, L.R., and S. Zola-Morgan (1983) The neurology of memory: The case for correspondence between the findings for humans nonhuman primate. In J.A. Deutsch (ed): The Physiological Basis of Memory. New York: Academic Press, pp. 199–268.

Tulving, E. (1985) On the classification problem in learning and memory. In L. Nilson, and T. Archer (eds): Perspectives On Learning and Memory. Hillsdale, NJ: Lawrence Erlbaum Associates, pp. 67–94.

Watanabe, T., and H. Niki (1985) Hippocampal unit activity and delayed-response in the monkey. Brain Res. *325*:241–254.

Wible, C.G., R.L. Findling, M. Shapiro, E.J. Lang, S. Crane, and D.S. Olton (1986) Mnemonic correlates of unit activity in the hippocampus. Brain Res. *399*:97–110.

Zola-Morgan, S., and L.R. Squire (1986) Memory impairments in monkeys following lesions limited to the hippocampus. Behav. Neurosci. *100*:155–160.

Zola-Morgan, S., L.R. Squire, and D. Amaral (1986) Human amnesia and the medial temporal region: Enduring memory impairment following a bilateral lesion limited to the CA1 field of the hippocampus. J. Neurosci. *6*:2950–2967.

The Hippocampus—New Vistas, pages 425–441
© 1989 Alan R. Liss, Inc.

27
Hippocampal Place Cells and Hippocampal Theories

A. SPEAKMAN AND J. O'KEEFE

MRC Cerebral Functions Group, Department of Anatomy and Developmental Biology, University College, London, England

INTRODUCTION

The hypothesis that the hippocampus is the site of a system of true allocentric spatial learning was expounded in detail by O'Keefe and Nadel (1978) in their book *The Hippocampus as a Cognitive Map*. An alternative hypothesis, that the hippocampus is the site of a system concerned with the temporary storage of all types of information, has been proposed in different forms by several investigators (Marr, 1971; Olton et al., 1979; Rawlins, 1985). The most influential of these latter theories is the proposal of Olton et al. (1979) that the hippocampus is the site of a system of working memory (as opposed to reference memory). Another important class of theory has recently been advanced by Sutherland and Rudy (1988). They proposed a configural association theory: The hippocampus is concerned with unique representations of conjunctions of several stimuli as opposed to simple associations between two individual events. A similar position is taken by Eichenbaum et al. (1988) who have proposed that the hippocampus mediates the storage of relations among multiple stimuli and their associations. The evidence for and against these rival hypotheses is controversial. In support of the "cognitive map" position, several studies have reported that animals with various forms of hippocampal and retrohippocampal damage perform badly when required to discriminate between "places" as opposed to visual or tactile "cues" (O'Keefe et al., 1975; Nadel and MacDonald, 1980; Morris et al., 1982; Jarrard, 1983, 1986; Sutherland et al., 1983; Schenk and Morris, 1985; Okaichi, 1987). In contradiction of the "working-reference memory" hypothesis, Aggleton et al. (1986) have shown that rats with hippocampal lesions can learn a nonspatial test of working memory involving behavioral choices delayed over periods of 60 s. Nevertheless, the other theorists can produce evidence in support of their positions: The results of experiments by Olton and Feustle (1981) and Olton and Papas (1979) support the "working-reference memory" theory; the experiments by Ross et

Abbreviations: CCE, cue-controlled environment; df, degrees of freedom; *P*, probability; S.E., standard error; SRR, stimulus-response-reinforcement; SWM, spatial working memory; SRM, spatial reference memory.

al. (1984) and Eichenbaum et al. (1988) support the "configural association" position.

The best evidence in favor of the cognitive map hypothesis comes from the study of complex spike cell activity in the hippocampus. Hippocampal complex spike cells fire at particular locations within an environment (O'Keefe and Dostrovsky, 1971) and have been christened *place cells* (O'Keefe, 1976). O'Keefe and Nadel (1978) proposed that these cells are the functional elements in a system representing the spatial features of an environment and all the interconnections between them. There has been a tendency for other theories of hippocampal function to neglect evidence concerning place cells. However, more recently, serious attempts have been made to evaluate the actions of complex spike cells in terms of those theories. Sutherland and Rudy (1988) reinterpreted complex spike activity in terms of configural associations—the unit firing represents the association of several arbitrary environmental events, either simultaneously occurring or temporally discontiguous. Olton (1987) proposed that complex spike units encode various temporal aspects of available spatial information; thus they signal to the brain the salient events that change or remain the same over time in a given spatial location.

Our aim in recent experiments has been to determine the controlling factors of place cell firing. The experiments have used a particular training environment (the cue-controlled environment [CCE]) first described by O'Keefe and Conway (1978). The important point about experiments conducted within the CCE is that the experimenters have the ability to identify, control, and manipulate the cues used by an animal to solve a spatial learning task. The manipulations take place at the same time as the monitoring of the cells' activity and the observation of the outcomes of behavioral choices. This chapter will summarize several of our most recent experiments using the CCE training apparatus and will also discuss some of the properties of place cells that have been established in our own and other laboratories. We believe that the phenomena to be discussed must be accounted for by all comprehensive hippocampal theories and that we can evaluate the theories by examining their treatment of this evidence.

CORRELATES OF COMPLEX SPIKE CELL ACTIVITY IN THE CCE: SPATIAL REFERENCE MEMORY

A schematic overhead view of the CCE environment is presented in Figure 1. It can be seen that the apparatus consists of an elevated plus-shaped maze set within a circular curtained enclosure. Six cues hang from the enclosure ceiling or are attached to the curtains. Rats are placed down in one of the arms of the plus maze, and their task is to run to one of the other three arms where they will find food. The task is designed so that the food can only be located by reference to the six cues. Thus, the food is found at a fixed position in relation to the cues, and the constellation of cues is rotated by multiples of 90° between trials so that all other external cues are made irrelevant. Rats readily learn this task and perform consistently at a high standard (O'Keefe and Conway, 1980). Using the operational definition of Olton et al. (1979), we can classify this task as a (spatial) reference memory procedure. The rat learns

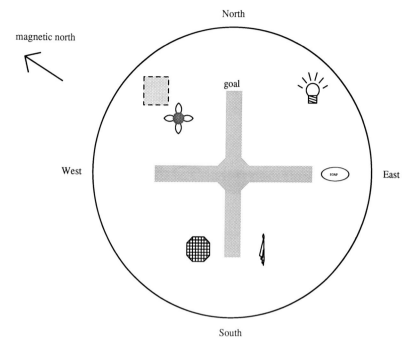

Fig. 1. Layout of the cue-controlled environment. An elevated plus maze is situated within a set of floor-length curtains. Six controlled cues are shown in this example: a light, a towel, a cage, a card, a fan, and a bar of soap. In other experiments we used different cues (for example a toilet air freshener instead of the bar of soap). The direction of magnetic north is shown as well as the arbitrary directions termed North, East, South, and West (in this particular instance the goal is in the North).

about the mutual relationships between the locations of the cues and the goal, the important aspect being that these learned relationships do not change from trial to trial.

Our recent experiments (O'Keefe and Speakman, 1987a) have confirmed the previous reports of various investigators (O'Keefe, 1976; Hill, 1976; Olton et al., 1978; Muller et al., 1987) that the principal correlate of hippocampal complex spike cell firing is the animal's location in an environment; that is, the cells fire in particular places and are therefore called *place cells*. Thus in the CCE the animal learned to define its location in relation to the controlled cues, and we therefore found that the place cells fired in a fixed spatial relationship to them. This relationship was clearly evident, because the four possible positions of the controlled cues corresponded to four distinct place field positions (see Fig. 2). The place cells were therefore firing at a fixed position in relation to the cues, but at four different places in relation to the outside world. Thus, if the four possible sets of place fields are rotated so that in each case the cues superimpose in the same orientation (with the goal at the top

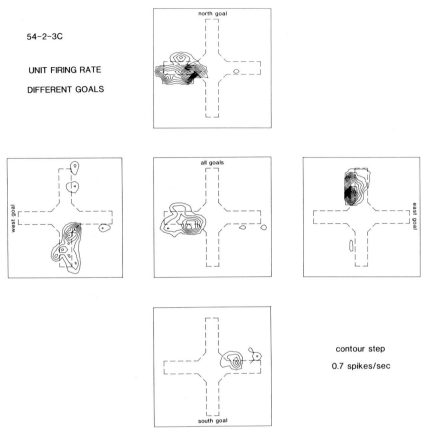

Fig. 2.   Place fields of unit 54-2-3c at different orientations of the controlled cues. Each plot represents data from several superimposed trials. In the central plot all the trials have been rotated (so that the rat's goal is at the top) before being superimposed. In all five cases the rat visited all parts of the elevated plus maze, and contour lines have been added to show the place field(s). Successive contours represent progressively higher firing rates (number of spikes in a location divided by the total time spent at that location); the contour step (spikes · s^{-1}) is 0.7. The numbers of trials at each goal orientation were North, 9; East, 10; South, 7; West, 10 (total, 36).

of the picture) then the fields are in exactly the same position in each case (see Fig. 2, central panel). This manipulation reveals that place cell firing is determined by a set of familiar landmarks, which can be controlled. After recent experiments, Muller and Kubie (1987) came to the same conclusion, although they used a single salient landmark.

Earlier experiments by Kubie and Ranck (1983) showed that, when an animal is exposed to several different environments, the pattern of unit activity is stable but unique in each case. Therefore, place cell activity seems to reflect an animal's learning about the spatial relationships between the landmarks in an environment and its ability to distinguish it from other environments. It seems likely that the place cell activity represents the output from a (reference) memory system that stores and retrieves the unique spatial characteristics of an environment. An alternative view is that the place cells are only related to the remembered arrangement of the cues in a secondary manner. Their job might simply be to learn about arbitrary and unique conjunctions of the impinging stimuli (as suggested by Sutherland and Rudy, 1988) and then feed this information forward for further analysis. Evidence against this contention was provided by the experiment of O'Keefe and Conway (1978) in which a rat was put into a cue-controlled environment in which any two of four controlled cues had been removed. The place fields remained in the same places, and the rat behaved as usual. This indicates that place cell firing is not signalling a unique conjunction of stimuli, because it is active when any of the constituent elements of a configuration are present. For example, if we consider any two of the four cues, the cell will fire when they are present simultaneously and separately and when both are absent. Furthermore, evidence to be presented in the following two sections suggests that place cells are not tied in any strict sense to the moment-to-moment state of the spatial surround. An example comes from reference memory trials in which the rat makes a mistake—the place fields then correspond to where the animal thinks the cues are (as evidenced by his behavioral choice) rather than to where they really are (see Fig. 9 in Speakman, 1987).

A statistical analysis of data from 55 units has added to our understanding of place cells (O'Keefe and Speakman, 1987a). As might be expected, we found that the largest amount of variance in unit firing rates could be accounted for by the animal's spatial location in relation to the controlled cues (37 out of the 55 firing patterns were significantly related to the position of the cues). However, in a small number of cells (16) the unit firing pattern was significantly related to the static background cues (the uncontrolled cues that did not define the goal and did not rotate between trials, e.g. smells on the maze, noises from the recording apparatus). A further interesting aspect of some cells (19) was an interaction between the controlled cues and the static background cues. One manifestation of this effect is illustrated in Figure 2. It can be seen that the place cell in this case always fired in a fixed location relative to the controlled cues (its place field). However, the amplitude of firing in the place field depended on the particular orientation of the controlled cue constellation within the real world. The firing was most intense when the controlled cues indicated that the food was to be found in the North or East and was much less intense when the goal was in the South or West. In some cases we found that these variations in firing rates at particular goal orientations were attributable to the different times at which firing began in the field. Thus, place firing began early in a trial when the goal was in the North or East but only began at a much later time when the goal was in the South or West. We have speculated that these variations in onset time represent different degrees of difficulty the animal may experience in retrieving the reference memory representation of the environment in each case. One possibility is that there is a serial search through separate representations for each of the four possible cue orientations. A more attractive possibility, given the similarity between the place cell firing patterns at each of the cue orientations, is that one representation has to be manipulated into a "best fit" form in each case. Thus it may be that there is a default representation for the environment with the cues in the North goal orientation (possibly including the static background cues). When the goal is not in the North the available representation may be adapted to fit (e.g. rotated, filtered, scaled). This idea is very speculative, but it fits well with the latest results reported by Muller and Kubie (1987). In their experiments direct changes in the size of an environment resulted, in some cases, in appropriate decreases or increases in the size of a place field (although the scaling was not exact).

Figure 3 illustrates the development of a place field over time and shows different aspects of the firing pattern of the single place cell shown in Figure 2. The periods either early or late within a trial and when the animal was either stationary or moving have been accumulated separately and displayed in the respective panels. The place field firing patterns under these different circumstances were very similar and found to be highly intercorrelated (mean correlation coefficient, 0.70 ± 0.03 S.E., all $Ps < 0.001$). In each case the region of high firing activity remained substantially in the same place. This occurred even though the rate of firing *within* the field showed certain variations: It was generally higher when the rat was moving as opposed to stationary, it also increased as time progressed. These results suggest that 1) the location and shape of a place field is not a function of the animal's behavior in that part of the environment, but equally that 2) nonspatial factors can influence the *firing rate* within the place field (see O'Keefe 1976, 1979; McNaughton et al., 1983a). Some of these nonspatial factors include the time since the animal entered the field, the speed with which the animal traverses the field, the direction in which the animal points in the field, and, as described in the previous paragraph, the orientation of the field relative to (unknown) background cues. In addition, some cells increase their activity during exploratory sniffing in the field either because an expected cue has been removed or because an unexpected cue has been added. Factors that do not influence the field firing rate are motivational levels or the presence of incentives such as rewards within the field (see Effects of Moving the Goal: Goal Relocation Trials, below).

Two proposals made by O'Keefe (1976, 1979) were also confirmed by the study of O'Keefe and Speakman (1987a). First, place fields do not cluster around significant regions in an environment, such as the goal. Rather they are distributed with equal density across the entire environmental surface. The recent study by Muller et al. (1987) reached the same conclusion (although a study by Eichenbaum et al. [1987] claimed that the place fields cluster around particular regions). Second, neighboring cells within the hippocampus have place

54-2-3C   UNIT FIRING RATE

PERCEPTUAL

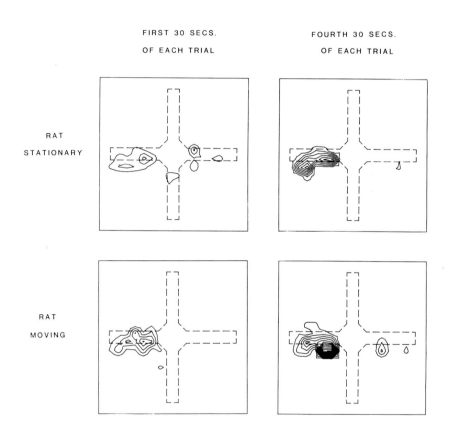

FIRST 30 SECS.   FOURTH 30 SECS.

OF EACH TRIAL   OF EACH TRIAL

RAT

STATIONARY

RAT

MOVING

contour step :- 0.7 spikes/sec

Fig. 3. Place fields for unit 54-2-3c displayed in the same manner as the central plot in Figure 2 (all trials superimposed with the goal rotated to the top). Each plot shows the place field during a different type of behavioral activity (stationary vs. moving) and temporal period within a trial (early vs. late). Data from the first 30 s of all 36 trials were used to form the left side "early" panels; the cues were present for the full 2 min for 24 of these trials, and the data from the last 30 s of these form the "late" panels.

fields that are as likely to be widely separated as they are to overlap. There is no topographical relationship between adjacent places in the environment and the place fields of neighboring units. Using the stereotrode technique of isolating single unit activity from multichannel multiunit activity (McNaughton et al., 1983b), we found that clusters of neighboring units have widely dispersed fields. One cluster of eight units produced place fields that covered almost the entire surface of the plus maze (Fig. 12 in O'Keefe and Speakman, 1987a). These findings suggest to us that the representation of an environment is distributed across the hippocampus and that any small hippocampal area will contain enough information to identify approximately an animal's location.

EFFECTS OF REMOVING THE CUES: SPATIAL WORKING MEMORY

We adapted the spatial reference memory trials described above to study working memory. During spatial working memory trials the rat was placed on the start arm of the plus maze with the cues present, but was not allowed to run to the goal. Then the six cues defining the position of the goal were removed, and, after a delay, the rat was required to run to the goal. The study of O'Keefe and Conway (1980) showed that rats perform this delayed response task well and that they do it without using residual cues such as odor markers. This is a working memory procedure as defined by Olton et al. (1979), because the information on which the animal's choice is based changes from trial to trial. We found that the place fields of complex spike cells remained in the same place during the delay (working memory) periods. That is, the fields established by a particular arrangement of cues persisted when the cues were removed. Of 30 place cells studied using this type of trial, 27 produced a significant correlation when the firing from the predelay and delay periods was compared. Fig 4 (upper panels) shows place fields both before ("perceptual") and after ("memory") the cues were removed. It can clearly be seen that there is no change in the location of the place fields from one period to the other, although there may be an increase in the firing rate.

It seems probable to us that the place fields during the delay periods of SWM trials represent the rat's remembered location within the spatial arrangement of the environment. We therefore believe that the place cells are the site of a spatial learning system or one of its immediate targets. We have described these learning trials, in terms used by Olton et al. (1979), as *working memory* and *reference memory* trials. However, the similarity between place cell activity during the reference and working memory periods (when the cues were present and absent, respectively) tends to imply that one unitary memory system is involved and this was used to get to the goal during both periods. In response, Olton (1987) has introduced a new concept to explain the results of SWM trials in this experiment. Place units are referred to as the substrate of "temporally constant spatial memory"—memory for the constant aspects of a spatial scene that persist despite substantial changes in its original appearance. Thus place

UNIT FIRING RATE   45-2-9

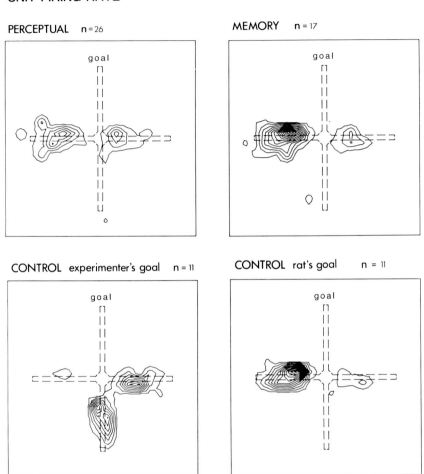

PERCEPTUAL   n = 26

MEMORY   n = 17

CONTROL experimenter's goal   n = 11

CONTROL rat's goal   n = 11

contour step = 1·5 spikes per sec

Fig. 4.   Place fields for unit 45-2-9 displayed in the same manner as the central plot of Figure 2. "Perceptual" represents those periods from SRM and SWM trials during which the cues were present. "Memory" represents the delay period of SWM trials after the cues were removed. "Control" represents the control trials superimposed in two different forms. On the lower left the trials are rotated and superimposed with the experimenter-chosen goal at the top of the panel. On the lower right the same trials are rotated and superimposed with the goal chosen by the rat at the top. In this and subsequent figures, "n" indicates the number of trials superimposed.

units reflect the rat's decision to treat a changed environment the same as before. Similarly, Sutherland and Rudy (1988) interpreted these results as "unit firing correlated with specific events [that] significantly outlast[s] the event."

EFFECTS OF NOT PRESENTING THE CUES: CONTROL TRIALS

Another type of trial, called a control trial, throws light on these rival interpretations. Control trials were conducted in exactly the same way as the spatial working memory trials described above; however, the rats were not put onto the plus maze until the delay period when the controlled cues had been removed. Thus the rats had not seen the original orientation of the controlled cues, and, as might be expected, they found it impossible to choose the goal correctly. These trials were designed to control for the effects of residual cues and experimenter effects in the experiment. However, they also provided important information about the place cell system, because we found that rats did usually choose to run to one of the maze arms, even though it was wrong. Furthermore, we found that the place cells were firing in an entirely consistent manner; that is, the place fields were related to the position of the chosen arm (intended goal) in the environment, but not to the position of the real goal. If the place cell fired in the maze arm opposite the goal when the cues were present, it would do so in the control case when the rat chose to run (erroneously) to the arm opposite the start arm. In other words, the place fields were consistent with where the rat *thought* the goal was, not with where it really was. Using this information we were often able to predict the rat's choice during a control trial before the rat was allowed to make it. Interestingly, Muller and Kubie (1987) reported a phenomenon that may have the same explanation. In their experiment, place field firing was controlled by a single polarizing card stimulus (on the cage wall). When this was removed, the place fields would sometimes rotate to unpredictable angular coordinates relative to the remaining environment.

Minimal numbers of control trials were presented because they often disrupted the subsequent learned performance of trained rats. Nevertheless, we managed to study eight units (from four animals) during this type of trial. We found that the mean correlation coefficient between the firing pattern on these trials and that during spatial reference memory trials was 0.11 ($\pm$ 0.05 S.E.; seven of the eight coefficients were not significant; one was significant, $0.05 > P > 0.01$). However, if the control trial data were reoriented to correspond to the rat's goal and not to the experimenter's goal, then the mean correlation rose to 0.58 ($\pm$ 0.06 S.E.; all $Ps < 0.01$). Figure 4 illustrates these findings. The lower left panel in Figure 4 shows the place cell firing relative to the goal defined by the experimenter. The lower right panel in Figure 4 shows the place fields when the trials were superimposed with the goal chosen by the rat rotated to the top of the picture. It can be seen that the picture of place field activity in the lower right panel of Figure 4 is very similar to that produced during a normal spatial reference memory trial (upper left panel).

We interpret the activity of place fields during control trials as the activation of a spatial map in the absence of the controlled cues. The rats tended to choose a particular arm in a decisive manner during these trials, and we believe that this represents the recall and use of a "preferred" representation of the environment. It seems plausible to assume that, following the initial exploration of an environment, a map of the environment is established that is at a particular orientation with respect to the background cues. When the animal enters the environment in the presence of the controlled cues the "preferred" representation is changed to correspond to the orientation of the stimulus configuration. However, if the controlled cues are not present, the "preferred" map orientation is still recalled by the background cues and is used in their absence.

Control trials are difficult to interpret within the schemes of both Olton (1987, 1988) and Sutherland and Rudy (1988). In both theories, the place cell firing is evoked or recalled by aspects of the spatial scene, and it can then persist during periods in which the original stimuli have been altered or removed. However, during control trials, the original stimulation, which is supposed to establish the place cell firing, is not experienced. For example, Olton (1987) suggested that place cells encode the temporally constant aspects of the spatial scene in a dynamic manner. Thus he explained the spatial working memory trials by proposing cells that fire in relation to the "temporally constant" controlled cues; these cells then recode their firing over time onto other unidentified but similarly constant background cues. This explains how the place fields persist when the controlled cues are removed. However, during control trials, the controlled cues were not seen at all, and therefore the firing cannot be related to the same temporally constant aspects of the scene (unless that constancy is provided by the goal location; see Effects of Moving the Goal: Goal Relocation Trials, below).

EFFECTS OF TRANSPOSING THE ANIMAL'S LOCATION DURING A TRIAL: DETOUR TRIALS

Another type of trial conducted by O'Keefe and Speakman (1987a) presents further difficulties for the two alternative theories considered here. Detour trials, based on the spatial working memory trial, were presented to one rat. During a detour trial, the rat was forced to enter a nongoal arm during the memory delay period. Only after this "detour" was the animal allowed to choose the goal. We found that the place fields that would normally be seen in any particular maze arm were also seen when the same arm was used as a detour arm. Figure 5 illustrates the place fields seen during spatial reference and working memory trials and the fields of the same cell when the detour periods of detour trials were examined. It can be seen that the fields are substantially the same, although there is a difference in firing rate. Eleven place units were studied using detour trials. The mean correlation coefficient when the unit firing activity during SRM trials was compared with that during detour trials was 0.52 ($\pm$ 0.06 S.E., all $Ps < 0.01$).

UNIT FIRING RATE   55-2-3A'

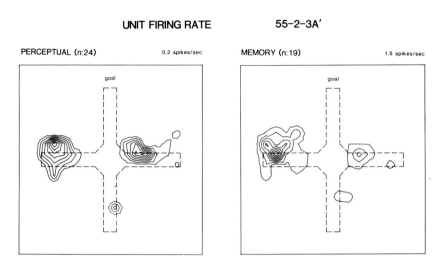

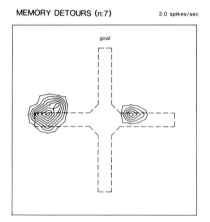

Fig. 5.   Place fields for unit 55-2-3a. The top two panels were formed in the same way as the comparable panels in Figure 4. The lower left panel represents data from detour periods: when the rat was forced to enter another arm during the delay period (in the absence of the cues). Note that the contour step is different in each of the three cases.

The importance of these findings stems, first, from the fact that the cues were absent throughout the detour period. The fields seen during the detour period cannot therefore be described as "outlasting" the stimulus configuration, because they were never evoked during the immediately preceding period when the cues were presented (the animal was in a different arm). Second, the unit firing during detour trials is important because the same place fields *were* seen on other occasions when the animal visited the arm with the cues present. This indicates that place field responses are not merely isolated responses to unique conjunctions of perceived stimuli. It is true that the place responses for each location in a particular environment can be evoked by presenting the animal with the cues that directly define its position. However, all the same place responses can spontaneously appear in the absence of direct sensory stimulation as the animal enters the same locations during a detour. Therefore, the detour trial indicates that place unit activity must correspond to an inter-connected set of representations of the spatial scene, the activation of one small part of which recalls the representation of the whole. We interpret this as the description of a map-like structure.

EFFECTS OF MOVING THE GOAL: GOAL RELOCATION TRIALS

One possible alternative explanation for the interdependent activity of place cells has been considered in a subsequent paper by O'Keefe and Speakman (1987b). The explanation is based on the fact that the controlled cues and the goal always bear a fixed topographical relationship to each other. Thus, to reach the goal from any particular place the rat always had to make a particular turn. The unit firing might therefore represent some intentional or motivational process that precedes a body turn or some other aspect of the rat's knowledge of where the goal is. For example, Hunter (1913) noted that his rats maintained a consistent orientation toward the goal in the original delayed reaction task. According to this hypothesis the similar pattern of firing during the presence or absence of the cues (see Effects of Removing the Cues: Spatial Working Memory, above) is no surprise, because it is related to something constant to the two situations and only indirectly to the cue constellation. Similarly, the unit firing that appears during the detour trials merely represents the animal's recalculation of which particular turn is required to reach the goal from a new location.

A similar point has been made recently by two groups, both starting from the observation that nonspatial variables appear to affect the activity of com-plex-spike units. Thus the study by Wible et al. (1986) demonstrated that com-plex spike cells fired maximally in two goal boxes only under certain conditions and phases of a visual discrimination task. Olton (1988) used this finding as the basis for his proposal that place fields are established by a spatial con-stellation of stimuli, but they then are sensitive to the temporal constancy of the stimulus-response-reinforcement (SRR) contingencies operating within an environment. With this idea in mind, he proposed that place fields persist at the same locations during the detour and spatial working memory trials de-scribed above because "the relatively major stimulus changes in the experi-ments of O'Keefe . . . reflected a continuity (rather than a change) in SRR con-tingencies (the correct arm was still in the same location and the way to get to that arm was still the same after the spatial stimuli were altered)."

A similar point has been made by Eichenbaum et al. (1987). In an odor dis-crimination task they found that 15% of hippocampal cells fired during the sam-pling of particular discriminative cues with learned significance. However, the majority of cells (60%) were classified as goal-approach cells: The cells were said to fire during locomotion or orientation toward either the goal or the cue sampling port. Eichenbaum et al. (1987) asserted that the goal-approach cells were equivalent to those classified as place cells by other investigators (p. 729). However, they proposed that the correlates of the cell firing could be characterized as "orientation movements with respect to specific targets of attention i.e. goals" (p. 730). With regard to the apparent spatial correlates of place/goal-approach cells, they conceded that the cells fire in relation to the absolute (allocentric) location of the target (not to the animal's egocentric perspective of it). However, they concluded that "the best description of goal-approach cells is that they fire during an act of orientation toward a target of attention, regardless of its immediate egocentric perspective or the movements required to obtain it" (p. 731).

We have listed many reasons for believing that these explanations are unlikely to be true (O'Keefe and Speakman, 1987a, p.23). However, we also undertook a direct test of the hypothesis by moving the location of the goal halfway through a series of spatial reference memory trials (O'Keefe and Speakman, 1987b). Place cells were recorded as three rats were initially trained with the goal in one place relative to the controlled cues; they were then retrained with the goal shifted by 180° relative to the cues. We found that place fields remained in the same position *relative to the controlled cues* whatever the location of the goal. They did not rotate by 180° relative to the controlled cues as one would expect if the fields were related to the goal location. Figure 6 presents illustrations of the same place field both before and after the goal was moved. In both diagrams the controlled cues are in the same orientation; only the position of the food location (goal) has changed. Figure 6 represents a powerful argument against the case for goal-approach cells made by Eichenbaum et al. (1987). It can be seen that the field illustrated in Figure 6 is initially found at the location occupied by the goal. However, the field remains in the same place (in relation to the cues) when the goal is moved to another location. Thus the place field is unaffected by the substantial changes that take place in the rat's orientation toward, attention toward, and intended movements toward the new learned target.

We performed a correlational analysis on similar data from 19 place cells. When place field firing in relation to the position of the controlled cues was compared before and after the goal was moved, the mean correlation coefficient was 0.40 ($\pm$ 0.05 S.E.). When place field activity in relation to the spatial position of the goal was compared before and after the goal was moved, the mean was significantly lower (0.14 $\pm$ 0.04 S.E., t test for correlated samples, $0.01 > P > 0.001$, df = 18). After further statistical and visual analysis, we classified the activity of 14 cells as being clearly related to the location of the controlled cues. Two cells were classified as "goal-related," and a further three cells were unclassified. We therefore concluded that the activity of the majority of place cells is unrelated to the goal or to the intended movements toward the goal. In Olton's terms (1988), we believe this experiment represents a major change in SRR contingencies that was not associated with a corresponding change in unit firing and that therefore the data do not support his contention.

72-2-5B   UNIT FIRING RATE

BEFORE (n:12)   AFTER (n:13)

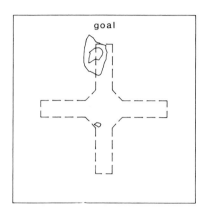
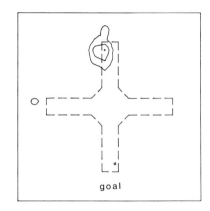

contour step — 0.8 spikes per sec

Fig. 6. Place fields of unit 72-2-5b. The two panels were formed in the same way as the "perceptual" plots in Figure 4. The left panel represents trials before the goal was moved. The right panel represents trials after the rat had learned the new location of the goal. The controlled cues are not shown but are in the same locations in each panel; only the goal changes position.

SUMMARY

The activity of an individual place cell reflects an animal's location in relation to the landmarks in an environment. As a population, therefore, place cells provide a representation of the spatial topography of a particular environment. The experiments described in Correlates of Complex Spike Cell Activity in the CCE: Spatial Reference Memory indicate that the representation has a distributed structure and that it can be subjected to various manipulations. In addition, place cells have a clear mnemonic role: In a familiar environment they can continue to represent an animal's remembered spatial position in the absence of the landmarks that initially defined it. The place cell activity under these circumstances is related to the animal's cognitive processes: It reliably predicts the animal's behavioral choice. We believe that these results support the cognitive map theory of hippocampal function (O'Keefe and Nadel, 1978). The results from control, detour, and goal relocation trials are also supportive and present three problems for rival interpretations of hippocampal function.

First, place cell activity is not bound to the state of the current stimulus array. Second, place cell actions are mutually interlinked and interdependent. Third, place fields are not related to any aspect of the learned goal or the animal's movements and motivation to reach it.

REFERENCES

Aggleton, J.P., P.R. Hunt, and J.N.P Rawlins (1986) The effects of hippocampal lesions upon spatial and non-spatial tests of working memory. Behav. Brain Res. *19*:133–146.

Eichenbaum, H., A. Fagan, P. Mathews and N.J. Cohen (1988) Hippocampal system dysfunction and odor discrimination learning in rats: Impairment or facilitation depending on representational demands. Behav. Neurosci. 102:331–339.

Eichenbaum, H., M. Kuperstein, A. Fagan, and J. Nagode (1987) Cue-sampling and goal-approach correlates of hippocampal unit activity in rats performing an odor discrimination task. J. Neurosci. *7*:716–732.

Hill, A.J. (1976) Neuronal activity in the hippocampus during a spatial alternation task. Soc. Neurosci. Abstr. *2*:388.

Hunter, W.S. (1913) The delayed reaction in animals and children. Behav. Monogr. *2*:1–86.

Jarrard, L.E. (1983) Selective hippocampal lesions and behaviour. Effects of kainic acid lesions on the performance of place and cue tasks. Behav. Neurosci. *97*:873–889.

Jarrard, L.E. (1986) Selective hippocampal lesions and behaviour: Implications for current research and theorizing. In R.L. Isaacson and K.H. Pribram (eds): The Hippocampus, Vol. 4. New York: Plenum Press, pp. 93–126.

Kubie, J.L., and J.B. Ranck (1983) Sensory-behavioural correlates in individual hippocampus neurons in three situations: Space and context. In W. Seifert (ed): Neurobiology of the Hippocampus. London: Academic Press, pp. 433–437.

Marr, D. (1971) Simple memory: A theory for archicortex. Philos. Trans. R. Soc. [Biol.] *262*:23–81.

McNaughton, B.L., C.A. Barnes, and J. O'Keefe (1983a) The contributions of position, direction and velocity to single unit activity in the hippocampus of freely-moving rats. Exp. Brain Res. *52*:41–49.

McNaughton, B.L., J. O'Keefe, and C.A. Barnes (1983b) The stereotrode, a new technique for simultaneous isolation of several single units in the central nervous system from multiple unit records. J. Neurosci. Methods *8*:391–397.

Morris, R.G.M., P. Garrud, J.N.P. Rawlins, and J. O'Keefe (1982) Place navigation impaired in rats with hippocampal lesions. Nature *297*:681–683.

Muller, R.U., and J.L Kubie (1987) The effects of changes in the environment on the spatial firing of hippocampal complex-spike cells. J. Neurosci. *7*:1951–1968.

Muller, R.U., J.L. Kubie, and J.B. Ranck (1987) Spatial firing patterns of hippocampal complex-spike cells in a fixed environment. J. Neurosci. *7*:1935–1950.

Nadel, L., and L. MacDonald (1980) Hippocampus: Cognitive map or working memory? Behav. Neural. Biol. *29*:405–409.

Okaichi, H. (1987) Performance and dominant strategies on place and cue tasks following hippocampal lesions in rats. Psychobiology *15*:58–63.

O'Keefe, J. (1976) Place units in the hippocampus of the freely moving rat. Exp. Neurol. *51*:78–109.

O'Keefe, J. (1979) A review of the hippocampal place cells. Prog. Neurobiol. *13*:419–439.

O'Keefe, J., and D.H. Conway (1978) Hippocampal place units in the freely moving rat: Why they fire where they fire. Exp. Brain Res. *31*:573–590.

O'Keefe, J., and D.H. Conway (1980) On the trail of the hippocampal engram. Physiol. Psychol. *8:*229–238.

O'Keefe, J., and J. Dostrovsky (1971) The hippocampus as a cognitive map. Preliminary evidence from unit activity in freely moving rats. Brain Res. *34:*171–175.

O'Keefe, J., and L. Nadel (1978) The Hippocampus as a Cognitive Map. Oxford: Clarendon Press.

O'Keefe, J., L. Nadel, S. Keightley, and D. Kill (1975) Fornix lesions selectively abolish place learning in the rat. Exp. Neurol. *48:*152–166.

O'Keefe, J., and A. Speakman (1987a) Single unit activity in the rat hippocampus during a spatial memory task. Exp. Brain Res. *68:*1–27.

O'Keefe, J., and A. Speakman (1987b) Hippocampal place field activity is not related to the location of the goal or the intended response in the cue-controlled environment. Neurosci. Lett. *29:*S96.

Olton, D.S. (1987) Temporally constant and temporally changing spatial memory: Single unit correlates in the hippocampus. In P. Ellen and C. Thinus-Blanc (eds): Cognitive Processes and Spatial Orientation in Animal and Man, Vol II. Neurophysiology and Developmental Aspects. Dordrecht, The Netherlands: Martinus Nijhoff, pp. 16–27.

Olton, D.S. (1988) Spatial perception: Behavioral and neural analyses. In W.C. Stebbins and M.A Berkley (eds): Comparative Perception (in press).

Olton, D.S., J.T. Becker, and G.E. Handelmann (1979) Hippocampus, space and memory. Behav. Brain Sci. *2:*313–365.

Olton, D.S., M. Branch, and P.J. Best (1978) Spatial correlates of hippocampal unit activity. Exp. Neurol. *58:*387–409.

Olton, D.S., and W.A. Feustle (1981) Hippocampal function required for non-spatial working memory. Exp. Brain Res. *41:*380–389.

Olton, D.S., and B.C. Papas (1979) Spatial memory and hippocampal function. Neuro-psychologia *17:*669–682.

Rawlins, J.N.P (1985) Associations across time: The hippocampus as a temporary memory store. Behav. Brain Sci. *8:*479–496.

Ross, R.T., W.B. Orr, P.C. Holland, and T.W. Berger (1984) Hippocampectomy disrupts acquisition and retention of learned conditional responding. Behav. Neurosci. *98:*211–225.

Schenk, F., and R.G.M. Morris (1985) Dissociation between components of spatial memory in rats after recovery from the effects of retrohippocampal lesions. Exp. Brain Res. *58:*11–28.

Speakman, A. (1987) Place cells in the brain: Evidence for a cognitive map. Sci. Prog. *71:*511–530.

Sutherland, R.J., and J.W. Rudy (1988) Configural association theory: The role of the hippocampal formation in learning, memory and amnesia. Submitted for publication.

Sutherland, R.J., I.Q. Whishaw, and B. Kolb (1983) A behavioural analysis of spatial localization following electrolytic, kainate- or colchine-induced damage to the hip-pocampal formation in the rat. Behav. Brain Res. *7:*133–153.

Wible, C.G., R.L. Findling, M. Shapiro, E.J. Lang, S. Crane, and D.S. Olton (1986) Mnemonic correlates of unit activity in the hippocampus. Brain Res. *399:*97–110.

The Hippocampus—New Vistas, pages 443–461

28
Chemically Defined Hippocampal Interneurons and Their Possible Relationship to Seizure Mechanisms

ROBERT S. SLOVITER

Neurology Research Center, Helen Hayes Hospital, New York State Department of Health, West Haverstraw, New York and Departments of Pharmacology and Neurology, College of Physicians and Surgeons, Columbia University, New York, New York

INTRODUCTION

The hippocampus is a subject of intense study for several reasons. Its laminar structure greatly facilitates anatomical studies of hippocampal afferent and efferent pathways, and its cell types exhibit differences in morphology, location, and chemical content that permit meaningful classification. In addition, the tightly clustered principal cell populations (granule and pyramidal cells) generate extracellular voltage shifts in response to afferent stimulation that reflect the state of hippocampal excitability and inhibition (Andersen et al., 1966; Lømo, 1971). Painstaking studies by hippocampal anatomists and physiologists have constructed a framework for experimental studies in which changes in hippocampal structure and function can be interpreted meaningfully. The studies described in this chapter have focused on experimentally induced changes in hippocampal morphology, excitability, and inhibition that are relevant to the epileptic state and possibly caused by the selective loss of particular hippocampal interneurons.

The experiments that led us to this subject began with an effort to determine the cause of the seizure-associated pattern of hippocampal damage seen in a high proportion of patients suffering from intractable, cryptogenic temporal lobe epilepsy (Meldrum and Corsellis, 1984). During the last decade, experimental studies in many laboratories suggested that seizure activity itself might be the causative factor in epileptic brain damage (Olney et al., 1979; Ben-Ari et al., 1979; Nadler and Cuthbertson, 1980; Meldrum and Corsellis, 1984). If so, how does excessive presynaptic activity alone cause postsynaptic damage? Olney (1983) hypothesized that excessive excitation results in the release and extracellular accumulation of "endogenous excitotoxin," possibly glutamate or aspartate, that if present at its receptors in a sufficient concentration for a critical period, is neurotoxic. According to this view (Olney's "excitotoxic hypothesis"), excitatory amino acid-containing neurons are inherently capable of destroying the cells they innervate.

PERFORANT PATHWAY STIMULATION AND HIPPOCAMPAL DAMAGE

It is difficult to test the intriguing hypothesis that excitatory activity alone can be neurotoxic if seizures are induced with a convulsant drug. Using this approach, it is impossible to determine which effects are due to an action of the drug, which changes are due to the seizures produced by the drug, or which effects are secondary to metabolic changes that accompany motor convulsions.

We attempted to solve the epileptic brain damage enigma by evoking seizure discharges from the hippocampal granule cells with electrical stimulation of the perforant pathway. This afferent pathway projects monosynaptically to the granule cells from the temporal neocortex (Andersen et al., 1966; Lømo, 1971). With focal stimulation, the seizure activity evoked from hippocampal granule cells is of a known cause and initiation site, and it can be controlled quite precisely. With stimulation in urethane-anesthetized animals, motor convulsions and physiological variables that change as a result of convulsions do not occur. By stimulating unilaterally, the unstimulated and relatively undamaged hippocampus of each animal serves as a control for anatomical and electrophysiological studies in which interanimal variability can be a significant problem. Using this experimental design, we reproduced the full pattern of seizure-associated hippocampal damage unilaterally with focal stimulation outside the hippocampus (Sloviter and Damiano, 1981; Sloviter, 1983). Interestingly, perforant pathway stimulation produced little damage to the dentate granule cells, which are directly innervated by the perforant pathway fibers, whereas it did damage dentate hilar cells and CA3 pyramidal cells, two cell populations innervated monosynaptically by the granule cells. In addition, the acute damage was produced in the exact region of area CA3 (stratum lucidum) where the mossy fibers (axons of the granule cells) innervate the CA3 pyramidal cells (Fig. 1).

Significantly, if perforant pathway stimulation evoked dendritic field excitatory postsynaptic potentials (EPSPs) but no granule cell population spikes, no damage to hilar neurons and CA3 pyramidal cells resulted (Sloviter, 1983). Therefore, damage to the cells innervated by the granule cells occurred only when granule cells generated synchronous discharges. Since the animals were anesthetized with urethane and did not convulse or stop breathing, the damage could not be due to factors secondary to motor convulsions. Also, granule cell seizure activity was recorded extracellularly throughout the period during which the damage occurred, suggesting that damage was not the result of generalized hippocampal anoxia since anoxia rapidly prevents evoked activity. The damage was also not due solely to blood-borne metabolic factors, i.e. altered pH, lactate, and so forth, since the hippocampus on the unstimulated side was relatively undamaged. The results of this experiment (Sloviter and Damiano, 1981; Sloviter, 1983) and another showing that intraventricular injection of glutamate or

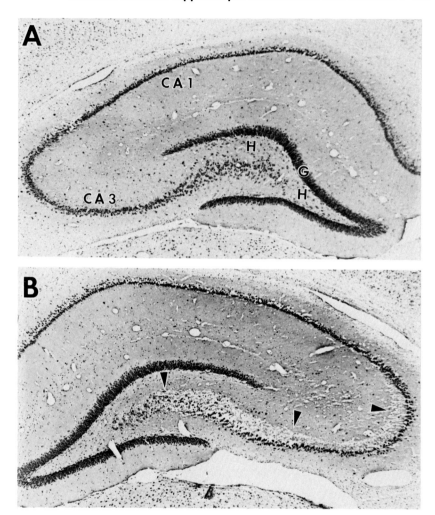

Fig. 1. Effect of 24 h intermittent perforant pathway stimulation on hippocampal morphology. **A:** Unstimulated side. **B:** Stimulated side. Perfusion fixation immediately after stimulation as described previously (Sloviter, 1983, 1987). Note acute reaction in hilus (H) and region of CA3 innervated by the mossy fibers (arrowheads), the axons of the dentate granule cells (G). Paraffin embedded; cresyl violet stain.

aspartate reproduced all of the morphological hippocampal effects of perforant pathway stimulation (Sloviter and Dempster, 1985) support Olney's excitotoxic hypothesis as it relates to experimental epileptic brain damage (Olney, 1983) and suggest that excessive presynaptic activity per se can produce postsynaptic damage.

INTERNEURON DAMAGE AND DECREASED RECURRENT INHIBITION

During the course of these initial experiments, we noted unexpectedly that, during the 24 h of intermittent perforant pathway stimulation, there was a gradual loss of granule cell recurrent inhibition as measured by the twin pulse method (Andersen et al., 1966). Even after a "rest" for several hours without stimulation, granule cell discharge no longer activated the recurrent inhibitory pathway. Since stimulation also caused extensive damage to hilar neurons, and it had been asserted that the majority of hilar cells are γ-aminobutyric acid (GABA) neurons (Seress and Ribak, 1983), we concluded that the loss of inhibition was probably the result of irreversible damage to inhibitory basket cells (Sloviter, 1983). This was a tentative conclusion, and we noted at the time that the seizure-induced loss of GABA-positive interneurons needed to be demonstrated using immunocytochemical methods since some interneurons of the hilus appeared to be undamaged by the seizure activity. The need to identify the damaged and undamaged interneurons in terms of their neuroactive chemical content led us to map the different interneuron populations in the normal hippocampus (Sloviter and Nilaver, 1987).

CHEMICAL ANATOMY OF THE NORMAL RAT DENTATE GYRUS

Three general points about the chemical anatomy of the normal hippocampus are clear. First, the two principal cell populations, the granule cells and the pyramidal cells, are devoid of GABA and most identified neuroactive peptides. Second, distinct subpopulations of nonprincipal cells (interneurons and similar cells with commissural projections), contain different neuroactive substances that are useful markers for the different cell types. Third, not all hippocampal nonprincipal cells are GABA- or glutamate decarboxylase (GAD)-immunoreactive. The locations and known features of the main cell types of the area dentata are presented in Figure 2.

The following section, which describes normal chemical anatomy and connections in the hippocampus, focuses on the rat area dentata, since this region is most relevant to the subsequently described experimental epilepsy studies.

Peptide-Immunoreactive Subpopulations of GABA-Containing Neurons

The most numerous chemically identified nonprincipal cells in the rat hippocampus are the GABA-immunoreactive neurons. They include morphologically heterogeneous cells of all hippocampal subregions, and their fibers surround virtually all other hippocampal cells and processes, principal and nonprincipal cells alike. When tissue is fixed with a high glutaraldehyde fixative that covalently captures the GABA present, it is apparent that GABA-immunoreactive fibers are everywhere, surrounding somata and dendrites, and no regions, except for white matter tracts, can be described as relatively lacking in GABA-immunoreactive fibers.

In the area dentata, GABA-positive cells are present in all three subregions—the molecular layer, the granule cell layer, and the hilus. On the basis of the available information, there appear to be at least three distinct subpopulations

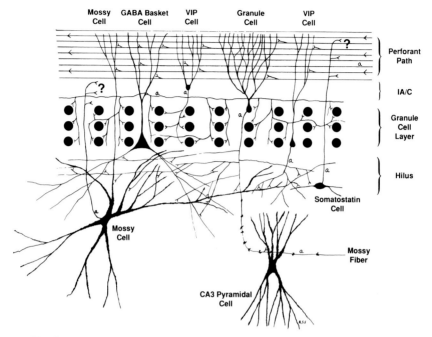

Fig. 2.   Anatomy of the rat dentate gyrus. a, axon. See text for discussion.

of dentate GABA- or GAD-positive cells, which are described in the sections below.

Cholecystokinin-Immunoreactive Neurons

Cholecystokinin (CCK)-like immunoreactive dentate neurons, virtually all of which are GAD positive (Kosaka et al., 1985), exhibit the morphology of the pyramidal-shaped type 1 and type 2 basket cells (Amaral, 1978) of the granule cell layer and hilus (Greenwood et al., 1981; Handelmann et al., 1981) but are fewer in number than the GABA-positive basket cell populations in adjacent sections (Sloviter and Nilaver, 1987). Kosaka et al. (1985) estimated that approximately 10% of GABA neurons are CCK immunoreactive. CCK-positive cells are rarely present in the molecular layer. The CCK-positive GABA neurons form a dense fiber plexus in the inner molecular and granule cell layers and an axosomatic innervation of CCK-negative hilar cells (Sloviter and Nilaver, 1987).

Vasoactive Intestinal Polypeptide-Immunoreactive Neurons

Vasoactive intestinal polypeptide (VIP)-immunoreactive dentate neurons, many of which are also GAD positive (Kosaka et al., 1985), are relatively few in number, usually five to ten per 50 μm thick section, smaller in somal size, and different from the CCK-positive basket cells in terms of somal and dendritic morphology. Unlike the far more numerous type 1 and 2 basket cells, which form a wide-ranging plexus in the inner molecular and granule cell layers, VIP-positive cells form a relatively dense plexus in the hilus around hilar neurons and around a small number of granule cells near each VIP-positive soma (Sloviter and Nilaver, 1987).

Somatostatin- and Neuropeptide Y-Immunoreactive Neurons

Somatostatin-immunoreactive neurons are, with few exceptions, restricted to the dentate hilus; very few cells of the granular or molecular layers exhibit somatostatin-like immunoreactivity (Köhler and Chan-Palay, 1982; Morrisson et al., 1982; Bakst et al., 1986; Sloviter and Nilaver, 1987). Many of the somatostatin-positive hilar cells also exhibit neuropeptide Y (NPY)-like immunoreactivity (Köhler et al., 1987). However, whereas few somatostatin-positive cells are present in the granule cell or molecular layers, many NPY-positive cells that apparently lack somatostatin immunoreactivity are present there and they have the morphological characteristics of the GABA-positive pyramidal-shaped basket cells of the granule cell layer (Fig. 3E). Unlike the basket cells, hilar somatostatin- and NPY-positive cells send an axonal plexus to the outer molecular layer (Bakst et al., 1986), and the somatostatin- and NPY-immunoreactive plexuses appear identical (Fig. 3A,E).

We formerly considered somatostatin-positive hilar cells to be mainly distinct from hilar GABA neurons (Sloviter, 1987; Sloviter and Nilaver, 1987) for two reasons. First, the GABA-immunoreactive cells are numerous in the granule cell layer, where somatostatin-immunoreactive cells are rare, and they are sparse in the hilus, where somatostatin-immunoreactive cells are numerous. Also, the number of hilar cells immunoreactive for GABA was always smaller than the number immunoreactive for somatostatin in adjacent sections. The relatively small number of GABA-immunoreactive cells in the hilus has also been reported by Gamrani et al. (1986) and by Woodson et al. (1989). Second, the colocalization study by Schmechel et al. (1984) indicated that a minority of hilar somatostatin-positive cells was immunoreactive for GAD. However, the recent study by Kosaka et al. (1988) indicated that 90% of hilar cells that exhibited somatostatin-immunoreactivity were also immunoreactive for GAD, suggests that somatostatin-immunoreactive cells are probably another subset of GABA neurons.

Since it appears that more GAD- than GABA-positive hilar cells are visualized by the immunocytochemical method, some GAD-immunoreactive cells may not synthesize GABA in the soma in immunocytochemically detectable concentrations. Conversely, differences in the number of cells stained using different antisera could be due to technical factors and therefore of no biological significance. If, however, some GAD-positive cells synthesize little GABA in their somata, it is important to determine if they synthesize GABA in their terminals and can therefore be considered to be "GABAergic," a term implying GABA-mediated physiological effects. The possibility that some GAD-positive

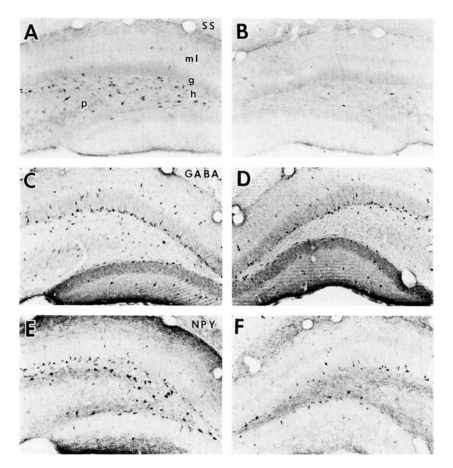

Fig. 3.   Somatostatin (SS)-, GABA-, and neuropeptide Y (NPY)-like immunoreactivity (LI) in the dentate gyrus 5 days after perforant pathway stimulation. Same animal as shown in Figure 4C,D. **A:** Unstimulated side, SS-LI. **B:** Stimulated side, SS-LI. Note loss of hilar cell staining. The SS-immunoreactive plexus in the outer molecular layer (ml) is faintly visible in A and lost in B. **C,D:** Unstimulated and stimulated, respectively; GABA-LI. Note relative survival of GABA-immunoreactive cells in all layers. **E,F:** Unstimulated and stimulated sides, respectively; NPY-LI. NPY-LI is present in the hilar SS-LI cells (Köhler et al., 1987) and also in some interneurons of the granule cell layer (g) that resemble the GABA-LI basket cells. Note loss of hilar NPY-LI cells and the NPY-immunoreactive plexus in the molecular layer but survival of the presumed basket cells in the same section. Fixative was 2% paraformaldehyde/0.01% glutaraldehyde as described previously (Sloviter and Nilaver, 1987). h:hilus; p:pyramidal cell layer.

cells suppress the synthesis of GABA and utilize another substance as a neurotransmitter (somatostatin or NPY?) may exist.

In summary then, there appear to be at least three mainly distinct subpopulations of GABA neurons in the rat area dentata. One is the GABA-positive, pyramidal-shaped basket cells of the granule cell layer and hilus (Amaral, 1978), which form the axosomatic, "basket-like" plexus around dentate granule cells. Some of these basket cells are also immunoreactive for CCK or NPY. A second subpopulation is the less numerous VIP-positive cells, which are smaller in somal diameter and form an axonal plexus mainly in the hilus. The third subpopulation consists of the somatostatin-, NPY-, and GAD-positive hilar cells that innervate unknown elements in the outer dentate molecular layer.

GABA-Negative Neurons

A large number of dentate hilar neurons appear to be devoid of GABA- and GAD-like immunoreactivity (Sloviter and Nilaver, 1987; Fig. 2 in Kosaka et al., 1987). The main hilar cell type is the "mossy" cell. Unlike most hippocampal nonprincipal cells, mossy cell dendrites exhibit an extensive spine apparatus (Amaral, 1978). Mossy cell axons innervate the inner dentate molecular layer where they form assymetric synapses (Ribak et al., 1985), a possibly distinguishing feature of excitatory terminals (Gray, 1959; Uchinozo, 1965). They are apparently not immunoreactive for GABA or any identified peptide (Ribak et al., 1985), but their terminals in the inner molecular layer do exhibit glutamate-like immunoreactivity (Storm-Mathisen et al., 1983; Fischer et al., 1986). Although hilar mossy cells and somatostatin/NPY-immunoreactive neurons are intermingled, these two populations are distinct; mossy cells do not exhibit somatostatin-like immunoreactivity, and each population innervates different strata of the molecular layer (Bakst et al., 1986).

ALTERED FUNCTION AND STRUCTURE AFTER SEIZURE ACTIVITY

Having considered the different immunoreactive cell populations in normal rats (Sloviter and Nilaver, 1987), we proceeded to evaluate inhibition electrophysiologically long after stimulation and determine precisely which hippocampal cells were irreversibly damaged by perforant pathway stimulation. This was done using both the silver impregnation method for degeneration (Nadler and Evenson, 1983) and the immunocytochemical approach described above.

In the first series of experiments, rats were silver stained to reveal degenerating neurons. Immediately, one, two, or three days after 24 h of intermittent perforant pathway stimulation, rats were re-evaluated electrophysiologically and then perfusion fixed (Sloviter, 1987). The 0–3 day period of recovery after an acute insult is optimal for showing, first, the stained cell bodies and dendrites of damaged cells and, later, both cell bodies and terminals.

Short-Term Recovery: Electrophysiology and Degeneration Stain

Extracellular recording of granule cell potentials evoked by twin pulses to the perforant pathway showed an obvious decrease in recurrent inhibition on the previously stimulated side compared with the unstimulated side of the same rat (Sloviter, 1983). Silver staining revealed a large number of hilar neuron somata and dendrites impregnated with silver immediately after stimulation (0 day recovery) but no evidence in the same sections of impregnated pyramidal-shaped basket cells (Fig. 4A). There was also no apparent damage to nongranule cells of the molecular layer, where GABA-positive neurons are common. Later in the 0–3 day recovery period, impregnated fibers characteristic of degenerating axon terminals were visible in the inner and outer dentate molecular layers, but they were rare in the granule cell layer where the GABA-positive basket cells form their axosomatic plexus (Fig. 4B). Plastic-embedded sections from each animal showed shrunken hilar neurons with pyknotic nuclei as well as some apparently unaffected hilar cells (data not shown). Several days later, Nissl-stained sections revealed that the hilus had narrowed and that most, but not all, hilar neurons had degenerated (Fig. 4C,D).

This pattern of degeneration is interpreted as follows. Intermittent perforant pathway stimulation for 24 h produces little or no damage to dentate granule

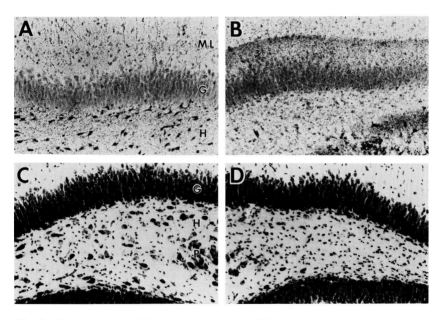

Fig. 4. Degeneration of dentate neurons after 24 h intermittent perforant pathway stimulation. **A:** Three hours after end of 24 h of stimulation. Note silver-impregnated hilar cells (H) and lack of impregnation of granule cells and basket cells of the granule cell layer (G). **B:** Three days after stimulation, silver-impregnated elements (terminals) appeared in the inner molecular layer (ML) innervated by hilar mossy cells. **C,D:** Nissl staining 5 days after stimulation. Note the normal appearance in previously unstimulated hippocampus (C) and shrinkage of the hilus and loss of hilar cells in the previously stimulated hippocampus (D) of the same animal. C and D are from the same animal as described in Figure 3. p:pyramidal cell layer.

cells or to GABA-positive interneurons of the molecular and granule cell layers despite their monosynaptic activation by the perforant pathway. The extensive damage to hilar neurons and CA3 pyramidal cells occurs in the exact location innervated by the mossy fibers and their hilar collaterals. The location of degenerating somata and terminals fits precisely the known morphology of two dentate cell populations. One is the hilar mossy cells. In all rats evaluated, degenerating terminals were present in the inner molecular layers of both hippocampi precisely where the mossy cells innervate the area dentata. The second population is the somatostatin/NPY-immunoreactive hilar cells. These cells project their axons to the outer molecular layer where they form a dense plexus (Bakst et al., 1986). Silver-stained sections of stimulated animals showed degenerating terminals in the outer molecular layer. However, these could also be degenerating terminals of perforant pathway fibers damaged by the stimulating electrode, since both the hilar somatostatin/NPY-positive cells and the perforant pathway fibers innervate the same region of the molecular layer.

Interpretive Problems With Regard to the Degeneration Stain

As stated above, degenerating terminals in the outer molecular layer cannot be taken as definitive evidence that somatostatin-positive cells have been damaged. Similarly, a lack of silver impregnation of basket cells is not evidence that basket cells have not been damaged. Conceivably, basket cells could be damaged and degenerating but not impregnated by the silver staining process. Since the chemical bases of some anatomical methods are unknown and the results sometimes seem capricious, it would be reckless to conclude that GABA-positive basket cells have not been damaged simply because none were seen to be silver-impregnated after stimulation. The experiments described below were designed to address the same question with an unrelated anatomical method (immunocytochemistry) to avoid basing a conclusion on only one, possibly fallible, method.

Long-Term Recovery: Electrophysiology and Immunocytochemistry

In the second series of experiments, rats were allowed to recover for up to 3 months after stimulation. They were re-evaluated electrophysiologically and perfusion fixed for subsequent immunocytochemical staining. Two questions were addressed. First, is the loss of recurrent inhibition long-lasting? If the decreased inhibition is a consequence of interneuron loss, then it should persist long after the animal has recovered from the acute insult. Second, exactly which hilar cells are damaged, and are the GABA-positive basket cells of the granule cell layer as resistant to seizure activity as the results of the degeneration experiments suggest?

The results of these experiments showed that the loss of recurrent inhibition lasts at least as long as 3 months after 24 h of intermittent perforant pathway stimulation, which is the longest period yet tested. As perforant pathway stimulus frequency is increased to 2 or 3 Hz, frequencies optimal for evoking twin pulse inhibition, the decreased seizure threshold in the previously stimulated granule cells becomes apparent. That is, stimuli that normally evoke single population spikes with evident inhibition (Fig. 5a,b, top traces) produce epileptiform discharges with little inhibition evident (Fig. 5a,b, lower traces).

It should be noted that all electrophysiological evaluations were performed by the author without knowledge of the previous treatment (control or left side–right side stimulated). All data were recorded and evaluated and a con-

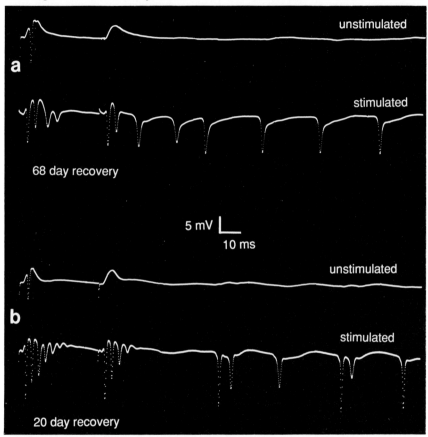

Fig. 5. Evoked potentials recorded in the granule cell layers in response to twin pulse, perforant pathway stimulation. **a:** 68 day recovery; **b:** 20 day recovery. Extracellular activity was recorded simultaneously in both hippocampi after animals underwent 24 h of intermittent perforant pathway stimulation (Sloviter, 1983, 1987). Note on the unstimulated side of each animal the large first population spike in response to the first of two identical pulses delivered 40 ms apart. Activation of the recurrent inhibitory pathway (Andersen et al., 1966) prevents the second spike, resulting only in the positive field "EPSP" in response to the second pulse. This is similar to the control response (not shown) except that the first spike is unusually large compared with the response evoked before stimulation. Note on the stimulated sides of the same animals that identical stimuli evoked epileptiform granule cell discharges and unsynchronized spikes occurred with little inhibition apparent. 3 Hz stimulation; 40 ms interpulse interval; positivity up.

clusion was made as to the previous treatment. Only then was the nature of the previous treatment compared with the conclusion based on blind evaluation. In more than 70 animals now studied, the loss of inhibition on the stimulated side has been so reproducible and obvious that conclusions made blindly as to which side had been previously stimulated have been made correctly without exception.

Selective Vulnerability of Immunoreactive Dentate Neurons

Immunocytochemical staining of alternate sections from each control and experimental animal with antisera to GABA, CCK, VIP, neuropeptide Y, and somatostatin revealed that, in addition to the damage to hilar mossy cells shown by the degeneration stain (Fig. 4), there was a nearly complete loss of hilar somatostatin/NPY cells (Fig. 3A,B). To conclude that cells have degenerated solely because immunoreactivity is absent is unwarranted since a loss of antigen without cell death would produce the same immunocytochemical result as cell death. Therefore, alternate sections of each brain were either mounted on glass slides and Nissl-stained or embedded in plastic. In this way, it could be determined if hilar cells were alive but immunocytochemically unstained or if they had degenerated. The latter was found to be the case (Sloviter, 1987) (Fig. 4D). The loss of hilar somatostatin/NPY-immunoreactive cells and mossy cells occurred throughout the dorsal hippocampus on the stimulated side with little obvious damage to the contralateral hippocampus. Accompanying the unilateral loss of somatostatin-positive somata was a unilateral loss of the somatostatin- and NPY-immunoreactive plexus in the outer dentate molecular layer (Fig. 3E,F). Interestingly, the NPY-immunoreactive cells of the granule cell layer that have the location and morphology of GABA-positive basket cells appeared to be unaffected by perforant pathway stimulation, whereas the immediately adjacent NPY-positive hilar cells and their fiber plexus in the molecular layer were absent (Fig. 3F).

Staining of alternate sections of the same brains with GABA antiserum revealed that the GABA-positive cells of the molecular layer and the GABA-positive basket cells of the granule cell layer appeared relatively unaffected (Figs. 3C,D, 6). Also apparently unchanged was the GABA-immunoreactive axosomatic plexus around the granule cells. Since the GABA-positive hilar neurons are scattered within the hilus, it cannot be stated that some GABA-positive hilar cells have not been lost. Cell counts show only that no statistically significant loss of dentate GABA-positive cells occurred (Sloviter, 1987). Nor was there any noticeable loss of VIP- or CCK-positive cells, which are subsets of GABA neurons (Kosaka et al., 1985). In addition, it should be noted that there was usually a loss of greater than 90% of hilar somatostatin-positive cells. In immediately adjacent sections, remaining hilar cells were usually found to be GABA positive (Fig. 6D).

Figure 6 shows the stimulated and unstimulated hippocampi of an animal stimulated 20 days previously, re-evaluated electrophysiologically (data shown in Fig. 5b), perfusion fixed with a high glutaraldehyde fixative (1.5% glutaraldehyde/1% paraformaldehyde), and processed for GABA immunocytochemistry as reported previously (Sloviter and Nilaver, 1987). The results show clearly

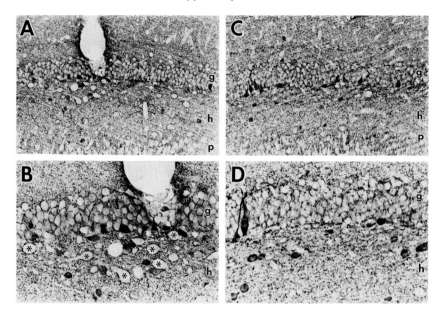

Fig. 6.   GABA immunoreactivity 20 days after perforant pathway stimulation. Same animal as shown in Figure 5b with decreased inhibition and epileptiform discharges. **A,B:** Previously unstimulated side. **C,D:** Stimulated side of same brain. Note uniformly dense GABA immunoreactivity surrounding unstained CA3 pyramidal cells (p) and dentate granule cells (g), as well as unstained hilar neurons surrounded by GABA-positive fibers (asterisks). In C and D, note similarly dense GABA immunoreactivity in neuropil, loss of unstained hilar cells, and survival of GABA-positive cells in the granule cell layer (g) and hilus (h). Fixative was 1.5% glutaraldehyde/1.0% paraformaldehyde as described previously (Sloviter and Nilaver, 1987).

that hilar GABA-negative neurons (Fig. 6B, asterisks) are selectively affected, whereas dentate GABA neurons and their immunoreactive fibers around the unstained granule cells appear relatively unaffected.

In summary, these electrophysiological and anatomical studies answer the two questions asked. First, the loss of inhibition and decreased seizure threshold is immediate and long-lasting. Second, hilar mossy cells and somatostatin/NPY-immunoreactive neurons are selectively vulnerable whereas GABA-positive dentate basket cells are clearly less vulnerable to the neurotoxic effects of granule cell discharge.

DISCUSSION
Seizures and Cell Death

Our current view of the process by which perforant pathway stimulation irreversibly damages hippocampal principal cells and interneurons supports Olney's "excitotoxic hypothesis" (Olney, 1983) and is summarized below.

1. Perforant pathway stimulation excites granule cells by releasing an excitatory amino acid, probably glutamate, from the terminals of perforant pathway fibers (Cotman and Nadler, 1981). The portion of the granule cell dendrites innervated by the perforant pathway develops spherical swellings, presumably as the result of ion and water influx (Sloviter, 1983; Olney et al., 1983). However, granule cells seldom die; the reason for this relative invulnerability is unknown.

2. Granule cell action potentials release an excitatory substance, probably glutamate, onto hilar cells and CA3 pyramidal cells, respectively (Crawford and Connor, 1973; Storm-Mathisen et al., 1983). If the extracellular concentration of transmitter reaches and maintains a critical level at their receptors for a sufficient period of time, irreversible damage to hilar neurons and CA3 pyramidal cells occurs. The postsynaptic processes that ultimately cause cell death are unknown. If stimulation evokes granule cell "field EPSPs" but no population spikes, no loss of inhibition or damage to hilar and CA3 pyramidal cells occurs, but granule cell dendrites still swell reversibly. Most or all GABA-positive basket cells survive excitation by granule cells despite extensive damage to immediately adjacent hilar neurons. The reason for the relative invulnerability of GABA-immunoreactive basket cells is unknown. One possible factor is that vulnerable cells lack calcium-binding proteins capable of decreasing the intracellular concentration of free calcium (Sloviter, 1989).

3. According to this scheme, other hippocampal and nonhippocampal damage to area CA1, lateral septum, dorsolateral thalamus, and amygdala (Sloviter, 1983) results from the propagation of excitatory activity polysynaptically with subsequent release of potentially lethal concentrations of excitatory transmitter (Sloviter and Dempster, 1985).

The Possible Relationship Between Decreased Inhibition, Decreased Seizure Threshold, and Interneuron Damage

The pattern of irreversible damage to hilar mossy cells and somatostatin/NPY neurons is accompanied by long-lasting changes in hippocampal granule cell excitability. Recurrent inhibition in granule cells is decreased for months after stimulation despite large amplitude granule cell population spikes that would normally activate the recurrent inhibitory pathway. Seizure threshold is similarly decreased after stimulation. This is a striking and highly reproducible effect of perforant pathway stimulation, and it only occurs if perforant pathway stimulation evokes granule cell population spikes. The issue that now needs to be clarified is whether the loss of these hilar cells is the cause of the decreased inhibition and the increased excitability, or if both effects are simply unrelated consequences of seizure activity.

HYPOTHESIS
What Do Hilar Mossy Cells and Somatostatin/NPY Neurons Do Normally?

Clearly, the pathophysiological significance of losing hilar somatostatin/NPY neurons and mossy cells depends entirely on what these cells do normally. Although physiological studies of dentate cell interactions have begun (Scharfman and Schwartzkroin, 1988), little definitive information is available. Nonetheless, inferences about the normal function of these cells can be drawn from the available anatomical and electrophysiological data. Hilar mossy cells innervate the inner molecular layers of both hippocampi via associational and commissural pathways (Blackstad, 1956; Gottlieb and Cowan, 1973) and their glutamate-like immunoreactive terminals (Storm-Mathisen et al., 1983; Fischer et al., 1986) form asymmetric synapses (Ribak et al., 1985). They are therefore probably excitatory cells. Hilar somatostatin/NPY/GAD-positive cells innervate the outer molecular layer of the ipsilateral area dentata, and there is little overlap between the regions innervated by these two cell populations. Since the somatostatin/GAD-positive interneurons of area CA1 have been shown to be inhibitory to other CA1 cells when depolarized directly (Lacaille et al., 1987), the somatostatin/NPY/GAD hilar neurons are also probably inhibitory.

If the mossy cells are excitatory and the somatostatin/NPY cells are inhibitory (this may be too simple a classification given the variety of neuroactive substances many interneurons contain), how are their actions manifested in terms of overall dentate function? Buzsáki and Eidelberg (1981, 1982) found that hilar stimulation excited contralateral dentate interneurons, possibly basket cells, and inhibited contralateral granule cell population spike amplitude concomitantly. A similar, primarily inhibitory effect of hilar stimulation on granule cell activity was reported by Douglas et al. (1983) and by Bilkey and Goddard (1987). Douglas et al. (1983) reported that hilar stimulation evoked a bicuculline-insensitive dentate potential and produced a bicuculline-sensitive inhibition of the granule cell population spike. When bicuculline blocked the inhibitory effect of hilar stimulation, a weak excitatory effect was revealed, suggesting that the primary influence of hilar cells on granule cells is inhibitory via excitation of GABA-containing basket cells (Douglas et al., 1983). If this effect of hilar stimulation is mediated by hilar neurons, and not fibers of passage or nearby cells, then the cells responsible are most likely the mossy cells, since, of the two main hilar cell populations, i.e. mossy cells and somatostatin/NPY cells, only the former have extensive commissural projections (Ribak et al., 1985; Bakst et al., 1986) that could convey the activity to the contralateral area dentata. If this is the case, the primary function of the mossy cells may be to regulate inhibitory basket cell excitability and thereby govern the excitability of the principal cell population.

This hypothesis raises another question. If surviving GABA neurons are functional but lack their normal excitatory input, why does not granule cell discharge alone activate the surviving basket cells directly and evoke recurrent inhibition. Why invoke or even have a basket cell-activating system if granule cells can activate basket cells directly? Assuming that all surviving connections are intact and capable of functioning after stimulation (this has not been demonstrated), it may be that the normal function of mossy cells is to provide a degree of tonic excitation that basket cells need to keep them near their threshold for discharge and thereby enable them to respond sensitively and rapidly to granule cell excitation and other inputs. This hypothesis would explain why, in the absence of mossy cell input, basket cells are unable to exert their normal inhibitory influence despite direct granule cell input. The existence of such a feed-forward excitation system might also be advantageous because it would provide an additional locus for the integration of activity from other inputs to the dentate region without all activity having to influence the basket cells directly.

Although even less is known about the hilar somatostatin/NPY neurons, their axon terminal location provides a clue. These cells form a dense somatostatin- and NPY-immunoreactive plexus in the outer two-thirds of the molecular layer, and loss of their cell bodies after perforant pathway stimulation is accompanied by the loss of this plexus (Fig. 3E,F). What cellular elements do these hilar cells innervate normally and what is their function? Although the dentate molecular layer contains granule cell and interneuron dendrites and afferent fibers, and the hilar somatostatin/NPY fiber plexus may innervate and influence any or all of these elements, the location of the somatostatin/NPY plexus is the same region of the molecular layer innervated by the perforant pathway. It is possible that one function of the hilar somatostatin-, NPY-, and GAD-immunoreactive projection may be to influence afferent excitatory input presynaptically. The results of several studies are relevant in this regard. $GABA_B$ binding sites are relatively dense in the outer molecular layer compared with other dentate strata (Bowery et al., 1987), and $GABA_B$ receptors are located presynaptically in several brain regions (Price et al., 1984a,b). In addition, Colmers and colleagues (1987) have concluded that NPY inhibits CA1 pyramidal cell activity by inhibiting afferent activity presynaptically. Thus, one function of these hilar neurons may be to reduce granule cell excitation by presynaptically inhibiting perforant pathway transmitter release.

These hypothetical roles for specific hilar cell types in governing overall dentate function, i.e. one population decreasing granule cell excitation by presynaptic inhibition of perforant pathway fibers and the other population increasing granule cell feed-forward and feedback inhibition by tonically exciting basket cells, are consistent with our experimental results. Accordingly, a loss of mossy cells would partially deafferent dentate basket cells, decreasing feed-forward and feedback inhibition, and loss of somatostatin/NPY-immunoreactive hilar cells would lead to an increase in perforant pathway excitation of granule cells. An alternate possibility that must be considered is that despite their survival, relatively normal appearance, and continued synthesis of GABA (an antiserum to GABA itself was used to visualize the surviving cells), the basket cells might be 1) incapable of discharging because of some long-lasting functional impairment; 2) discharging but unable to release GABA, or 3) releasing GABA but the GABA receptors and postsynaptic mechanisms may be dysfunctional or subsensitive.

Future studies will undoubtedly focus on the roles that different neuron populations play in hippocampal function, why basket cells survive but adjacent interneurons do not, whether surviving basket cells are capable of mediating inhibition, and, if so, how they might be induced pharmacologically to reassert their influence and thereby correct deficits possibly relevant to the human epileptic state.

ACKNOWLEDGMENTS

I thank Drs. D.G. Amaral and P.A. Schwartzkroin for invaluable discussions and Drs. G. Nilaver and E.A. Zimmerman for training me in the method and interpretation of immunocytochemistry. This work was supported by an equipment grant from the Citizen's Advisory Council of Helen Hayes Hospital and by NINCDS grant NS18201.

REFERENCES

Amaral, D.G. (1978) A Golgi study of cell types in the hilar region of the hippocampus in the rat. J. Comp. Neurol. 182:851–914.

Andersen, P., B. Holmqvist and P.E. Voorhoeve (1966) Entorhinal activation of dentate granule cells. Acta Physiol. Scand. 66:448–460.

Bakst, I., C. Avendano, J.H. Morrison, and D.G. Amaral (1986) An experimental analysis of the origins of somatostatin-like immunoreactivity in the dentate gyrus of the rat. J. Neurosci. 6:1452–1462.

Ben-Ari, Y., E. Tremblay, O.P. Ottersen, and R. Naquet (1979) Evidence suggesting secondary epileptogenic lesions after kainic acid lesions: Pretreatment with diazepam reduces distant but not local brain damage. Brain Res. 165:362–365.

Bilkey, D.K., and G.V. Goddard (1987) Septohippocampal and commissural pathways antagonistically control inhibitory interneurons in the dentate gyrus. Brain Res. 405:320–325.

Blackstad, T.W. (1956) Commissural connections of the hippocampal region in the rat, with special reference to their mode of termination. J. Comp. Neurol. 105:417–538.

Bowery, N.G., A.L. Hudson, and G.W. Price (1987) $GABA_A$ and $GABA_B$ receptor site distribution in the rat central nervous system. Neuroscience 20:365–383.

Buzsáki, G., and E. Eidelberg (1981) Commissural projection to the dentate gyrus of the rat: Evidence for feed-forward inhibition. Brain Res. 230:346–350.

Buzsáki, G., and E. Eidelberg (1982) Direct afferent excitation and long-term potentiation of hippocampal interneurons. J. Neurophysiol. 48:597–607.

Colmers, W.F., K. Lukowiak, and Q.J. Pittman (1987) Presynaptic action of neuropeptide Y in area CA1 of the rat hippocampal slice. J. Physiol. 383:285–299.

Cotman, C.W., and J.V. Nadler (1981) Glutamate and aspartate as hippocampal transmitters: Biochemical and pharmacological evidence. In P.J. Roberts, J. Storm-Mathisen, and G.A.R. Johnston (eds): Glutamate: Transmitter in the Nervous System. New York: Wiley, pp. 117–154.

Crawford, I.L., and J.D. Connor (1973) Localization and release of glutamic acid in relation to the hippocampal mossy fiber pathway. Nature 244:442–443.

Douglas, R.M., B.L. McNaughton, and G.V. Goddard (1983) Commissural inhibition and facilitation of granule cell discharge in fascia dentata. J. Comp. Neurol. 219:285–294.

Fischer, B.O., O.P. Ottersen, and J. Storm-Mathisen (1986) Implantation of D-[^{3}H] aspartate loaded gel particles permits restricted uptake sites for transmitter-selective axonal transport. Exp. Brain Res. 63:620–626.

Gamrani, H., B. Onteniente, P. Seguela, M. Geffard, and A. Calas (1986) Gamma-aminobutyric acid-immunoreactivity in the rat hippocampus. A light and electron microscopic study with anti-GABA antibodies. Brain Res. 364:30–38.

Gottlieb, D.I., and W.M. Cowan (1973) Autoradiographic studies of the commissural and associational connections of the hippocampus and dentate gyrus of the rat. I. The commissural connections. J. Comp. Neurol. 149:383–422.

Gray, E.C. (1959) Axo-somatic and axo-dendritic synapses of cerebral cortex: An electron microscopic study. J. Anat. *93*:420–433.

Greenwood, R.S., S.E. Godar, T.A. Reaves, and J.N. Hayward (1981) Cholecystokinin in hippocampal pathways. J. Comp. Neurol. *203*:335–350.

Handelmann, G.E., D.K. Meyer, M.C. Beinfeld, and W.H. Oertel (1981) CCK-containing terminals in the hippocampus are derived from intrinsic neurons: An immunohistochemical and radioimmunological study. Brain Res. *224*:180–184.

Köhler, C., and V. Chan-Palay (1982) Somatostatin-like immunoreactive neurons in the hippocampus: An immunocytochemical study in the rat. Neurosci. Lett. *34*:259–264.

Köhler, C., L.G. Eriksson, S. Davies, and V. Chan-Palay (1987) Co-localization of neuropeptide tyrosine and somatostatin immunoreactivity in neurons of individual subfields of the rat hippocampal region. Neurosci. Lett. *78*:1–6.

Kosaka, T., H. Katsumaru, K. Hama, J.-Y. Wu, and C.W. Heizmann (1987) GABAergic neurons containing the Ca^{2+}-binding protein parvalbumin in the rat hippocampus and dentate gyrus. Brain Res. *419*:119–130.

Kosaka, T., K. Kosaka, K. Tateishi, Y. Hamaoka, N. Yanaihara, J.-Y. Wu, and K. Hama (1985) GABAergic neurons containing CCK-8-like and/or VIP-like immunoreactivities in the rat hippocampus and dentate gyrus. J. Comp. Neurol. *239*:420–430.

Kosaka, T., J.-Y. Wu, and R. Benoit (1988) GABAergic neurons containing somatostatin-like immunoreactivity in the rat hippocampus and dentate gyrus. Exp. Brain Res. *71*:388–398.

Lacaille, J.-C., A.L. Mueller, D.D. Kunkel, and P.A. Schwartzkroin (1987) Local circuit interactions between oriens/alveus interneurons and CA1 pyramidal cells in hippocampal slices: Electrophysiology and morphology. J. Neurosci. *7*:1979–1993.

Lømo, T. (1971) Patterns of activation in a monosynaptic cortical pathway: The perforant path input to the dentate area of the hippocampal formation. Exp. Brain Res. *12*:18–45.

Meldrum, B.S., and J.A.N. Corsellis (1984) Epilepsy. In J.A.N. Corsellis and L.W. Duchen (eds): Greenfield's Neuropathology. New York: Wiley, pp. 921–950.

Morrison, J.H., R. Benoit, P.J. Magistretti, N. Ling, and F.E. Bloom (1982) Immunohistochemical distribution of pro-somatostatin-related peptides in hippocampus. Neurosci. Lett. *34*:137–142.

Nadler, J.V., and G.J. Cuthbertson (1980) Kainic acid neurotoxicity toward hippocampus: Dependence on specific excitatory pathways. Brain Res. *195*:47–56.

Nadler, J.V., and D.A. Evenson (1983) Use of excitatory amino acids to make axon-sparing lesions of hypothalamus. Methods Enzymol. *103*:393–400.

Olney, J.W. (1983) Excitotoxins: An overview. In K. Fuxe, P. Roberts, and R. Schwarcz (eds): Excitotoxins. London: Macmillan, pp. 82–96.

Olney, J.W., T. deGubareff, and R.S. Sloviter (1983) "Epileptic" brain damage in rats induced by sustained electrical stimulation of the perforant path. II. Ultrastructural analysis of acute pathology. Brain Res. Bull. *10*:699–712.

Olney, J.W., T. Fuller, and T. deGubareff (1979) Acute dendrotoxic changes in the hippocampus of kainate treated rats. Brain Res. *76*:91–100.

Price, G.W., T.P. Blackburn, A.L. Hudson, and N.G. Bowery (1984a) Presynaptic $GABA_B$ sites in the interpeduncular nucleus. Neuropharmacology *23*:861–862.

Price, G.W., G.P. Wilkin, M.J. Turnbull, and N.G. Bowery (1984b) Are baclofen-sensitive $GABA_B$ receptors present on primary afferent terminals of the spinal cord? Nature *307*:71–74.

Ribak, C.E., L. Seress, and D.G. Amaral (1985) The development, ultrastructure and synaptic connections of the mossy cells of the dentate gyrus. J. Neurocytol. *14*:835–857.

Scharfman, H.E., and P.A. Schwartzkroin (1988) Electrophysiology of morphologically identified mossy cells of the dentate hilus recorded in guinea pig hippocampal slices. J. Neurosci. 8:3812–3821.

Schmechel, D.E., B.G., Vickrey, D., Fitzpatrick, and R.P. Elde (1984) GABAergic neurons of mammalian cerebral cortex: widespread subclass defined by somatostatin content. Neurosci. Lett. 47:227–232.

Seress, L., and C.E. Ribak (1983) GABAergic cells in the dentate gyrus appear to be local circuit and projection neurons. Exp. Brain Res. 50:173–182.

Sloviter, R.S. (1983) "Epileptic" brain damage in rats induced by sustained electrical stimulation of the perforant path. I. Acute electrophysiological and light microscopic studies. Brain Res. Bull. 10:675–697.

Sloviter, R.S. (1987) Decreased hippocampal inhibition and a selective loss of interneurons in experimental epilepsy. Science 235:73–76.

Sloviter, R.S. (1989) Calcium binding protein (Calbindin-$_{D28K}$) and parvalbumin immunocytochemistry: Localization in the rat hippocampus with specific reference to the selective vulnerability of hippocampal neurons to seizure activity. J. Comp. Neurol. 280:183–196.

Sloviter, R.S., and B.P. Damiano (1981) Sustained electrical stimulation of the perforant path duplicates kainate-induced electrophysiological effects and hippocampal damage in rats. Neurosci. Lett. 24:279–284.

Sloviter, R.S., and D.W. Dempster (1985) "Epileptic" brain damage is replicated qualitatively in the rat hippocampus by central injection of glutamate or aspartate but not by GABA or acetylcholine. Brain Res. Bull. 15:39–60.

Sloviter, R.S., and G. Nilaver (1987) Immunocytochemical localization of GABA-, cholecystokinin-, vasoactive intestinal polypeptide- and somatostatin-like immunoreactivity in the area dentata and hippocampus of the rat. J. Comp. Neurol. 256:42–60.

Storm-Mathisen, J., A.K. Leknes, A.T. Bore, J.L. Vaaland, P. Edminson, F.-M.S. Haug, and O.P. Ottersen (1983) First visualization of glutamate and GABA in neurons by immunocytochemistry. Nature 301:517–520.

Uchinozo, K. (1965) Characteristics of excitatory and inhibitory synapses in the central nervous system of the cat. Nature 207:642–643.

Woodson, W., L. Nitecka, and Y. Ben-Ari (1989) Organization of the GABAergic system in the rat hippocampal formation: a quantitative immunocytochemical study. J. Comp. Neurol. 280:254–271.

The Hippocampus—New Vistas, pages 463–481
© 1989 Alan R. Liss, Inc.

29
Seizures and Neuronal Cell Death in the Hippocampus

J. VICTOR NADLER

Department of Pharmacology, Duke University Medical Center, Durham, North Carolina

INTRODUCTION

Hippocampal damage was first noted in epileptic patients by Bouchet and Cazauvieilh in 1825. The relationship between seizures, on the one hand, and atrophy and/or hardening (sclerosis) of the hippocampus, on the other, does not appear to have been appreciated, however, until Sommer's classic paper of 1880. Reviewing the available postmortem neuropathological evaluations of epileptics, Sommer concluded that the hippocampus is easily damaged by all manner of insults and diseases, that this damage is ultimately expressed as a loss of principal neurons, and that hippocampal pathology is an important etiological factor in the subsequent development of seizures. Upon histological examination, the classic "Ammon's horn sclerosis (AHS)" was found to involve extensive loss of pyramidal cells from area CA1 (h_1, regiosuperior), a somewhat less extensive loss of neurons from the CA3b,c–CA4 area (h_{3-5}, endfolium), and usually some loss of dentate granule cells (Fig. 1). Characteristically, the h_2 (CA2–CA3a) pyramidal cells were relatively spared. The loss of CA1 hippocampal pyramidal cells is such an obvious feature of AHS that the CA1 has been given the special name *Sommer sector*.

During the century since Sommer's report, a number of neuropathologists have confirmed and extended his observations. After temporal lobectomy was introduced as a treatment for pharmacologically intractable complex partial (limbic, temporal lobe, psychomotor) epilepsy, histopathological studies of resected temporal lobes enlarged the available data base. Findings from some of the more notable reports are summarized in Table I. Neuronal loss in one or both hippocampi could be demonstrated in the majority of patients examined. Although the same range of hippocampal damage has been noted in autopsy and surgically resected material, it may be said in general that CA1 damage, often regarded as the central feature of epileptic damage, appears more frequently in resected temporal lobes. In contrast, CA3–CA4 damage is nearly

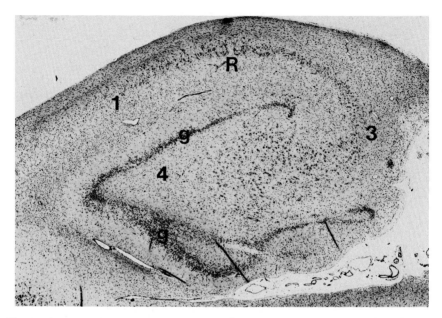

Fig. 1. Section cut from a hippocampal formation resected for pharmacologically intractable complex partial epilepsy and stained with Cresyl violet. Note loss of neurons in areas CA1 (1), CA3b,c (3), and CA4 (4). Pyramidal cells in the "resistant zone" (R; area CA2 and immediately adjacent portion of area CA3a) and granule cells of the fascia dentata (g) are *relatively* spared. (Courtesy of Dr. B. J. Crain.)

always observed in both types of material. Prominent cell loss in the CA3–CA4 area may be present without obvious damage to area CA1, but the converse has only infrequently been observed. Thus there is reason to believe that the most vulnerable hippocampal neurons are the CA3 pyramidal cells and the morphologically diverse neurons of area CA4. Lesions of the CA3–CA4 area without involvement of area CA1 have been termed *endfolium sclerosis* (EFS) (Margerison and Corsellis, 1966). In addition to the different hippocampal pathology, AHS and EFS differ in the associated damage to regions outside the hippocampal area. AHS, but not EFS, is nearly always accompanied by cell loss and gliosis in other brain regions. The regions most commonly include the cerebellar cortex, thalamus, somatosensory neocortex, and amygdala. The terms *hippocampal sclerosis* and *mesial temporal sclerosis* (Falconer et al., 1964) refer to neuronal loss and gliosis anywhere in the hippocampal formation and thus include both AHS and EFS. With respect to the incidence of AHS and EFS in complex partial epilepsy, it must be emphasized that nearly all studies to date have been limited to patients whose condition had either become pharmacologically intractable or had reached a state of severity that necessitated long-term hospitalization. It is unclear to what extent the high incidence of these lesions in clinical studies applies to less seriously afflicted individuals.

TABLE I. Some Neuropathological Studies of the Hippocampal Formation in Epileptic Patients[a]

Reference	Material	No. of patients studied	Findings
Sano and Malamud (1953)	PM	50	Hippocampal sclerosis, 29; AHS (on at least one side), 13; incomplete damage usually involved CA3–CA4 alone, not CA1 alone
Cavanagh and Meyer (1956)	S	27	AHS, 70%; history of SE, 64%; mean age at onset of seizures, 4 years
Margerison and Corsellis (1966)	PM	55	Hippocampal sclerosis, 36; AHS bilateral, 4, unilateral, 10; EFS bilateral, 5, unilateral, 9; EFS on one side, AHS on the other, 8; no CA1 damage without CA3–CA4 damage; mean age at onset of seizures, AHS, 6 years and EFS, 16 years
Falconer (1971)	S	200	Hippocampal sclerosis, 47%; of the 47%, 60% had seizure onset before age 10, 13% had family history of epilepsy, and 30–40% had had febrile convulsion that approached or reached SE
Brown (1973)	S	45	Hippocampal sclerosis, 65%, ranging from small CA3–CA4 lesion to complete loss of neurons; lesion never exclusive to CA1
Falconer (1974)	S	30[b]	Hippocampal sclerosis, 20; febrile convulsions, 75%
Mouritzen Dam (1980)	PM	20	AHS, 2; for others greatest cell loss in CA3 and fascia dentata; cell loss related to duration of seizure history; CA1 damage related to early age of seizure onset and number of generalized seizures
Babb et al. (1984a)	S	45	Varying degree of hippocampal sclerosis; neuronal density reduced in all hippocampal regions; granule cell decline correlated with age of seizure onset; otherwise no correlation with age, laterality, duration of seizure history, seizure frequency, or total number of seizures; little damage when focus was outside hippocampal formation
Sagar and Oxbury (1987)	S	32	Onset of generalized seizures at age 3 or before: AHS, 11/13; NSHS, 1/13. Onset of generalized seizures after age 3: AHS, 1/12; NSHS, 5/12. Complex partial seizures only: AHS, 0/7; NSHS, 4/7

[a]Abbreviations: AHS, Ammon's horn sclerosis; EFS, endfolium sclerosis; NSHS; nonspecific hippocampal sclerosis; PM, postmortem; S, surgical; SE, status epilepticus.
[b]Children.

The relation between hippocampal damage and complex partial seizures has been debated since the time of Sommer, yet even today the issue remains unresolved. Detailed discussions of this controversy have been published (e.g. Meldrum and Corsellis, 1984). Some clinical investigators have supported Sommer's unequivocal position that hippocampal sclerosis leads to epileptic attacks, whereas others have, with equal vehemence, advanced the view that the damage resulted from seizure activity occurring over a period of years.

In favor of hippocampal sclerosis as a cause of seizures is evidence from some studies that the extent of hippocampal cell loss correlates poorly with seizure history (Gastaut et al., 1959; Falconer and Taylor, 1968; Babb et al., 1984a), suggesting that the pathology may have been present before the seizures began. Although much of the brain is involved in seizures, removal of only the damaged portion of hippocampal formation is sufficient to reduce the incidence of or abolish further seizures (Falconer et al., 1964; Falconer and Taylor, 1968; Babb et al., 1984b). Electrophysiological recordings suggest that the sclerotic hippocampal formation, although relatively silent, contains hyperexcitable neurons that generate spontaneous bursts (Babb, 1986). The damaged region is therefore presumed to serve as the primary seizure focus. Seizures that appear from EEG recordings to originate elsewhere in the brain and to propagate throughout the hippocampal circuitry are associated with much less cell loss than seizures that appear to originate in the sclerotic hippocampus (Babb et al., 1984a).

As to the origin of the hippocampal damage, Falconer (1971, 1974) reported that a large percentage of his surgical patients testified to a history of febrile convulsions during the first few years of life. In many cases, the febrile convulsions had progressed to status epilepticus. His data also indicated that 13% of surgical patients with hippocampal sclerosis had a positive family history of epilepsy, compared with less then 1% of the general population. On the basis of these observations, Falconer theorized that some individuals are genetically predisposed to develop convulsions at a given body temperature and that these convulsions, when prolonged or frequently repeated at a vulnerable time during development, lead to neuronal cell death. By some unexplained mechanism, the region of damage later develops into a seizure focus. Other workers, however, have rejected any role whatever for seizures in the etiology of hippocampal sclerosis (Gastaut et al., 1959).

In support of the contrary view, the Scheibels noted morphological features in hippocampal neurons from the brains of epileptics, which suggested that neuronal deterioration and death result from an ongoing process presumably related to the repeated seizures (Scheibel et al., 1974). Along the same lines, one detailed study of autopsy material suggested a relation between the severity of cell loss in the hippocampal formation and the duration of seizure history (Mouritzen Dam, 1980). Furthermore, if prolonged seizures are damaging in early life, it is unclear why they should later become benign. In fact, status epilepticus can lead to acute hippocampal sclerosis in adults, as well as in children (Corsellis and Bruton, 1983).

With respect to the mechanism by which seizures might lead to neuronal degeneration, Spielmeyer (1927) emphasized the rake-like vascularization of the CA1 area and suggested that neuronal cell death resulted from partial hindrance of the blood supply from vasospasm during seizures. In other words, AHS was postulated to result from focal ischemia. A somewhat different version of this hypothesis was promoted by Scholz (1959), eliminating the mistaken idea of vasospasm, but supporting the view that cell death in the epileptic brain results from focal ischemia. This idea is consistent with the well-known vulnerability of CA1 pyramidal cells to ischemic damage (Brierley and Graham, 1984). Of course, systemic hypoxia, hypotension, and other concomitants of generalized seizures could also contribute to neuronal degeneration. Only recently, on the basis of work with animal models, have the potentially damaging effects of seizures per se been appreciated (see below).

A formulation recently proposed by Sagar and Oxbury (1987) appears to accomodate these seemingly irreconcilable hypotheses. These investigators were able to separate surgical epilepsy patients with hippocampal lesions into two distinct groups. One group presented with a long history of generalized seizures, which had its onset at the age of 3 years or earlier. Nearly all of these patients had developed full-blown AHS, as defined by a significant loss of principal neurons in the CA1 and CA3–CA4 areas and in the fascia dentata. The second group of patients presented with an equally long seizure history, but no history of an early childhood convulsion. In some cases they had experienced only complex partial seizures that did not generalize. The hippocampi of these patients were characterized by a lesser neuronal loss in area CA1 and/or area CA3–CA4 than in the first group, and there was no significant loss of granule cells. This histological pattern was termed *nonspecific hippocampal sclerosis* (NSHS). Thus AHS was suggested to result in many cases from a severe convulsion or status epilepticus early in life and to be associated with a history of generalized seizures. In contrast to AHS, the severity of NSHS tends to correlate with age and with the duration of the epileptic condition, but not with convulsions in early childhood or with a history of generalized seizures. Thus NSHS was suggested to arise from seizure activity repeated over a long period of time.

Although more will undoubtedly be learned from studies of human material, it seems unlikely that such studies could precisely define the relationship between seizures and neuronal cell death or explain these phenomena at the cellular and molecular levels. For this purpose, animal models are needed. The earliest studies of animal models were conducted by Meldrum and his colleagues in the 1970s (Meldrum and Brierley, 1972, 1973; Meldrum et al., 1973, 1974; Blennow et al., 1978). Their work with baboons and rodents treated with convulsant drugs demonstrated for the first time that, although secondary systemic effects of generalized seizures (hypotension, hyperthermia, hypoxia, and so forth) contribute to neuronal degeneration in the brain, sustained seizures in and of themselves can produce the pattern of epileptic brain damage observed in humans. However, the convulsants employed in those studies lack specificity for the limbic system and thus do not provide an ideal model of partial complex seizures. In addition, further experimentation was needed to evaluate other hypotheses generated by the clinical data, such as the idea that the sclerotic hippocampal formation evolves into a focus for spontaneous complex partial seizures.

The efforts of my laboratory to understand the relation between hippocampal damage and seizures have utilized two animal models: kainic acid (KA) and stimulation-induced status epilepticus. These studies have supported both the ability of seizures to destroy brain neurons and the ability of the lesions so created to facilitate the development of further seizure activity.

STUDIES OF THE KAINIC ACID MODEL

KA is the active principle of the red marine alga *Digenea simplex*, extracts of which have long been used in Japan as a treatment for ascariasis (Takemoto, 1978). Because of its structural resemblance to glutamate and related amino acids, KA was tested in the early 1970s for neuroexcitatory (Shinozaki and Konishi, 1970; Johnston et al., 1974) and neurotoxic (Olney et al., 1974, 1975) activity in the mammalian brain and was found to be extremely potent in both respects. The latter studies also provided behavioral evidence of its potent convulsant properties. Subsequent electrographic, metabolic, histologic, pharmacologic, and behavioral investigations established that KA can provide a useful and unique animal model of hippocampal sclerosis (Nadler, 1981; Collins et al., 1983a; Ben-Ari, 1985).

KA has proved especially useful as a tool with which to investigate the conditions under which complex partial seizures lead to neuronal degeneration. KA provokes in experimental animals electrographic seizures that appear to originate in and remain largely confined to the limbic system (Ben-Ari et al., 1980, 1981; Menini et al., 1980; Lothman and Collins, 1981). The behavioral expression of these seizures is generally quite mild, closely resembling the behaviors described in amygdaloid kindled rats (Ben-Ari et al., 1981; Ault et al., 1986). Thus systemic changes are minimal unless relatively high doses are given. At the same time, KA destroys brain neurons by two mechanisms that are at least partially distinct. One type of damage develops after intracerebroventricular (i.c.v.) or parenteral administration of the convulsant and at a distance from the site of a focal injection into the brain. This "distant" or "remote" damage results from prolonged seizure activity and not from a direct interaction of the affected neurons with KA (Nadler, 1981; Ben-Ari, 1985). The second type of damage develops after focal administration of KA into the brain. Neurons in the immediate vicinity of the injection site are killed by a direct "excitotoxic" mechanism that does not involve seizure activity (Coyle, 1983). Finally, several laboratories have noted that rats treated with sufficient KA to produce extensive brain damage often develop spontaneous seizures (Pisa et al., 1980; Cavalheiro et al., 1982; Tanaka et al., 1985; Nitecka and Tremblay, 1986; Whishaw, 1987). This observation has helped to generate new ideas about the possible mechanisms by which a pre-existing hippocampal sclerosis might lead to the development of epilepsy.

Although they differ somewhat according to the route of administration, all distant KA lesions bear some resemblance to forms of hippocampal sclerosis in humans. Intracerebroventricular KA preferentially destroys the CA3–CA4 neurons of the hippocampus (Nadler et al., 1978). These lesions resemble EFS, especially when the doses used are low enough to avoid much extrahippocampal damage. In our hands, lesions made by parenteral KA tend to involve hippocampal pyramidal cells somewhat indiscriminately, showing no obvious preference for those in area CA3 over those in area CA1. These lesions most closely resemble NSHS. At doses sufficient to provoke many hours of status epilepticus, KA administered by either route can produce a lesion that resembles AHS. Hence each route of administration appears to provide a useful model of the clinical pathology.

The idea that brain lesions made by i.c.v. KA result from excessive limbic seizure activity implies that other convulsants administered by the same route will produce similar lesions, provided that they elicit seizure activity within the limbic circuit for the same duration. A comparison of i.c.v. KA and i.c.v. bicuculline methiodide (BMI) supported this view (Gruenthal et al., 1986). The electrographic and behavioral seizures evoked by the two convulsants were quite different, indicating that KA and BMI seizures originate at different sites within the brain. Despite these differences, however, i.c.v. KA and BMI proved capable of producing a similar pattern of brain damage for a given total limbic seizure duration (Fig. 2A,B). In particular, the CA3–CA4 neurons of the rostral hippocampal formation were most vulnerable in both instances.

With the use of silver impregnation (Nadler and Evenson, 1983), we demonstrated a clear relationship between the total duration of electrographic limbic seizures (sum of the durations of each temporally discrete ictal episode) induced by i.c.v. BMI and the extent of neuronal cell death. A similar relationship emerged when the dose of i.c.v. KA was varied (Sater and Nadler, 1988). The extent of neuronal cell death varied with the total duration of limbic seizure activity, not with the dose of KA. In addition, phenobarbital and baclofen, which have anticonvulsant activity in the KA model, reduced the total duration of electrographic seizures and the extent of brain damage in parallel (Ault et al., 1986). Thus the total duration of electrographic seizure activity within the limbic system was identified as one of the critical factors that determine the probability that seizures will lead to cell death.

Different neuronal populations, of course, differ in their ability to withstand seizure activity. Extrahippocampal neurons and hippocampal neurons contralateral to the KA infusion were usually destroyed only when the animal developed electrographic status epilepticus (Fig. 3). In contrast, at least some ipsilateral CA3–CA4 neurons were always killed when the total seizure duration exceeded 27 min. More surprising was the finding that at least a few of these neurons were sometimes killed even when the animal experienced only a few brief electrographic seizures totalling less than 10 min. This extreme vulnerability could not be explained by systemic effects of the behavioral seizures nor by any focal toxicity of the convulsant, but suggested instead that KA (and possibly also BMI) sensitizes CA3–CA4 neurons to the destructive effect of

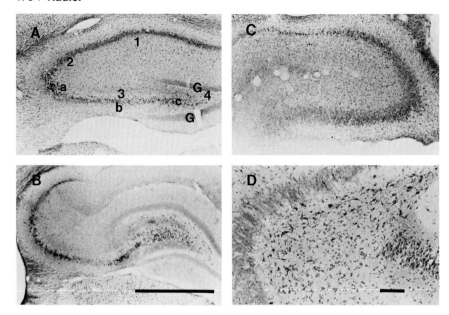

Fig. 2.   Neuronal degeneration in the rat hippocampal formation after status epilepticus. Silver impregnation. **A:** Neuronal degeneration in areas CA3 (3a,b,c) and CA4 (4) after i.c.v. KA (940 pmol). Pyramidal cells in areas CA1 (1) and CA2 (2) and dentate granule cells (G) were spared. **B:** Similar neuronal degeneration after i.c.v. BMI (5–6 nmol). Bar = 1 mm for A–C. **C:** Prior destruction of dentate granule cells with colchicine protects CA3–CA4 neurons from i.c.v. KA (1.41 nmol). **D:** The dentate hilus after 360 min of stimulation-induced status epilepticus. Note extensive degeneration of CA3c and CA4 neurons. Scale bar = 0.1 mm. Data are based on results of Gruenthal et al. (1986), Vicedomini and Nadler (1987a), and Okazaki and Nadler (1988). Part A adapted from Gruenthal et al. (1986), with permission of Academic Press, Inc.; B reproduced from Gruenthal et al. (1986), with permission of Academic Press, Inc.; C reproduced from Okazaki and Nadler (1988), with permission of Pergamon Press, Inc.; D reproduced from Vicedomini and Nadler (1987a), with permission of Academic Press, Inc.

seizure activity. If this is so, then seizure-related neuronal degeneration cannot depend solely on the total duration of seizure activity. This point was reinforced by the far greater damage suffered by the ipsilateral than by the contralateral hippocampal formation, even though the contralateral hippocampal formation experienced nearly as much electrographic seizure activity as the ipsilateral. This difference may be accounted for in part by the higher concentration of KA present on the ipsilateral side, but seems more importantly to involve the different anatomical pathways that support and/or convey seizure discharge in the two regions.

When selective lesions of various hippocampal pathways were tested for their effect on the neurotoxic action of KA, only destruction of the mossy fibers (by transection or with focal injections of colchicine) protected CA3–CA4 neurons from i.c.v. KA (Nadler and Cuthbertson, 1980; Nadler et al., 1981).

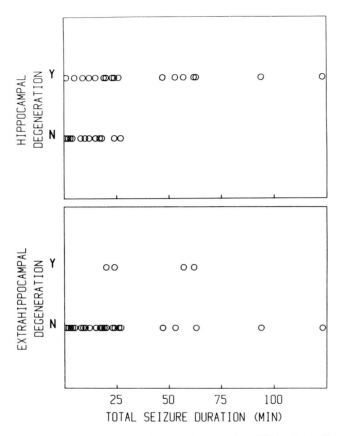

Fig. 3. Neuronal degeneration (Y) or lack of degeneration (N) in the ipsilateral hippocampal formation (top) or elsewhere in the brain (bottom) after i.c.v. administration of BMI (5–6 nmol) alone, BMI (5–6 nmol) with baclofen (5 mg/kg, i.p.), KA (117–820 pmol) alone, KA (940 pmol) with baclofen (5 mg/kg, i.p.), or KA (940 pmol) with phenobarbital (40 mg/kg, i.p.). Total seizure duration was calculated by summing the durations of each temporally discrete ictal episode. Each circle represents results from one animal; N = 37. Animals that developed status epilepticus have been excluded. Data are based on results of Ault et al. (1986), Gruenthal et al. (1986), Sater and Nadler (1988), and unpublished studies.

Mossy fiber lesions were effective immediately, suggesting that the destruction of CA3 pyramidal cells depends on impulse flow within the mossy fiber pathway. These results were initially interpreted to suggest that KA-induced degeneration of CA3–CA4 neurons requires a functional mossy fiber pathway simply because the mossy fibers serve as an obligatory link in the generation of hippocampal seizures. Subsequent investigations failed to bear out this idea, however. When tested in unanesthetized rats that had been chronically implanted with depth electrodes to record EEG, mossy fiber lesions were confirmed to protect the denervated CA3–CA4 neurons from i.c.v. KA (Fig. 2C) (Okazaki and Nadler, 1988). However, they did not usually attenuate seizure activity recorded from the denervated CA3 area; the development of status epilepticus was prevented in only 26% of subjects. Thus neuronal cell death could be dissociated from seizure activity, in the sense that seizures were insufficient by themselves to assure cell death. Death of CA3–CA4 neurons must also require some specific influence of or interaction with the mossy fiber pathway. These results further implied that seizures that do not involve the mossy fibers are less damaging than those that do (see also Nitecka et al., 1984). Thus neuronal cell death in the ipsilateral CA3–CA4 area depended on 1) seizure activity, 2) a sensitizing effect of KA, and 3) mossy fiber activity.

STUDIES OF STIMULATION-INDUCED STATUS EPILEPTICUS

As useful as animal models based on the administration of convulsant drugs have been, they present several interpretive problems. It can be difficult, for example, to relate cell death directly to neuronal activity and to separate effects of seizure activity from effects of the specific convulsant. In particular, the evidence that a specific interaction between KA (and perhaps BMI) with the mossy fiber pathway potentiated the destructive effects of seizures on CA3–CA4 hippocampal neurons motivated us to determine whether such an interaction was selective to convulsant-induced damage or might be involved in seizure-related damage of any origin. One approach that avoids these potential ambiguities is to stimulate selected brain pathways electrically in such a way as to evoke seizure activity. Sloviter (1983) demonstrated that prolonged intermittent or continuous stimulation of the entorhinohippocampal fibers in rats anesthetized with urethane essentially replicates the pattern of brain damage obtained with parenteral KA. Thus this type of damage does not result simply from systemic effects associated with behavioral seizures. By systematically varying the parameters for stimulating excitatory afferent pathways to the hippocampal formation of unanesthetized rats, we were able to develop a model of status epilepticus that allowed for activation of preselected excitatory pathways, continuous EEG recording, monitoring of synaptic responses in a neuronal population vulnerable to seizure activity, and behavioral monitoring (Vicedomini and Nadler, 1987a).

Studies of stimulation-induced status epilepticus revealed a clear correlation between the overall extent of neuronal cell death and the duration of self-sustained seizure activity. In general, the pattern of neuronal cell death, as revealed by silver impregnation, resembled lesions that result from angular bundle stimulation in animals anesthetized with urethane (Sloviter, 1983) and from parenteral administration of KA (Ben-Ari et al., 1980; Sloviter and Damiano, 1981). The first neurons to die were those in hippocampal area CA4 (Fig. 2D) and in layers 3 and 5 of the entorhinal cortex ipsilateral to angular bundle stimulation or contralateral to fimbrial stimulation. These neurons can be destroyed with as little as 13–17 min of self-sustained seizure activity (Fig. 4). If the afterdischarges recorded from the CA3 area are added to the self-sustained seizure, then the threshold for neuronal degeneration in this model is about

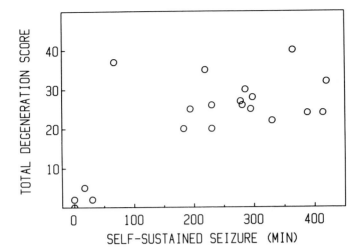

Fig. 4. Neuronal degeneration or lack of degeneration in the rat brain after various durations of self-sustained seizure induced by stimulation of the angular bundle or fimbria. Each circle represents results from one animal; N = 23. Self-sustained seizure is the electrographic seizure recorded after electrical stimulation ceased. In addition, all animals generated some hippocampal afterdischarge before this time. Data are based on results of Vicedomini and Nadler (1987a) and unpublished studies.

20–25 min of total seizure activity. This figure is consistent with our studies of convulsant-induced damage and with a neuropathological study of flurothyl-induced seizures (Nevander et al., 1985). In addition, we have observed that some CA4 and entorhinal cortical neurons degenerated in a few, but not all, animals whose afterdischarges totalled 25 min or more in a 6–7 h period, even if there were no self-sustained seizures. An important point is that the destruction of even a single neuron, as judged by silver impregnation, depended on the development of seizure activity, not on electrical stimulation per se. More than 700 10 s periods of synaptic activity could be evoked without evidence of neuronal degeneration, provided that seizure activity was minimal. Thus the neuronal hyperactivity associated with tetanic stimulation can lead to cell death only if it provokes seizure activity of some minimum duration.

It should be noted that our ability to detect this minimal degeneration depended on the use of a sensitive silver impregnation technique. Even considerably greater damage than this may have gone undetected if our histological analysis had been limited to the use of the routine stains employed by clinical neuropathologists or if we had relied on cell counting with its considerable errors. It is possible that even relatively prolonged complex partial seizures in humans destroy too few neurons to be detected at autopsy years later. Unfortunately, because silver impregnation labels degenerating neurons for no more than a few days after their death, this approach would be of little help in analyzing clinical material.

With the use of stimulation-induced status epilepticus, we were able to test the hypothesis that seizures that involve the mossy fibers are inherently more damaging than seizures that do not. Rats received a unilateral mossy fiber transection or colchicine lesion and were later subjected to stimulation of the contralateral fimbria (Vicedomini and Nadler, 1987b). The results suggested that at least some mossy fibers must be intact for contralateral fimbrial stimulation to evoke status epilepticus. Hence the mossy fiber pathway appears to be a more essential component of the seizure circuit in this model than in the KA model. Conversely, the mossy fibers appeared to be less crucial for the degeneration of CA3–CA4 neurons in the stimulation model. The special interaction between chemical convulsants, such as KA, and the mossy fibers evidently has no counterpart in this model. Thus seizures that involve the mossy fibers are not necessarily much more damaging than seizures that do not.

HOW COULD HIPPOCAMPAL SCLEROSIS LEAD TO EPILEPSY?

Although many clinicians have for over a century asserted their belief that complex partial epilepsy arises from hippocampal sclerosis, it was difficult until recently to propose a convincing mechanism by which neuronal degeneration could facilitate seizure discharge. During the last few years, however, several plausible mechanisms have been proposed based on evidence from animal models. Two that have attracted recent attention may be termed the *sprouting mechanism* and the *disinhibition mechanism*. Only the sprouting mechanism will be considered here. Sloviter (Chapter 28, this volume) has discussed the disinhibition mechanism, and data from studies of KA-induced hippocampal sclerosis that are relevant to this mechanism have been summarized by Franck et al. (1988).

The sprouting mechanism suggests that aberrant synaptic connections formed in response to the loss of hippocampal neurons produce a state of hyperexcitability that either provokes or facilitates abnormal discharge. Synaptic rearrangements almost inevitably follow brain damage in experimental animals (Cotman et al., 1981). Degeneration of neural pathways evokes growth in nearby undamaged pathways that reoccupies the vacated synaptic space. This process, termed *sprouting* or *reactive synaptogenesis*, has been extensively studied in the rat hippocampal formation and is likely to operate also in the hippocampal formation of complex partial epileptics (de Lorenzo and Glaser, 1981; de Lorenzo et al., 1982).

In KA-treated rats, degeneration of the axons of CA3–CA4 neurons leads to a substantial loss of synapses in regions innervated by these axons. This degenerative phase is followed by replacement of these synapses (Nadler et al., 1980b). Several of the projections that contribute to this reinnervation have been identified (Nadler et al., 1980a). The most intriguing finding was that mossy fibers in the dentate hilus sprout axon collaterals, which grow through the granule cell layer of the fascia dentata and form a terminal plexus within the inner third of the molecular layer (Fig. 5B), that is, in the zone vacated by degenerated axon terminals of associational-commissural CA4 neurons. This type of axonal growth is of special interest for three reasons. 1) Few mossy fiber axon collaterals enter the molecular layer normally. Supragranular mossy fibers can be demonstrated at the ends and apex of the granule cell arch, but in between they are rare. Thus the moderate-to-dense projection that develops in many KA-treated animals is clearly aberrant. 2) This reactive growth creates a recurrent excitatory circuit that could support repetitive discharge of granule cells in response to a single stimulus. In light of evidence that the fascia dentata normally serves to dampen high-frequency discharges in the limbic circuit (Collins et al., 1983b), one might expect that the formation of recurrent mossy fibers would lead to a reduction in seizure threshold. 3) Loss of CA4 neurons is a consistent feature of hippocampal sclerosis. Thus the stimulus for recurrent mossy fiber sprouting is present in a large percentage of epileptic patients. It was of obvious importance then to determine whether these connections were electrophysiologically functional.

Studies on hippocampal slices prepared from KA-treated rats suggested that the recurrent mossy fibers did indeed form aberrant excitatory connections (Tauck and Nadler, 1985). Most notably, antidromic activation of the mossy fibers evoked multiple granule cell population spikes in some cases, whereas antidromic activation in slices from control rats evoked only a single spike (Fig. 5A). The second and succeeding population spikes in the complex behaved as though they were synaptically driven. Multiple firing could not be explained by loss of inhibition. This abnormal response developed only in slices from those animals that had both lost a high percentage of CA4 neurons (Fig. 5C) and had subsequently grown a moderate-to-dense supragranular mossy fiber projection (Fig. 5D). These results suggested that mossy fiber sprouting formed a type of excitatory circuit that could facilitate the development and spread of limbic seizure activity. In line with this idea, recent evidence has linked this sprouting response to an enhanced susceptibility to kindling (Feldblum and Ackermann, 1987; Sutula et al., 1987). It seems likely that recurrent mossy fibers and other nascent excitatory circuits account, in part, for the spontaneous seizures that develop after a KA lesion.

In view of these results, it would be important to determine the incidence of recurrent mossy fiber sprouting and other synaptic rearrangements in epilepsy patients. It is possible that much of the functional impairment in complex partial epileptics, as well as their recurring seizures, derives from aberrant reactive growth.

Although the formation of aberrant circuitry provides a reasonable explanation for the epileptogenic potential of hippocampal sclerosis, some cautionary statements are in order. First, lesions similar to clinical and experimentally induced hippocampal sclerosis have been described after insults, such as cerebral ischemia (Brierley and Graham, 1984), that do not necessarily lead to epilepsy. In fact, aberrant supragranular mossy fibers have been demonstrated in hippocampi from aged, but nonepileptic, patients (Cassell and Brown, 1984). Thus factors other than the mere presence of CA4 damage and/or recurrent mossy fibers are necessary to support seizure discharge. Second, the spontaneous seizures that follow KA-induced hippocampal sclerosis tend to remit after a period of months (Cavalheiro et al., 1982), despite the persistence of

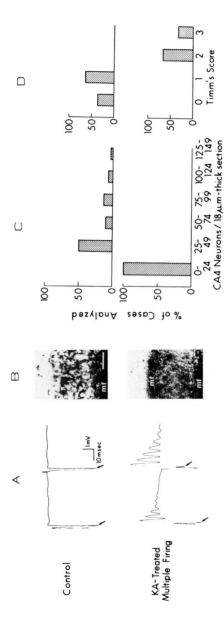

Fig. 5. Mossy fiber sprouting and dentate granule cell electrophysiology 12–21 days after intravenous KA (11 mg/kg). **A**: Responses of dentate granule cells to antidromic stimulation of the mossy fibers. A pair of identical submaximal electrical pulses was delivered with an interstimulus interval of 50 ms. Arrows indicate the antidromic population spike. **B**: Timm's sulfide silver staining to reveal the localization of mossy fibers (mf) in relation to the granule cell layer. Cresyl violet counterstain. Only subgranular mossy fibers are present in the control, but the KA-treated animal developed a supragranular mossy fiber band. Bar = 0.03 mm. **C**: Number of CA4 neurons in sections cut from temporal hippocampal slices. **D**: Timm's score (density of supragranular mossy fiber projection). Data are based on results of Tauck and Nadler (1985). Reproduced from Tauck and Nadler (1985), with permission of Oxford University Press.

recurrent mossy fibers. This observation again suggests that some additional factor, critical but transient, is required to induce spontaneous seizures. Alternatively, the effects of mossy fiber sprouting may eventually be compensated by some slowly developing change in the tissue. Third, mossy fiber sprouting can be provoked in experimental animals by electrical stimulation of the perforant path that does not noticeably damage area CA4 (Sutula et al., 1988). Thus degeneration of CA4 neurons is not the only stimulus for mossy fiber growth. Perforant path stimulation by itself appears to induce much less growth than CA4 degeneration, however. Judging from our studies of KA-treated rats, the stimulation protocols employed by Sutula et al. (1988) produce too little sprouting to induce the multiple firing of granule cells. It would be interesting to know whether a denser supragranular mossy fiber projection could be created by stimulating the perforant path to the point of spontaneous seizures. Fourth, there is still no direct evidence linking the recurrent mossy fibers to hyperexcitability in the hippocampal formation. Further studies of this issue would require a means of selectively blocking mossy fiber transmission and the use of intracellular recording techniques.

CONCLUSIONS

Investigations of animal models and detailed analyses of epilepsy patients have led to a tentative understanding of the relationship between complex partial seizures and neuronal cell death in the hippocampal formation. A subset of patients, whose condition often progresses to a pharmacologically intractable state, develops AHS or severe EFS early in childhood. Extrahippocampal damage is likely to be present also. In many cases, the lesion probably arises from prolonged febrile convulsions/status epilepticus, but other etiologies may exist. Whatever the original cause of the sclerotic lesion, the damage serves as a focus for hyperexcitability followed eventually by spontaneous seizures. Two factors that might link hippocampal damage to the subsequent development of an epileptic focus are the formation of aberrant excitatory circuitry through axon sprouting and permanently depressed synaptic inhibition.

A second group of patients, at least as numerous as the first, develops NSHS. In these cases, the etiology of their epileptic condition is uncertain. Epilepsy tends to develop over a more prolonged time course and may less often progress to a pharmacologically intractable state. In many of these cases, especially those in which the lesion involves mainly the CA3–CA4 area, the damage probably arises as a result of repeated seizures. Each seizure that lasts for at least a certain minimum duration destroys some hippocampal neurons. If the patient sustains enough of these relatively prolonged seizure episodes, the cumulative histopathology will become obvious by conventional staining methods. Widespread damage outside the hippocampal formation would not be expected unless one or more episodes of status epilepticus had occurred. If there are few prolonged seizures, then hippocampal damage will be minor and conventional staining methods may not pick it up. This may explain why some patients with complex partial epilepsy, especially those whose seizures originate outside the hippocampus, exhibit no obvious hippocampal pathology. No damage would be expected if the hippocampal seizures are all quite brief. In the rat, 20–25 min of seizure activity appears sufficient to destroy at least a few of the most vulnerable hippocampal neurons, but it not clear to what seizure duration this figure would correspond in humans. Regardless, experimental data reinforce the view that seizures are damaging to the brain and should be controlled whenever possible before a clinically significant number of neurons is lost (Engel, 1983).

ACKNOWLEDGMENTS

Special thanks are due to my collaborators, especially Maxine Okazaki, Debra Evenson, Michael Gruenthal, John Vicedomini, David Tauck, David Armstrong, Brian Ault, Richard Sater, Gil Cuthbertson and Michael Smith. I also wish to acknowledge the generous support of our research provided by grants NS 17771 and NS 06233 from the National Institutes of Health.

REFERENCES

Ault, B., M. Gruenthal, D.R. Armstrong, and J.V. Nadler (1986) Efficacy of baclofen and phenobarbital against the kainic acid limbic seizure-brain damage syndrome. J. Pharmacol. Exp. Ther. *239:*612–617.

Babb, T.L. (1986) Metabolic, morphologic and electrophysiologic profiles of human temporal lobe foci: An attempt at correlation. In R. Schwarcz and Y. Ben-Ari (eds): Excitatory Amino Acids and Epilepsy. New York: Plenum Press, pp. 115–125.

Babb, T.L., W.J. Brown, J. Pretorius, C. Davenport, J.P. Lieb, and P.H. Crandall (1984a) Temporal lobe volumetric cell densities in temporal lobe epilepsy. Epilepsia *25:*729–740.

Babb, T.L., J.P. Lieb, W.J. Brown, J. Pretorius, and P.H. Crandall (1984b) Distribution of pyramidal cell density and hyperexcitability in the epileptic human hippocampal formation. Epilepsia *25:*721–728.

Ben-Ari, Y. (1985) Limbic seizure and brain damage produced by kainic acid: Mechanisms and revelance to human temporal lobe epilepsy. Neuroscience *14:*375–403.

Ben-Ari, Y., E. Tremblay, O.P. Ottersen, and B.S. Meldrum (1980) The role of epileptic activity in the hippocampal and "remote" certebral lesions induced by kainic acid. Brain Res. *191:*79–97.

Ben-Ari, Y., E. Tremblay, D. Riche, G. Ghilini, and R. Naquet (1981) Electrographic, clinical and pathological alterations following systemic administration of kainic acid, bicuculline or pentetrazole: Metabolic mapping using the deoxyglucose method with special reference to the pathology of epilepsy. Neuroscience *6:*1361–1391.

Blennow, G., J.B. Brierley, B.S. Meldrum, and B.K. Siesjö (1978) Epileptic brain damage: The role of systemic factors that modify cerebral energy metabolism. Brain *101:*687–700.

Bouchet and Cazauvieilh (1825) De l'épilepsie considerée dans ses rapports avec l'alienation mentale. Arch. Gen. Med. *9:*510–542.

Brierley, J.B., and D.I. Graham (1984) Hypoxia and vascular disorders of the central nervous system. In J.H. Adams, J.A.N. Corsellis, and L.W. Duchen (eds): Greenfield's Neuropathology. New York: John Wiley & Sons, pp. 125–207.

Brown, W.J. (1973) Structural substrates of seizure foci in the human temporal lobe. In M.A.B. Brazier (ed): Epilepsy: Its Phenomena in Man. New York: Academic Press, pp. 339–374.

Cassell, M.D., and M.W. Brown (1984) The distribution of Timm's stain in the nonsulphide-perfused human hippocampal formation. J. Comp. Neurol. *222:*461–471.

Cavalheiro, E.A., D.A. Riche, and G. Le Gal La Salle (1982) Long-term effects of intrahippocampal kainic acid injection in rats: A method for inducing spontaneous recurrent seizures. Electroencephalogr. Clin. Neurophysiol. 53:581–589.

Cavanagh, J.B., and A. Meyer (1956) Aetiological aspects of Ammon's horn sclerosis associated with temporal lobe epilepsy. Br. Med. J. 2:1403–1407.

Collins, R.C., E.W. Lothman, and J.W. Olney (1983a) Status epilepticus in the limbic system: Biochemical and pathological changes. In A.V. Delgado-Escueta, C.G. Wasterlain, D.M. Treiman, and R.J. Porter (eds): Advances in Neurology, Vol. 34: Status Epilepticus. New York: Raven Press, pp. 277–288.

Collins, R.C., R.G. Tearse, and E.W. Lothman (1983b) Functional anatomy of limbic seizures: Focal discharges from medial entorhinal cortex in rat. Brain Res., 280: 25–40.

Corsellis, J.A.N., and C.J. Bruton (1983) Neuropathology of status epilepticus in humans. In A.V. Delgado-Escueta, C.G. Wasterlain, D.M. Treiman, and R.J. Porter (eds): Advances in Neurology, Vol. 34, Status Epilepticus. New York: Raven Press, pp. 129–139.

Cotman, C.W., M. Nieto-Sampedro, and E.W. Harris (1981) Synapse replacement in the nervous system of adult vertebrates. Physiol. Rev. 61:684–784.

Coyle, J.T. (1983) Neurotoxic action of kainic acid. J. Neurochem. 41:1–11.

de Lorenzo, R.J., and G.H. Glaser (1981) Neuropathologic changes and neuronal plasticity in temporal lobe-limbic epilepsy. Neurology 31:114.

de Lorenzo, R.J., G.H. Glaser, P. De Lucia, and D. Schwartz (1982) The role of neuronal plasticity in epilepsy. Neurology 32:A92.

Engel, J. (1983) Epileptic brain damage: How much excitement can a limbic neuron take? Trends Neurosci. 6:356–357.

Falconer, M.A. (1971) Genetic and related aetiological factors in temporal lobe epilepsy: A review. Epilepsia 12:13–31.

Falconer, M.A. (1974) Mesial temporal (Ammon's horn) sclerosis as a common cause of epilepsy: Aetiology, treatment and prevention. Lancet 2:767–770.

Falconer, M.A., E.A. Serafetinides, and J.A.N. Corsellis (1964) Etiology and pathogenesis of temporal lobe epilepsy. Arch. Neurol. 10:233–248.

Falconer, M.A., and D.C. Taylor (1968) Surgical treatment of drug-resistant epilepsy due to mesial temporal sclerosis. Arch. Neurol. 19:353–361.

Feldblum, S., and R.F. Ackermann (1987) Increased susceptibility to hippocampal and amygdala kindling following intrahippocampal kainic acid. Exp. Neurol. 97:255–269.

Franck, J.E., D.D. Kunkel, D.G. Baskin, and P.A. Schwartzkroin (1988) Inhibition in kainate-lesioned hyperexcitable hippocampi: Physiologic, autoradiographic, and immunocytochemical observations. J. Neurosci. 8:1991–2002.

Gastaut, H., M. Toga, J. Roger, and W.C. Gibson (1959) A correlation of clinical electroencephalographic and anatomical findings in nine autopsied cases of "temporal lobe epilepsy." Epilepsia 1:56–85.

Gruenthal, M., D.R. Armstrong, B. Ault, and J.V. Nadler (1986) Comparison of seizures and brain lesions produced by intracerebroventricular kainic acid and bicuculline methiodide. Exp. Neurol. 93:621–630.

Johnston, G.A.R., D.R. Curtis, J. Davies, and R.M. McCulloch (1974) Excitation of spinal interneurones by some conformationally restricted analogues of L-glutamic acid. Nature 248:804–805.

Lothman, E.W., and R.C. Collins (1981) Kainic acid induced limbic seizures: Metabolic, behavioral, electrographic, and neuropathological correlates. Brain Res. 218:299–318.

Margerison, J.H., and J.A.N. Corsellis (1966) Epilepsy and the temporal lobes. Brain 89:499–530.

Meldrum, B.S., and J.B. Brierley (1972) Neuronal loss and gliosis in the hippocampus following repetitive epileptic seizures induced in adolescent baboons by allylglycine. Brain Res. *48*:361–365.

Meldrum, B.S., and J.B. Brierley (1973) Prolonged epileptic seizures in primates: Ischemic cell change and its relation to ictal physiological events. Arch. Neurol. *28*:10–17.

Meldrum, B.S., and J.A.N. Corsellis (1984) Epilepsy. In J.H. Adams, J.A.N. Corsellis, and L.W. Duchen (eds): Greenfield's Neuropathology. New York: John Wiley & Sons, pp. 921–950.

Meldrum, B.S., R.W. Horton, and J.B. Brierley (1974) Epileptic brain damage in adolescent baboons following seizures induced by allylglycine. Brain *97*:407–418.

Meldrum, B.S., R.A. Vigouroux, and J.B. Brierley (1973) Systemic factors and epileptic brain damage. Arch. Neurol. *29*:82–87.

Menini, C., B.S. Meldrum, D. Riche, C. Silva-Comte, and J.M. Stutzmann (1980) Sustained limbic seizures induced by intraamygdaloid kainic acid in the baboon: Symptomatology and neuropathological consequences. Ann. Neurol. *8*:501–509.

Mouritzen Dam, A. (1980) Epilepsy and neuron loss in the hippocampus. Epilepsia *21*:617–629.

Nadler, J.V. (1981) Kainic acid as a tool for the study of temporal lobe epilepsy. Life Sci. *29*:2031–2042.

Nadler, J.V., and G.J. Cuthbertson (1980) Kainic acid neurotoxicity toward hippocampal formation: Dependence on specific excitatory pathways. Brain Res. *195*:47–56.

Nadler, J.V., and D.A. Evenson (1983) Use of excitatory amino acids to make axon-sparing lesions of hypothalamus. Methods Enzymol. *103*:393–400.

Nadler, J.V., D.A. Evenson, and E.M. Smith (1981) Evidence from lesion studies for epileptogenic and non-epileptogenic neurotoxic interactions between kainic acid and excitatory innervation. Brain Res. *205*:405–410.

Nadler, J.V., B.W. Perry, and C.W. Cotman (1978) Intraventricular kainic acid preferentially destroys hippocampal pyramidal cells. Nature *271*:676–677.

Nadler, J.V., B.W. Perry, and C.W. Cotman (1980a) Selective reinnervation of hippocampal area CA1 and the fascia dentata after destruction of CA3-CA4 afferents with kainic acid. Brain Res. *182*:1–9.

Nadler, J.V., B.W. Perry, C. Gentry, and C.W. Cotman (1980b) Loss and reacquisition of hippocampal synapses after selective destruction of CA3-CA4 afferents with kainic acid. Brain Res. *191*:387–403.

Nevander, G., M. Ingvar, R. Auer, and B.K. Siesjö (1985) Status epilepticus in well-oxygenated rats causes neuronal necrosis. Ann. Neurol. *18*:281–290.

Nitecka, L., and E. Tremblay (1986) Long term sequelae of parenteral administration of kainic acid. In R. Schwarcz, and Y. Ben-Ari (eds): Excitatory Amino Acids and Epilepsy. New York: Plenum Press, pp. 147–155.

Nitecka, L., E. Tremblay, G. Charton, J.P. Bouillot, M.L. Berger, and Y. Ben-Ari (1984) Maturation of kainic acid seizure-brain damage syndrome in the rat. II. Histopathological sequelae. Neuroscience *13*:1073–1094.

Okazaki, M.M., and J.V. Nadler (1988) Protective effects of mossy fiber lesions against kainic acid-induced seizures and neuronal degeneration. Neuroscience *26*:763–781.

Olney, J.W., V. Rhee, and O.L. Ho (1974) Kainic acid: A powerful neurotoxic analogue of glutamate. Brain Res. *77*:507–512.

Olney, J.W., L.G. Sharpe, and T. de Gubareff (1975) Excitotoxic amino acids. Soc. Neurosci. Abstr. *1*:371.

Pisa, M., P.R. Sanberg, M.E. Corcoran, and H.C. Fibiger (1980) Spontaneous recurrent seizures after intracerebral injections of kainic acid in rats: A possible model of human temporal lobe epilepsy. Brain Res. *200*:481–487.

Sagar, H.J., and J.M. Oxbury (1987) Hippocampal neuron loss in temporal lobe epilepsy: Correlation with early childhood convulsions. Ann. Neurol. *22:*334–340.

Sano, K., and N. Malamud (1953) Clinical significance of sclerosis of the cornu Ammonis. Arch. Neurol. Psychiatry *70:*40–53.

Sater, R.A., and J.V. Nadler (1988) On the relation between seizures and brain lesions after intracerebroventricular kainic acid. Neurosci. Lett. *84:*73–78.

Scheibel, M.E., P.H. Crandall, and A.B. Scheibel (1974) The hippocampal-dentate complex in temporal lobe epilepsy: A Golgi study. Epilepsia *15:*55–80.

Scholz, W. (1959) The contribution of patho-anatomical research to the problem of epilepsy. Epilepsia *1:*36–55.

Shinozaki, H., and S. Konishi (1970) Actions of several anthelmintics and insecticides on rat cortical neurones. Brain Res. *24:*368–371.

Sloviter, R.S. (1983) "Epileptic" brain damage in rats induced by sustained electrical stimulation of the perforant path. I. Acute electrophysiological and light microscopic studies. Brain Res. Bull. *10:*675–697.

Sloviter, R.S., and B.P. Damiano (1981) On the relationship between kainic acid-induced epileptiform activity and hippocampal neuronal damage. Neuropharmacology *20:*1003–1011.

Sommer, W. (1880) Erkrankung des Ammonshorns als aetiologisches Moment der Epilepsie. Arch. Psychiat. Nervenkr. *10:*631–675.

Spielmeyer, W. (1927) Die Pathogenese des epileptischen Krampfes. Histopathologischer Teil. Z. Neurol. Psychiat. *109:*501–520.

Sutula, T., X.-X. He, J. Cavazos, and G. Scott (1988) Synaptic reorganization in the hippocampus induced by abnormal functional activity. Science *239:*1147–1150.

Sutula, T., X. He, and C. Hurtenbach (1987) Facilitation of kindling by CA3 lesions: Potential of lesion-induced sprouting and synaptic reorganization. Epilepsia *28:*593.

Takemoto, T. (1978) Isolation and identification of naturally occurring excitatory amino acids. In E.G. McGeer, J.W. Olney, and P.L. McGeer (eds): Kainic acid as a Tool in Neurobiology. New York: Raven Press, pp. 1–15.

Tanaka, T., M. Kaijima, Y. Yonemasu, and C. Cepeda (1985) Spontaneous secondarily generalized seizures induced by a single microinjection of kainic acid into unilateral amygdala in cats. Electroencephalogr. Clin. Neurophysiol. *61:*422–429.

Tauck, D.L., and J.V. Nadler (1985) Evidence of functional mossy fiber sprouting in hippocampal formation of kainic acid-treated rats. J. Neurosci. *5:*1016–1022.

Vicedomini, J.P., and J.V. Nadler (1987a) A model of status epilepticus based on electrical stimulation of hippocampal afferent pathways. Exp. Neurol. *96:*681–691.

Vicedomini, J.P., and J.V. Nadler (1987b) Stimulation-induced status epilepticus: Role of the hippocampal mossy fiber projection. Soc. Neurosci. Abstr. *13:*1155.

Whishaw, I.Q. (1987) Hippocampal, granule cell and CA_{3-4} lesions impair formation of a place learning-set in the rat and induce reflex epilepsy. Behav. Brain Res. *24:*59–72.

The Hippocampus—New Vistas, pages 483–497
© 1989 Alan R. Liss, Inc.

30
Relationship of the Hippocampal GABAergic System and Genetic Epilepsy in the Seizure-Sensitive Gerbil

GARY M. PETERSON AND CHARLES E. RIBAK

Department of Anatomy and Cell Biology, East Carolina University, Greenville, North Carolina (G.M.P.); Department of Anatomy and Neurobiology, University of California, Irvine, California College of Medicine, Irvine, California (C.E.R)

INTRODUCTION

The role of cortical γ-aminobutyric acidergic (GABAergic) neurons in focal epilepsy and the involvement of the hippocampus in the etiology and expression of epilepsy are both well established. Numerous studies have demonstrated specific defects in the cortical GABAergic neuronal system in certain experimental models of epilepsy. For example, a specific reduction in the number of GABAergic neurons (Ribak et al., 1986) and axon terminals (Ribak, 1985; Ribak et al., 1979, 1982) has been observed in the monkey alumina gel model of post-traumatic epilepsy. These findings are consistent with results from biochemical studies that have shown a reduction in glutamate decarboxylase (GAD) activity as well as in concentrations of GABA at epileptic foci in the same model (Bakay and Harris, 1981) and in tumor patients (Lloyd et al., 1981). The involvement of the hippocampal formation in epilepsy has been known since 1880, when Sommer reported a loss of hippocampal pyramidal cells associated with temporal lobe epilepsy. This finding has been repeated and extended by many subsequent studies (Brown, 1973; Hughes and Adams, 1984; Meldrum and Brierly, 1972; Mouritzen Dam, 1980; Scheibel et al., 1974). In addition, the tendency of the hippocampus toward seizure activity is one of its best documented electrophysiological characteristics (Kandel and Spencer, 1961; Prince, 1983). This sensitivity has been demonstrated in several species, including man, and is particularly interesting because seizures in the human hippocampus and surrounding temporal cortex account for about one-half of all focal cortical seizures and one-fifth of all epileptic attacks (DeJong, 1957; Jasper, 1961). The sensitivity of the hippocampus to seizure-induced damage and its propensity for seizure activity are further demonstrated by its response to excitatory agents such as kainic acid (Ben-Ari et al., 1979; Franck, 1984; Nadler et al., 1978, 1980; Ruth, 1982; Schwarcz et al., 1978; Sloviter and Damiano, 1981) as well as by its ability to be kindled (Goddard et al., 1969; Pinel et al., 1975; Wada and Sato, 1973; Wada et al., 1974).

The role of hippocampal GABAergic neurons in epilepsy has only recently been investigated. In animal models of experimentally induced seizure activity the involvement of the hippocampal GABAergic system is equivocal. GABAergic neurons are apparently not damaged by kainic acid-induced seizures (Davies et al., 1985). More recently, it was claimed that GABAergic hilar neurons were not significantly decreased in number by prolonged electrical stimulation of the perforant pathway (Sloviter, 1987) even though an earlier report suggested damage to GABAergic-type basket cells and indicated a loss of recurrent inhibition in this model (Sloviter, 1983). In contrast, kindling of the hippocampus has been shown to be related to a reduction in the number of GABAergic neurons in the CA1 region (Kamphuis et al., 1986). In our work we have used an animal model of epilepsy in which the seizures are related to genetic causes rather than to experimentally induced changes. Our data from the seizure-sensitive Mongolian gerbil suggest a direct relationship between the GABAergic system in the hippocampus and the existence of epileptic seizures.

THE GENETICALLY SEIZURE-SENSITIVE GERBIL

Mongolian gerbils *(Meriones unguiculatus)* are a particularly useful animal model for the study of epilepsy because the animals exhibit spontaneous clonic-tonic seizures that resemble human generalized seizures (Loskota et al., 1974; Thiessen et al., 1968). Seizures are induced by a number of sensory stimuli, including exposure to a novel environment (Loskota et al., 1974). The intensity of the seizures varies within the gerbil population but is constant for individual animals so that it is therefore possible to correlate a known history of seizure intensity with morphological observations. The animals used in our studies had been bred phenotypically over 10 to 15 generations to produce two strains, one that is seizure sensitive (SS) and one that is seizure resistant (SR). Since the onset of seizure activity does not begin until about 50 days of age (Loskota et al., 1974), it is possible to examine the brains of young "seizure-predisposed" (SP) progeny of SS animals prior to the occurrence of seizure activity to determine whether the differences between SS and SR brains occur prior to seizure onset or are the result of seizure activity.

Abnormalities in the GABAergic system of SS gerbils have been shown to be related to seizure sensitivity. For example, when GABA levels are increased in SS gerbils by the administration of GABA agonist drugs, seizure susceptibility is reduced and the dose required for this effect is significantly smaller than that required for other genetically predisposed animals or animals with chemically or electrically induced seizures (Löscher, 1984; Löscher et al., 1983). Olsen et al. (1984, 1985) have demonstrated reduced benzodiazepine receptor binding in the substantia nigra of SS gerbils as well as a parallel deficit of bicuculline binding to low-affinity GABA receptors. However, forebrain regions, including the hippocampus and dentate gyrus, do not show any differences between SS and SR gerbils for these receptors.

The hippocampus of SS gerbils is known to be involved in seizures. For example, epileptic EEG activity has been recorded from the ventral hippocampus during seizures (Majkowski and Donadio, 1984). In addition, two anatomical studies have indicated morphological alterations in the hippocampus. Paul et al. (1981) have demonstrated a reduction in the number of dendritic spines on the apical dendrites of CA3 pyramidal cells, whereas Mouritzen Dam et al. (1981) have shown a loss of pyramidal cells restricted to the CA2 region.

Using immunocytochemical, histochemical, and Golgi techniques we have morphometrically examined both the dentate gyrus and hippocampus as well as other brain regions that are either rich in GABAergic neurons or thought to be involved in seizure activity (Peterson et al., 1985; Peterson and Ribak, 1987). The major morphological differences observed between SS and SR gerbils were in the GABAergic system of the hippocampal formation (Peterson and Ribak, 1987). Therefore, we will discuss in the following section only those data that are directly related to the GABAergic neurons in the hippocampal formation of genetically epileptic gerbils.

HIPPOCAMPAL GABAergic NEURONS IN GENETICALLY EPILEPTIC GERBILS

In the experiments to be discussed, GABAergic somata and terminals were identified immunocytochemically using a polyclonal antiserum to glutamate decarboxylase (GAD), the synthesizing enzyme for GABA. The antiserum was kindly provided by Drs. Wolfgang H. Oertel and Donald E. Schmechel, and its characterization and use have been previously described (Oertel et al., 1981a,b). Quantitative analysis involved counting and measuring the size of GABAergic neurons in the dentate gyrus and hippocampus proper in both cerebral hemispheres of six SS, four SR, and three SP brains. Every fifth section (40 μm thick) throughout the septotemporal extent of the hippocampal formation was analyzed. Within the dentate gyrus five subregions were analyzed for somata size and number: the hilar region, the infra- and suprapyramidal blades of stratum granulosum, and the infra- and suprapyramidal blades of the stratum moleculare. GABAergic terminal density was measured in the infra- and suprapyramidal blades of stratum granulosum. Within the hippocampus proper, counts were made in six subdivisions: three in regio superior (CA1; strata oriens, pyramidale, and radiatum-lacunosum-moleculare) and three in regio inferior (CA2,3; strata oriens, pyramidale, and lucidum-radiatum-lacunosum-moleculare). The density of GABAergic terminals was qualitatively assessed in all regions. To standardize the data for variations in the sizes of strata granulosum and moleculare of the dentate gyrus, area measurements were made by tracing each of the laminae onto the digitizing tablet of a Bioquant Image Analysis System (R & M Biometrics, Nashville, Tennessee), and relative cell counts were converted to cell densities. Since these data were not used to estimate the total number of neurons in any of the brain regions studied, but rather the relative number per section, it was not necessary to use a split-cell correction factor.

GABAergic Neurons in the Dentate Gyrus

The GABAergic neurons of the hippocampal formation have been studied best in the rat brain. For this reason the morphology of the GABAergic cells in the dentate gyrus and hippocampus of the SR gerbil (the presumed "normal") brain will first be compared with that of the rat brain, and then comparisons will be made between the SR and SS gerbil brains. The normal rat dentate gyrus contains several types of GABAergic cells (Ribak et al., 1978; Seress and Ribak, 1983), and the most numerous and heterogenous population is found in the hilar region. Seress and Ribak (1983) have characterized four distinct types of GABAergic basket cells within or immediately subjacent to the stratum granulosum: the pyramidal basket, large fusiform, horizontal basket, and inverted fusiform cells. A fifth type of basket cell is present in the stratum moleculare. These cells all have a multipolar configuration. Each of these cell types gives rise to a pericellular axonal plexus that contacts granule cells (Ribak and Seress, 1983). The somata of the basket cells are substantially larger than the somata of the granule cells, which are not GABAergic (Ribak et al., 1978; Seress and Ribak, 1983). All five types of basket cell were found in the dentate gyrus of the SR gerbil. The size and distribution of GABAergic neurons and the density of terminals in the dentate gyrus of the SR gerbil were also found to be similar to that which has been reported in the rat (Barber and Saito, 1976; Goldowitz et al., 1982; Ribak et al., 1978; Seress and Ribak, 1983). Thus the somata of GABAergic basket cells in the SR stratum granulosum were usually spaced 80 to 140 μm apart and were only rarely found in close proximity to one another (Fig. 1A). In contrast, GABAergic somata in the SS dentate gyrus were more numerous and often formed groups of three or four where some appeared to contact each other (Fig. 1B). In addition, the average size of the GABAergic somata in the SS dentate gyrus was 30% smaller than in SR brains ($\bar{X}_{SS}$ = 112.6 μm^2, $\bar{X}_{SR}$ = 144.1 μm^2, $P < 0.01$, Student's t test). The distribution of somal areas in the SS brains was bimodal, indicating that there are two sizes of GABAergic neurons in the SS dentate gyrus, one small and the other comparable in size to those in the SR dentate gyrus. Each of the five types of GABAergic basket cell found in the rat and SR gerbil dentate gyrus was also found in the dentate gyrus of SS gerbils. The pyramidal basket cell was the most common cell type in the dentate gyrus of both SR and SS gerbils, as has been described previously for the rat (Seress and Pokorny, 1981).

The qualitative differences in the number of GABAergic somata between the SR and SS dentate gyri were confirmed in the quantitative analysis ($P < 0.05$, Kruskal-Wallis method, H = 7.053). A statistically significant 35% increase in the total number of GABAergic neurons occurred in the suprapyramidal blade of stratum granulosum of SS brains as compared with SR brains ($P < 0.05$, Mann-Whitney U test). The difference was most substantial and consistent in the septal half of the dentate gyrus (Fig. 1D) in which significant differences were also observed (unpaired t test, SS vs. SR, $P < 0.05$). In contrast, the number of GABAergic neurons in the infrapyramidal blade of SS brains was not significantly different from that in the infrapyramidal blade of SR brains

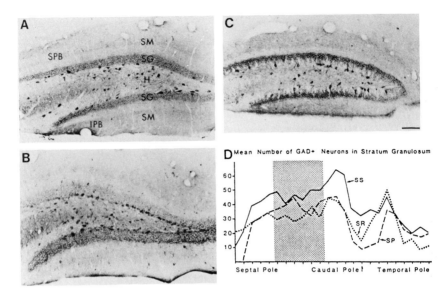

Fig. 1. Coronal sections that were incubated in antiserum to GAD show the somal distribution of GABAergic neurons in the gerbil dentate gyrus. GABAergic pyramidal basket cells in the SR dentate gyrus (**A**) are found at the border between the stratum granulosum (SG) and the hilus (H) in both the suprapyramidal (SPB) and infrapyramidal (IPB) blades. SM, stratum moleculare. Both SS (**B**) and SP (**C**) dentate gyri display more GABAergic neurons at this location than those from SR brains. Counts from the hilus and stratum moleculare also showed increases in the SS brains (see text). Bar = 100 μm. **D:** Graphic representation of the mean number of GAD-immunoreactive neurons in the dentate gyrus of SS, SR, and SP gerbils. The septotemporal axis has been displayed in a linear fashion so that variations in cell number along this axis can be identified. The position of the septal, caudal, and temporal poles of the dentate gyrus are indicated. Only the data for the suprapyramidal blade are shown. The shading indicates the septal region where the differences between SS and SR gerbils were most substantial. A, B, and C are reproduced from Peterson et al., 1985, with permission of the publisher. D is reproduced from Peterson and Ribak, 1987, with permission of the publisher.

(Table I). In addition, a trend appeared in that gerbils with the highest average seizure ratings displayed the largest number of GABAergic neurons in this part of the dentate gyrus (Table I). The stratum moleculare also displayed more GABAergic neurons in SS brains as compared with SR brains, and, again, the difference was most marked in the suprapyramidal blade. Within the hilus the number of GABAergic neurons in SS brains outnumbered those in the SR brains by approximately 20%.

In general, the brains of the young offspring of SS gerbils, the SP group, displayed more GABAergic neurons than the SR brains but somewhat less

TABLE I. Number of GAD-Immunoreactive Neurons in Stratum Granulosum
of Dentate Gyrus

Animal[a]	Seizure intensity	Total count[b]		Regional count[c]	
		SPB	IPB	SPB	IPB
SR3722	0	508	515	169	123
SR3616	0	607	382	146	101
SR0040	0	787	476	288	134
SR00CH	0	824	542	290	135
		X̄ = 681.5 ± 74.8	478.8 ± 35.0	223.3 ± 38.3	123.3 ± 7.9
SS3703	4.81	1,096	784	393	209
SS3699	4.83	926	676	339	174
SS3670	3.66	847	515	303	125
SS3666	3.87	837	528	292	144
SS0033[d]	1.44	(773)	(552)	—	—
		X̄ = 926.5 ± 59.9	625.8 ± 64.2	331.8 ± 22.8	163.0 ± 18.4
SP0037	—[e]	675	476	258	137
SP0041	—[e]	518	443	238	134
SP0042	—[e]	751	586	292	177
		X̄ = 648.0 ± 68.6	501.7 ± 43.2	262.7 ± 15.8	149.3 ± 13.9

[a]SR, seizure-resistant; SS, seizure-sensitive; SP, seizure-predisposed.
[b]Total count represents the total number of GAD-immunoreactive neurons in every fifth section throughout the entire septotemporal extent of the dentate gyrus. SPB, suprapyramidal blade; IPB, infrapyramidal blade.
[c]Regional count represents the number of GAD-immunoreactive neurons in every fifth section throughout the septal third of the dentate gyrus.
[d]This SS gerbil was not included in the mean because its seizure record was uncharacteristically low compared with the main group.
[e]These SP gerbils were analyzed prior to the age when seizures begin.
Reproduced from Peterson and Ribak, 1987, with permission from the publisher.

than the SS brains (see Fig. 1C,D and Table I). After correcting for differences in size by converting raw cell counts to cell densities, some of the SP brains were found to have GABAergic neuronal densities similar to the SS brains. Furthermore, with this calculation, all SP brains had densities greater than the SR brains. The variation in SP data may reflect the variation that is known to occur in the seizure records of different mature offspring of SS gerbils.

GABAergic Terminals in the Dentate Gyrus

The distribution of GABAergic puncta (presumed terminals) within the dentate gyrus of the SR gerbil was similar to that reported in the rat (Barber and Saito, 1976; Goldowitz et al., 1982; Ribak et al., 1978; Seress and Ribak, 1983). Thus the outer third of the stratum moleculare was moderately dense, and the density of puncta in the stratum granulosum was uniform between the infra- and suprapyramidal blades. These GABAergic puncta were closely apposed to the surfaces of granule cell somata (Fig. 2a). In contrast to the SR dentate gyrus, the density of GABAergic puncta in the SS dentate gyrus was approximately three times greater in the infrapyramidal blade of the stratum granulosum than in the suprapyramidal blade. The terminal density in both blades of the SS dentate gyrus was significantly greater than in the SR ($P < 0.01$; Student's t test), and the GABAergic puncta appeared to be both larger and more densely stained in the SS brains, especially in the infrapyramidal blade (Fig. 2b,c). The increased density of GABAergic puncta was found to be specifically related to GABAergic somata within or immediately subjacent to the stratum granulosum. GABAergic somata in the SS dentate gyrus generally had two to three times more GABAergic puncta apposed to them than did the GABAergic somata in the dentate gyrus of SR gerbils (Peterson and Ribak, 1985). Consistent with this light microscopic finding was the ultrastructural observation of increased numbers of axosomatic symmetric synapses onto basket cell somata.

GABAergic Neurons in the Hippocampus

Within the hippocampus, GABAergic neurons were found in all subregions except the alveus, and they varied in size, ranging from 13 to 20 µm in diameter. Those cells that showed staining of the proximal dendrites could be characterized as either multipolar or fusiform. The major difference in the number of GABAergic somata in the hippocampus was observed in the CA2,3 region, where an overall increase of 42% was observed in SS gerbils as compared with SR gerbils. The most pronounced difference and the only one that was statistically significant between groups ($P < 0.05$, Kruskal-Wallis method) occurred between SS and SR gerbils (65%, $P < 0.05$, unpaired t test) and was observed in the CA2,3 apical dendritic field, which consisted of the strata lucidum, radiatum, and lacunosum-moleculare (Fig. 3). The CA1 region of SS brains showed a small (10–15%) increase in the number of GABAergic cells (Fig. 3). Thus, every region of the hippocampus of the SS gerbil displayed greater numbers of GABAergic neurons than the corresponding region of the SR gerbil. In SP gerbil brains an overall increase of 10% was observed in the number of GABAergic neurons in all regions of the hippocampus when compared with SR brains. This difference was not statistically significant. Again, the greatest difference (23%) was noted in the apical dendritic field of the CA2,3 pyramidal cells. In general, the numbers for SP gerbils were intermediate between the counts for SS and SR gerbils.

GABAergic Terminals in the Hippocampus

Presumed GABAergic terminals were most dense within stratum pyramidale, where they surrounded the perikarya of pyramidal cells. No differences between SR and SS brains were detected in the density of these light microscopic correlates of GABAergic terminals.

OTHER EVIDENCE FOR HIPPOCAMPAL INVOLVEMENT IN GERBIL SEIZURE ACTIVITY

In addition to the data that show differences in the GABAergic system in the dentate gyrus and hippocampus of SS gerbils as compared with SR gerbils, other evidence exists to demonstrate hippocampal involvement in gerbil seizure

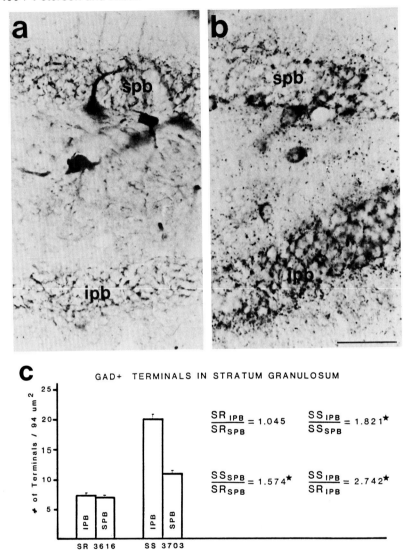

Fig. 2. Density and location of GAD-immunoreactive terminals in the dentate gyrus. **a,b:** Photomicrographs of the supra- and infrapyramidal blades (SPB and IPB, respectively) of stratum granulosum showing GAD-immunoreactive puncta. The densely packed puncta are most numerous and clearly visible in the infrapyramidal blade of the SS dentate gyrus (b). The suprapyramidal blade of the SS dentate gyrus has a slightly higher terminal density compared with either blade of the SR dentate gyrus (a). Bar = 50 μm. **c:** Histogram showing the increase in the density of GAD-immunoreactive puncta in stratum granulosum of a representative SS gerbil as compared with an SR animal. The largest increase is found in the infrapyramidal blade (IPB) of the SS gerbil, where the ratios indicate that terminal density is larger than in either blade of the SR and sub-

activity. We have shown that, immediately following seizures, the ultrastructural morphology of the mossy fiber tufts (the synaptic terminals of granule cells) in SS gerbils is indicative of a high rate of synaptic activity as compared with those in SR brains (Peterson et al., 1985). The mossy tufts of SR brains display a normal appearance in that they are filled with round synaptic vesicles and form typical asymmetric axospinous synapses as described for mossy tufts in other rodents (Amaral, 1979; Amaral and Dent, 1981; Frotscher, 1985; Nitsch and Rinne, 1981). In contrast, many mossy tufts in the SS brains showed 1) a depletion of synaptic vesicles, 2) an increase in the number of cisternae of agranular reticulum, 3) mitochondria located close to synaptic active zones, and 4) a high degree of infolding of the plasma membrane which in some cases was attached to cisternae (Peterson et al., 1985). The observed decrease in the number of vesicles in these tufts and the increased number of smooth cisternae have been observed in other systems following high rates of synaptic activity (Nitsch and Rinne, 1981). These data indicate that the granule cells in the SS dentate gyrus are more active than those in the SR dentate gyrus.

To determine better the role of the hippocampal formation in seizure activity, the effects of lesions of hippocampal afferents and efferents has been analyzed behaviorally. Bilateral transection of the perforant pathway, which provides the hippocampal formation with its primary excitatory input from the entorhinal cortex, results in the abolition of the behavioral expression of seizure activity, whereas unilateral transection of the perforant pathway or bilateral transection of the fornix resulted in no change or in an increase in seizure intensity (Ribak and Khan, 1987).

Taken together, these data suggest that the hippocampal formation has an abnormal circuitry that is involved in the generation and/or propagation of epileptic activity. The differences between the SS and SR hippocampi do not appear to be the result of compensatory changes following seizure activity, because the hippocampus of young SS progeny (SP) that had not had seizures also showed increased numbers of GABAergic cells. Thus, it would appear that the differences found in the hippocampal formation between the two strains are related to seizure activity. We have proposed a disinhibition hypothesis to explain the apparent contradiction between the occurrence of seizure activity and the increased numbers of inhibitory structures (GABAergic somata and terminals) in the hippocampal formation.

HIPPOCAMPAL DISINHIBITION HYPOTHESIS

GABAergic basket cells in the hippocampal formation receive collateral input from excitatory granule cells (Frotscher, 1985; Ribak and Seress, 1983). The GABAergic cells in turn form pericellular basket plexuses around the granule and pyramidal cell somata, where they form axosomatic synapses (Ribak and Seress, 1983; Seress and Ribak, 1985). Thus, the GABAergic cells have been

---

stantially larger than its own suprapyramidal blade (SPB). Stars indicate a statistically significant difference ($P < 0.01$, Student's t test). (Reproduced from Peterson and Ribak, 1987, with permission of the publisher.)

GAD+ NEURONS IN HIPPOCAMPUS PROPER

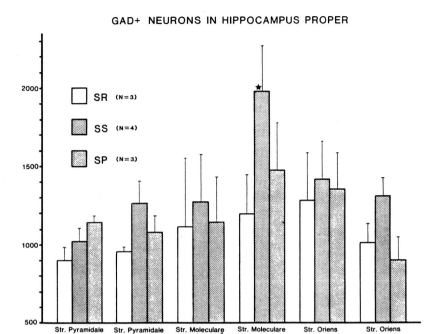

Fig. 3. Histogram showing the mean number of GAD-immunoreactive cells in the hippocampus proper of four SS, three SR, and three SP gerbils. The cell counts are from the three principal laminae in CA1 and CA2,3: stratum oriens, stratum pyramidale, and the apical dendritic field of the pyramidal cells (referred to here as *stratum moleculare* and includes strata lucidum, radiatum, and lacunosum-moleculare). The GAD-immunoreactive neurons are more numerous throughout the CA2,3 fields of the SS gerbils as compared with the number for SR gerbils, and this increase is most dramatic and statistically significant (star, $P < 0.05$, Student's t test) in the stratum moleculare of CA2,3. The error bars indicate standard deviations. (Reproduced from Peterson and Ribak, 1987, with permission of the publisher.)

shown to have a circuitry that may underlie their functional role in feedback inhibition (Andersen, 1975). In the nonepileptic hippocampal formation, feedback inhibition is responsible for controlling the output of the granule and pyramidal cells. Our morphological observations have shown that there is an increased number of GABAergic neurons in both the dentate gyrus and hippocampus in the genetically epileptic SS gerbil and that there is an increased number of inhibitory synaptic connections with GABAergic basket cell bodies in the dentate gyrus. The normal feedback circuit and our proposed abnormal circuitry is illustrated in Figure 4. Activation of the abnormal circuit found in SS gerbils by axon collaterals of excitatory granule cells would cause one of the inhibitory neurons to inhibit the other, thereby effectively blocking the

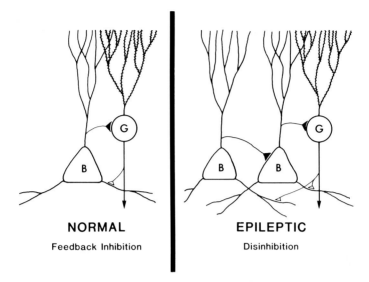

Fig. 4. Schematic diagram of the proposed differences in circuitry between granule and basket (GABAergic) cells in the dentate gyrus from SR (left) and SS (right) gerbils. In SR gerbils, axon collaterals of granule cells (G) form excitatory synapses with the basal dendrites of basket cells (B), which send inhibitory axons to the soma of the granule cell. This circuitry provides a normal feedback inhibition. In contrast, the SS gerbils have additional basket cells that inhibit other basket cells that contact the granule cells, thereby resulting in disinhibition of the granule cells. (Reproduced from Ribak, 1986, with permission of the publisher.)

feedback inhibition or inducing *dis*inhibition. Thus, it appears that the basic mechanism of genetic epilepsy in this model is different from that found in post-traumatic epilepsy in monkeys in that one displays increased numbers of GABAergic neurons that may cause disinhibition, whereas the other shows reduced numbers of GABAergic neurons and decreased inhibition.

SUMMARY

Focal, post-traumatic epilepsy has been shown to be related to a decrease in the number of GABAergic neurons and terminals in the cerebral cortex. We have studied the hippocampal GABAergic system in an animal model of genetic epilepsy using seizure-sensitive and seizure-resistant gerbils to determine whether a defect exists in the GABAergic inhibitory system. A major difference between the SS and SR strains of gerbils was found in the number of GABAergic neurons in the hippocampal formation. In contrast to the results from the model of post-traumatic epilepsy, an increase in the number of glutamate decarboxylase-immunoreactive neurons was observed within the dentate gyrus and the CA3 region of the hippocampus of the SS gerbils as compared with the SR gerbils. The density of GAD-immunoreactive puncta, the light microscopic correlates of synaptic boutons, was also greater in the SS animals. An ultrastructural analysis showed evidence of high synaptic activity in the terminals of the granule cells in the SS gerbils in that many mossy fibers displayed partial depletion of synaptic vesicles. An increase in the number of symmetric axosomatic synapses was also found for GABAergic-type basket cells in SS gerbils. Taken together, these data suggest that many of the supernumerary GABAergic basket cells in the SS gerbil are making inhibitory connections onto other GABAergic basket cells, thereby producing disinhibition by effectively removing the granule cells from feedback inhibition.

ACKNOWLEDGMENTS

The authors gratefully acknowledge Drs. Wolfgang H. Oertel and Donald E. Schmechel for the GAD antiserum, Kim Andersen, Sana Khan, and Debbie Rau for technical assistance, and Margot Brundage and Yashoda Jhurani for assistance with the photography. This work was supported by NIH grant NS-15669 and by a fellowship from the Klingenstein Foundation (C.E.R.).

REFERENCES

Amaral, D.G. (1979) Synaptic extensions from the mossy fibers of the fascia dentata. Anat. Embryol. *155*:241–251.

Amaral, D.G., and J. Dent (1981) Development of the mossy fibers of the dentate gyrus: I. A light and electron microscopic study of the mossy fibers and their expansions. J. Comp. Neurol. *195*:51–86.

Andersen, P. (1975) Organization of hippocampal neurons and their connections. In R.L. Isaacson and K.H. Pribram (eds): The Hippocampus. New York: Plenum Press, pp. 155–175.

Bakay, R.A.E., and A.B. Harris (1981) Neurotransmitter, receptor and biochemical changes in monkey cortical epileptic foci. Brain Res. *206*:387–404.

Barber, R., and K. Saito (1976) Light microscopic visualization of GAD and GABA-T in immunocytochemical preparations of rodent C.N.S. In E. Roberts, T.N. Chase, and D.B. Tower (eds): GABA in Nervous System Function. New York: Raven Press, pp. 113–132.

Ben-Ari, Y., E. Tremblay, and O.P. Otterson (1979) Lesions cerebrales primaires et secondaires produites par des injections d'acide kainique chez le Rat. C.R. Acad. Sci. (Paris) *288*:991–994.

Brown, W.J. (1973) Structural substrates of seizure foci in the human temporal lobe. In M.A.B. Brazier (ed): Epilepsy, Its Phenomena in Man. New York: Academic Press, pp. 339–374.

Davies, S.W., T.J. Ashwood, H.V. Wheal, and C. Köhler (1985) Glutamate decarboxylase (GAD) and GAD immunoreactivity (GADI) in the CA1 region of the kainic acid-lesioned rat hippocampus. Neurosci. Lett. *21*:S43.

DeJong, R.N. (1957) "Psychomotor" or "temporal lobe" epilepsy. Neurology *7*:1–14.

Franck, J.E. (1984) Dynamic alterations in hippocampal morphology following intraventricular kainic acid. Acta Neuropathol. *62*:242–253.

Frotscher, M. (1985) Mossy fibres form synapses with identified pyramidal basket cells in the CA3 region of the guinea pig hippocampus: A combined Golgi-electron microscope study. J. Neurocytol. *14*:245–259.

Goddard, G.V., D.C. McIntyre, and C.K. Leech (1969) A permanent change in brain function, resulting from daily electrical stimulation. Exp. Neurol. *5*:295–330.

Goldowitz, D., S.R. Vincent, J.-Y. Wu, and T. Hökfelt (1982) Immunohistochemical demonstration of plasticity in GABA neurons of the adult rat dentate gyrus. Brain Res. *238*:413–420.

Hughes, J.T., and C.B.T. Adams (1984) Pathological findings in 50 cases of temporal lobe epilepsy (partial complex seizures) treated by anterior temporal lobectomy. In R.J. Porter, R.H. Mattson, A.A. Ward, and M. Dam (eds): Advances in Epileptology: XVth Epilepsy International Symposium. New York: Raven Press, pp. 457–462.

Jasper, H. (1961) General summary of "Basic Mechanisms of the Epileptic Discharge." Epilepsia *2*:91–99.

Kamphuis, W., W.J. Wadman, R.M. Buijs, and F.H. Lopes da Silva (1986) Decrease in number of hippocampal gamma-aminobutyric acid (GABA) immunoreactive cells in the rat kindling model of epilepsy. Exp Brain Res. *64*:491–495.

Kandel, E.R., and W.A. Spencer (1961) Excitation and inhibition of single pyramidal cells during hippocampal seizure. Exp. Neurol. *4*:162–179.

Lloyd, K.G., C. Munari, L. Bossi, J. Bancaud, J. Talairach, and P.L. Morselli (1981) Biochemical evidence for the alterations of GABA-mediated synaptic transmission in human epileptic foci. In P.L. Morselli, K.G. Lloyd, W. Löscher, B. Meldrum, and E.H. Reynolds (eds): Neurotransmitters, Seizures and Epilepsy. New York: Raven Press, pp. 331–354.

Löscher, W. (1984) Evidence for abnormal sensitivity of the GABA system in gerbils with genetically determined epilepsy. In R.G. Fariello, K.G. Lloyd, P.L. Morselli, L.F. Quesney, and J. Engel (eds): Neurotransmitters, Seizures and Epilepsy II. New York: Raven Press, pp. 179–188.

Löscher, W., H.-H. Frey, R. Reiche, and D. Schultz (1983) High anticonvulsant potency of γ-aminobutyric acid (GABA) mimetic drugs in gerbils with genetically determined epilepsy. J. Pharmacol. Exp. Ther. *226*:839–844.

Loskota, W.J., P. Lomax, and S.T. Rich (1974) The gerbil as a model for the study of the epilepsies. Epilepsia *15*:109–119.

Majkowski, J., and M. Donadio (1984) Electro-clinical studies of epileptic seizures in Mongolian gerbils. Electroencephalogr. Clin. Neurophysiol. *57*:369–377.

Meldrum, B.S., and J.B. Brierly (1972) Neuronal loss and gliosis in the hippocampus following repetitive epileptic seizures induced in adolescent baboons by allylglycine. Brain Res. *48*:361–365.

Mouritzen Dam, A. (1980) Epilepsy and neuron loss in the hippocampus. Epilepsia *21*:617–629.

Mouritzen Dam, A., J.C. Bajorek, and P. Lomax (1981) Hippocampal neuron density and seizures in the Mongolian gerbil. Epilepsia *22*:667–674.

Nadler, J.V., B.W. Perry, and C.W. Cotman (1978) Intraventricular kainic acid preferentially destroys hippocampal pyramidal cells. Nature *271*:676–677.

Nadler, J.V., B.W. Perry, C. Gentry, and C.W. Cotman (1980) Degeneration of hippocampal CA3 pyramidal cells induced by intraventricular kainic acid. J. Comp. Neurol. *192*:333–359.

Nitsch, C., and U. Rinne (1981) Large dense-core vesicle exocytosis and membrane recycling in the mossy fibre synapses of the rabbit hippocampus during epileptiform seizures. J. Neurocytol. *57*:201–219.

Oertel, W.H., D.E. Schmechel, E. Mugnaini, M.L. Tappaz, and I.J. Kopin (1981a) Immunocytochemical localization of glutamate decarboxylase in rat cerebellum with a new antiserum. Neuroscience *6*:2715–2735.

Oertel, W.H., D.E. Schmechel, V.K. Weise, D.H. Ranson, M.L. Tappaz, H.C. Krutzsch, and I.J. Kopin (1981b) Comparison of cysteine sulphinic acid decarboxylase isoenzymes and glutamic acid decarboxylase in rat liver and brain. Neuroscience 6:2701–2714.

Olsen, R.W., J.K. Wamsley, R. Lee, and P. Lomax (1984) Alterations in the benzodiazepine/GABA receptor-chloride ion channel complex in the seizure-sensitive Mongolian gerbil. In R.G. Fariello, K.G. Lloyd, P.L. Morselli, L.F. Quesney, J. Engel (eds): Neurotransmitters, Seizure and Epilepsy II. New York: Raven Press, pp. 210–213.

Olsen R.W., J.K. Wamsley, R.T. McCabe, R.J. Lee, and P. Lomax (1985) Benzodiazepine/γ-aminobutyric acid receptor deficit in the midbrain of the seizure-susceptible gerbil. Proc. Natl. Acad. Sci. U.S.A. 82:6701–6705.

Paul, L.A., I. Fried, K. Watanabe, A.B. Forsythe, and A.B. Scheibel (1981) Structural correlates of seizure behavior in the Mongolian gerbil. Science 213:924–926.

Peterson, G.M., and C.E. Ribak (1985) Morphological evidence for increased inhibition of basket cells in the dentate gyrus of Mongolian gerbils. Soc. Neurosci. Abstr. 11:1321.

Peterson, G.M., and C.E. Ribak (1987) Hippocampus of the seizure-sensitive gerbil is a specific site for anatomical changes in the GABAergic system. J. Comp. Neurol. 261:405–422.

Peterson, G.M., C.E. Ribak, and W.H. Oertel (1985) A regional increase in the number of hippocampal GABAergic neurons and terminals in the seizure-sensitive gerbil. Brain Res. 340:384–389.

Pinel, J.P.J., R.F. Mucha, and A.G. Phillips (1975) Spontaneous seizures generated in rats by kindling: A preliminary report. Physiol. Psychol. 3:127–129.

Prince, D.A. (1983) Mechanisms of epileptogenesis in brain-slice model systems. In A.A. Ward, Jr., J.K. Penry, and D. Purpura (eds): Epilepsy. New York: Raven Press, pp. 29–52.

Ribak, C.E. (1985) Axon terminals of GABAergic chandelier cells are lost at epileptic foci. Brain Res. 326:251–260.

Ribak, C.E. (1986) Contemporary methods in neurocytology and their application to the study of epilepsy. In A.V. Delgado-Escueta, A.A. Ward, Jr., D.M. Woodbury, and R.J. Porter (eds): Basic Mechanisms of the Epilepsies. New York: Raven Press, pp. 739–764.

Ribak, C.E., R.M. Bradburne, and A.B Harris (1982) A preferential loss of GABAergic, symmetric synapses in epileptic foci: A quantitative ultrastructural analysis of monkey neocortex. J. Neurosci. 2:1725–1735.

Ribak, C.E., A.B. Harris, J.E. Vaughn, and E. Roberts (1979) Inhibitory, GABAergic nerve terminals decrease at sites of focal epilepsy. Science 205:211–214.

Ribak, C.E., C.A. Hunt, R.A.E. Bakay, and W.H. Oertel (1986) A decrease in the number of GABAergic somata is associated with the preferential loss of GABAergic terminals at epileptic foci. Brain Res. 363:78–90.

Ribak, C.E., and S.U. Khan (1987) The effects of knife cuts of hippocampal pathways on epileptic activity in the seizure-sensitive gerbil. Brain Res. 418:146–151.

Ribak, C.E., and L. Seress (1983) Five types of basket cell in the hippocampal dentate gyrus: A combined Golgi and electron microscopic study. J. Neurocytol. 12:577–597.

Ribak, C.E., J.E. Vaughn, and K. Saito (1978) Immunocytochemical localization of glutamic acid decarboxylase in neuronal somata following colchicine inhibition of axonal transport. Brain Res. 140:315–332.

Ruth, R.E. (1982) Kainic-acid lesions of hippocampus produced iontophoretically: The problem of distant damage. Exp. Neurol. 76:508–527.

Scheibel, M.E., P.H. Crandall, and A.B. Scheibel (1974) The hippocampal-dentate complex in temporal lobe epilepsy. Epilepsia 15:55–80.

Schwarcz, R., R. Zaczek, and J.T. Coyle (1978) Microinjection of kainic acid into the rat hippocampus. Eur. J. Pharmacol. *50*:209–220.

Seress, L., and J. Pokorny (1981) Structure of the granular layer of the rat dentate gyrus. A light microscopic and Golgi study. J. Anat. *133*:181–195.

Seress, L., and C.E. Ribak (1983) GABAergic cells in the dentate gyrus appear to be local circuit and projection neurons. Exp. Brain Res. *50*:173–182.

Seress, L., and C.E. Ribak (1985) A combined Golgi-electron microscopic study of nonpyramidal neurons in the CA1 area of the hippocampus. J. Neurocytol. *14*:717–730.

Sloviter, R.S. (1983) "Epileptic" brain damage in rats induced by sustained electrical stimulation of the perforant path. I. Acute electrophysiological and light microscopic studies. Brain Res. Bull. *10*:675–697.

Sloviter, R.S. (1987) Decreased hippocampal inhibition and a selective loss of interneurons in experimental epilepsy. Science *235*:73–76.

Sloviter, R.S., and B.P. Damiano (1981) Sustained electrical stimulation of the perforant path duplicates kainate-induced electrophysiological effects and hippocampal damage in rats. Neurosci. Lett. *24*:279–284.

Sommer, W. (1880) Erkrankung des Ammonshorns als aetiologisches Moment der Epilepsie. Arch. Psychiatr. Neurvenkrankh. *10*:631–675.

Thiessen, D.D., G. Lindzey, and H.D. Friend (1968) Spontaneous seizures in the Mongolian gerbil. Psychon. Sci. *11*:227–228.

Wada, J.A., and M. Sato (1973) Recurrent spontaneous epileptic seizure state induced by localized brain stimulation. Neurology *23*:447.

Wada, J.A., M. Sato, and M.E. Corcoran (1974) Persistent seizure susceptibility and recurrent spontaneous seizures in kindled cats. Epilepsia *15*:465–478.

The Hippocampus—New Vistas, pages 499–512

31
Hippocampal and Entorhinal Cortex Cellular Pathology in Alzheimer's Disease

BRADLEY T. HYMAN and GARY W. VAN HOESEN

Departments of Neurology and Anatomy, University of Iowa College of Medicine, Iowa City, Iowa

INTRODUCTION

The hippocampal formation[1] and parahippocampal gyrus[2] have long been known to be sites of predilection for the pathologic alterations of Alzheimer's disease (2,3,5,6,8,11,15,27). However, a full appreciation of the importance of their vulnerability has been impossible without an understanding of the anatomical, physiological, and behavioral correlates of the hippocampus. Considerable progress has occurred in the last two decades in gaining knowledge of all of these areas. Thus, it is our goal to re-examine the pathologic alterations seen in the hippocampal formation in Alzheimer's disease in the context of the new findings. On the basis of our results, we have concluded that Alzheimer pathology specifically and selectively affects certain hippocampal and parahippocampal neurons while consistently sparing others in adjacent lamina or cytoarchitectural fields. The neurons affected are projection neurons responsible for the majority of hippocampocortical and corticohippocampal interconnections. Their loss suggests that the hippocampus is functionally isolated from the remainder of the cortex in Alzheimer's disease and that this contributes to the memory impairment characteristic of the disorder. These alterations, in our estimation, are a major correlate of Alzheimer's disease and foci for

---

[1]The hippocampal formation refers to the combined allocortical fields that form the dentate gyrus, hippocampus (CA1–CA4), and the subicular cortices.

[2]The parahippocampal gyrus is composed of five major cytoarchitectural fields: the olfactory cortex, the cortical nuclei of the amygdala, the entorhinal cortex, or Brodmann's area 28, the posterior parahippocampal cortex, or Brodmann's area 36, and the perirhinal cortex, or Brodmann's area 35. These all lie largely medial to the rhinal and collateral sulci in the human brain and the rhinal and occipitotemporal sulci in the nonhuman primate brain.

early changes in both pathology and behavior. A brief perspective on the neurobiology of Alzheimer's disease is essential to develop our argument.

Dementia of the Alzheimer type[3] is the major form of dementia in the United States (49). It is characterized by profound memory dysfunction. An anterograde impairment is usually the inaugural feature of the disease and remains at its core. This is joined later by impairments in the retrograde compartment, in both contextual and generic memory. Problem-solving skills and language difficulty often supervene, with loss of lexical knowledge. By its end stages, perhaps 6 to 10 years after clinical onset, the patient has profound cognitive failure, loses the ability to remember and communicate, and finally even loses self-identity (52).

Alzheimer's disease is used here to refer to the pathologic process that accompanies the clinical syndrome described above. Alzheimer's disease is marked by neuronal loss, neurofibrillary tangles, neuritic plaques, granulovacuolar degeneration, and Hirano bodies, which are present to a much greater extent than in control tissue from age-compatible normals (49). In addition, a new abnormality in Alzheimer brain tissue has recently been described using a monoclonal antibody and immunocytochemical techniques. An antigen, called *A68*, recognized by Alz-50 antibody, is present to at least a 20-fold excess in Alzheimer's disease brain tissue as compared with control tissue (20,60). The diagnosis of Alzheimer's disease rests on the pathologic confirmation of these abnormalities.

The pathologic changes of Alzheimer's disease occur both within neurons (neurofibrillary tangles, Alz-50 immunoreactivity, granulovacuolar degeneration) and within the neuropil (neuritic plaques, Alz-50 immunoreactivity, Hirano bodies). However, these are not distributed uniformly throughout the brain. Granulovacuolar degeneration and Hirano bodies are found almost entirely in the hippocampal formation (2). Neurofibrillary tangles are located primarily in specific neurons of the hippocampal formation, amygdala, basal forebrain, association (but not primary sensory or motor) cortices, and certain diencephalic and brainstem structures (for review, see 52). Neuritic plaques are found in the neuropil in a widespread distribution, involving primary and association cortices and limbic structures including the hippocampal formation (35,36). Alz-50 immunoreactivity largely reflects that of neurofibrillary tangles and neuritic plaques, but, in addition, often reveals more widespread alterations within specific and, in most instances, the same neuronal populations and the neuropil (20,21).

The importance of specific sets of neurons being affected in Alzheimer's disease is, of course, linked to the function and connectivity of those neurons.

---

[3]Although in this chapter we make a distinction between the *clinical dementia of the Alzheimer type* and the pathologically proven diagnosis of *Alzheimer's disease*, it should be noted that these terms, as well as *senile dementia of the Alzheimer type* (SDAT), are sometimes used interchangeably. However, in clinical-pathologic correlation studies, it appears that Alzheimer's disease accounts for approximately 50–80% of all cases of clinical dementia in the elderly, suggesting that the linguistic caution is justified.

Therefore, neuroanatomical considerations are crucial to draw specific comparisons between the pattern of pathology in Alzheimer's disease and neural correlates of memory. The hippocampal formation is an integral component of several forebrain neural systems thought to play a role in memory processes (1,40,50,51). In higher mammals, a stereotypical picture of corticocortical and corticolimbic connections joins the hippocampal formation to other limbic structures, to subcortical structures, and to sensory-specific and multimodal association cortices (12–14,25,26,28–30,37,38,41–48,54–59) (Fig. 1). Converging information from telencephalic sources is directed from these structures to the entorhinal cortex. This area, in particular the large neurons that make up the clusters in layer II of entorhinal cortex, gives rise to a massive projection that terminates on the distal dendrites of the granule cells of the dentate gyrus and of the hippocampal pyramidal cells. This projection, the perforant pathway, is therefore a final common route and carries corticohippocampal input. After a series of intrinsic connections, hippocampal output directed toward telencephalic and diencephalic targets arises primarily from the subiculum and the

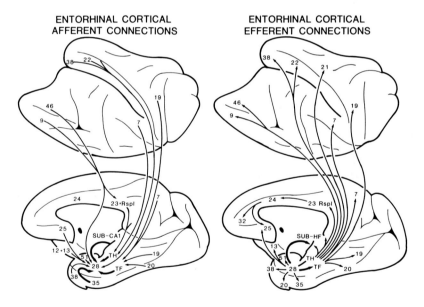

Fig. 1. This illustration summarizes the major cortical afferent and efferent neural systems of the entorhinal cortex in the rhesus monkey on medial and lateral views of the cerebral hemisphere. Identification of cortical areas correspond to those of Brodmann and Bonin and Bailey. Note that cortical neural systems from the frontal, parietal, occipital, temporal, and limbic lobes converge on Brodmann's area 28, the entorhinal cortex. Layer IV of the entorhinal cortex receives a powerful output from the subiculum (SUB) and CA1 parts of the hippocampal formation (HF) and gives rise to neural systems that feedback to widespread limbic and association cortical areas. (Redrawn from 50.)

portion of the hippocampus adjacent to it, the CA1 area. Of interest, one of the strongest projections of the subiculum is to layer IV of entorhinal cortex, which in turn projects to widespread cortical and subcortical targets (31,39,40,46,50). Our results suggest that the major projection neurons of this system are affected in Alzheimer's disease.

METHODS

For these studies, series of sections were prepared from a temporal lobe block from 50 cases of pathologically confirmed Alzheimer's disease. The block usually contained the entire anteroposterior extent of the hippocampal formation. Adjacent series of sections were stained for Nissl substance and for neurofibrillary tangles and neuritic plaques with thioflavin S (for details, see 16). A series from approximately half of these cases was available for Alz-50 immunocytochemistry (20,21,60). We also prepared material from ten age-compatible controls who had died of non-neurologic disease and seven controls with dementia but without Alzheimer's pathology (three Pick's disease, one Creutzfeldt-Jakob's disease, one multi-infarct dementia, one Huntington's disease, and one pseudodementia [depression]).

RESULTS

The hippocampal formation from all cases of Alzheimer's disease contained numerous neurofibrillary tangles and neuritic plaques when stained with Congo red or thioflavin S. Neither the non-neurologic disease controls nor the dementia controls contained this pathology.

Distribution of Neurofibrillary Tangles

Of most importance, the distribution of pathology was remarkably consistent in all cases. Neurofibrillary tangles occurred primarily in layers II and IV of entorhinal cortex, layers III and V of perirhinal cortex, and in the CA1/subiculum and parasubiculum fields of the hippocampus. Neuron layers III, V, and VI of entorhinal cortex, layers II, IV, and VI of perirhinal cortex, and the dentate gyrus and other subfields of the hippocampal formation (CA3-4, presubiculum) are, by contrast, relatively spared (see Fig. 2). This hierarchical pattern was evident through the entire extent of the anterior portion of the hippocampal formation.

The pattern changes in the cortex posterior to the entorhinal cortex, at approximately the level of the lateral geniculate, in Brodmann's areas 36 and 37 (posterior parahippocampal gyrus). Neurofibrillary tangles are again present in a laminar distribution, but here, in the posterior parahippocampal gyrus, occupy layers II, III, and V to a much greater extent than layers IV and VI. In the hippocampal formation neurofibrillary pathology is located primarily in the CA1/subicular fields (Fig. 2). These specific neuronal lamina and cytoarchitectonic fields were invested by neurofibrillary tangles in each case of Alzheimer's disease examined. With minimal variation, the same hierarchical pattern was consistently present.

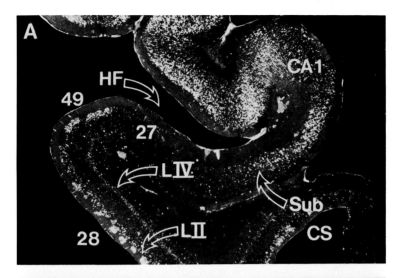

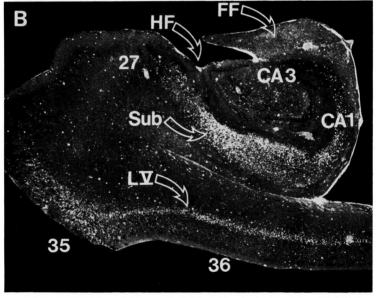

Fig. 2. The hippocampal formation in a case of Alzheimer's disease is illustrated in these low-power photomicrographs. The tissue is stained with Congo red and viewed under cross-polarized light so that neurofibrillary tangles are bright against a dark background. The anterior hippocampal formation at the level of the uncus (**A**) and a more posterior level of the hippocampal formation at the level of the lateral geniculate (**B**) are shown. Discrete areas such as the subicular/CA1 field and layers II and IV of entorhinal cortex are severely affected, with relative sparing of other cell lamina and areas. CS, collateral sulcus; FF, fimbria-fornix; HF, hippocampal fissure; L, layer; Sub, subiculum.

Distribution of Neuritic Plaques

The distribution of neuritic plaques also consistently respects cytoarchitectural features. Within the hippocampus, neuritic plaques often were located in the middle third of the molecular layer of the dentate gyrus (the terminal zone of the perforant pathway) and in the molecular layer and pyramidal cell layer of the CA1/subicular zone. Neuritic plaques are sparse in the more medial aspects of the subiculum and presubiculum.

Distribution of Alz-50 Immunoreactivity

Alz-50 immunocytochemistry dramatically amplifies the impression of lamina and cell-specific pathologic alterations. Alz-50 immunoreactivity occurs both in neurons that contain neurofibrillary tangles as well as some neurons "at risk" that do not contain neurofibrillary tangles (Fig. 3) (20,60). In addition, Alz-50 recognizes the neuritic portion of neuritic plaques and a dense plexus of fibers, which in many instances appear to be the dendritic arborization and terminal fields of affected neurons (21,53). The result of this combination of staining is a set of dense fields of immunoreactivity located in specific regions and lamina that is obvious even to the naked eye.

Within entorhinal cortex, layers II and IV are vividly stained, demonstrating the normal clusters of neurons within layer II of entorhinal cortex. This pattern is consistent in all instances, with a single interesting caveat. In severely affected cases, neurofibrillary tangles in layer II are primarily "ghost tangles," i.e. neurofibrillary tangles no longer associated with appreciable Nissl-staining substance, thus marking the site of a once-viable neuron. These tangles are not recognized by Alz-50, presumably because the antigen, like other cellular proteins in these "ghosts," is no longer associated with the tangles (16,20).

In adjacent perirhinal cortex, the merging of lamina in this cytoarchitectural transition zone (5) can be appreciated by the distinctive pattern of Alz-50 immunoreactivity. Again a bilaminar distribution of affected neurons is obvious. Of note, in some cases a definite columnar distribution of neuropil staining can be appreciated, perhaps reflecting the terminal zone of affected projection neurons. In posterior parahippocampal areas, a bilaminar distribution of Alz-50 immunoreactivity is seen, involving primarily cell layers II, III, and V.

In the hippocampal formation, a dense area of immunoreactivity occurs over the pyramidal cell layer in the CA1/subicular field and the parasubiculum (layer II). In addition, the molecular layer of the CA1/subicular field and the outer two-thirds of the molecular layer of the dentate gyrus contain distinct staining. The latter corresponds exactly to the terminal zone of the perforant pathway (16,21).

The pattern of Alz-50 immunohistochemistry in the hippocampal formation can be predicted accurately by assessing the relevant connectional anatomy. For example, there is a strong projection from the subiculum to layer IV of entorhinal cortex (31). The subiculum is severely affected, and layer IV of entorhinal cortex contains a fine stippling of immunoreactivity reminiscent of terminal staining (53). The converse argument applies as well. The dentate

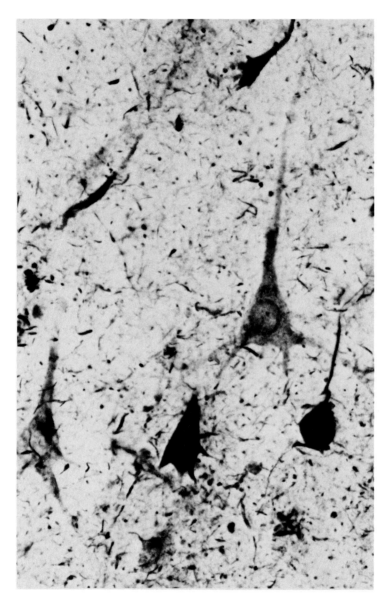

Fig. 3. Alz-50 immunocytochemistry from the hippocampus of a patient with Alzheimer's disease. Shrunken neurons that contain neurofibrillary tangles stain darkly, whereas some neurons appear morphologically normal but nonetheless have immunoreactivity. The latter may represent a "preneurofibrillary tangle" stage of degeneration.

gyrus granule cells are not usually affected, and their terminal area, in the mossy fiber zone, is conspicuously free of Alz-50 immunoreactivity. These results support the contention that Alz-50 immunoreactivity is present in the cytoplasm, dendritic tree, and axonal processes of affected neurons.

In general, the degree of pathological alterations observed by Alz-50 immunoreactivity is substantially greater than that appreciated using conventional stains such as thioflavin S. However, in essentially every instance, the same pattern of hierarchically ordered cell, lamina, and cytoarchitectonic involvement by pathological change is seen with Alz-50. This result is consistent with the hypothesis that Alz-50 immunoreactivity precedes and accompanies neurofibrillary tangle formation (20).

Tissue for Alz-50 immunohistochemistry was available in three non-Alzheimer's dementia controls (two Pick's, one Creutzfeldt-Jakob's) and two age-compatible non-neurologic disease controls. The remarkably heavy neuronal and neuropil staining seen uniformly in Alzheimer's disease was not present in any of these cases. The Creutzfeldt-Jakob's tissue and one of the non-neurologic controls contained essentially no immunoreactivity. Alz-50 immunoreactivity in the case of Pick's disease (33) was limited to a rare neuronal inclusion, similar to Pick's bodies.[4] The cytoplasmic and neuropil staining characteristic of Alzheimer's disease was absent in these cases. Finally, one non-neurologic control that did not contain neurofibrillary tangles or neuritic plaques had several neurons that contained Alz-50 immunoreactivity. These were located in layer II of the entorhinal cortex, layer III of the perirhinal cortex, and the CA1/subicular area. It is tempting to speculate that these alterations represent the first changes of a "preclinical" Alzheimer's disease (23).

DISCUSSION

The hippocampal formation is severely affected by pathology in Alzheimer's disease. Yet, even within severely affected areas, certain neurons appear to be consistently vulnerable, while others, even those immediately adjacent, are consistently spared. Of particular interest, those neurons that are most likely to be destroyed in Alzheimer's disease are precisely those neurons responsible for interconnections between the hippocampus and other parts of the cerebral cortex. Afferents to the hippocampus are funneled through the perforant pathway. The cells of origin of the perforant pathway, layer II of the entorhinal cortex, are consistently invested by neurofibrillary tangles (15,16) (Fig. 2).

The terminal zone of the perforant pathway, in the outer portion of the molecular layer of the dentate gyrus, contains neuritic plaques (16) and Alz-50 immunoreactivity (21). This combination of lesions must interfere with information obtaining access to the hippocampus.

Hippocampal efferents are similarly and severely affected. The CA1/subicular field gives rise to hippocampal output to both cortical and subcortical targets.

[4]We have not proven identity of these inclusions with Pick bodies in our material, but Love et al. (33) suggest that Pick bodies do contain Alz-50 immunoreactive material. Whether this is A68 or a cross-reactive protein is unknown.

These neurons are severely affected by neurofibrillary tangles. One of the primary projections of these neurons is to layer IV of the entorhinal cortex, which in turn projects to widespread cortical areas, as well as to basal forebrain subcortical areas. The terminal zone of the subicular to layer IV projection contains Alz-50 immunoreactivity, and the neurons of layer IV contain neurofibrillary tangles (15,53). These alterations would greatly compromise the output of the hippocampus.

Together, the destruction of afferents and efferents functionally isolates the hippocampus from the other cortical and subcortical areas known to be important for memory. One would predict a clinical syndrome of memory deficit based on this pattern of pathology alone. In combination with the known pathology in other areas (19,22,24,32) (e.g. amygdala, nucleus basalis, midline thalamic nuclei), a memory deficit based on destruction of the anatomic substrate of mnemonic processing is an inescapable conclusion.

These results are useful to establish a clinicopathologic correlation between memory dysfunction and certain structural alterations. In addition, the selective and consistent nature of the pathology can be used to make predictions. For example, a well-established experimental model of neuroplasticity events is the destruction of the perforant pathway (7). Deafferentation of the dentate gyrus granule cell leads to a reorganization of remaining, intact afferent systems in the zone of synaptic deafferentation. In Alzheimer's disease, a severe deafferentation of the dentate gyrus granule cells occurs as a result of the pathologic changes described above. A robust reorganization response can be identified in Alzheimer's disease using either glutamate receptor techniques (9) or acetylcholinesterase histochemistry (17). This is the first demonstration of neuroplasticity in the human and has implications for understanding plasticity on the one hand and for treatment strategies for Alzheimer's disease on the other.

A second observation that follows directly from the anatomic analysis of lesions in Alzheimer's disease is the question of which neurotransmitters are likely to be involved. Again the perforant pathway is a useful system, in that the most likely neurotransmitter in this system is the excitatory amino acid glutamate (34). To assess whether glutamate was diminished as a result of the lesions of Alzheimer's disease, we isolated the "transmitter" pool of glutamate by microdissection of the terminal zone of the perforant pathway. As one would predict, there was an 83% decrease in the level of free glutamate in the perforant pathway terminal zone in subjects with Alzheimer's disease as compared with controls (18). This provides a neurochemical correlate to the destruction of this major hippocampal afferent.

Our observations with regard to Alz-50 immunohistochemistry, together with our observations on the hierarchy of affected neurons, suggest that Alz-50 immunoreactivity is present in neurons that are "at risk" to develop neurofibrillary tangles as well as in neurons that contain neurofibrillary tangles (20). One prediction from this is that cases that are "early" in the disease process will have Alz-50 immunoreactivity in neurons that are the "most vulnerable." We have now examined ten cases of dementia that, by standard staining techniques, do not meet quantitative pathologic criteria for Alzheimer's disease. Nonetheless, these cases all contain substantial numbers of neurons that contain Alz-50 immunoreactivity. These include layer II of the entorhinal cortex, layer III of the perirhinal cortex, and the CA1/subiculum field of the hippocampus. It is thus possible that these neurons (especially those in layer II of entorhinal cortex) are the most vulnerable to Alzheimer-type degeneration (23).

Alz-50 immunoreactivity is also apparently present in the dendritic tree and axonal processes of affected neurons. This fact can be used to advantage in defining the terminal zone of affected neuron's projections. For example, the cells of origin of the perforant pathway (layer II of the entorhinal cortex) are affected in Alzheimer's disease and contain Alz-50 immunoreactivity. Based on studies in the primate, the predicted terminal zone of these cells is in the outer two-thirds of the molecular layer of the dentate gyrus. In Alzheimer's disease, this exact portion of the molecular layer of the dentate gyrus contains a fine pattern of Alz-50 staining (21). Thus, by taking advantage of a naturally occurring lesion, we are able to demonstrate directly some basic connectional anatomy in the human hippocampal formation.

In summary, there are several reasons to believe that pathology in the hippocampal formation is central to the disease process in Alzheimer's disease. 1) The hippocampal formation bears the brunt of the different types of pathologic alterations, and pathologic alterations are consistently present in the hippocampal formation (15,16). Our experience with over 50 such cases suggests that it is the most uniformly affected brain area. 2) The hippocampus or temporal lobe is commonly the site of the most severe changes in neurochemical parameters (10). 3) The hippocampal formation is the site of a robust "plasticity" phenomenon, likely in response to massive deafferentation (9,17). 4) Cases that appear to be "early" in the disease process consistently have pathologic alterations and Alz-50 immunoreactivity in entorhinal cortex and hippocampus (23). 5) If hippocampal pathology contributes to memory impairment in dementia of the Alzheimer type, as seems certainly to be the case, this pathology lies at the heart of the clinical syndrome (3,15,52).

These points should not, of course, be taken to indicate that the only site of pathology in Alzheimer's disease is in the hippocampal formation. Neurofibrillary tangles and neuritic plaques occur in multiple (although predictable and consistent) areas (for review, see 52). There is a laminar pattern of neuronal involvement in association cortices (19,24,35,36), a consistent pattern in certain nuclei of the amygdala (32) and specific subcortical, diencephalic, and brain stem structures. Neurochemical alterations have been noted in multiple transmitter systems, again in multiple brain regions (4,10). Nonetheless, alterations in the hippocampal formation are clearly among the most severe, and possibly among the first, that occur in Alzheimer's disease.

SUMMARY

Certain cells in the hippocampal formation are specifically and selectively affected by pathologic changes in Alzheimer's disease. Both neurons responsible for hippocampal input from the cortex (layer II of the entorhinal cortex, the major source of the perforant pathway) and those responsible for hippocampal output to the cortex (the CA1/subicular zone and layer IV of the entorhinal cortex) contain neurofibrillary tangles. Moreover, the terminal zone of the perforant pathway in the outer part of the molecular layer of the dentate gyrus contains neuritic plaques, is the site of a sprouting phenomenon, and contains a decreased amount of the excitatory amino acid glutamate in Alzheimer's disease. These results suggest that the hippocampal formation is effectively deafferented and de-efferented from the cortex in Alzheimer's disease. It is likely that these pathologic changes preclude normal hippocampal function, thereby contributing to the memory dysfunction in Alzheimer's disease.

REFERENCES

1. Amaral, D.G. (1987) Memory: Anatomical Organization of Candidate Brain Regions. In F. Plum (ed): Handbook of Physiology, Section 1, The Nervous System, Vol. V, part 2. Bethesda, MD: American Physiological Society, pp. 211–294.
2. Ball, M.J. (1978) Topographic distribution of neurofibrillary tangles and granulovacuolar degeneration in hippocampal cortex of aging and demented patients: A quantitative study. Acta Neuropathol. (Berl.) *74:*173–178.
3. Ball, M.J., V. Hachinski, A. Fox, et al. (1985) A new definition of Alzheimer's disease: A hippocampal dementia. Lancet *1:*14–16.
4. Beal, M.F., and J.B. Martin (1986) Neuropeptides in neurological disease. Ann. Neurol. *20:*547–565.
5. Braak, H., and E. Braak (1985) On areas of transition between entorhinal allocortex and temporal isocortex in the human brain. Normal morphology and lamina-specific pathology in Alzheimer's disease. Acta Neuropathol. *68:*325–332.
6. Brun, A., and L. Gustafson (1976) Distribution of cerebral degeneration in Alzheimer's disease. Arch. Psychiatr. Nervenkr. *223:*15–33.
7. Cotman, C.W., D.A. Mathews, P. Taylor, and G. Lynch (1973) Synaptic rearrangement in the dentate gyrus: Histochemical evidence of adjustments after lesions in immature and adult rats. Proc. Natl. Acad. Sci. U.S.A. *70:*3473–3477.
8. Fuller, S.C. (1911) Alzheimer's disease (senium praecox): The report of a case and review of published cases. J. Nerv. Ment. Dis. *39:*440–455, 536–557.
9. Geddes, J.W., D.T. Monaghan, C.W. Cotman, et al. (1985) Plasticity of hippocampal circuitry in Alzheimer's disease. Science *230:*1179–1181.
10. Hardy, J., R. Adolfsson, I. Alafuzoff, et al. (1985) Transmitter deficits in Alzheimer's disease. Neurochem. Int. *7:*545–563.
11. Hirano, A., and H.M. Zimmerman (1962) Alzheimer's neurofibrillary changes: A topograhic study. Arch. Neurol. *7:*73–88.
12. Hjörth-Simonsen, A. (1973) Some intrinsic connections of the hippocampus in the rat: An experimental analysis. J. Comp. Neurol. *147:*145–161.
13. Hjörth-Simonsen, A. (1972) Projections of the lateral part of the entorhinal area to the hippocampus and fascia dentata. J. Comp. Neurol. *146:*219–232.
14. Hjörth-Simonsen, A., and B. Jeune (1973) Origin and termination of the hippocampal perforant path in the rat studied by silver impregnation. J. Comp. Neurol. *147:*145–161.
15. Hyman, B.T., A.R. Damasio, G.W. Van Hoesen, and C.L. Barnes (1984) Cell specific pathology isolates the hippocampal formation in Alzheimer's disease. Science *225:*1168–1170.
16. Hyman, B.T., G.W. Van Hoesen, L.J. Kromer, and A.R. Damasio (1986) Perforant pathway changes and the memory impairment of Alzheimer's disease. Ann. Neurol. *20:*472–482.

17. Hyman, B.T., L.J. Kromer, and G.W. Van Hoesen (1987) Reinnervation of the hippocampal perforant pathway zone in Alzheimer's disease. Ann. Neurol. *21:*259–267.

18. Hyman, B.T., G.W. Van Hoesen, and A.R. Damasio (1987) Alzheimer's disease: Glutamate depletion in perforant pathway terminals. Ann. Neurol. *22:*37–40.

19. Hyman, B.T., K. Maskey, G.W. Van Hoesen, L.J. Kromer, and A.R. Damasio (1987) Pathological changes in the multimodal association areas of the superior temporal sulcus in Alzheimer's disease. Neurology (Suppl. 1) *37:*168.

20. Hyman, B.T., G.W. Van Hoesen, B. Wolozin, P. Davies, and A.R. Damasio (1988) Alz-50 antibody recognizes Alzheimer-related neuronal changes. Ann. Neurol. *23:*371–379.

21. Hyman, B.T., L.J. Kromer, and G.W. Van Hoesen (1988) A direct demonstration of the perforant pathway terminal zone in Alzheimer's disease using the monoclonal antibody Alz-50. Brain Res. *450:*392–397.

22. Hyman, B.T., L.J. Kromer, G.W. Van Hoesen, and A.R. Damasio (1988) Disruption of amygdala-hippocampal connections demonstrated by Alz-50 immunoreactivity in Alzheimer's disease. Neurology (Suppl. 1) *38:*319.

23. Hyman, B.T., and G.W. Van Hoesen (1988) Sites of early Alzheimer-type pathologic changes in enthorhinal cortex and hippocampus visualized by Alz-50 immunocytochemistry. Soc. Neurosci. *14:*1084.

24. Hyman, B.T., K.P. Maskey, G.W. Van Hoesen, and A.R. Damasio (1988) The auditory system in Alzheimer's disease (AD): Hierarchical pattern of pathology. Neurology (Suppl. 1) *38:*133.

25. Insausti, R., D.G. Amaral, and W.M. Cowan (1987) The entorhinal cortex of the monkey: II. Cortical afferents. J. Comp. Neurol. *264:*356–395.

26. Insausti, R., D.G. Amaral, and W.M. Cowan (1987) The entorhinal cortex of the monkey: III. Subcortical afferents. J. Comp. Neurol. *264:*396–408.

27. Kemper, T.L. (1978) Senile dementia: A focal disease in the temporal lobe. In K. Nandy (ed): Senile Dementia: A Biomedical Approach. Amsterdam: Elsevier, North Holland, pp. 105–113.

28. Köhler, C. (1985) Intrinsic projections of the retrohippocampal region in the rat brain. I. The subicular complex. J. Comp. Neurol. *236:*504–522.

29. Köhler, C. (1986) Intrinsic connections of the retrohippocampal region in the rat brain. II. The medial entorhinal area. J. Comp. Neurol. *246:*149–169.

30. Köhler, C., and V. Chan-Palay (1983) Somatostatin and vasoactive intestinal polypeptide-like immunoreactive cells and terminals in the retrohippocampal region of the rat brain. Anat. Embryol. *167:*151–172.

31. Kosel, K.C., G.W. Van Hoesen, and D.L. Rosene (1982) Non-hippocampal cortical projections from the entorhinal cortex in the rat and rhesus monkey. Brain Res. *244:*201–213.

32. Kromer, L.J., B.T. Hyman, G.W. Van Hoesen, and A.R. Damasio (1987) Pathological alterations in the basolateral amygdala in Alzheimer's disease. Soc. Neurosci. *13:*1067.

33. Love, S., P. Burrola, R.D. Terry, and C.A. Wiley (1988) Immunoelectron microscopy of Alzheimer's and Pick brains with the monoclonal antibody Alz-50. J. Neuropathol. Exp. Neurol. *47:*333.

34. Nadler, J.V., and E.M. Smith (1981) Perforant path lesion depletes glutamate content of fasica detata synaptosomes. Neurosci. Lett. *25:*275–280.

35. Pearson, R.C.A., M.M. Esiri, R.W. Hiorns, et al. (1985) Anatomical correlates of the distribution of pathological changes in the neocortex in Alzheimer's disease. Proc. Natl. Acad. Sci. U.S.A. *83:*4531–4534.

36. Rogers, J., and J.H. Morrison (1985) Quantitative morphology and regional and laminar distributions of senile plaques in Alzheimer's disease. J. Neurosci. *5*:2801–2808.
37. Room, P., and H.J. Groenewegen (1986) Connections of the parahippocampal cortex. I. Cortical afferents. J. Comp. Neurol. *251*:415–450.
38. Room, P., and H.J. Groenewegen (1986) Connections of the parahippocampal cortex in cat. II. Subcortical afferents. J. Comp. Neurol. *251*:451–473.
39. Rosene, D.L., and G.W. Van Hoesen (1977) Hippocampal efferents reach widespread areas of the cerebral cortex and amygdala in the rhesus monkey. Science *198*:315–317.
40. Rosene, D.L., and G.W. Van Hoesen (1987) The Hippocampal formation of the primate brain. In E.G. Jones and A. Peters (eds): Cerebral Cortex, Vol. 6. New York Plenum, pp. 345–455.
41. Sorensen, K.E. (1985) Projections of the entorhinal area to the striatum, nucleus accumbens, and cerebral cortex in the guinea pig. J. Comp. Neurol. *238*:308–322.
42. Sorensen, K.E., and M.T. Shipley (1979) Projections from the subiculum to the deep layers of the ipsilateral presubicular and entorhinal cortices in the guinea pig. J. Comp. Neurol. *188*:313–334.
43. Steward, O. (1976) Topographic organization of the projections from the entorhinal area to the hippocampal formation in the rat. J. Comp. Neurol. *167*:285–314.
44. Steward, O., and S.A. Scoville (1976) Cells of origin of entorhinal cortical afferents to the hippocampus and fascia dentata of the rat. J. Comp. Neurol. *169*:347–370.
45. Storm-Mathisen, J. (1977) Glutamic acid and excitatory nerve endings: Reduction in glutamic acid uptake after axotomy. Brain Res. *120*:379–386.
46. Swanson, L.W., and C. Köhler (1986) Anatomical evidence for direct projections from the entorhinal area to the entire cortical mantle in the rat. J. Neurosci. *6*:3010–3023.
47. Swanson, L.W., J.M. Wyss, and W.M. Cowan (1978) An autoradiographic study of the organization of intra-hippocampal association pathways in the rat. J. Comp. Neurol. *181*:681–716.
48. Swanson, L.W., and W.M. Cowan (1977) An autoradiographic study of the organization of the afferent connections of the hippocampus formation in the rat. J. Comp. Neurol. *172*:49–84.
49. Terry, R.D., and R. Katzman (1983) Senile dementia of the Alzheimer type. Ann. Neurol. *14*:497–506.
50. Van Hoesen, G.W. (1982) The primate parahippocampal gyrus: New insights regarding its cortical connections. Trends Neurosci. *5*:345–350.
51. Van Hoesen, G.W. (1985) Neural systems of the nonhuman primate forebrain in monkey. Ann. N.Y. Acad. Sci. *444*:97–112.
52. Van Hoesen, G.W., and A.R. Damasio (1987) Neural correlates of cognitive impairment in Alzheimer's disease. In F. Plum (ed): Handbook of Physiology, Vol. 5. Bethesda, MD: American Physiological Society, pp. 872–898.
53. Van Hoesen, G.W., B.T. Hyman, P. Wolozin, P. Davies, and A.R. Damasio (1987) A direct demonstration of the involvement of cortico-cortical pathways in Alzheimer's disease. Neurology (Suppl. 1) *37*:332.
54. Van Hoesen, G.W., D.N. Pandya, and N. Butters (1972) Cortical afferents to the entorhinal cortex in the rhesus monkey. Science *175*:1471–1473.
55. Van Hoesen, G.W., and D.N. Pandya (1975) Some connections of the entorhinal (area 28) and perirhinal (area 35) cortices in the rhesus monkey. I. Temporal lobe afferents. Brain Res. *95*:1–24.

56. Van Hoesen, G.W., D.N. Pandya, and N. Butters (1975) Some connections of the entorhinal (area 28) and perirhinal (area 35) cortices in the rhesus monkey. II. Frontal lobe afferents. Brain Res. *95*:25–38.

57. Van Hoesen, G.W., and D.N. Pandya (1975) Some connections of the entorhinal (area 28) and perirhinal (area 35) cortices in the rhesus monkey. III. Entorhinal cortex efferents. Brain Res. *95*:39–59.

58. Witter, M.P., and H.J. Groenewegen (1986) Connections of the parahippocampal cortex in the cat. III. Cortical and thalamic efferents. J. Comp. Neurol. *252*:1–31.

59. Witter, M.P., and H.J. Groenewegen (1986) Connections of the parahippocampal cortex in the cat. IV. Subcortical efferents. J. Comp. Neurol. *251*:51–77.

60. Wolozin, B.L., A. Pruchnicki, D.W. Dickson, and P. Davies (1986) A neuronal antigen in the brains of Alzheimer's patients. Science *232*:648–650.

The Hippocampus—New Vistas, pages 513–534

32
Coexistence of Somatostatin and Neuropeptide Y in the Hippocampus of Patients With Alzheimer's and Parkinson's Dementia Compared With Age-Matched Controls

VICTORIA CHAN-PALAY, CHRISTER KÖHLER, and MATHIAS HÖCHLI

Neurology Clinic, University Hospital, Zürich, Switzerland (V.C.-P., M.H.); Astra Research Center, Södertälje, Sweden (C.K.)

INTRODUCTION

Senile dementia of the Alzheimer type (SDAT) is characterized clinically by dementia and histologically by the presence of numerous neuritic or senile plaques and neurofibrillary tangles in the neocortex and hippocampus (Tomlinson et al., 1970; Tomlinson and Corsellis, 1984). The degree of dementia is reported to be positively correlated with the number of cortical plaques (Blessed et al., 1968; Perry et al., 1978) and cortical and hippocampal neurofibrillary tangles (Wilcock and Esiri, 1982). Of the numerous neurotransmitter systems studied in postmortem brains of patients with SDAT, reduction of choline acetyltransferase activity has been most consistently found (Bowen et al., 1976; Davies and Maloney, 1976; Perry et al., 1977; Rossor et al., 1982). This decrease of cortical and hippocampal cholinergic activity has been attributed to a loss of cholinergic innervation from the basal forebrain, the septal nuclei, and the nucleus of Meynert (Whitehouse et al., 1982; Rossor et al., 1982; Coyle et al., 1983; Henke and Lang, 1983; McGeer et al., 1984). In addition to these well-documented cholinergic abnormalities, noradrenergic and serotonin deficits (Carlsson et al., 1980; Cross et al., 1983; Gottfries et al., 1983; Hardy et al., 1985) have also been reported, indicating degeneration of projections from the locus coeruleus and the raphe nuclei. More recently, reductions of somatostatin concentrations have been demonstrated in the cerebral cortex (Davies et al., 1980; Davies and Terry, 1981; Rossor et al., 1982; Ferrier et al., 1983; Hardy et al., 1985), and somatostatin immunoreactive axons have been shown to participate in the formation of neuritic plaques (Armstrong et al., 1985; Morrison et al., 1985; Nakamura and Vincent, 1986) and neurofibrillary tangles (Roberts et al., 1985). However, reports of somatostatin reduction or loss in the hippocampus are less consistent; some studies report no change in SDAT compared with normals (Ferrier et al., 1983) and others a dramatic reduction in the SDAT condition (Davies et al., 1980; Chan-Palay, 1987a–c).

Another peptide, neuropeptide Y (NPY), has also been studied in relation to possible changes in SDAT. NPY concentrations are unchanged or even increased in the substantia innominata (Allen et al., 1984). Studies in the cerebral cortex of SDAT patients indicated that the greatest severity of NPY loss parallels histopathological abnormalities shown by plaques and tangles. Of the areas studied, the temporal cortex was most severely involved (Chan-Palay et al., 1985a,b). NPY axons contribute to neuritic plaque formations (Dawbarn et al., 1984; Chan-Palay et al., 1985b). The hippocampal regions from the brains of SDAT patients have been shown (Chan-Palay et al., 1986a,b) to have afflictions in NPY immunoreactive (NPY-i) networks in the hilus, CA1, the parasubiculum, and the entorhinal cortex. Parallel semiquantitative estimates made of the numbers of neuritic plaques and neurofibrillary tangles in the other hippocampi of the brains in every SDAT case showed that the areas of heaviest pathological change by these indices are CA1 and the entorhinal cortex, the subicular complex CA3, and the area dentata being less affected. NPY-i axons were shown to participate in neuritic plaques. Thus areas with the most severe loss of NPY-i neurons and axons, CA1 and the entorhinal cortex, are synonymous with those areas most severely affected by the other indices of SDAT, thus confirming that NPY-i networks are involved in the SDAT disease process. However, other NPY-i neurons survive in some subfields better than others. The cumulative evidence suggests a population of hippocampal peptide neurons that are remarkably resistant in terminal neurological disease. The present study aims to clarify the changes encountered in somatostatin neurons in severe SDAT and to compare them with changes of NPY cells and fibers.

Studies of the possible coexistence of neuropeptides in the forebrain and cortex of animals and humans show that NPY and somatostatin (SOM) may be colocalized (Hendry et al., 1984; Köhler et al., 1987; Chan-Palay, 1987c). There has been some suggestion that this overlap between immunoreactive NPY and SOM in rat and mouse hypothalamic and cortical neurons may be high (Chronwall et al., 1985) in pyramidal and nonpyramidal neurons. However, their description of NPY-i neurons as being of the pyramidal type throws some doubt onto these observations because they do not conform to those in most other reports of cortical NPY-i neurons in animal or human brains, which describe NPY-i neurons as of the nonpyramidal type (Allen et al., 1983; Chan-Palay et al., 1985a,b, 1986a,b; Dawbarn et al., 1984; Chan-Palay and Yasargil, 1986). The question whether or not immunoreactive SOM and NPY coexist in human hippocampal neurons has been recently investigated (Chan-Palay, 1987a–c, 1988). We include in this chapter studies by double label immunocytochemistry that demonstrate the coexistence of immunoreactive SOM and NPY in hippocampal neurons, and their extent and regional differences, in the normal aged human brain and in the brains of patients with senile dementia of the Alzheimer type (SDAT) and a patient with Parkinson's disease with progressive dementia symptoms.

CASE SELECTION

The objective of the study was to compare the distribution of SOM-i neurons in SDAT in the hippocampus and the temporal cortex with those of age-matched controls. The patients were selected according to clinical and neuropathological criteria established at the outset, prior to collection of the material for this study. The study included two cases of severe SDAT and two control cases. The control subjects had no clinical history of neurological disease. All subjects were matched for age. The SDAT subjects had documented clinical histories of progressive dementia, and their therapeutic management included symptomatic treatment and prolonged hospitalization. One patient with parkinsonismus with fulminant dementia and motor symptoms not responsive to L-dopa treatment (PARK +D, dopa−) was also included for comparison. All patients and controls used in this study did not include any with a history of stroke, cerebral tumors, or brain-related infections. Patients with evidence of vascular disease at gross neuropathological examination were eliminated. Patients with histories of hypertension were included, but not those with a history of cerebral infarcts. All six patients, SDAT and controls, had gross neuropathological examination and microscopic examination of the brain. Gross examination of the brain included assessment of cortical atrophy and ventricular dilation. One hemisphere was then removed for neuropathological examination and the other for immunocytochemistry. The question of laterality was avoided by taking alternating hemispheres in chronological order—first case on the left, next on the right, and so forth. Microscopic examination for neuropathological assessment included routine hematoxylin and eosin stain, Nissl stain, and Bodian silver stain performed on paraffin-embedded tissue, 10 μm thick. Neuritic plaque and neurofibrillary tangle counts indicated minimal indices in controls and PARK +D cases but numerous in the SDAT cases.

DOUBLE LABELING: IMMUNOREACTIVE SOM AND NPY COEXISTENCE

Cryostat sections 10 μm thick or Vibratome sections not more than 20 μm thick were prepared as pairs of sections. Strict attention was paid to keep track of the adjacent surfaces between the two sections. The exposure of the two adjacent surfaces was achieved by inverting one of the sections. Thus the exposed surfaces represent the two facing surfaces of one sectioning procedure. For studying coexistence in the light microscope, cells lying in the plane of section could be cut into two parts, one part remaining within the exposed surface of the first section face and the other part remaining in the second exposed face. However, other cells could remain unsectioned in one or the other face.

Each section was then treated separately but simultaneously in individual wells with either a somatostatin or NPY antiserum to examine the coexistence of the two immunoreactivities in neurons. The following procedures were used. Pairs of sections were floated onto 1% hydrogen peroxide in phosphate-buffered saline for 2 h to reduce or eliminate endogenous peroxidase reactions, reacted sequentially with the primary antibody (1:1,000 NPY or 1:1,500 somatostatin) overnight (goat antirabbit antibodies, peroxidase, and diaminobenzidine [DAB]) as previously described (Chan-Palay, 1987a–c; Chan-Palay et al., 1985a,b, 1986a,b; Chan-Palay and Yasargil, 1986). Alternatively, the immunogold/silver reaction described in the above section was also used on paired sections with one antibody on each of the pairs, or one of a pair of sections was treated with the immunogold/silver method and the other with the peroxidase-anti-peroxidase method. In another group of double label experiments, pairs of sections were simultaneously incubated with both antibodies on the same section in a mixture of the polyclonal NPY (1:1,000) and the monoclonal somatostatin (1:1,500). Subsequently fluorescein (FITC) conjugated with goat antirabbit immunoglobulins and rhodamine-conjugated antimouse immuno-globulins were applied. The preparations were mounted in a glycerine buffer mixture.

To localize the neuronal elements accurately in the different hippocampal regions, maps were made of all the specimens, charting the lamination of the regions in relation to stained neurons. Identified SOM-i neurons were counted with attention to their specific location in the hippocampal layers, regions, and the major fiber bundles. Because of the difficulty of maintaining consistent section thickness, these counts were considered only semiquantitative. Black-and-white and color photomicrographs were made with a Zeiss photomicroscope fitted with Nomarski optics. The nomenclature for the hippocampal regions follows that used by Schaltenbrand and Bailey (1959), Braak (1974), and Kemper (1984).

For the double staining SOM-i NPY-i coexistence studies, all neurons immunoreactive to either NPY or SOM from pairs of adjacent peroxidase-stained sections were plotted with the aid of an interactive computer program (Biometrics) and IBM-AT2 computer system. The outlines of the NPY-i section and every immunostained neuron were plotted. Thereafter the adjacent SOM-i section in the pair was drawn and every immunostained neuron then plotted as well. The two maps were then superimposed to locate the NPY-i and SOM-i cells. Coincident neurons were then selected for examination at greater magnifications and for camera lucida mapping at ×360 to confirm that the two neuron faces with immunoreactive NPY and SOM indeed belonged to one single neuron. These neurons were then considered to store both NPY and SOM. Counts of the total numbers of immunoreactive NPY and SOM and those considered to store both peptides were made. Pairs of double labeled neurons were photographed with a Zeiss photomicroscope or with a fluorescence microscope equipped to distinguish rhodamine and fluorescein emission wavelengths. Because of the variations in section thickness and technique, the assessments of the amount of coexistence of the two peptides are probably minimal estimates. There could be more coexistence demonstrable on thinner sections because of the small size of many NPY-i and SOM-i neurons.

These results were compiled from a comparison between the SDAT cases and their age-matched controls and the PARK +D (dopa−) case. Each case when carefully examined revealed some differences in the degree of involvement of SOM-i neurons in the SDAT process. However, by the criterion of the numbers of neuritic plaques and filamentous tangles, all cases were classified as severe. However, both of the SDAT cases had hippocampal gyri that were atrophied to almost one-third of the normal volume, and with all of the SOM-i neurons no longer persisting in the severely atrophied parts.

In general, SDAT material immunostained with SOM antisera is readily distinguished from the control material on the basis of the particular morphology of the individual SOM neurons and networks. SOM-i neurons of the SDAT type have a dense, intense immunoreactive character; the deposit of silver enhancement grains is smooth and fills the neuron. Dendrites are foreshortened, and axonal fibers are wispy and fragile in appearance, if present at all. The varicosities are larger than in the control material, and the intervaricose segments are difficult to follow except for the occasional very thick ones and for short distances. All observed SOM-i neurons were of the nonpyramidal type, multipolar or bitufted in shape, and of various sizes. The locations of SOM-i neurons (See Fig. 6) affected by SDAT were charted onto a schema with the various subfields indicated (black dots for surviving SOM-i SDAT neurons). The schema also indicates by open circles the relative number of NPY-i neurons remaining in the same subfields. The data concerning the NPY-i neurons in SDAT have been previously described in detail (Chan-Palay et al., 1986b) and are included here for comparative purposes. Fundamentally, the whole Ammon's horn, but particularly the area dentata and the subfield CA, are most severely affected by SDAT. The few SOM-i neurons that remain are vestiges, with few processes and misshapen perikarya. The rest are gone altogether, as severe regional atrophy has occurred.

In the subicular region SDAT has less effect on SOM-i neurons. The entorhinal cortex and perirhinal cortex, however, are sites of serious SOM-i neuron loss. Compared with the controls, the numbers of surviving SOM-i neurons are considerably reduced. There are stratification differences in this reduction in the cortical regions. The upper layers (I and II) are basically devoid of the few SOM-i neurons that might normally be found there. The middle layers have a few neurons, sometimes found in pairs or small groups of middle-sized SOM-i cells. In the deepest layers one finds the best survival of SOM-i neurons. This coincides with the fact that the deeper layers are also where the largest numbers of SOM-i neurons occur. The larger SOM-i cells survive well, and middle-sized cells and a few of the small fusiform bipolar neurons in the white matter also remain.

Comparatively, in the same subfields in these cases of SDAT, NPY-i neurons survive in greater numbers than the SOM-i neurons. This is particularly significant, as there are more SOM-i neurons, as detected by the NPY and SOM-28 antibodies that we used consistently in these studies. Nevertheless, one may have to consider that the proportional relationship between numbers of neurons revealed by NPY and by SOM immunoreactivity may reflect the specifities of these two antibodies for their respective antigens under the technical constraints imposed by fixation as much as the biological activities and states of the neurons.

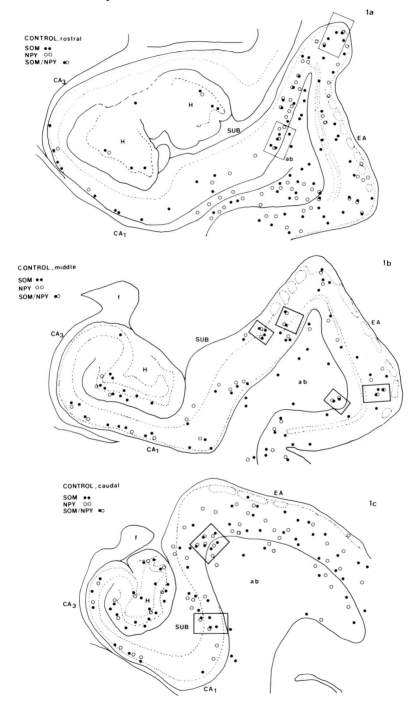

SOM-i neurons are most abundant in the hilus of the area dentata, in strata oriens and pyramidale in the CA1 subfield, and in the deeper layers of the entorhinal cortex (II through VI and white matter) and the perirhinal cortex. Small fusiform neurons occur in the white matter, fimbria, alveus, and angular bundle and in the white matter in the hippocampus, retrohippocampus, and temporal cortex. NPY-i neurons are most abundant in the area dentata and the strata oriens and pyramidale of CA1. The subicular complex, entorhinal cortex, and the temporal cortex have numerous NPY-i neurons. Most prominent are the small fusiform neurons of the white matter in fimbria, alveus, and the angular bundle (Chan-Palay et al., 1986a,b). It is clear at this point that the distributions of these two peptide immunoreactivities are remarkably similar, and the superimposition of the maps compiled from the rostral hippocampus—one showing NPY-i neurons and axons and the other showing SOM-i neurons and axons—supports this impression. The major similarities of the two groups are those of like cell morphology and cell size and parallel locations of neuron distribution. The fact that neither cell population includes pyramidal neurons in our material is also relevant.

Several minor differences exist as well between these two neuronal immunoreactivities. The SOM-i neuron population by and large in every region of hippocampus and cortex is more numerous than the NPY-i population. This is especially evident in the hilar regions and in the entorhinal and temporal cortex. However, the reverse is true of the small, fusiform neurons in the white matter. Although common to both, these cells have a distinctly higher incidence in NPY-i material. In terms of regional distribution, there are more SOM-i neurons caudally than rostrally in the hippocampus. With NPY-i neurons, the reverse relationship appears to be true.

The parallel distribution of SOM-i and NPY-i cells raises the question of whether these neurons are separate neuron populations or whether immunoreactive SOM and NPY coexist in some neurons. If immunoreactive SOM and NPY coexistence occurs, then to what extent, and what are the differences in their regional distribution?

The parallel distributions of SOM-i and NPY-i neurons underscore the impression that these two peptides occur in similar neuronal populations in comparable subfields of the hippocampus and cortex. The results of the double labeling experiments demonstrate that about 30% of the SOM-i neurons in the hilus of the area dentata are also NPY immunoreactive. However, since, numerically, more SOM-i neurons are visualized by our methods than NPY-i neu-

---

Fig. 1. Schematic representation of the rostral (**a**), middle (**b**), and caudal (**c**) hippocampus with sites of SOM-i neurons (black dots) and NPY neurons (open circles). Both peptides have comparable distributions and exhibit a significant proportion of SOM-i/NPY-i coexistence (see text). Control brains. Immunogold/silver method. The areas enclosed within boxes are regions with multiple examples of neurons with NPY/SOM coexistence, some of which are shown in the photomicrographs in Figures 2–5. ab, angular bundle; Ca_1, CA_3, subfields of Ammon's horn; EA, entorhinal area; f, fimbria; H, hilus of area dentata; SUB, subiculum.

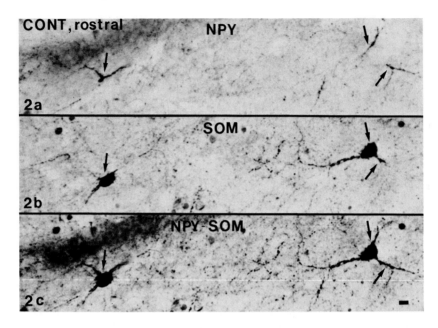

Fig. 2. NPY and SOM immunoreactivities in two hippocampal neurons. Two adjacent facing surfaces of two neurons in the hippocampus are exposed by the sectioning procedure, and one face has been reacted specifically for NPY antibodies (**a**) and the other for SOM (**b**), indicating that the neurons have both SOM and NPY in coexistence. **c:** Photographic exposition of the two labeled neuron surfaces to demonstrate the fact that they belong to one and the same cell. Bar = 100 μm. Control case, rostral hippocampus, CA1 region. ×260. Single arrows (left) and double arrows (right) indicate the origins of primary dendrites from the somata.

rons, the coexistence population constitutes approximately 50% of all NPY-i neurons. NPY-i coexistence was found in several SOM-i neurons in CA1, the dentate hilus, and particularly in the subicular complex. The highest coexistence coefficients were found in the deep layers of the entorhinal cortices, where more than 50% of the SOM-i neurons were NPY immunoreactive as well. The neurons occurred individually or in small groups. Large neurons of the retrohippocampal areas and small neurons in the white matter were particularly noted as frequent examples of NPY-i and SOM-i coexistence (see Figs. 1–5 for controls, Figs. 6–10 for SDAT, and Figs. 11–14 for PARK + D, dopa –).

In the SDAT cases, both NPY and SOM immunoreactivities in neurons and axons were seriously affected, with a numerically higher survival of NPY-i neurons and axons than SOM-i neurons and axons in the cortical areas and equally severe destruction of both peptide neurons in the area dentata and

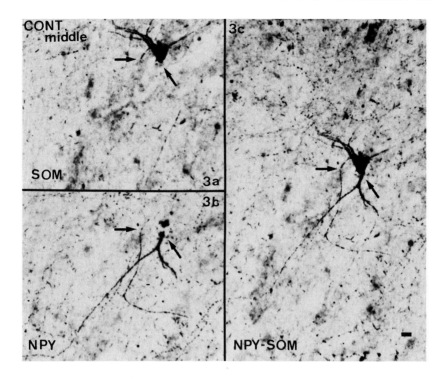

Fig. 3. NPY and SOM immunoreactivities in a single human hippocampal neuron are exposed by the sectioning procedure, and one face has been reacted specifically for SOM antibodies **(a)** and the other for NPY **(b),** indicating that this neuron has both SOM reactivity and NPY in coexistence. **c:** Photographic exposition of the two labeled neuron surfaces to demonstrate the fact that they belong to one and the same cell. Bar = 100 μm. Control case, middle hippocampus, entorhinal cortex. ×260. Double arrows indicate the emergence of primary dendrites from the soma.

CA1. Neurons with coexistence of NPY and SOM immunoreactivities appear to be more readily detected and may be better protected against SDAT than the neurons with SOM immunoreactivity alone or NPY immunoreactivity alone. Because of the techniques that we used for the demonstrations of coexistence, we anticipate that our estimates are generally lower than might otherwise be found. Thus the numerical estimates given here can be considered minimal rather than maximal.

Although SOM-i axons within plaques are readily recognized, as previously reported (Armstrong et al., 1985; Nakamura and Vincent, 1986), SOM-i neurons/ perikarya do not occur within the neuritic plaques themselves, despite the fact that well-preserved labeled neurons appear on the periphery of neuritic plaques.

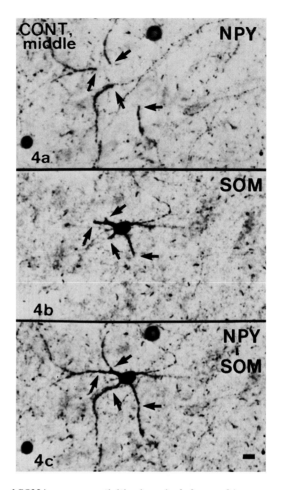

Fig. 4. NPY and SOM immunoreactivities in a single human hippocampal neuron. Two adjacent facing surfaces of one neuron are exposed by the sectioning procedure, and one face has been reacted specifically for NPY antibodies (a) and the other for SOM (b), indicating that this neuron has both NPY reactivity and SOM in coexistence. c: Photgraphic exposition of the two labeled neuron surfaces to demonstrate the fact that they belong to one and the same cell. Bar = 100 μm. Control case, middle hippocampus, subiculum. ×320. Arrows indicate primary dendrites.

Fig. 5. NPY and SOM immunoreactivities in a single hippocampal neuron. Two adjacent facing surfaces of one neuron are exposed by the sectioning procedure, and one face has been reacted specifically for NPY antibodies (a) and the other for SOM (b), indicating that this neuron has both NPY reactivity and SOM in coexistence. c: Photographic exposition of the two labeled neuron surfaces to demonstrate the fact that they belong to one and the same cell. Bar = 100 μm. Control case, caudal hippocampus, entorhinal cortex. ×320. Arrows indicate primary dendrites.

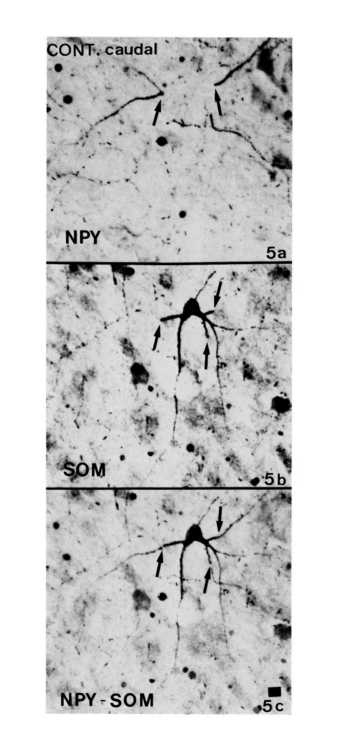

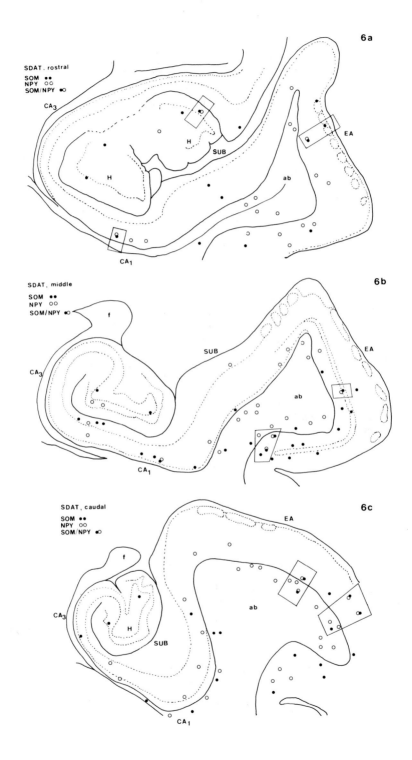

6a

SDAT, rostral
SOM ●●
NPY ○○
SOM/NPY ●○

CA₃

H

H

SUB

EA

ab

CA₁

6b

SDAT, middle
SOM ●●
NPY ○○
SOM/NPY ●○

f

CA₃

SUB

EA

ab

CA₁

6c

SDAT, caudal
SOM ●●
NPY ○○
SOM/NPY ●○

f

CA₃

H

SUB

EA

ab

CA₁

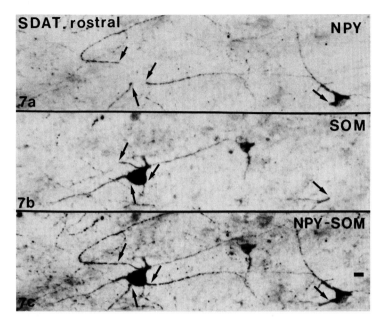

Fig. 7. NPY and SOM immunoreactivities in two hippocampal neurons. Two adjacent facing surfaces of the two neurons are exposed by the sectioning procedure, and one face has been reacted specifically for NPY antibodies (a) and the other for SOM (b), indicating that these neurons have both NPY reactivity and SOM in coexistence. c: Photographic exposition of the two labeled neuron surfaces to demonstrate the fact that they belong to one and the same cell. Bar = 100 μm. Alzheimer case (SDAT), rostral hippocampus, entorhinal region. × 260. Arrows indicate primary dendrites.

Fig. 6. Schematic representation of the rostral (a), middle (b), and caudal (c) hippocampus with sites of SOM-i neurons (black dots) and NPY-i neurons (open circles). Both peptides have comparable distributions and exhibit a significant proportion of SOM-i/NPY-i coexistence (see text). SOM/NPY neurons are also indicated. Immunogold/silver method. The areas enclosed within boxes are regions with multiple examples of neurons with NPY/SOM coexistence, some of which are shown in the photomicrographs in Figures 7–10. Alzheimer case (SDAT). Note the severe loss of neurons of both neuropeptide types compared with the control case (Fig. 3a–c). The neurons with NPY/SOM coexistence are readily found because of the scarcity of the remaining neurons in the atrophic hippocampus. ab, angular bundle; Ca$_1$, CA$_3$, subfields of Ammon's horn; EA, entorhinal area; f, fimbria, H, hilus of area dentata; SUB, subiculum.

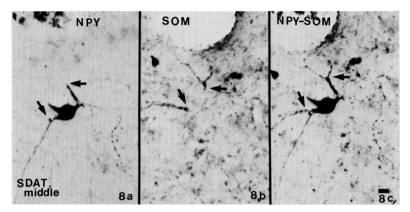

Fig. 8. NPY and SOM immunoreactivities in a single human hippocampal neuron. Two adjacent facing surfaces of one neuron are exposed by the sectioning procedure, and one face has been reacted specifically for NPY antibodies (a) and the other for SOM (b), indicating that this neuron has both NPY reactivity and SOM in coexistence. c: Photographic exposition of the two labeled neuron surfaces to demonstrate the fact that they belong to one and the same cell. Bar = 100 μm. Alzheimer case (SDAT), middle hippocampus, CA1. ×280. Arrows indicate primary dendrites.

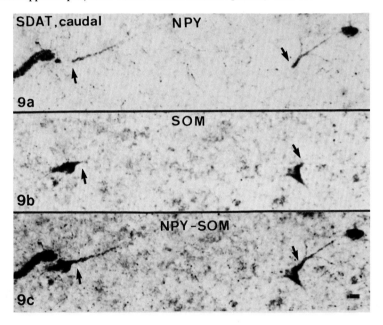

Fig. 9. NPY and SOM immunoreactivities in two hippocampal neurons. Two adjacent facing surfaces of two neurons are exposed by the sectioning procedure, and one face has been reacted specifically for NPY antibodies (a) and the other for SOM (b), indicating that this neuron has both NPY reactivity and SOM in coexistence. c: Photographic exposition of the two labeled neuron surfaces to demonstrate the fact that they belong to one and the same cell. Bar = 100 μm. Alzheimer case (SDAT), caudal hippocampus, subiculum. ×260. Arrows indicate primary dendrites.

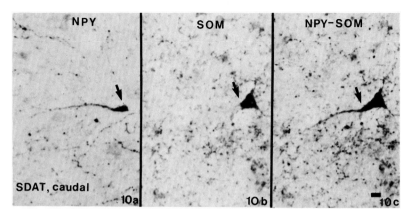

Fig. 10. NPY and SOM immunoreactivities in a single human hippocampal neuron. Two adjacent facing surfaces of one neuron are exposed by the sectioning procedure, and one face has been reacted specifically for NPY antibodies **(a)** and the other for SOM **(b)**, indicating that this neuron has both NPY reactivity and SOM in coexistence. **c:** Photographic exposition of the two labeled neuron surfaces to demonstrate the fact that they belong to one and the same cell. Black scale indicator is 100 μm. Alzheimer case (SDAT), caudal hippocampus, entorhinal cortex. ×280. Arrows indicate primary dendrites.

We have no information on the coexistence of SOM-i neurons and neurofibrillary tangles, since we have been unable to replicate the experiments of Roberts et al. (1985) with double labeling using immunocytochemistry and silver stains on the same preparation.

Table I summarizes the details of the cases and the counts of neuritic plaques and neurofibrillary tangles in the hippocampal CA1, parietal cortex, and temporal cortex in the two SDAT cases, two controls, and the parkinsonism with dementia (dopa−) case. The areas with the highest densities of plaques and tangles are the hilus of the area dentata, the CA1, and the entorhinal and temporal cortices. The numbers of neuritic plaques and neurofibrillary tangles reported in these cases are in accordance with the guidelines recently established for the diagnosis of SDAT (Katchaturian, 1985), and CA and the entorhinal cortex are known to be sites of predilection for SDAT morphological changes (Hooper and Vogel, 1976; Ball, 1978; Wilcock and Esiri, 1982; Hyman et al., 1984; Tomlinson and Corsellis, 1984).

Table II lists the numbers of NPY-i and SOM-i neurons in single selected sections through the rostral, middle, and caudal areas of hippocampus in the controls, SDAT, and PARK +D (dopa−) cases. Note that the numbers of neurons immunoreactive for these two peptides are basically comparable in the age-matched control case and the PARK +D (dopa−) case, but are severely reduced in the SDAT cases.

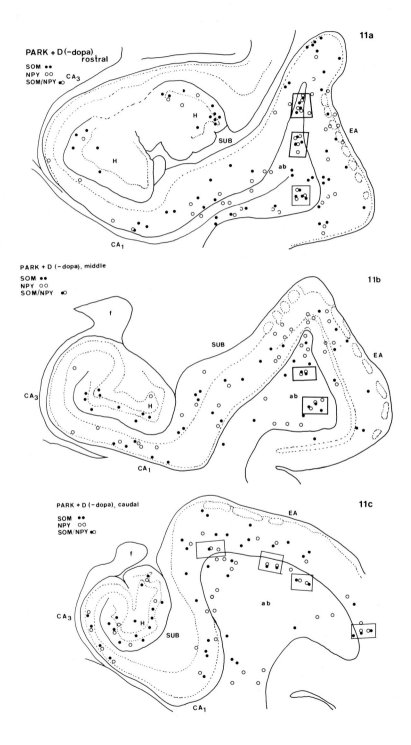

PARK + D (–dopa)
rostral

SOM ●●
NPY ○○
SOM/NPY ◐○

CA₃

H

H

SUB

ab

CA₁

EA

11a

PARK + D (–dopa), middle

SOM ●●
NPY ○○
SOM/NPY ◐

f

SUB

EA

CA₃

H

ab

CA₁

11b

PARK + D (–dopa), caudal

SOM ●●
NPY ○○
SOM/NPY ◐○

f

EA

CA₃

H

SUB

ab

CA₁

11c

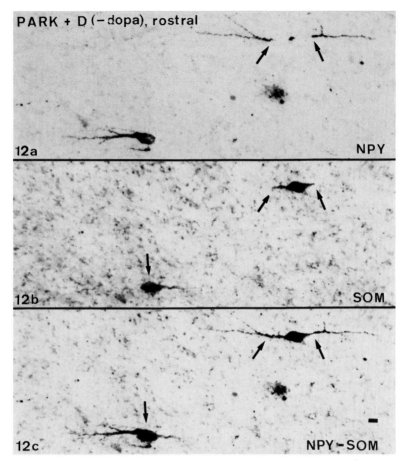

PARK + D (−dopa), rostral

12a   NPY

12b   SOM

12c   NPY−SOM

Fig. 12. NPY and SOM immunoreactivities in two hippocampal neurons. Two adjacent facing surfaces of two neurons are exposed by sectioning procedure, and one face has been reacted specifically for NPY antibodies (a) and the other for SOM (b), indicating that these neurons have both NPY reactivity and SOM in coexistence. c: Photographic exposition of the two labeled neuron surfaces to demonstrate the fact that they belong to one and the same cell. The single arrows (b,c) indicate the cell body of the neuron on the left, the double arrows point to the dendrites of the neuron on the right. Bar = 100 μm. Parkinson's disease with dementia, dopa-nonresponsive case, rostral hippocampus, entorhinal cortex. ×260.

Fig. 11. Schematic representation of the rostral (a), middle (b), and caudal (c) hippocampus with sites of SOM-i neurons (black dots) and NPY-i neurons (open circles) superimposed. Both peptides have comparable distributions and exhibit a significant proportion of SOM-i/NPY-i coexistence (indicated by both dots and circles). Immunogold/silver method. The areas enclosed within boxes are regions with multiple examples of neurons with NPY/SOM coexistence, some of which are shown in the micrographs in Figures 12–14. Parkinson's disease with dementia, nonresponsive to L-dopa treatment, PARK +D (dopa−). Note that the numbers of neuropeptide-reactive neurons of both types are about equivalent to the control case (Fig. 1a–c). ab, angular bundle; CA_1, CA_3, subfields of Ammon's horn; EA, entorhinal area; f, fimbria; H, hilus of area dentata; SUB, subiculum.

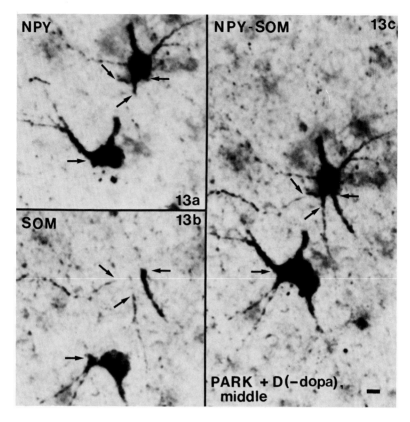

Fig. 13.   NPY and SOM immunoreactivities in two hippocampal neurons. Two adjacent facing surfaces of two neurons are exposed by the sectioning procedure, and one face has been reacted specifically for NPY antibodies (a) and the other for SOM (b), indicating that this neuron has both NPY reactivity and SOM in coexistence. c: Photographic exposition of two labeled neuron surfaces to demonstrate the fact that they belong to one and the same cell. The single arrow (lower neuron) and the group of three arrows (upper neuron) indicate the primary dendrites of these neurons and recur in a, b, and c as indications of coexistence. Bar = 100 μm. Parkinson's disease with dementia, dopa-nonresponsive case, middle hippocampus, CA1 region. ×450.

In the SDAT cases there is a more severe reduction in SOM neurons than in NPY neurons. However, the numbers of neurons with NPY and SOM in coexistence are comparable in the PARK + D (dopa −) cases with the normal cases but are more readily found in the SDAT cases.

Thus, the present study clearly indicates that in severe SDAT, the predilection sites for the highest incidence of neuritic plaques and neurofibrillary tangles are the sites of the severest loss of SOM-i neurons and networks. These regions are also the sites of the most severe loss and alterations in NPY-i neurons and

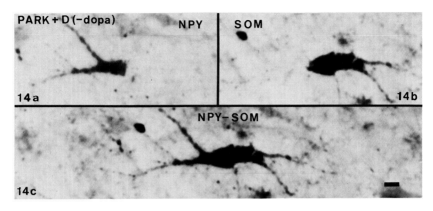

Fig. 14. NPY and SOM immunoreactivities in a single hippocampal neuron. Two adjacent facing surfaces of one neuron are exposed by the sectioning procedure, and one face has been reacted specifically for NPY antibodies (**a**) and the other for SOM (**b**), indicating that this neuron has both NPY reactivity and SOM in coexistence. **c:** Photographic exposition of the two labeled neuron surfaces to demonstrate the fact that they belong to one and the same cell. Bar = 100 μm. Parkinson's disease with dementia, dopa-nonresponsive case, caudal hippocampus, entorhinal cortex. ×450.

networks (Chan-Palay et al., 1985a,b, 1986a,b), implicating both peptide neuron systems in the disease process.

The fact that NPY and SOM neurons in coexistence are found in all three types of cases in our studies indicates that they are readily detectable and survive the neurogenerative disease processes involved in both Parkinson's

TABLE I. List of Brains Used in This Study, With Data on Neurological Disease, Ages, Sex, Clinical Diagnosis, Postmortem Delays, and Causes of Death[a]

Diagnosis	Age (years)	Sex	Cause of death	Post mortem delay (hours)	Brain weight (grams)
Control	54	M	Leukemia	11	1,410
Control	86	F	Pulmonary embolism	5	1,022
Alzheimer	74	F	Pulmonary embolism	9.5	1,091
Alzheimer	78	F	Bronchopneumonia	5	1,103
PARK+D (dopa−)	79	M	Bronchopneumonia	5.5	1,241

[a]The mini-mental test scores were 22–28 out of 30 for the controls, 0–5 of a possible 30 for SDAT cases, and 0–11 for the Parkinson's disease with dementia case.

TABLE II. List of Total Number of Neurons Labeled With NPY or SOM
Immunoreactivity in the Rostral, Middle, and Caudal Aspects of the
Hippocampus

	Rostral		Middle		Caudal	
	NPY	SOM	NPY	SOM	NPY	SOM
Control	139	121	180	154	165	166
SDAT	24	10	50	38	36	20
PARK +D (dopa−)	145	147	117	109	124	124

disease with dementia and the late-onset senile dementia of the Alzheimer
type. The fact that NPY and SOM coexistent neurons are found very readily
in the SDAT cases suggest that there may be a predilection for their survival
in atrophied hippocampi where there is severe destruction of other NPY-i and
SOM-i neurons.

ACKNOWLEDGMENTS

We are grateful to U. Haesler and B. Jentsch for their meticulous assistance
during this study.

REFERENCES

Allen, J.M., I.N. Fernier, G.W. Roberts, A.J. Cross, T.E. Adrian, T.J. Crow, and S.R. Bloom
(1984) Elevation of neuropeptide Y in substantia innominata in Alzheimer's type
dementia. J. Neurol. Sci. 64:325–331

Allen, Y.S., T.E. Adrian, J.M. Allen, K. Tatemoto, T.J. Crow, S.R. Bloom, and J.M. Polak
(1983) Neuropeptide Y distribution in the rat brain. Science 221:877–879.

Armstrong, D.M., S. LeRoy, D. Shields, and R.D. Terry (1985) Somatostatin like immunoreactivities within neuritic plaques. Brain Res. 338:71–79.

Ball, M.J. (1978) Topographic distribution of neurofibrillary tangles and grano-vacular
degeneration in hippocampal cortex of aging and demented patients. Acta Neuropathol. 42:73–80.

Blessed, G., B.E. Tomlinson, and M. Roth (1968) The association between quantitative
measurements of dementia and senile changes in the cerebral grey matter of elderly
subjects. Br. J. Psychiatry 114:797–811.

Bowen, D.M., C.B. Smith, B. White, and A.N. Davison (1976) Neurotransmitter related
enzymes and indices of hypoxia in senile dementia and other abiotrophies. Brain
99:459–466.

Braak, H. (1974) On the Structure of the human archicortex. Cell Tissue Res. 152:349–
383.

Carlsson, A., R. Adolfsson, S.M. Aquilonius, C. Gottfries, L. Oreland, L. Svennerholm,
and B. Winblad (1980) Biogenic amines in human brain in normal aging, senile dementia and chronic alcoholism. In M. Goldstein, A. Lieberman, D.B. Calne, and M.O.
Thorner (eds): Ergot Compounds and Brain Functions: Neuroendocrine and Neu-
ropsychiatric Aspects. New York: Raven Press, pp. 295–304.

Chan-Palay, V. (1987a) Neuropeptide Y and somatostatin neurons in normal and Alzheimer hippocampi with special attention to their colocalisation in single neurons.

In R.J. Wurtman, S.H. Corkin, and J.H. Growdon (eds): Alzheimer's Disease: Advances in Basic Research and Therapies. Cambridge, USA: Center for Brain Sciences and Metabolism Charitable Trust, pp. 367–369.

Chan-Palay, V. (1987b) Somatostatin and neuropeptide Y: Alterations and coexistence in the Alzheimer's dementia hippocampus. In J. Ulrich (ed): Histology and Histopathology of the Ageing Brain (Gerontoloy Series). Basel: Karger Verlag, pp. 17–38.

Chan-Palay, V. (1987c) Somatostatin immunoreactive neurons in the human hippocampus and cortex shown by immunogold silver intensification on vibratome sections: Coexistence with neuropeptide Y neurons. J. Comp. Neurol. *257*:208–215.

Chan-Palay, V. (1988) Somatostatin and neuropeptide Y coexistence in the hippocampus and alteration in Alzheimer's disease. In B.T. Pickering, A.J.S. Summerlee, and J.B. Waverly (eds): Neurosecretion: Cellular Aspects of the Production and Release of Neuropeptides. New York: Plenum Press, pp. 89–97.

Chan-Palay, V., Y.S. Allen, W. Lang, U. Hasler, and J.M. Polak (1985a) I. Cytology and distribution in normal human cerebral cortex of neurons immunoreactive with antisera against neuropeptide Y. J. Comp. Neurol. *238*:382–389.

Chan-Palay, V., W. Lang, Y.S. Allen, U. Haesler, and J.M. Polak J.M. (1985b) II. Cortical neurons immunoreactive with antisera against neuropeptide Y are altered in Alzheimer's-type dementia. J. Comp. Neurol. *238*:390–400.

Chan-Palay, V., C. Köhler, U. Haesler, W. Lang, and G. Yasargil (1986a) Distribution of neurons and axons immunoreactive with antisera against neuropeptide Y in the normal human hippocampus. J. Comp. Neurol. *248*:360–375.

Chan-Palay, V., W. Lang, U. Haesler, C. Köhler, and G. Yasargil (1986b) Hippocampal neurons and axons immunoreactive with antisera against neuropeptide Y in Alzheimer's type dementia. J. Comp. Neurol. *248*:376–394.

Chan-Palay, V., and G. Yasargil (1986) Immunocytochemistry of human brain tissue with a polyclonal antiserum against neuropeptide Y. Anat. Embryol. *174*:27–33.

Chronwall, B.M., D.A. DiMaggio, V.J. Massari, V.M. Pickel, D.A. Ruggiero, and T.L. O'-Donohue (1985) The anatomy of neuropeptide-Y-containing neurons in rat brain. Neuroscience *15*:1159–1181.

Coyle, J.T., D.L. Price, and M.R. DeLong (1983) Alzheimer's disease: A disorder of cortical cholinergic innervation. Science *219*:1184–1190.

Cross, A.J., T.J. Crow, J.A. Johnson, E.K. Perry, G. Blessed, and B.E. Tomlinson (1983) Monoamine metabolism in senile dementia of Alzheimer's typ. J. Neurol. Sci. *60*:383–392.

Davies, P., R. Katzmann, and R.D. Terry (1980) Reduced somatostatin-like immunoreactivity in cases of Alzheimer's disease and Alzheimer senile dementia. Nature *288*:279–280.

Davies, P., and A.J. Maloney (1976) Selective loss of central cholinergic neurons in Alzheimer's disease. Lancet *ii:*1043.

Davies, P., and R.D. Terry (1981) Cortical somatostatin-like immunoreactivity in cases of Alzeimer's and senile dementia of Alzheimer type. Neurobiol. Aging *2*:9–14.

Dawbarn, D., S.P. Hunt, and P.C. Emson (1984) Neuropeptide Y: Regional distribution, chromatographic characterization and immunohistochemical demonstration in post mortem human brain. Brain Res. *296*:168–173.

Ferrier, I.N., J.A. Cross, J.A. Johnson, G.W. Robers, T.J. Crow, J.A.N. Carsellis, Y.C. Lee, A.T.E. O'Shangoressey, G.P. McGregor, A.J. Bacarese-Hamilton, and S.R. Bloom (1983) Neuropeptides in Alzheimer type dementia. J. Neurol. *62*:152–170.

Gottfries, C.G., R. Adolfsson, S.M. Aquilonius, A. Carlsson, S.A. Ecernas, A. Norberg, L. Oveland, L.E. Svennerholm, A. Wiberg and B. Winbald (1983) Biochemical changes in dementia disorder of Alzheimer type (AS/SDAT). Neurobiol. Aging *4*:261–271.

Hardy, J., R. Adolfsson, I. Alafusoff, G. Bucht, J. Marcosson, P. Nyberg, E. Perdahl, P. Wester, and P. Winblad (1985) Transmitter deficits in Alzheimer's disease. Neurochem. Int. 7:545–562.

Hendry, S.H.C., E.G. Jones, and P.C. Emson (1984) Morphology, distribution and synaptic relations of somatostatin and neuropeptide Y-immunoreactive neurons in rat monkey neocortex. J. Neurosci. 4:2497–2517.

Henke, H., and W. Lang (1983) Cholinergic enzymes in neocortex, hippocampus and basal forebrain of non-neurological and senile dementia of Alzheimer type patients. Brain Res. 267:281–291.

Hooper, W.M., and F.S. Vogel (1976) The limbic system in Alzheimer's disease. Am. J. Pathol. 85:1–19.

Hyman, B.T., A.R. Damasio, G.W. van Hoesen, and C.L. Barnes (1984) Cell specific pathology isolates the hippocampal formation in Alzheimer's disease. Science 225:1168–1170.

Katchaturian. Z.S. (1985) Diagnosis of Alzheimer's disease. Arch. Neurol. 42:1097–1105.

Kemper, T.L. (1978) Senile dementia: A focal disease in the temporal lobe. In K. Nandy (ed): Senile Dementia: A Biomedical Approach. Amsterdam: Elsevier, pp. 105–113.

Köhler, C., L.G. Eriksson, S. Davies, and V. Chan-Palay (1987) Colocalisation of neuropeptide tyrosine and somatostatin immunoreactivities in neurons of individual hippocampal subfields in rat. Neurosci. Lett. 78:1–6.

McGeer, P.I., E.G. McGeer, J. Suzuki, C.E. Dolman, and T. Nagai (1984) Aging, Alzheimer's disease and the cholinergic system of the basal forbrain. Neurology 34:741–734.

Morrison, J.H., J. Rogers, S. Scherr, R. Benoit, and F.E. Bloom (1985) Somatostatin in neuritic plaques of Alzheimer's patients. Nature 314:90–92.

Nakamura, S., and S.R. Vincent (1986) Somatostatin and neuropeptide Y-immunoreactive neurons in the neocortex in senile dementia of Alzheimer's type. Brain Res. 370:11–20.

Perry, E.K., R.H. Perry, G. Blessed and B.E. Tomlinson (1977) Necropsy evidence of central cholinergic deficits in senile dementia. Lancet i:189.

Perry, E.K., B.E. Tomlinson, G. Blessed, K. Bergman, P.H. Gibson, and R.H. Perry (1978) Correlation of cholinergic abnormalities with senile plaques and mental test scores in senile dementia. Br. Med. J. II:1457–1459.

Roberts, G.W., T.W., Crow, and J.M. Polak (1985) Location of neuronal tangles in somatostatin neurons in Alzheimer's disease. Nature 314:92–94.

Rossor, M.N., C. Svendsen, S.P. Hunt, C.Q. Mountjoy, M. Roth, and L.L. Iversen (1982) The substantia innominata in Alzheimer's disease: A histochemical and biochemical study of cholinergic marker enzyme. Neurosci. Lett. 28:217–222.

Schaltenbrand, G., and P. Bailey (1959) Introduction to Stereotaxis With an Atlas of the Human Brain. Stuttgart: Georg Thieme Verlag.

Tomlinson, B.E., G. Blessed, and M. Roth. (1970) Observations on the brains of demented old people. J. Neurol. Sci. II:205–242.

Tomlinson, B.E., and J.A.N. Corsellis (1984) Ageing and the dementias. In Hume-Adams, J.A.N. Corsellis, L.W. Duchen, and Greenfield (eds): Neuropathology. London: Arnold, pp. 951–1025.

Whitehouse, P.J., D.L. Price, R.G. Struble, A.W. Clark, and M.R. DeLong (1982) Alzheimer's disease and senile dementia: Loss of neurons in the central forebrain. Science 215:1237–1239.

Wilcock, G.K., and M.M. Esiri (1982) Plaques, tangles and dementia: A quantitative study. J. Neurol. Sci. 56:343–356.

Index